Clinical Nephrology

Clinical Nephrology

Editor: Valentina Houston

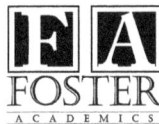

FA FOSTER ACADEMICS

www.fosteracademics.com

www.fosteracademics.com

FA FOSTER
ACADEMICS

Cataloging-in-Publication Data

Clinical nephrology / edited by Valentina Houston.
    p. cm.
Includes bibliographical references and index.
ISBN 978-1-63242-705-2
1. Kidneys--Diseases. 2. Nephrology. 3. Clinical medicine. I. Houston, Valentina.
RC902 .C55 2019
616.61--dc23

Foster Academics,
118-35 Queens Blvd., Suite 400,
Forest Hills, NY 11375, USA

ISBN 978-1-63242-705-2 (Hardback)

Contents

Permissions

List of Contributors

Index

Preface

This book has been an outcome of determined endeavour from a group of educationists in the field. The primary objective was to involve a broad spectrum of professionals from diverse cultural background involved in the field for developing new researches. The book not only targets students but also scholars pursuing higher research for further enhancement of the theoretical and practical applications of the subject.

The specialty of medicine that deals with the functions and diseases related to kidneys is known as nephrology. It is also related to the diverse aspects concerned with kidney health and its preservation. The treatment of kidney diseases along with replacement also falls under this domain. Some common conditions treated under nephrology include polycystic kidney disease, autoimmune diseases such as lupus, ANCA vasculitis, etc. A physician who specializes in the treatment and care of the diseases related to kidneys is known as a nephrologist. This book unfolds the innovative aspects of nephrology, which will be crucial for the progress of this field in future. It presents researches and studies performed by experts across the globe. This book is appropriate for medical students seeking detailed information in the field of nephrology as well as for experts.

It was an honour to edit such a profound book and also a challenging task to compile and examine all the relevant data for accuracy and originality. I wish to acknowledge the efforts of the contributors for submitting such brilliant and diverse chapters in the field and for endlessly working for the completion of the book. Last, but not the least; I thank my family for being a constant source of support in all my research endeavours.

Editor

Impact of reduced exposure to calcineurin inhibitors on the development of de novo DSA: a cohort of non-immunized first kidney graft recipients between 2007 and 2014

S. Girerd [1,2*], J. Schikowski[1], N. Girerd[2], K. Duarte[2], H. Busby[3], N. Gambier[4], M. Ladrière[1], M. Kessler[1], L. Frimat[1] and A. Aarnink[5]

Abstract

Background: In low-immunological risk kidney transplant recipients (KTRs), reduced exposure to calcineurin inhibitor (CNI) appears particularly attractive for avoiding adverse events, but may increase the risk of developing de novo Donor Specific Antibodies (dnDSA).

Methods: CNI exposure was retrospectively analyzed in 247 non-HLA immunized first KTRs by taking into account trough levels (C0) collected during follow-up. Reduced exposure to CNI was defined as follows: C0 less than the lower limit of the international targets for $\geq$50% of follow-up.

Results: During a mean follow-up of 5.0 ± 2.0 years, 39 patients (15.8%) developed dnDSA (MFI $\geq$1000). Patients with DSA were significantly younger (46.6 ± 13.8 vs. 51.7 ± 14.0 years, $p = 0.039$), received more frequently poorly-matched grafts (59% with 6–8 A-B-DR-DQ HLA mismatches vs. 34.6%, $p = 0.016$) and had more frequently a reduced exposure to CNI (92.3% vs. 62.0%, $p = 0.0002$). Reduced exposure to CNI was associated with an increased risk of dnDSA (multivariable HR = 9.77, $p = 0.002$). Reduced exposure to CNI had no effect on patient survival, graft loss from any cause including death, or post-transplant cancer.

Conclusions: Even in a low-immunological risk population, reduced exposure to CNI is associated with increased risk of dnDSA. Benefits and risks of under-immunosuppression must be carefully evaluated before deciding on CNI minimization.

Keywords: Kidney transplantation, Calcineurin inhibitors, Donor specific antibodies, Under immunosuppression

Background

Calcineurin inhibitors (CNI) were first introduced in the 1980s and have led to dramatic improvements in short-term kidney transplantation outcomes. Nevertheless, CNI were traditionally thought to be the major contributors of chronic kidney graft dysfunction due to nephrotoxicity [1]. This historical view was challenged during the past decades [2, 3], given that chronic graft nephropathy was largely related to humoral chronic rejection [4–6] and not only CNI nephrotoxicity [7].

Nevertheless, the overall level of immunosuppressive therapy obviously increases the risk of infectious or neoplastic complications [8]. Therefore, clinicians continue to attempt numerous protocols to reduce exposure to CNI, including primary avoidance, dose reduction, and switching to other drug classes, namely mTOR inhibitors or belatacept [9–12].

There is now a large body of evidence whereby antibody-mediated rejection (ABMR) is the major cause of late kidney allograft failure [4–6]. CNI minimization may fail to improve long-term outcomes due to the development of Donor Specific Antibodies (DSA) and chronic rejection despite less chronic nephrotoxicity. Thus, nephrotoxicity prevention by CNI minimization may be counterbalanced by an increased risk of DSA development, leading to

* Correspondence: s.girerd@chru-nancy.fr
[1]Service de Néphrologie et Transplantation rénale, CHRU Nancy Brabois, Vandoeuvre-les-, Nancy, France
[2]INSERM, Centre d'Investigations Cliniques Plurithématique 1433, Université de Lorraine, CHRU de Nancy and F-CRIN INI-CRCT, Nancy, France
Full list of author information is available at the end of the article

non-significant improvements in long-term graft prognosis. In low immunological risk populations, the impact of reduced exposure to CNI is of particular interest, considering that the benefit/risk balance is, a priori, in disfavor of strong immunosuppressive therapy.

The present study aimed to assess the impact of reduced exposure to CNI (i.e. CNI trough level reduction without avoidance or switch) on the development of de novo DSA (dnDSA) among a cohort of low-immunological risk patients, i.e. first kidney transplant recipients (KTRs) with negative class I and class II anti-HLA antibodies prior to transplantation.

Methods

Study population

This observational single-center cohort study included all non-immunized first KTRs in the University Hospital of Nancy between 01/01/2007 and 31/12/2014. Exclusion criteria consisted of patients aged < 18 years, receiving a combined non-renal graft, or followed in another center after the transplantation. Patients who did not receive CNI or had CNI discontinuation during follow-up were also excluded. Patients with more than 50% of missing values of CNI trough levels ($n = 7$) were also excluded. The study population flowchart is presented in Fig. 1. Non-immunization was defined by the absence of both class I and class II anti-HLA antibodies before transplantation as assessed by Luminex technique, as described hereafter.

Immunosuppressive therapy consisted in an induction therapy (anti-thymocyte globulins or anti-IL2 monoclonal antibody), steroid pulses, followed by maintenance therapy generally including long-term oral corticotherapy (5 mg/day), an antimetabolite (mycophenolic acid or azathioprine) and CNI (either tacrolimus or cyclosporine). The usual initial dosage of tacrolimus was 0.15 mg/kg/day for tacrolimus and 6 mg/kg/day for cyclosporine. The initial dosage of mycophenolic acid was 1000 mg/day when associated with tacrolimus and 2000 mg/day when associated with cyclosporine.

Data collection

Data were extracted from the prospective French database of transplanted patients DIVAT (computerized and VAlidated data in Transplantation) (www.divat.fr). Written informed consent was obtained from all participants and The "Comité National de l'Informatique et des Libertés" approved the study (CNIL no. 891735). Data were entered in a computerized database on day 0, at 3 months and 12 months, and subsequently updated annually thereafter. Patients were followed annually until June 2016.

Characteristics collected at baseline included: age, gender, body mass index, comorbidities, causal nephropathy, dialysis method and time on dialysis prior to kidney transplantation, as well as duration on waiting list. Transplantation

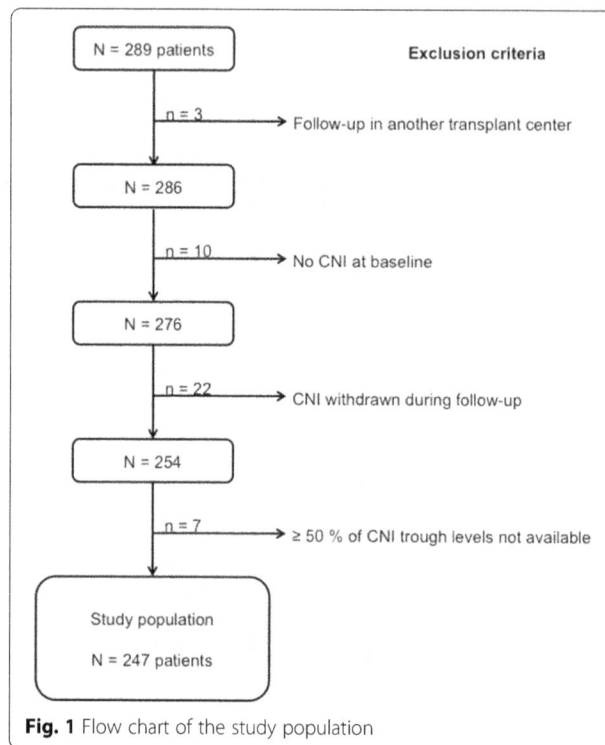

Fig. 1 Flow chart of the study population

parameters included: donor type (living donors; standard criteria donors (SCD); expanded criteria donors (ECD) defined as follows: donors aged ≥60 years, or donors aged 50–59 years with ≥2 of the following conditions: history of hypertension, cerebrovascular cause of death, serum creatinine greater than 1.5 mg/dL), cold ischemia time, HLA A-B-DR-DQ incompatibilities, induction therapy and maintenance immunosuppressive regimen, as well as delayed graft function defined by the necessity of one or more dialysis sessions in the first week after transplantation. Data collected during follow-up included: dnDSA detection, acute rejection, return to dialysis and death before return to dialysis. Post-transplant cancers were also recorded. Patients were followed until death, return to dialysis or last follow-up visit up until March 2016. Mean follow-up was 5.0 ± 2.0 years.

Anti-HLA immunization and DSA detection

All patients included in the study cohort underwent a search for anti-HLA class I and class II antibodies that was negative prior to transplantation. The monitoring of anti-HLA immunization after transplantation was performed at 3, 6 and 12 months after the graft and annually thereafter, as well as at the time of biopsy when clinically warranted (presence of graft dysfunction or suspicion of rejection). The sera were screened for HLA-specific antibodies using solid-phase Luminex HLA antibody-detection beads (LABScreen™ Mixed, One Lambda Inc., Canoga Park) and selected HLA-specific antibody-positive samples were analyzed using Luminex single-antigen HLA class I and class II antibody-detection beads (LABScreen™ Single Antigen HLA Class I and Class II, One Lambda Inc., Canoga Park). Antibodies were considered as Donor Specific Antibodies if the MFI (Mean Fluorescence Intensity) of antibodies directed against a donor antigen (HLA-A, -B, -C, –DR, –DR51, –DR52, –DR53, –DQ or -DP) was greater than 1000. For each serum, the sum of MFI DSA(s) was also studied. In instances where the recipient had DSA directed against a homozygous donor antigen, the MFI was doubled.

Exposure to CNI

The blood concentration of CNI were measured by the antibody-conjugated magnetic immunoassay (ACMIA) method using an Dimension® system (Siemens). The lower limit of quantification was 25 ng/mL and 2 ng/mL for cyclosporine and tacrolimus, respectively. Trough levels were measured at month 3, month 6, month 12, and annually thereafter. For every patient and every outcome, the number of time intervals of CNI exposure before the event was established considering that the event itself could lead to a modification in CNI posology (the next trough level may be the consequence of the event). For example, in the case of first DSA detection at month 30 (Fig. 2), the time intervals M0-M3 (trough level measured at month 3), M3-M6 (trough level measured at month 6), M6-M12 (trough level measured at month 12) and M12-M24 (trough level measured at month 24) were taken into account.

Trough levels less than the lower limit of the international targets [13–15] for ≥50% of time intervals defined the reduced exposure to CNI. In case of a missing value, the time interval was not considered, and the total number of intervals decreased accordingly.

Post transplant delay	Cyclosporine trough level (ng/mL)	Tacrolimus trough level (ng/mL)
0–3 months	250–350	10–15
3–6 months	150–250	8–10
6–12 months	125–200	6–8
> 12 months	100–150	5–8

Consequently, patients were classified into two groups according to the presence or the absence of a reduced exposure to CNI. Patients having developed dnDSA or not during follow-up were also compared.

The distribution of CNI trough levels at each visit is presented in Fig. 3 a-d. The number of patients recieving tacrolimus increased over time while the number of patients receiving cyclosporin decreased, because some patients were switched from cyclosporin to tacrolimus during follow-up (Fig. 3).

Statistical methods

All analyses were performed using R software (the R foundation for Statistical Computing). The two-tailed significance level was set at $p < 0.05$. Continuous variables are described as means ± standard deviation, categorical

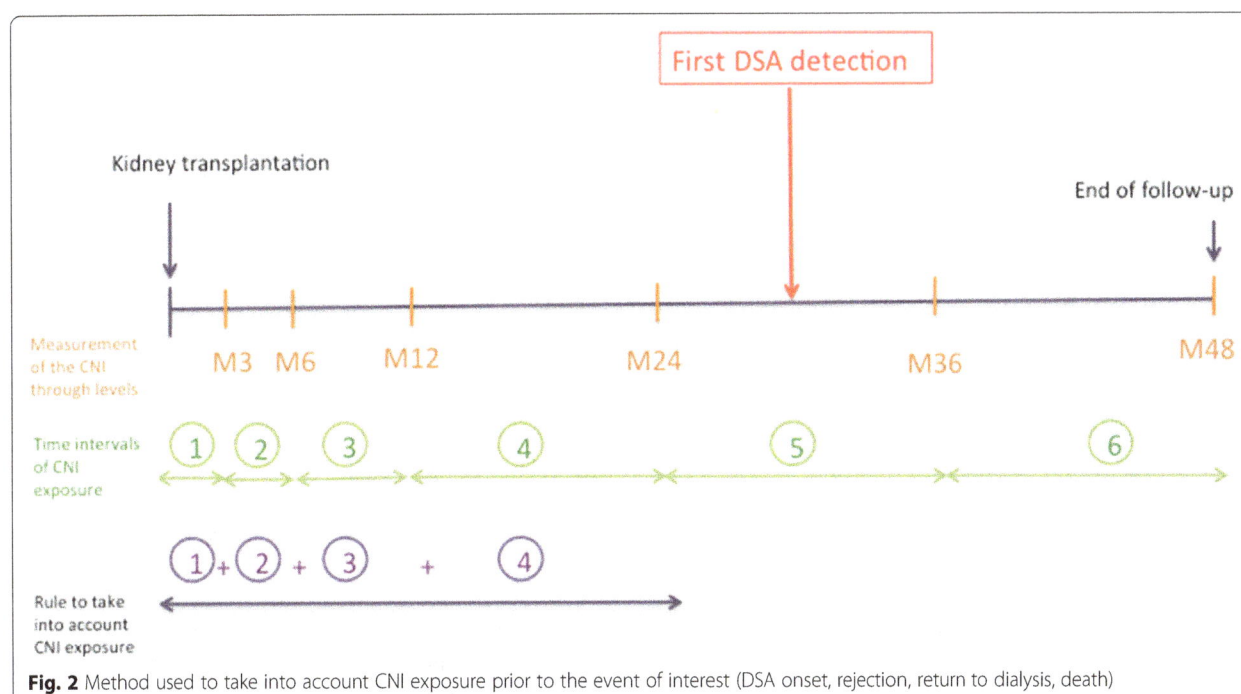

Fig. 2 Method used to take into account CNI exposure prior to the event of interest (DSA onset, rejection, return to dialysis, death)

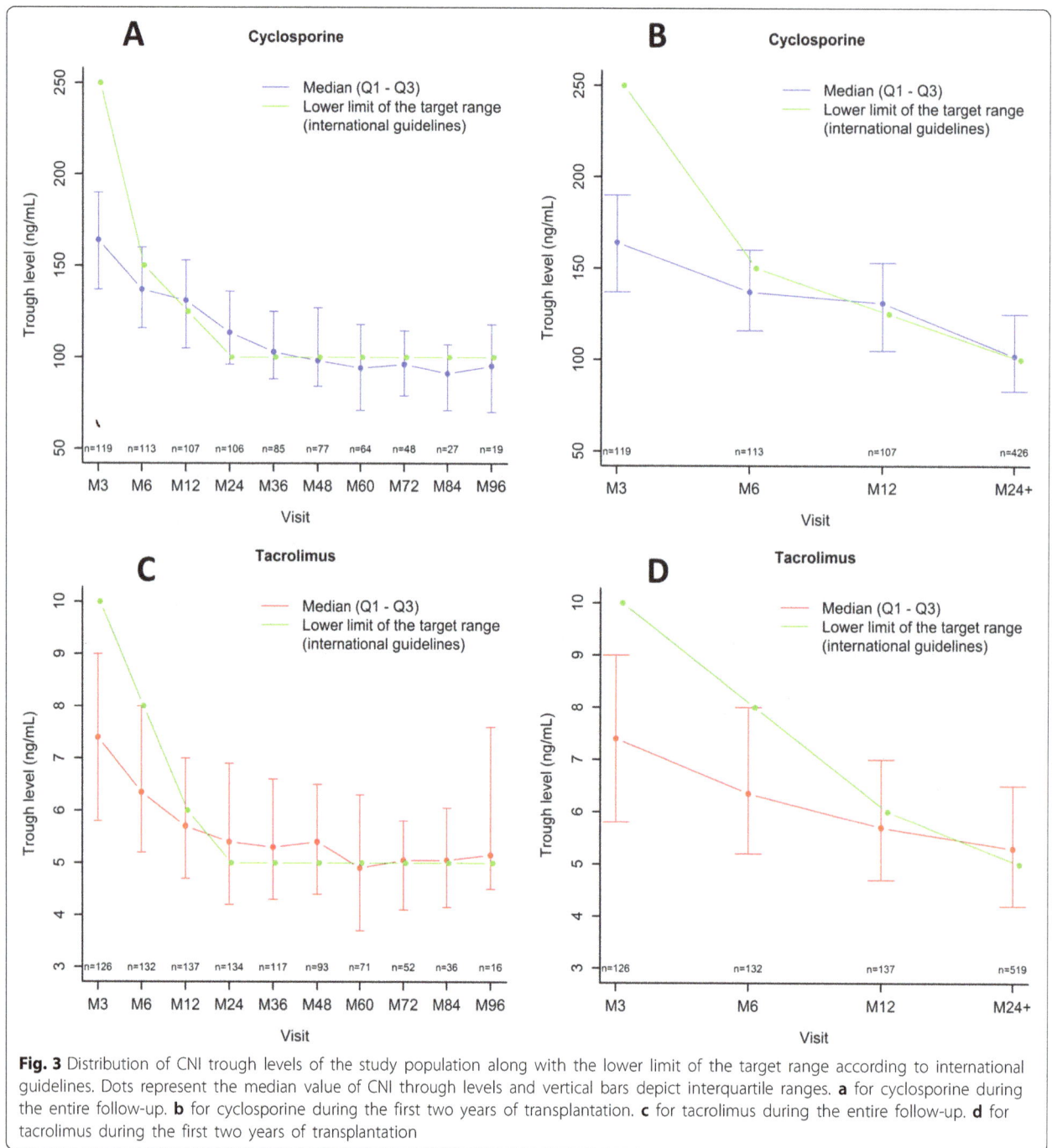

Fig. 3 Distribution of CNI trough levels of the study population along with the lower limit of the target range according to international guidelines. Dots represent the median value of CNI through levels and vertical bars depict interquartile ranges. **a** for cyclosporine during the entire follow-up. **b** for cyclosporine during the first two years of transplantation. **c** for tacrolimus during the entire follow-up. **d** for tacrolimus during the first two years of transplantation

variables as frequencies (percentages). Hazard ratios are presented with their 95% confidence intervals as HR (CI 95%). Comparisons of baseline characteristics according to reduced exposure to CNI or not or DSA detection were carried out using the non parametric Mann-Whitney test for continuous variables and chi-square or Fisher's exact test for categorical variables. Time-to-event analyses using Cox regression models were performed to assess the associations between reduced exposure to CNI and outcomes (DSA detection, return to dialysis, death before return to

dialysis, return to dialysis or death before return to dialysis). Proportional hazard assumption was thoroughly verified using the Schoenfeld residuals test. Multivariable analyses were performed using iterative backward selection ($p < 0.05$), by forcing "reduced exposure to CNI" in the Cox model, with the following variables as candidate covariates: number of HLA mismatches, donor type, age and gender of the recipient, mycofenolic acid cessation, delayed graft function and induction therapy. Survival rates are illustrated using Kaplan Meier analyses.

Differences between survival curves were analyzed using the log-rank test. Intra-patient variability (IPV) of CNI trough levels was calculated. As others [16], C0 blood levels of cyclosporine to C0 tacrolimus equivalents were converted using an empiric 1/20 correction factor, based on the limits of the international targets.

Intra-patient variability (IPV) in CNI exposure was also studied and defined as the fluctuation in CNI blood concentrations within an individual over a given period. The mean absolute deviation percent (MAD%) formula was used as previously described [17]:

$$MAD\% = \frac{1}{n} \sum \frac{abs(X_j - \overline{X})}{\overline{X}} * 100.$$

where:

- $\overline{X}$ represents the average of all available samples (in the case of tacrolimus IPV, the average of all tacrolimus trough levels measured for time period j), X_j represents an individual data point (a single tacrolimus trough level measurement) and n the number of all available data points (the total number of all available tacrolimus trough levels during period j)

- Abs (...) denotes the absolute value function, such that the quantitative value $abs(X_j - \overline{X})$ is always a non-negative value. The obtained tacrolimus trough level (C0) must be corrected to the corresponding daily tacrolimus dose (C0/D)

Results

Baseline characteristics of the entire population

A total of 247 KTRs were included. Mean age of graft recipients was 50.9 ± 14.1 years. The proportion of living donors was 27.5% while 15.4% of patients received preemptive kidney transplantation. With regard to HLA compatibility, 24.7% patients had 0–3 mismatches (A-B-DR-DQ), 36.8% had 4–5 mismatches and 38.5% had 6–8 mismatches. An induction treatment was administered in 95.1% of patients (70.2% with lymphocyte-depletive agent and 29.8% with anti-interleukin-2 receptor antibodies), while 49.0% received cyclosporine as maintenance therapy with the remaining 51.0% receiving tacrolimus. Other baseline data are provided in Table 1.

Baseline characteristics of patients according to "exposure to CNI" status

Patient characteristics according to the presence or the absence of a reduced exposure to CNI are presented in Table 1. Patients did not differ in terms of age, causal nephropathy or medical history (cancer or infectious disease prior to transplantation as well as cardiovascular history). Of note, the proportion of living donors and the proportion of expanded criteria donors were higher in the group with reduced exposure to CNI (respectively 33.3% vs. 15.9 and 27.9% vs. 20.7%, $p = 0.0008$). Moreover, the number of HLA A-B-DR-DQ incompatibilities differed according to the two groups with a higher proportion of very well matched patients as well as very poorly matched patients in the group with reduced exposure to CNI (26.7% vs. 20.7 and 41.8% vs. 31.7%, $p = 0.048$ for 0–3 mismatches and 6–8 mismatches, respectively). The proportion of induction treatment was similar in the two groups, as well as the proportion of mycofenolic acid cessation during follow-up. The proportion of patients with high CNI IPV was similar in the two groups (for IPV > 30%: 12.1% vs. 14.6%, $p = 0.58$).

Follow-up data: DSA detection and impact of reduced exposure to CNI on DSA appearance

During follow-up, 39 patients (15.8%) developed dnDSA (with MFI ≥ 1000). The proportion of KTRs who developed DSA during follow-up was higher in the group of patients with reduced exposure to CNI (21.1% (35/166) vs 2.5% (2/81), $p < 0.0001$) (Fig. 4). Patients who developed dnDSA were significantly younger (46.6 ± 13.8 vs. 51.7 ± 14.0, $p = 0.039$) (Table 2), received more frequently poorly-matched grafts (59% with 6–8 HLA mismatches in the group with DSA vs. 34.6% in the group without DSA, $p = 0.016$), and have more frequently a reduced exposure to CNI (92.3% vs. 62.0%, $p = 0.0002$). The proportion of induction therapy was similar in both groups, as well as mycofenolic acid cessation during follow-up, or IPV. Of note, no patient had mycofenolic acid cessation before the first DSA detection in the group with DSA (Table 2). In a multivariate analysis adjusted for the number of HLA mismatches, donor type, age and gender of the recipient, mycofenolic acid cessation, delayed graft function and induction therapy, reduced exposure to CNI was associated with an increased risk of DSA development (for first detection of one DSA with MFI > 1000, HR in multivariable analysis 9.77 (2.34–40.77), $p = 0.002$; for first detection of DSAs with total MFI (sum MFI) > 6000 HR = 12.02 (1.62–89.25), $p = 0.015$) (Table 3). When adjusting, as a sensitivity analysis, on number HLA mismatches, donor type and induction treatment (without iterative backward selection) we found similar results (*data not shown*). When adjusting, as a sensitivity analysis, on number HLA mismatches, donor type and induction treatment (without iterative backward selection) we found similar results (*data not shown*). In addition, when adjusting on body mass index and cold ischemia time (without selection, based on the univariable analysis) we found similar associations and p-values (*data not shown*).

Only 3 ABMR were diagnosed during follow-up. A reduced exposure to CNI tended to be associated with an increased risk of all-type graft rejections (HR = 5.65 (0.73–43.74), $p = 0.097$).

Table 1 Baseline and follow-up data of patients according to the absence or presence of a reduced exposure to CNI

	Total ($n = 247$)	Controls ($n = 82$)	Reduced exposure to CNI ($n = 165$)	p-value
DEMOGRAPHICS				
Age (years)	50.9 ± 14.1	51.1 ± 13.1	50.8 ± 14.6	0.91
Male (n, %)	173 (70.0%)	62 (75.6%)	111 (67.3%)	0.18
BMI (kg/m^2)	25.5 ± 4.8	26.2 ± 4.3	25.1 ± 4.9	0.026
COMORBIDITIES				
Hypertension (n, %)	235 (95.1%)	77 (93.9%)	158 (95.8%)	0.54
No smoker (n, %)	122 (49.4%)	44 (53.7%)	78 (47.3%)	
Former smoker (n, %)	93 (37.7%)	28 (34.1%)	65 (39.4%)	
Active smoker (n, %)	32 (13.0%)	10 (12.2%)	22 (13.3%)	
Stroke (n, %)	11 (4.5%)	5 (6.1%)	6 (3.6%)	0.51
Diabetes (n, %)	55 (22.3%)	20 (24.4%)	35 (21.2%)	0.57
Type 1 diabetes	13 (23.6%)	3 (15.0%)	10 (28.6%)	
Type 2 diabetes (with insulin)	40 (72.7%)	17 (85.0%)	23 (65.7%)	
Type 2 diabetes (no insulin)	2 (3.6%)	0 (0.0%)	2 (5.7%)	
History of coronary disease (n, %)	25 (10.1%)	9 (11.0%)	16 (9.7%)	0.75
Heart failure (n, %)	41 (16.6%)	17 (20.7%)	24 (14.5%)	0.22
Peripheral artery disease (n, %)	19 (7.7%)	4 (4.9%)	15 (9.1%)	0.24
Chronic obstructive pulmonary disease (n, %)	8 (3.2%)	5 (6.1%)	3 (1.8%)	0.12
Pre-transplant cancer (n, %)	10 (4.0%)	4 (4.9%)	6 (3.6%)	0.73
Causal nephropathy (n, %)				
Other	25 (10.1%)	4 (4.9%)	21 (12.7%)	0.27
Chronic glomerulonephritis	63 (25.5%)	21 (25.6%)	42 (25.5%)	
Toxic	2 (0.8%)	1 (1.2%)	1 (0.6%)	
Diabetic nephropathy	37 (15.0%)	10 (12.2%)	27 (16.4%)	
Vascular nephropathy	20 (8.1%)	9 (11.0%)	11 (6.7%)	
Unknown	37 (15.0%)	14 (17.1%)	23 (13.9%)	
Polycystic disease	45 (18.2%)	13 (15.9%)	32 (19.4%)	
Nephrectomy	2 (0.8%)	1 (1.2%)	1 (0.6%)	
Malformative uropathy	12 (4.9%)	6 (7.3%)	6 (3.6%)	
Vasculitis	4 (1.6%)	3 (3.7%)	1 (0.6%)	
Dialysis prior to transplantation (n, %)	209 (84.6%)	73 (89.0%)	136 (82.4%)	0.18
Peritoneal dialysis	38 (18.2%)	15 (20.5%)	23 (16.9%)	
Hemodialysis	171 (81.8%)	58 (79.5%)	113 (83.1%)	
Pre-transplant dialysis time (years)	2.1 ± 2.0	2.1 ± 2.0	2.2 ± 2.0	0.73
TRANSPLANTATION DATA				
Viral status CMV donor/recipient (n, %)				0.51
D−/R−	59 (23.9%)	22 (26.8%)	37 (22.4%)	
D−/R+	57 (23.1%)	18 (22.0%)	39 (23.6%)	
D+/R−	64 (25.9%)	17 (20.7%)	47 (28.5%)	
D+/R+	67 (27.1%)	25 (30.5%)	42 (25.5%)	
Donor type (n, %)				**0.0008**
Expanded criteria donor	63 (25.5%)	17 (20.7%)	46 (27.9%)	
Standard criteria donor	116 (47.0%)	52 (63.4%)	64 (38.8%)	
Living donor	68 (27.5%)	13 (15.9%)	55 (33.3%)	

Table 1 Baseline and follow-up data of patients according to the absence or presence of a reduced exposure to CNI *(Continued)*

	Total (*n* = 247)	Controls (*n* = 82)	Reduced exposure to CNI (*n* = 165)	*p*-value
Cold ischemia time (hours)	13.1 ± 8.9	14.5 ± 8.0	12.4 ± 9.3	**0.023**
HLA A-B-DR-DQ incompatibilities (n, %)				
0–3	61 (24.7%)	17 (20.7%)	44 (26.7%)	**0.048**
4–5	91 (36.8%)	39 (47.6%)	52 (31.5%)	
6–8	95 (38.5%)	26 (31.7%)	69 (41.8%)	
Induction treatment (n, %)	235 (95.1%)	77 (93.9%)	158 (95.8%)	0.54
Lymphocyte-depletive agent	165 (70.2%)	56 (72.7%)	109 (69.0%)	
Anti-interleukin-2 receptor antibodies	70 (29.8%)	21 (27.3%)	49 (31.0%)	
Mycofenolic acid cessation during follow-up	28 (11.3%)	9 (11.0%)	19 (11.5%)	0.90
POST-TRANSPLANTATION EVENTS				
Delayed graft function (n, %)	72 (29.1%)	30 (36.6%)	42 (25.5%)	0.070
Rejection (n, %)	42 (17.0%)	9 (11.0%)	33 (20.0%)	0.075
T cell mediated rejection	40 (16.2%)	8 (9.8%)	32 (19.4%)	
Antibody mediated rejection	3 (1.2%)	1 (1.2%)	2 (1.2%)	
Time to first rejection (years)	0.5 ± 1.0	0.9 ± 1.2	0.4 ± 0.9	
Post-transplant cancer (n, %)	29 (11.7%)	9 (11.0%)	20 (12.1%)	0.79
Skin cancer	11 (37.9%)	2 (22.2%)	9 (45.0%)	
Hemopathy	3 (10.3%)	1 (11.1%)	2 (10.0%)	
Solid cancer	15 (51.7%)	6 (66.7%)	9 (45.0%)	
Time to post-transplant cancer (years)	3.2 ± 1.9	4.0 ± 2.0	2.9 ± 1.8	0.15
Return in dialysis (n, %)	18 (7.3%)	3 (3.7%)	15 (9.1%)	0.12
Death with a functioning graft (n, %)	22 (8.9%)	9 (11.0%)	13 (7.9%)	0.42
Graft failure from any cause including death (n, %)	40 (16.2%)	12 (14.6%)	28 (17.0%)	0.64
CNI Mean Absolute Deviation (%)				
Continuous	19.9 ± 9.6	19.2 ± 10.3	20.3 ± 9.3	0.21
< 5%	6 (2.4%)	2 (2.4%)	4 (2.4%)	1.00
< 15%	87 (35.2%)	36 (43.9%)	51 (30.9%)	**0.044**
> 30%	32 (13.0%)	12 (14.6%)	20 (12.1%)	0.58
> 50%	2 (0.8%)	1 (1.2%)	1 (0.6%)	1.00

BMI Body Mass Index, *DSA* Donor Specific Antibody, *D–/R-* Donor negative/Recipient negative, *D–/R+* Donor negative/Recipient positive, *D+/R-* Donor positive/ Recipient negative, *CNI* Calcineurin inhibitors. Results with *p* value less than 5% were emphasized using bold letters

During follow-up, 18 KTRs returned to dialysis and 22 patients died with a functioning graft. A reduced exposure to CNI tended to be associated with an increased risk of return to dialysis (HR = 3.22 (0.93–11.22), *p* = 0.066) (Table 3). There was no effect on patient survival or graft loss from any cause including death. Of note, there was no significant association between a reduced exposure to CNI and post-transplant cancer (HR = 1.20 (0.55–2.62), *p* = 0.64) (Table 3). Similar results were also found after exclusion of skin cancers.

Discussion
Main findings
In the present study, we demonstrate that even in a low-immunological risk population of kidney graft recipients, reduced exposure to CNI was associated with an increased risk of development of de novo DSA, known to be related to poor long-term graft outcomes. Long-term CNI exposure was assessed by taking into account different time intervals for the purpose of longitudinal pharmacological follow-up. Considering that the first detection of DSA frequently compels physicians to modify immunosuppressive treatment as well as the CNI target level, we deemed of value to take into account CNI exposure only in the period preceding DSA detection. Of note, a low exposure to CNI only tended in our cohort to be associated with increased risk of graft rejection, as well as increased risk of return to dialysis.

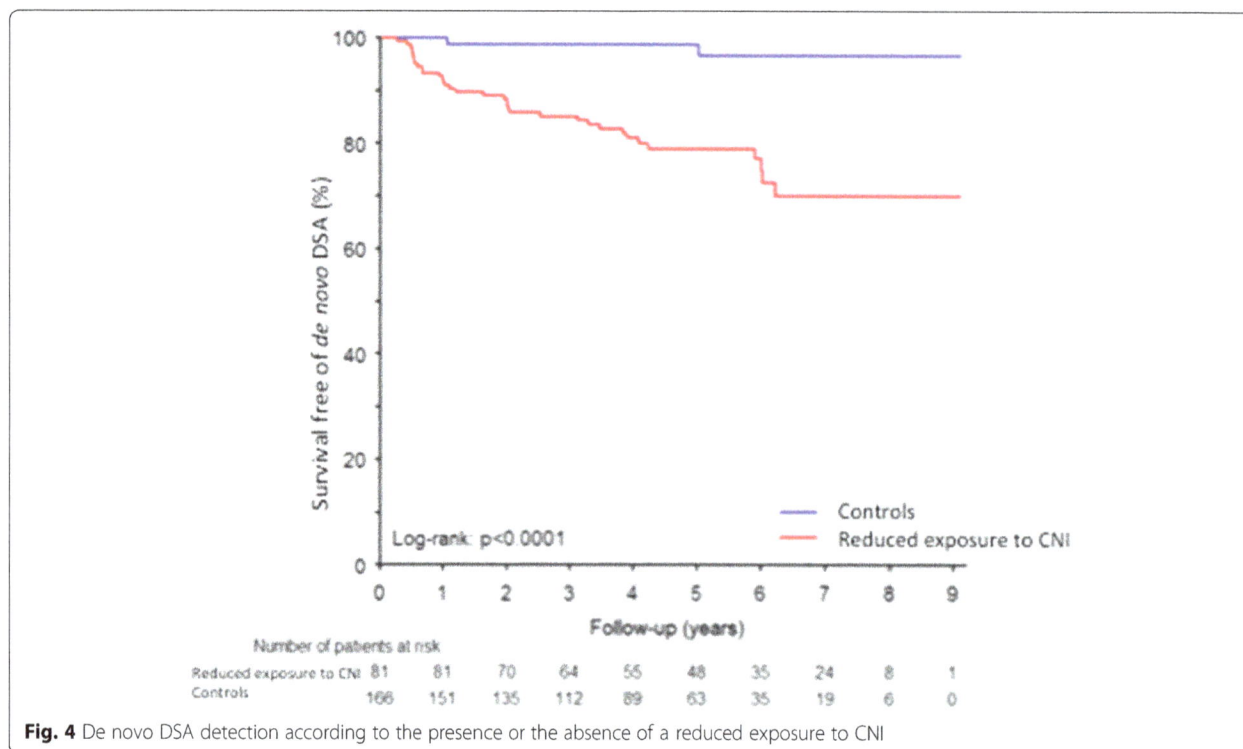

Fig. 4 De novo DSA detection according to the presence or the absence of a reduced exposure to CNI

CNI minimization and graft or patient prognosis

It is currently extremely difficult to draw definitive conclusions from the multiplicity of studies on CNI minimization given that strategies may vary in terms of: 1) the study population (baseline immunological risk), 2) CNI minimization strategy (withdrawn; long term maintenance with dose reduction; complete avoidance), 3) time of minimization (de novo; in case of graft function deterioration), 4) combination with an induction therapy, 5) combination with (or replacement with) maintenance therapy based on mycophenolic acid, mTOR inhibitors or belatacept. In a recent meta-analysis, Sawinski et al. assessed the impact on patient and allograft survival of four strategies of reduced-exposure to CNI (minimization, conversion, withdrawal and avoidance) [12]. The analysis of the 19 studies in which CNI minimization was associated with mycophenolic acid formulations reported reduced graft loss with this strategy, with a high level of evidence. In the most recent Cochrane meta-analysis (including randomized controlled trials (RCTs) with CNI withdrawal, tapering or low dose) [18], low dose CNI with induction regimens reduced acute rejection and graft loss, also in the short-term. The authors indicate that these conclusions must be tempered by the lack of long-term data in most of the studies, particularly with regards to chronic ABMR.

Deleterious impact of DSA on graft prognosis

Among sensitized patients, the deleterious impact on graft survival of preformed DSA is well established [19–21],

with increased risk of ABMR and graft loss. Among non-sensitized patients, dnDSA may also develop after transplantation in 15% of kidney recipients [22–24], leading to increased risk of acute rejection [23, 25] and graft loss [24, 25]. The incidence of acute rejection in kidney allograft recipients with dnDSA can reach 50%, with up to 30% subclinical acute rejection [23–25]. ABMR represents a substantial proportion of these 50% rejections [23–25], which constitutes the principal risk factor of graft loss [23–25]. dnDSA are also associated with subclinical histological lesions [26], which are an important determinant of graft survival [27, 28].

CNI minimization and DSA development in the literature

A few previous studies have assessed the impact of CNI minimization on dnDSA development. In a recent RCT, Gatault et al. [29] evaluated the efficacy and safety of two different doses of tacrolimus in KTRs between 4 and 12 months after transplantation. Stable steroid-free patients were randomized after 4 months: Group A had a 50% reduction in tacrolimus dose with a targeted trough level > 3 ng/mL while group B had no change in tacrolimus dose (C0 7–12 ng/mL). The primary outcome was eGFR at 1 year. Estimated GFR was similar in both groups at 12 months, while dnDSA appeared only in group A (6 vs. 0 patients, $p = 0.008$). The authors concluded that tacrolimus trough levels should be maintained > 7 ng/mL during the first year after transplantation in low-immunological risk, steroid-free patients receiving mycophenolic acid.

Table 2 Baseline and follow-up data of patients according to the absence or presence of de novo DSA during follow-up

	Population ($n = 247$)	No DSA ($n = 208$)	De novo DSA ($n = 39$)	p-value
DEMOGRAPHICS				
Age (years)	50.9 ± 14.1	51.7 ± 14.0	46.6 ± 13.8	**0.039**
Male (n, %)	173 (70.0%)	142 (68.3%)	31 (79.5%)	0.16
BMI (kg/m^2)	25.5 ± 4.8	25.3 ± 4.9	26.4 ± 4.1	0.16
COMORBIDITIES				
No smoker (n, %)	122 (49.4%)	101 (48.6%)	21 (53.8%)	0.81
Former smoker (n, %)	93 (37.7%)	80 (38.5%)	13 (33.3%)	
Current smoker (n, %)	32 (13.0%)	27 (13.0%)	5 (12.8%)	
Stroke (n, %)	11 (4.5%)	11 (5.3%)	0 (0.0%)	0.22
Diabetes (n, %)	55 (22.3%)	44 (21.2%)	11 (28.2%)	0.33
Type 1 diabetes	13 (23.6%)	9 (20.5%)	4 (36.4%)	
Type 2 diabetes (with insulin)	40 (72.7%)	34 (77.3%)	6 (54.5%)	
Type 2 diabetes (no insulin)	2 (3.6%)	1 (2.3%)	1 (9.1%)	
History of coronary disease (n, %)	25 (10.1%)	21 (10.1%)	4 (10.3%)	1.00
Heart failure (n, %)	41 (16.6%)	33 (15.9%)	8 (20.5%)	0.47
Peripheral artery disease (n, %)	19 (7.7%)	16 (7.7%)	3 (7.7%)	1.00
Pre-transplant cancer (n, %)	10 (4.0%)	9 (4.3%)	1 (2.6%)	1.00
Causal nephropathy (n, %)				0.24
Other	25 (10.1%)	20 (9.6%)	5 (12.8%)	
Chronic glomerulonephritis	63 (25.5%)	52 (25.0%)	11 (28.2%)	
Toxic	2 (0.8%)	2 (1.0%)	0 (0.0%)	
Diabetic nephropathy	37 (15.0%)	27 (13.0%)	10 (25.6%)	
Vascular nephropathy	20 (8.1%)	19 (9.1%)	1 (2.6%)	
Unknown	37 (15.0%)	35 (16.8%)	2 (5.1%)	
Polycystic disease	45 (18.2%)	38 (18.3%)	7 (17.9%)	
Nephrectomy	2 (0.8%)	1 (0.5%)	1 (2.6%)	
Malformative uropathy	12 (4.9%)	10 (4.8%)	2 (5.1%)	
Vasculitis	4 (1.6%)	4 (1.9%)	0 (0.0%)	
Dialysis prior to transplantation (n, %)	209 (84.6%)	174 (83.7%)	35 (89.7%)	0.33
Peritoneal dialysis	38 (18.2%)	32 (18.4%)	6 (17.1%)	
Hemodialysis	171 (81.8%)	142 (81.6%)	29 (82.9%)	
Pre-transplant dialysis time (years)	2.1 ± 2.0	2.1 ± 1.9	2.2 ± 2.1	0.78
TRANSPLANTATION DATA				
Viral status CMV donor/recipient (n, %)				0.72
D−/R-	59 (23.9%)	47 (22.6%)	12 (30.8%)	
D−/R+	57 (23.1%)	48 (23.1%)	9 (23.1%)	
D+/R-	64 (25.9%)	55 (26.4%)	9 (23.1%)	
D+/R+	67 (27.1%)	58 (27.9%)	9 (23.1%)	
Donor type (n, %)				
Expanded criteria donor	63 (25.5%)	55 (26.4%)	8 (20.5%)	0.72
Standard criteria donor	116 (47.0%)	97 (46.6%)	19 (48.7%)	
Living donor	68 (27.5%)	56 (26.9%)	12 (30.8%)	
Cold ischemia time (hours)	13.1 ± 8.9	13.1 ± 8.5	12.8 ± 10.9	0.38
HLA A-B-DR-DQ incompatibilities (n, %)				**0.016**

Table 2 Baseline and follow-up data of patients according to the absence or presence of de novo DSA during follow-up *(Continued)*

	Population (n = 247)	No DSA (n = 208)	De novo DSA (n = 39)	p-value
0–3	61 (24.7%)	55 (26.4%)	6 (15.4%)	
4–5	91 (36.8%)	81 (38.9%)	10 (25.6%)	
6–8	95 (38.5%)	72 (34.6%)	23 (59.0%)	
Induction treatment (n, %)	235 (95.1%)	196 (94.2%)	39 (100.0%)	0.22
Lymphocyte-depletive agent	165 (70.2%)	136 (69.4%)	29 (74.4%)	
Anti-interleukin-2 receptor antibodies	70 (29.8%)	60 (30.6%)	10 (25.6%)	
Reduced exposure to CNI (n, %)	165 (66.8%)	129 (62.0%)	36 (92.3%)	**0.0002**
Mycophenolic acid cessation				
During the entire follow-up	28 (11.3%)	26 (12.5%)	2 (5.1%)	0.27
Before the first detection of DSA[a]	26 (10.5%)	26 (12.5%)	0 (0.0%)	**0.019**
POST-TRANSPLANTATION EVENTS				
Delayed graft function (n, %)	72 (29.1%)	62 (29.8%)	10 (25.6%)	0.60
Rejection (n, %)	42 (17.0%)	30 (14.4%)	12 (30.8%)	**0.013**
T cell mediated rejection	40 (16.2%)	30 (14.4%)	10 (25.6%)	
Antibody mediated rejection	3 (1.2%)	0 (0.0%)	3 (7.7%)	
Time to first rejection (years)	0.5 ± 1.0	0.3 ± 0.6	1.1 ± 1.6	
Post-transplant neoplasia (n, %)	29 (11.7%)	26 (12.5%)	3 (7.7%)	0.59
Skin cancer	11 (37.9%)	11 (42.3%)	0 (0.0%)	
Hemopathy	3 (10.3%)	3 (11.5%)	0 (0.0%)	
Solid cancer	15 (51.7%)	12 (46.2%)	3 (100.0%)	
Time to post-transplant cancer (years)	3.2 ± 1.9	3.1 ± 1.9	4.0 ± 1.8	0.44
Return in dialysis (n, %)	18 (7.3%)	10 (4.8%)	8 (20.5%)	**0.003**
Death with a functioning graft (n, %)	22 (8.9%)	19 (9.1%)	3 (7.7%)	1.00
Graft failure from any cause including death (n, %)	40 (16.2%)	29 (13.9%)	11 (28.2%)	**0.027**
Mean Absolute Deviation (%)				
Continuous	19.9 ± 9.6	19.8 ± 9.3	20.7 ± 11.5	0.99
< 5%	6 (2.4%)	5 (2.4%)	1 (2.6%)	1.00
< 15%	87 (35.2%)	76 (36.5%)	11 (28.2%)	0.32
> 30%	32 (13.0%)	26 (12.5%)	6 (15.4%)	0.62
> 50%	2 (0.8%)	1 (0.5%)	1 (2.6%)	0.29

BMI Body Mass Index, *DSA* Donor Specific Antibody, *D–/R-* Donor negative/Recipient negative, *D–/R+* Donor negative/Recipient positive, *D+/R-* Donor positive/Recipient negative, *CNI* Calcineurin inhibitors. Results with *p* value less than 5% were emphasized using bold letters
[a]Number of patients (%) with mycophenolic acid cessation during the follow-up restricted to the period before the first DSA detection in the group "de novo DSA" and during the entire follow-up in the group "no DSA"

In patients highly selected for a low immunological risk of rejection (long-term stable KTRs with no histological abnormality and absence of anti-HLA immunization), Dugast et al. conducted a double-blind RCT to analyze the benefits and risks of tacrolimus weaning [30]. Fifty-two patients were scheduled in each treatment arm, although only 10 patients were eligible and thus randomized. In the tacrolimus maintenance arm, graft function remains stable in all patients with no occurrence of graft rejection or anti-HLA immunization. In contrast, all the five patients of the placebo group developed either an acute graft rejection (humoral or not) or anti-HLA antibodies (DSA or not).

In a recent work, Béland et al. observed that among KTRs with dnDSA, higher CNI levels predicted better kidney graft survival, with a threshold of 5.3 ng/mL seemingly predictive of graft loss [16].

Optimal trough levels of CNI / CNI target levels: Literature data

The optimal CNI trough target level remains to be defined. The KDIGO guideline suggests that maintenance immunosuppressive medication should be administered at the lowest planned dose by 2–4 months after transplantation if no rejection has occurred, although no target levels were proposed [31]. Over time, tacrolimus exposure levels have

Table 3 Impact of reduced exposure to CNI on the occurrence of de novo DSA in a multivariable[a] Cox adjusted model

Event	Reduced exposure to CNI	Nb events/Nb patients	Univariate model		Multivariate model[a]	
			HR (CI 95%)	p	HR (CI 95%)	p
First detection of one DSA with MFI > 1000	No	2/81 (2.5%)	1.00		1.00	
	Yes	35/166 (21.1%)	10.43 (2.50–43.46)	**0.001**	9.77 (2.34–40.77)	**0.002**
First detection of one DSA with MFI > 6000	No	1/82 (1.2%)	1.00		1.00	
	Yes	22/165 (13.3%)	12.31 (1.66–91.47)	**0.014**	11.54 (1.55–85.93)	**0.017**
First detection of one DSA with MFI > 10,000	No	1/84 (1.2%)	1.00		1.00	
	Yes	16/163 (9.8%)	8.86 (1.17–66.92)	**0.034**	7.40 (0.97–56.31)	0.053
First detection of DSA(s) with total MFI > 6000	No	1/82 (1.2%)	1.00		1.00	
	Yes	23/165 (13.9%)	12.81 (1.73–94.97)	**0.013**	12.02 (1.62–89.25)	**0.015**
First detection of DSA(s) with total MFI > 10,000	No	1/83 (1.2%)	1.00		1.00	
	Yes	19/164 (11.6%)	10.75 (1.44–80.43)	**0.021**	9.50 (1.26–71.43)	**0.029**
First rejection	No	1/83 (1.2%)	1.00		1.00	
	Yes	11/164 (6.7%)	5.65 (0.73–43.74)	0.097	5.65 (0.73–43.74)	0.097
Post-transplant neoplasia	No	10/88 (11.4%)	1.00		1.00	
	Yes	18/159 (11.3%)	1.16 (0.53–2.52)	0.71	1.20 (0.55–2.62)	0.64
Post-transplant neoplasia (excluding skin neoplasia)	No	8/88 (9.1%)	1.00		1.00	
	Yes	10/159 (6.3%)	0.75 (0.30–1.91)	0.55	0.75 (0.30–1.91)	0.55
Return in dialysis	No	3/87 (3.4%)	1.00		1.00	
	Yes	15/160 (9.4%)	3.22 (0.93–11.22)	0.066	3.22 (0.93–11.22)	0.066
Patient survival	No	9/87 (10.3%)	1.00		1.00	
	Yes	13/160 (8.1%)	1.01 (0.43–2.38)	0.97	1.03 (0.44–2.43)	0.94
Graft survival	No	12/87 (13.8%)	1.00		1.00	
	Yes	28/160 (17.5%)	1.57 (0.80–3.11)	0.19	1.64 (0.82–3.28)	0.16

DSA: Donor Specific Antibody, *MFI* Mean Fluorescence Intensity. Results with *p* value less than 5% were emphasized using bold letters
[a]Multivariable analyses were performed using iterative backward selection, by forcing "reduced exposure to CNI" in the Cox model, with the following variables as candidate covariates: number of HLA mismatches, donor type (living, deceased -standard or extended criteria-), age and gender of the recipient, mycofenolic acid cessation, delayed graft function and induction therapy

declined [31]. In more recent RCTs, the standard tacrolimus trough level 6 months after transplantation was defined between 5 and 10 ng/mL [32] or 6–9 ng/mL [33] although lower exposure ranges have been tested [34, 35]. In the present study, we consequently endeavored to encompass the latter with the term "international targets" comprised of a tacrolimus trough level between 6 and 8 ng/mL after 6 months and between 5 and 8 ng/mL after 12 months.

Certain authors have attempted to combine the data [36] of three large RCTs (the FDCC [37], Elite-Symphony [34] and OptiCept [38] trials) in order to determine the optimal tacrolimus C0 to prevent acute rejection during the first year of kidney transplantation. In general, these patients had a low-to-medium immunological risk. In the FDCC study, the mean tacrolimus C0 was 10–14 ng/mL in the first month, and tapered gradually thereafter. In the Elite-Symphony study, tacrolimus trough levels were 3-7 ng/mL during the study period. In the OptiCept trial, the tacrolimus trough levels were 8–12 ng/mL during the first month, 4–6 or 8–10 ng/mL until the end of the third months, and 3–5 or 6–8 ng/mL from the fourth month

thereafter, according to the randomization groups (reduced or standard CNI dosing). Despite this pooled analysis, the authors failed to find any significant correlations between tacrolimus trough levels and the incidence of acute rejection at the different time points.

In a recent study reporting on the pooled data [39] of four RCTs [40–43] (*n* = 528) in which patients received reduced tacrolimus dosing combined with mycofenolic acid, the authors concluded that tacrolimus levels < 4 ng/mL should be avoided during the first 12 months post-transplantation when tacrolimus is used in combination with fixed-dose mycofenolic acid with or without corticosteroids and induction therapy.

Study limitations
Certain limitations of this study should be acknowledged, the first of which being its observational single-center design. Second, protocol biopsies were not performed, nor was a biopsy systematically performed in instances of dnDSA detection. Consequently, the low number of ABMR should be taken with caution. Third, although IPV was

used herein as a proxy of patient adherence [44], it remains quite difficult to distinguish true minimization from non-adherence. Nevertheless, patients with > 50% non available trough levels were excluded from the analysis, with is also a well-known marker of non-adherence among KTRs. Consequently, it would appear reasonable to assume that the proportion of non-adherent patients was low in this study. Moreover, we discuss in this study the impact of reduced exposure to CNI, irrespective of its cause. Of note only 7 patients were excluded from study population because they had ≥50% of CNI trough levels non-available. And among these patients, only one developed dnDSA during follow-up. Due to this very small number of patients, it seems unreasonable to add a third group "non-adherence" in this study. Indeed, the addition of this third group is unlikely to allow us drawing reliable conclusion. Fourth, certain other factors potentially contributing to dnDSA development were not taking into account in this study, namely post-transplant pregnancies and transfusions [45]. Finally, while multivariable analyses were adjusted according to induction treatment and mycofenolic acid cessation during follow-up, mycofenolic acid dosage (area under curve) was not taken into account.

Clinical implications

In kidney graft recipients with low immunological risk, it is generally acknowledged that immunosuppressive treatment should be minimized given the low risk of graft rejection, and thus avoid exposing these patients to an accrued risk of neoplastic or infectious complications, as well as nephrotoxicity. As a result, clinicians frequently target low CNI trough levels in these cases. However, it should be kept in mind that such strategy is not without challenges in terms of risk of dnDSA development even in non-sensitized patients. At the very least, patients should be carefully monitored for DSA detection, in order to readjust treatment. Nevertheless, a low exposure to CNI only tended in our cohort to be associated with increased risk of graft rejection, as well as increased risk of return to dialysis. Although this absence of significant associations may be partly due to the size of our cohort, it also suggests that conflicting effects of CNI minimization might result in overall neutral effect. Despite an increased risk of dnDSA development, CNI minimization may well be beneficial for long-term graft prognosis by the way of nephrotoxicity avoidance among low-immunological risk patients [12, 18]. There are promising alternative strategies, such as the use of belatacept, which is a nonnephrotoxic drug, with no reported increased risk of DSA development [46]. The association of low-dose CNI with mTOR inhibitors could also be interesting, and has to be evaluated in regards to the risk of dnDSA development. In the recent multicenter non-inferiority trial

TRANSFORM [47], 2037 de novo kidney transplant recipients were randomized to receive, everolimus with reduced-exposure CNI or mycophenolic acid with standard-exposure CNI. DnDSA incidence at 12 months and ABMR rate did not differ between the two arms. Long-term results of the studies TRANSFORM [47] and ATHENA [48] will provide useful data.

Conclusions

Even in a low-immunological risk population, reduced exposure to CNI is associated with increased risk of dnDSA. Benefits and risks of under-immunosuppression must be carefully evaluated before deciding on CNI minimization.

Abbreviations
ABMR: Acute antibody-mediated rejection; C0: Trough level; CNI: Calcineurin inhibitors; dnDSA: De novo Donor Specific Antibodies; ECD: Expanded criteria donors; eGFR: Estimated Glomerular Filtration Rate; HLA: Human Leukocyte Antigen; HR: Hazard Ratio; IPV: Intra-patient variability; KTR: Kidney transplant recipients; MAD%: Mean absolute deviation percent; RCT: Randomized Controlled Trial; SCD: Standard criteria donors

Authors' contributions
SG: participated in research design, in the collection of the data, in the writing of the manuscript, in data analysis and data interpretation. JS: participated in research design, in the collection of the data, in the writing of the manuscript, in data interpretation. NG: participated in research design, in the reviewing of the manuscript, in data analysis and data interpretation. KD: participated in research design, in the reviewing of the manuscript, in data analysis and data interpretation. HB: participated in the collection of the data, in the reviewing of the manuscript, and data interpretation. NG: participated in the collection of the data, in the reviewing of the manuscript. ML: participated in the collection of the data, in the reviewing of the manuscript, and data interpretation. MK: participated in the collection of the data, in the reviewing of the manuscript, and in data interpretation. LF: participated in research design, in the reviewing of the manuscript, and data interpretation. AA: participated in research design, in the collection of the data, in the reviewing of the manuscript, in data analysis and data interpretation. All authors read and approved the final manuscript.

Competing interests
The authors declare that they have no competing interests.

Author details
[1]Service de Néphrologie et Transplantation rénale, CHRU Nancy Brabois, Vandoeuvre-les-, Nancy, France. [2]INSERM, Centre d'Investigations Cliniques Plurithématique 1433, Université de Lorraine, CHRU de Nancy and F-CRIN INI-CRCT, Nancy, France. [3]Service d'Anatomie pathologique, CHRU Nancy Brabois, Vandoeuvre-lès-Nancy, France. [4]Service de Pharmacologie-Toxicologie, CHRU Nancy Brabois, Vandoeuvre-lès-Nancy, France. [5]Laboratoire d'Histocompatibilité, CHRU Nancy Brabois, Vandoeuvre-lès-Nancy, France.

References
1. Naesens M, Kuypers DR, Sarwal M. Calcineurin inhibitor nephrotoxicity. Clinical journal of the American Society of Nephrology : CJASN. 2009;4(2):481–508.
2. Gaston RS. Chronic calcineurin inhibitor nephrotoxicity: reflections on an evolving paradigm. Clinical journal of the American Society of Nephrology : CJASN. 2009;4(12):2029–34.

3. Matas AJ. Chronic progressive calcineurin nephrotoxicity: an overstated concept. Am J Transplant Off J Am Soc Transplant Am Soc Transplant Surg. 2011;11(4):687–92.

4. Einecke G, Sis B, Reeve J, et al. Antibody-mediated microcirculation injury is the major cause of late kidney transplant failure. Am J Transplant Off J Am Soc Transplant Am Soc Transplant Surg. 2009;9(11):2520–31.

5. Gaston RS, Cecka JM, Kasiske BL, et al. Evidence for antibody-mediated injury as a major determinant of late kidney allograft failure. Transplantation. 2010;90(1):68–74.

6. Loupy A, Hill GS, Jordan SC. The impact of donor-specific anti-HLA antibodies on late kidney allograft failure. Nat Rev Nephrol. 2012;8(6):348–57.

7. Gourishankar S, Leduc R, Connett J, et al. Pathological and clinical characterization of the 'troubled transplant': data from the DeKAF study. Am J Transplant Off J Am Soc Transplant Am Soc Transplant Surg. 2010;10(2):324–30.

8. Bamoulid J, Staeck O, Halleck F, et al. The need for minimization strategies: current problems of immunosuppression. Transplant international : official journal of the European Society for Organ Transplantation. 2015;28(8):891–900.

9. Prashar R, Venkat KK. Immunosuppression minimization and avoidance protocols: when less is not more. Adv Chronic Kidney Dis. 2016;23(5): 295–300.

10. Sharif A, Shabir S, Chand S, Cockwell P, Ball S, Borrows R. Meta-analysis of calcineurin-inhibitor-sparing regimens in kidney transplantation. Journal of the American Society of Nephrology : JASN. 2011;22(11):2107–18.

11. Moore J, Middleton L, Cockwell P, et al. Calcineurin inhibitor sparing with mycophenolate in kidney transplantation: a systematic review and meta-analysis. Transplantation. 2009;87(4):591–605.

12. Sawinski D, Trofe-Clark J, Leas B, et al. Calcineurin inhibitor minimization, conversion, withdrawal, and avoidance strategies in renal transplantation: a systematic review and meta-analysis. Am J Transplant Off J Am Soc Transplant Am Soc Transplant Surg. 2016;16(7):2117–38.

13. Clinical Guidelines for Transpant Medications. 2018. http://www.transplant.bc.ca/Documents/Health%20Professionals/Clinical%20guidelines/Clinical%20Guidelines%20for%20Transplant%20Medications%20-%20June%202018.pdf.

14. Schiff J, Cole E, Cantarovich M. Therapeutic monitoring of calcineurin inhibitors for the nephrologist. Clinical journal of the American Society of Nephrology : CJASN. 2007;2(2):374–84.

15. Wallemacq P, Armstrong VW, Brunet M, et al. Opportunities to optimize tacrolimus therapy in solid organ transplantation: report of the European consensus conference. Ther Drug Monit. 2009;31(2):139–52.

16. Beland MA, Lapointe I, Noel R, et al. Higher calcineurin inhibitor levels predict better kidney graft survival in patients with de novo donor-specific anti-HLA antibodies: a cohort study. Transplant international : official journal of the European Society for Organ Transplantation. 2017;30(5):502–9.

17. Shuker N, van Gelder T, Hesselink DA. Intra-patient variability in tacrolimus exposure: causes, consequences for clinical management. Transplant Rev (Orlando). 2015;29(2):78–84.

18. Karpe KM, Talaulikar GS, Walters GD. Calcineurin inhibitor withdrawal or tapering for kidney transplant recipients. Cochrane Database Syst Rev. 2017; 7:CD006750.

19. Lefaucheur C, Loupy A, Hill GS, et al. Preexisting donor-specific HLA antibodies predict outcome in kidney transplantation. Journal of the American Society of Nephrology : JASN. 2010;21(8):1398–406.

20. Mohan S, Palanisamy A, Tsapepas D, et al. Donor-specific antibodies adversely affect kidney allograft outcomes. Journal of the American Society of Nephrology : JASN. 2012;23(12):2061–71.

21. Vo AA, Peng A, Toyoda M, et al. Use of intravenous immune globulin and rituximab for desensitization of highly HLA-sensitized patients awaiting kidney transplantation. Transplantation. 2010;89(9):1095–102.

22. Hidalgo LG, Campbell PM, Sis B, et al. De novo donor-specific antibody at the time of kidney transplant biopsy associates with microvascular pathology and late graft failure. Am J Transplant Off J Am Soc Transplant Am Soc Transplant Surg. 2009;9(11):2532–41.

23. Heilman RL, Nijim A, Desmarteau YM, et al. De novo donor-specific human leukocyte antigen antibodies early after kidney transplantation. Transplantation. 2014;98(12):1310–5.

24. Cooper JE, Gralla J, Cagle L, Goldberg R, Chan L, Wiseman AC. Inferior kidney allograft outcomes in patients with de novo donor-specific antibodies are due to acute rejection episodes. Transplantation. 2011;91(10):1103–9.

25. Devos JM, Gaber AO, Teeter LD, et al. Intermediate-term graft loss after renal transplantation is associated with both donor-specific antibody and acute rejection. Transplantation. 2014;97(5):534–40.

26. Wiebe C, Gibson IW, Blydt-Hansen TD, et al. Evolution and clinical pathologic correlations of de novo donor-specific HLA antibody post kidney transplant. Am J Transplant Off J Am Soc Transplant Am Soc Transplant Surg. 2012;12(5):1157–67.

27. Moreso F, Ibernon M, Goma M, et al. Subclinical rejection associated with chronic allograft nephropathy in protocol biopsies as a risk factor for late graft loss. Am J Transplant Off J Am Soc Transplant Am Soc Transplant Surg. 2006;6(4):747–52.

28. Moreso F, Carrera M, Goma M, et al. Early subclinical rejection as a risk factor for late chronic humoral rejection. Transplantation. 2012;93(1):41–6.

29. Gatault P, Kamar N, Buchler M, et al. Reduction of extended-release tacrolimus dose in low-immunological-risk kidney transplant recipients increases risk of rejection and appearance of donor-specific antibodies: a randomized study. Am J Transplant Off J Am Soc Transplant Am Soc Transplant Surg. 2017;17(5):1370–9.

30. Dugast E, Soulillou JP, Foucher Y, et al. Failure of Calcineurin inhibitor (tacrolimus) weaning randomized trial in long-term stable kidney transplant recipients. Am J Transplant Off J Am Soc Transplant Am Soc Transplant Surg. 2016;16(11):3255–61.

31. KDIGO clinical practice guideline for the care of kidney transplant recipients. Am J Transplant : official journal of the American Society of Transplantation and the American Society of Transplant Surgeons. 2009;9 Suppl 3:S1–155.

32. Ferguson R, Grinyo J, Vincenti F, et al. Immunosuppression with belatacept-based, corticosteroid-avoiding regimens in de novo kidney transplant recipients. Am J Transplant Off J Am Soc Transplant Am Soc Transplant Surg. 2011;11(1):66–76.

33. Bolin P Jr, Shihab FS, Mulloy L, et al. Optimizing tacrolimus therapy in the maintenance of renal allografts: 12-month results. Transplantation. 2008; 86(1):88–95.

34. Ekberg H, Tedesco-Silva H, Demirbas A, et al. Reduced exposure to calcineurin inhibitors in renal transplantation. N Engl J Med. 2007;357(25):2562–75.

35. Kamar N, Rostaing L, Cassuto E, et al. A multicenter, randomized trial of increased mycophenolic acid dose using enteric-coated mycophenolate sodium with reduced tacrolimus exposure in maintenance kidney transplant recipients. Clin Nephrol. 2012;77(2):126–36.

36. Bouamar R, Shuker N, Hesselink DA, et al. Tacrolimus predose concentrations do not predict the risk of acute rejection after renal transplantation: a pooled analysis from three randomized-controlled clinical trials(dagger). Am J Transplant Off J Am Soc Transplant Am Soc Transplant Surg. 2013;13(5):1253–61.

37. van Gelder T, Silva HT, de Fijter JW, et al. Comparing mycophenolate mofetil regimens for de novo renal transplant recipients: the fixed-dose concentration-controlled trial. Transplantation. 2008;86(8):1043–51.

38. Gaston RS, Kaplan B, Shah T, et al. Fixed- or controlled-dose mycophenolate mofetil with standard- or reduced-dose calcineurin inhibitors: the Opticept trial. Am J Transplant Off J Am Soc Transplant Am Soc Transplant Surg. 2009;9(7):1607–19.

39. Gaynor JJ, Ciancio G, Guerra G, et al. Lower tacrolimus trough levels are associated with subsequently higher acute rejection risk during the first 12 months after kidney transplantation. Transplant international : official journal of the European Society for Organ Transplantation. 2016;29(2):216–26.

40. Ciancio G, Burke GW, Gaynor JJ, et al. A randomized long-term trial of tacrolimus/sirolimus versus tacrolimus/mycophenolate mofetil versus cyclosporine (NEORAL)/sirolimus in renal transplantation. II. Survival, function, and protocol compliance at 1 year. Transplantation. 2004;77(2):252–8.

41. Ciancio G, Burke GW, Gaynor JJ, et al. A randomized trial of three renal transplant induction antibodies: early comparison of tacrolimus, mycophenolate mofetil, and steroid dosing, and newer immune-monitoring. Transplantation. 2005;80(4):457–65.

42. Ciancio G, Gaynor JJ, Roth D, et al. Randomized trial of thymoglobulin versus alemtuzumab (with lower dose maintenance immunosuppression) versus daclizumab in living donor renal transplantation. Transplant Proc. 2010;42(9):3503–6.

43. Ciancio G, Burke GW, Gaynor JJ, et al. Randomized trial of mycophenolate mofetil versus enteric-coated mycophenolate sodium in primary renal transplant recipients given tacrolimus and daclizumab/thymoglobulin: one year follow-up. Transplantation. 2008;86(1):67–74.

44. Neuberger JM, Bechstein WO, Kuypers DR, et al. Practical recommendations for long-term Management of Modifiable Risks in kidney and liver transplant recipients: a guidance report and clinical checklist by the consensus on managing modifiable risk in transplantation (COMMIT) group. Transplantation. 2017;101(4S Suppl 2):S1–S56.

45. Ferrandiz I, Congy-Jolivet N, Del Bello A, et al. Impact of early blood transfusion after kidney transplantation on the incidence of donor-specific anti-HLA antibodies. Am J Transplant Off J Am Soc Transplant Am Soc Transplant Surg. 2016;16(9):2661–9.

46. Bray RA, Gebel HM, Townsend R, et al. De novo donor-specific antibodies in belatacept-treated vs cyclosporine-treated kidney-transplant recipients: post hoc analyses of the randomized phase III BENEFIT and BENEFIT-EXT studies. Am J Transplant Off J Am Soc Transplant Am Soc Transplant Surg. 2018; 18(7):1783–9.

47. Pascual J, Berger SP, Witzke O, et al. Everolimus with reduced Calcineurin inhibitor exposure in renal transplantation. Journal of the American Society of Nephrology : JASN. 2018;29(7):1979–91.

48. Sommerer C, Suwelack B, Dragun D, et al. Design and rationale of the ATHENA study--a 12-month, multicentre, prospective study evaluating the outcomes of a de novo everolimus-based regimen in combination with reduced cyclosporine or tacrolimus versus a standard regimen in kidney transplant patients: study protocol for a randomised controlled trial. Trials. 2016;17:92.

2

Outcomes of bisphosphonate and its supplements for bone loss in kidney transplant recipients: a systematic review and network meta-analysis

Yan Yang[1,2†], Shi Qiu[3†], Linghui Deng[4], Xi Tang[1], Xinrui Li[1], Qiang Wei[3] and Ping Fu[1*] (iD)

Abstract

Background: Mineral bone disease constitutes a common complication of post-kidney transplantation, leading to great disability. As there is no consensus on the optimal treatment for post-kidney transplant recipients (KTRs), we aimed to evaluate the efficacy and safety of bisphosphonate and its combined therapies.

Methods: We incorporated relevant trials to perform a network meta-analysis from direct and indirect comparisons. We searched PubMed, Embase and the CENTRAL and the reference lists of relevant articles up to August 1, 2017, for randomized controlled trials. The primary outcome was bone mineral density (BMD) change at the femoral neck and the lumbar spine.

Results: From a total of 864 citations, 18 randomized controlled trials with a total of 1200 participants were included. Five different regimens were considered. Bisphosphonate plus calcium revealed a significant gain in percent BMD change than calcium alone at the femoral neck (mean difference (MD), 5.83; 95% credible interval (CrI), 1.61 to 9.27). No significant difference was detected when restricting to absolute terms. At the lumbar spine, bisphosphonate and calcium with or without vitamin D analogs outperformed calcium solely (MD, 0.07; 95% CrI, 0.00 to 0.13; MD, 0.06; 95% CrI, 0.02 to 0.09). Compared to calcium with vitamin D analogs, adding bisphosphonate was associated with marked improvement (MD, 0.03; 95% CrI, 0.00 to 0.05). Considering percent terms, combination of bisphosphonate with calcium and vitamin D analogs showed greater beneficial effects than calcium alone or with either vitamin D analogs or calcitonin (MD, 10.51; 95% CrI, 5.92 to 15.34; MD, 5.48; 95% CrI, 2.57 to 8.42; MD, 6.39; 95% CrI, 0.55 to 12.89). Both bisphosphonate and vitamin D analogs combined with calcium displayed a notable improvement compared to calcium alone (MD, 7.24; 95% CrI, 3.73 to 10.69; MD, 5.02; 95% CrI, 1.20 to 8.84).

Conclusions: Our study suggested that additional use of bisphosphonate was well-tolerated and more favorable in KTRs to improve BMD.

Keywords: Kidney transplant, Bisphosphonates, Bone mineral density, Network meta-analysis

* Correspondence: fupinghx@163.com
†Yan Yang and Shi Qiu contributed equally to this work.
[1]Kidney Research Laboratory, Division of Nephrology, National Clinical Research Center for Geriatrics, West China Hospital, Sichuan University, No. 37, Guoxue Alley, Chengdu, Sichuan, People's Republic of China610041
Full list of author information is available at the end of the article

Background

Since kidney transplantation (KT) became an effective treatment of patients with end-stage renal disease (ESRD), clinicians have paid more attention to complications of kidney transplant recipients (KTRs). Post-transplantation bone disease which can result in serious disabilities and fractures has been observed among a large proportion of KTRs [1]. According to Naylor and colleagues [2], the 5-year cumulative incidence of fracture ranged from 0.85 to 27% after KT. Hence, prevention and treatment of bone disorders are of great importance to improve high-quality long-term survival of KTRs.

The etiology of transplant bone disease is multifactorial and most KTRs have preexisting chronic kidney disease-mineral and bone disorders (CKD-MBD) [3]. Apart from these, glucocorticoid-induced suppression of bone formation, calcineurin inhibitors (CNIs) and persistent hyperparathyroidism are the most important risk factors for bone loss [4–6]. Postmenopausal status, prolonged immobilization, duration of CKD stage 5, smoking and presence of diabetes may also contribute to bone loss [4]. The Kidney Disease Improving Global Outcomes (KDIGO) guideline [7] suggested that "vitamin D, calcitriol/alfacalcidol, or bisphosphonates be considered for low BMD patients with stable graft function", but it was derived from the very low quality of evidence.

Previous meta-analyses [8, 9] have demonstrated that bisphosphonates have favorable efficacy on bone mineral density (BMD), but questionable effect on the fracture risk. However, these studies did not examine the effect of co-intervention with calcium and/or vitamin D. Moreover, it is still uncertain that the optimal approach to prevent bone loss and whether it is need to use combined therapy. To obtain a better understanding on this issue, we performed a network meta-analysis (NMA). In this NMA, we systematically reviewed the literature and estimated relative treatment effects for all possible comparisons including bisphosphonates and co-intervention.

Methods

Search strategy

This systematic review is performed in keeping with Preferred Reporting Items for Systematic Reviews and Meta-analyses (PRISMA) guideline [10]. A comprehensive search was conducted in PubMed, Embase and the Cochrane Library Central Register of Controlled Trials (CENTRAL) by two independent investigators up to August 1st, 2017. The full search parameters for each database was outlined in Additional file 1. Referenced articles and systematic reviews were screened to maximize inclusion of pertinent data.

Selection criteria

Only randomized controlled trials (RCTs) comparing bisphosphonate-treated and control groups of adult KTRs were included. The full-text original article with at least one interest outcome was finally involved. Two independent investigators (YY, QS) initially screened the citation titles and abstracts. Studies were excluded because of non-English text, combined transplantation. If duplicate studies from the identical authors were found, the reports were grouped together and only the publication with a complete data was used. Any discrepancies in the study inclusion were resolved by consulting the senior authors (TX).

Data extraction and quality assessment

The independent reviewers (YY, SQ) used a standardized form to extract information from each eligible study. Data regarding study-, patient- and treatment-related characteristics and outcomes were extracted simultaneously. When relevant information was unclear or needed data was unavailable, attempts were made to obtain eligible data from the first or corresponding author of such studies. We assessed the validity of the NMA through a qualitative appraisal of study designs and methods. We executed the tool recommended by the Cochrane Collaboration to evaluate the risk of bias [11].

Outcomes

The primary outcome was the BMD change (percent change and absolute change [in g/cm^2]) at the lumbar spine and the femoral neck after successful KT. The secondary outcomes were overall fractures, all-cause mortality, graft loss, acute renal rejection, adverse events. The fractures occurred during reported follow-up time that identified by radiographs were used to calculate fracture incidence. Graft loss was regarded as a doubling of the baseline serum creatinine level or progressing to ESRD again. We used data from the longest complete follow-up, when the outcomes of different follow-up intervals were reported. If investigators published more than one report addressing the same population, we included the most comprehensive report.

Data synthesis and statistical analysis

The pair-wise meta-analysis by the random-effects model was performed initially [12]. Results were expressed as mean difference (MD) with 95% confidence intervals (CI) for continuous outcomes (percent change and absolute change in BMD), while the odds ratio (OR) was used for dichotomous variables (fracture, all-cause mortality, graft loss, acute renal rejection, adverse events). The level of statistical significance was set at $P < 0.05$ and all statistical tests were two-sided. The statistical heterogeneity among studies was evaluated by the Cochran's Q test and the I^2

statistic. A P value of 0.05 or less for the Q test or an I^2 greater than 50% was suggestive of substantial study heterogeneity.

We performed random-effects Bayesian network meta-analyses for indirect and mixed comparisons using Markov chain Monte Carlo methods in Win-BUGS version 1.4.3 (MRC Biostatistics Unit) [13]. A Bayesian fixed-effect framework was deemed appropriate because of the limited number of studies supporting each edge in the network [13, 14]. We report the resultant effect as OR or MD with corresponding 95% credibility intervals (CrIs), which are the Bayesian analogue of 95% CIs. We estimated the relative ranking probability of each strategy and obtained the hierarchy of competing interventions using rankograms and surface under the cumulative ranking curve (SUCRA) [15]. The SUCRA index ranges between 0 (or 0%) and 1 (or 100%), where the treatments with highest and lowest SUCRA are considered to be the best and worst treatments, respectively.

To assess the presence of the inconsistency, we employed the node-splitting method, excluding one direct comparison at a time and estimating the indirect treatment effect for the excluded comparison. To check the assumption of consistency in the entire network, the design-by-treatment model was conducted [14]. If the total residual deviance and the effective number of parameters (pD) are almost the same, the network consistency is considered to be satisfied. We then performed sensitivity analysis and meta-regressions to explore important network inconsistency.

Quality of evidence

The quality of evidence was rated according to the Grading of Recommendations, Assessment, Development and Evaluation (GRADE) methodology [16]. In this approach, direct evidence from RCTs starts at high quality and can be downgraded based on the risk of bias, indirectness, imprecision, inconsistency (or heterogeneity) and publication bias to levels of moderate, low and relatively low quality [17].

Results

Study characteristics

The PRISMA [10] flowchart depicting the electronic searching process is presented in Fig. 1. There are 864 potentially relevant articles identified through electronic and reference searches. According to title and abstract, 821 publications were excluded after the initial screening. A further 26 studies were excluded because they were not RCT, without available data of interest outcomes and lack of full-text. Overall, 18 RCTs (19 publications) [18–36] involving 1200 participants were included in this NMA. The studies were published between October 1998 and March 2015. The details of the

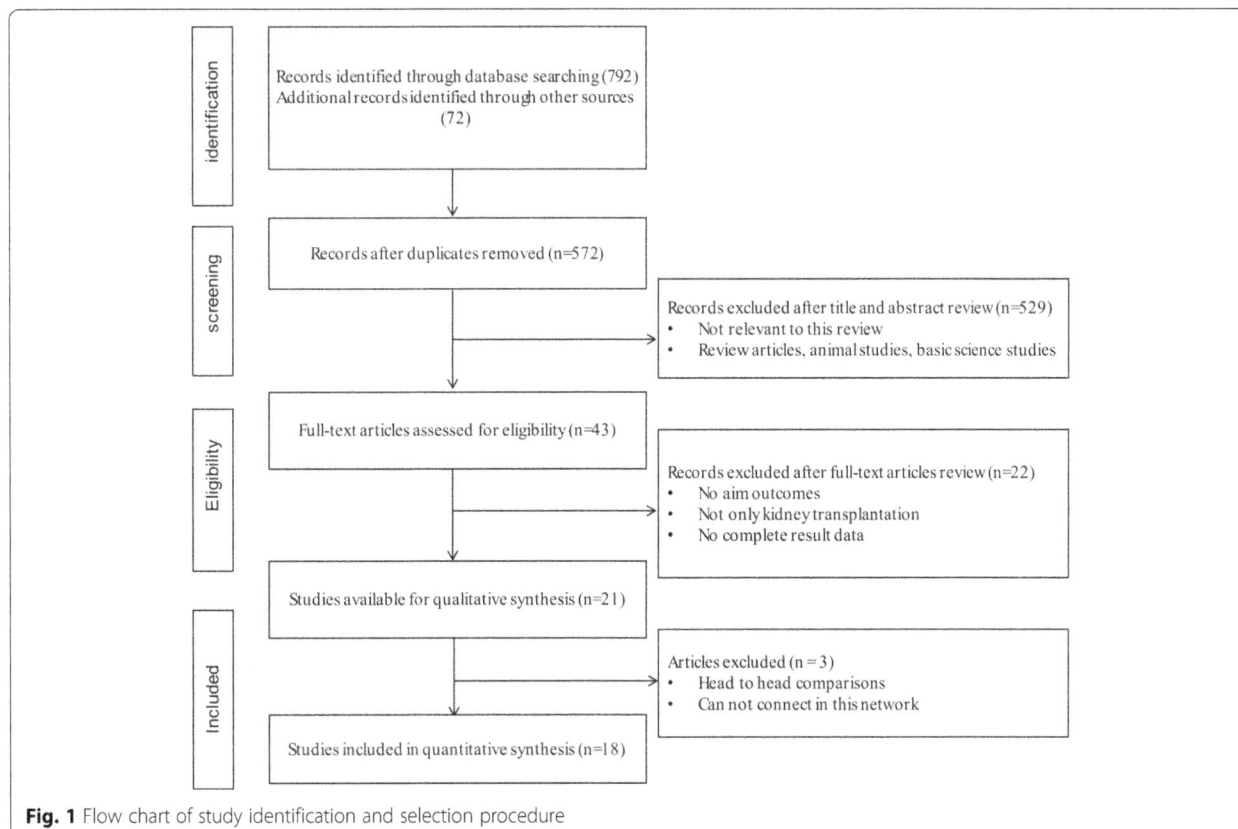

Fig. 1 Flow chart of study identification and selection procedure

interventions, baseline characteristics of the populations, follow-up period were outlined for NMA in Table 1. Most of the RCTs included both sexes, except one study [26] only included male patients and two studies [25, 27] did not mention. The number of patients allocated to each treatment ranged from 8 to 66, whereas patient follow-up duration ranged from 6 months to 3 years after first administration.

As expected, most studies compared bisphosphonate with vitamin D analogs (cholecalciferol, alfacalcidol, calcitriol) or placebo. All patients in the trials included received co-intervention including calcium [24, 26–28, 30–33, 35], vitamin D analogs [19], or both. Bisphosphonate interventions encompassed pamidronate [21, 22, 29, 32], zoledronic acid [27, 30] and ibandronate [18, 31] that were administered intravenously, while clodronate [33], alendronate [23–26, 28, 34, 35] and risedronate [19, 20, 36] were given orally.

Risk of Bias assessment result

The results from the risk of bias assessment are provided in Additional file 2. Details regarding trial methodology were unsatisfactory or incomplete for the majority of studies. Overall, there were 6 (32%) studies regarded as high risk of bias. Only 10 (53%) studies performed randomized sequence generation adequately. Furthermore, the risk of bias for concealment of treatment allocation was unclear in 10 (53%) studies. Only 4 (33%) studies explicitly reported blinding of participants and investigators, whereas the remaining studies were at high or unclear risk in this regard. The investigators attempted to blind outcome assessors in 6 (32%) studies, 3 studies did not make an effort to blind assessors, and the residual studies were unclear. When the results were summarized from at least 10 studies, the publication bias accessed via funnel plot. Comparison adjusted funnel plot showed no evidence of asymmetry (Additional file 2).

Pairwise meta-analysis

Primary results of pairwise meta-analysis (direct comparisons) are summarized in Table 2. In terms of absolute change for the longest follow-up, adding bisphosphonate was associated with a marginal improvement compared to the combination of calcium and vitamin D analogs (femoral neck: MD, 0.36; 95% CI, 0.08 to 0.64; lumbar spine: MD, 0.38; 95% CI, 0.19 to 0.57). Bisphosphonate combined with calcium was significantly better than calcium alone (femoral neck: MD, 1.30; 95% CI, 0.92 to 1.68; lumbar spine: MD, 0.51; 95% CI, 0.20 to 0.82). Treatments with calcium alone displayed significantly lower absolute change at the femoral neck than combining with vitamin D analogs or calcitonin (MD, – 0.74; 95% CI, – 1.34 to – 0.14; MD, – 0.55; 95% CI, – 1.07 to – 0.03). When measured in percent terms, additional use

of vitamin D analogs or bisphosphonate was significantly better than solely calcium (femoral neck: MD 1.53; 95% CI, 0.88 to 2.18; MD 1.14; 95% CI, 0.78 to 1.51; lumbar spine: MD 2.73; 95% CI, 1.95 to 3.51; MD 1.17; 95% CI, 0.80 to 1.54). Compared to calcium and vitamin D analogs, the combination of bisphosphonate and calcium showed significant improvement (femoral neck: MD, 1.55; 95% CI, 0.76 to 2.35; lumbar spine: MD, 1.53; 95% CI, 0.79 to 2.27). Bisphosphonate with calcium and vitamin D analogs also showed a significant gain at the lumbar spine compared to calcium and vitamin D analogs (MD, 1.32; 95% CI, 1.02 to 1.62).

Network meta-analysis— Primary outcome
Change of BMD at the femoral neck

Ten RCTs involving 536 adults evaluated the absolute change in BMD at the femoral neck. Figure 2 summarizes the network of direct evidence available for this outcome. No statistically significant difference was detected between each treatment groups. The SUCRA value for the regimens were 88%, 53%, 52%, 29%, 28% for bisphosphonate with calcium, bisphosphonate with calcium and vitamin D analogs, calcium with vitamin D analogs, calcitonin with calcium and calcium (Fig. 3a).

The result of percent terms was reported by 5 RCTs including 284 patients. Only bisphosphonate plus calcium revealed a significant gain in percent BMD change than calcium alone (MD, 5.83; 95% CrI, 1.61 to 9.27). No statistical difference was observed between other groups. Bisphosphonate combined with calcium and vitamin D analogs had the highest SUCRA value (97% Fig. 3b), followed by calcitonin with calcium (66%), bisphosphonate plus calcium (38%), calcium with vitamin D analogs (27%), and calcium only (22%).

Change of BMD at the lumbar spine

14 RCTs including 814 participants provided data for comparison of absolute change in BMD at the lumbar spine. Bisphosphonate and calcium with or without vitamin D analogs outperformed calcium solely (MD, 0.07; 95% CrI, 0.00 to 0.13; MD, 0.06; 95% CrI, 0.02 to 0.09). We also observed that compared to calcium with vitamin D analogs, adding bisphosphonate was associated with marked improvement (MD, 0.03; 95% CrI, 0.00 to 0.05). The SUCRA value for each treatment formulations were as follows (Fig. 3c): bisphosphonate with calcium and vitamin D analogs (87%), bisphosphonate with calcium (81%), calcium plus vitamin D analogs (48%), calcitonin with calcium (24%) and calcium solely (10%).

Considering percent terms, the result analyzed using data from 7 trials (466 patients). Combination of bisphosphonate with calcium and vitamin D analogs showed greater beneficial effects than calcium alone or with either vitamin D analogs or calcitonin (MD, 10.51;

Table 1 Study characteristics

Study	Follow-up	Country	No. of Patients	Female/Male	Intervention	Bisphosphonate Administration	N	Co-intervention	Immunosuppression
Smerud 2012 [18]	12 months	Norway	129	30/99	ibandronate	3 mg i.v. (every 3 months)	66	PO calcium 500 mg twice daily+ calcitriol 0.25 mcg daily	corticosteroids, MMF, CsA or FK506
					placebo		63		
Coco 2012 [19]	12 months	USA	42	15/27	risedronate	35 mg p.o. (weekly)	20	PO calcitriol 0.25 µg daily (with or without calcium)	corticosteroids, MMF, FK506, rapamycin
					placebo		22		
Torregrosa 2010 [20]	12 months	Spain	101	34/67	risedronate	35 mg p.o. (weekly)	52	PO calcium 1.5 g daily + vitamin D 400 IU daily	corticosteroids, FK506 with or without MMF
					no treatment		49		
Torregrosa 2011 [21]	12 months	Spain	39	13/26	pamidronate	30 mg iv (between day 7 and 10 after KT and 3 months post-KT)	24	PO calcium 1 g daily + cholecalciferol 800 IU daily	corticosteroids, MMF, CsA
					placebo		15		
Walsh 2009 [22]	24 months	UK	125	24/69	pamidronate	1 mg/kg i.v. (perioperatively and at month 1, 4, 8, 12)	65	PO calcium 500 mg daily + vitamin D 400 IU daily	corticosteroids, CsA
					no treatment		60		
Lan 2008 [23]	6 months	China	46	27/19	alendronate	70 mg p.o. (weekly)	23	PO calcium 800 mg daily + calcitriol 0.25 µg daily	corticosteroids, MMF, CsA
					no treatment		23		
Trabulus 2008 [24]	12 months	Turkey	64	19/40	alendronate	10 mg p.o. (daily)	13	PO calcium 1 g daily	corticosteroids, azathioprin or MMF, CsA or FK506
					alfacalcidol	0.5 µg p.o. (daily)	25		
					alendronate + alfacalcidol		17		
					no treatment		9		
Nayak 2007 [25]	6 months	India	50	NA	alendronate	35 mg p.o. (weekly)	27	PO calcium 1 g daily + vitamin D	NA
					no treatment		23		
El-Agroudy 2005 [26]	12 months	Egypt	60	0/60	alendronate	5 mg p.o. (daily)	15	PO calcium 500 mg daily	corticosteroids, CsA
					alfacalcidol	0.5 µg p.o. (daily)	15		
					calcitonin	100 µl intranasally (p.o.d and stopped for 1 month every 3 month)	15		
					no treatment		15		
Schwarz 2004 [27]	36 months	Austria	20	8/12	zoledronic acid	4 mg i.v. (week 2, month 3)	9	PO calcium 1 g daily	corticosteroids, MMF, CsA
					placebo		10		
Jeffery 2003 [28]	12 months	Canada	117	26/71	alendronate	10 mg p.o. (daily)	57	PO calcium 500 mg daily	corticosteroids, CsA, azathioprin or MMF
					calcitriol	0.25 µg p.o. (daily)	60		
Coco 2003 [29]	12 months	USA	72	28/31	pamidronate	60 mg i.v. (<48 h after KT, 30 mg i.v. at months 1, 2, 3, 6)	36	calcium + calcitriol	corticosteroids, CsA or FK506
					no treatment		36		

Table 1 Study characteristics (*Continued*)

Study	Follow-up	Country	No. of Patients	Female/Male	Intervention	Bisphosphonate Administration	N	Co-intervention	Immunosuppression
Hass 2003 [30]	6 months	Austria	20	8/12	zoledronic acid	4 mg i.v. (week 2, month 3)	10	PO calcium 1 g daily	corticosteroids, MMF, CsA
					placebo		10		
Grotz 2001 [31]	12 months	Germany	80	24/48	ibandronate	1 mg i.v. (just before KT, 2 mg i.v. at month 3, 6, 9)	36	PO calcium 500 mg daily	corticosteroids, MMF, CsA
					no treatment		36		
Nam 2000 [32]	6 months	South Kore	50	21/29	pamidronate	30 mg i.v. (every 4 weeks)	15	PO calcium 500 mg daily	NA
					calcitriol	0.5 µg p.o. (daily)	15		
					no treatment		20		
Grotz 1998 [33]	12 months	Germany	46	17/29	clodronate	800 mg p.o. (daily) for 14 days, each followed by 75 days without treatment	15	PO calcium 500 mg daily	corticosteroids, CsA
					calcitonin	100 IU intranasally twice a day	16		
					no treatment		15		
Giannini 2001 [34]	12 months	Italy	40	13/27	alendronate	10 mg p.o. (daily)	20	PO calcium 500 mg daily + calcitriol 0.5 µg daily	corticosteroids, CsA with or without azathioprin
					no treatment		20		
Koc 2002 [35]	12 months	Turkey	35	10/25	alendronate	10 mg p.o. (daily)	8	PO calcium 1 g daily	corticosteroids, azathioprin, CsA
					calcitriol	0.5 µg p.o. (daily)	8		
					no treatment		8		
Torregrosa 2007 [36]	12 months	Spain	84	42/42	risedronate	35 mg p.o. (weekly)	39	PO calcium 2.5 g daily + vitamin D	corticosteroids, CsA or FK506, with or without MMF
					no treatment		45		

KT: kidney transplantation; i.v.: intravenous; p.o., PO: peros; p.o.d: per other day; N: numbers; NA: not available; MMF: mycophenolate mofetil; CsA: cyclosporine; FK506: tacrolimus; AZA: azathioprine; mTOR: mammalian target of rapamycin

Table 2 Summary effect size of pairwise and network meta-analysis

Comparisons	No. of directed trials (participants)	Pairwise meta-analysis mean differences (95% CI)	Network meta-analysis mean differences (95% CrI)	Heterogeneity I²	P-Value	Quality of evidence
Absolute BMD change at the femoral neck (536)						
Bis+Ca vs. Bis+Ca + Vit D	1 (29)	–	− 0.01 (− 0.32, 0.29)	–	–	Low
Bis+Ca vs. Ca	5 (167)	**1.3 (0.92, 1.68)**	0.19 (− 0.01, 0.38)	94.70%	0.000	Low
Bis+Ca vs. Ca + Vit D	2 (176)	0.26 (−0.04, 0.56)	0.06 (− 0.15, 0.26)	38.10%	0.184	Moderate
Bis+Ca vs. Ca + Calcitonin	2 (61)	0.21 (−0.29, 0.72)	0.06 (− 0.22, 0.36)	24.60%	0.249	Moderate
Bis+Ca + Vit D vs. Ca	–	–	0.20 (−0.14, 0.53)	–	–	Very low
Bis+Ca + Vit D vs. Ca + Vit D	4 (206)	**0.36 (0.08, 0.64)**	0.07 (−0.18, 0.30)	67.60%	0.026	Low
Bis+Ca + Vit D vs. Ca + Calcitonin	–	–	0.07 (−0.34, 0.46)	–	–	Very low
Ca vs. Ca + Vit D	2 (46)	**−0.74 (−1.34, − 0.14)**	−0.13 (− 0.38, 0.13)	0.00%	0.403	Low
Ca vs. Ca + Calcitonin	2 (60)	**−0.55 (−1.07, − 0.03)**	−0.12 (− 0.41, 0.19)	60.20%	0.113	Low
Ca + Vit D vs. Ca + Calcitonin	1 (30)	–	0.00 (−0.30, 0.34)	–	–	Low
Percent BMD change at the femoral neck (284)						
Bis+Ca vs. Bis+Ca + Vit D	1 (29)	–	−4.60 (−18.07, 7.67)	–	–	Low
Bis+Ca vs. Ca	4 (152)	**1.14 (0.78, 1.51)**	**5.83 (1.61, 9.27)**	91.10%	0.000	Moderate
Bis+Ca vs. Ca + Vit D	4 (46)	**1.55 (0.76, 2.35)**	−0.24 (5.62, 9.79)	96.10%	0.000	Low
Bis+Ca vs. Ca + Calcitonin	1 (31)	–	−0.04 (−19.65, 18.12)	–	–	Low
Bis+Ca + Vit D vs. Ca	–	–	10.43 (−2.64, 23.31)	–	–	Very low
Bis+Ca + Vit D vs. Ca + Vit D	–	–	4.35 (−2.29, 11.37)	–	–	Very low
Bis+Ca + Vit D vs. Ca + Calcitonin	–	–	4.56 (−18.36, 19.16)	–	–	Very low
Ca vs. Ca + Vit D	3 (51)	**−1.53 (−2.18, −0.88)**	−6.07 (− 17.09, 4.47)	79.30%	0.028	Low
Ca vs. Ca + Calcitonin	1 (30)	–	−5.87 (−20.01, 18.60)	–	–	Low
Ca + Vit D vs. Ca + Calcitonin	1 (30)	–	0.20 (−19.15, 19.61)	–	–	Low
Absolute BMD change at the lumbar spine (814)						
Bis+Ca vs. Bis+Ca + Vit D	1 (29)	–	−0.01 (−0.06, 0.04)	–	–	Low
Bis+Ca vs. Ca	5 (167)	**0.51 (0.20, 0.82)**	**0.06 (0.02, 0.09)**	0.00%	0.571	Moderate
Bis+Ca vs. Ca + Vit D	4 (176)	0.19 (−0.11, 0.49)	0.01 (−0.03, 0.06)	0.00%	0.866	Moderate
Bis+Ca vs. Ca + Calcitonin	2 (61)	0.49 (−0.02, 1.00)	0.05 (−0.01, 0.11)	24.60%	0.250	Moderate
Bis+Ca + Vit D vs. Ca	1 (30)	–	**0.07 (0.00, 0.13)**	–	–	Low
Bis+Ca + Vit D vs. Ca + Vit D	8 (484)	**0.38 (0.19, 0.57)**	**0.03 (0.00, 0.05)**	92.10%	0.000	Moderate
Bis+Ca + Vit D vs. Ca + Calcitonin	–	–	0.06 (−0.01, 0.15)	–	–	Very low
Ca vs. Ca + Vit D	2 (46)	−0.40 (− 0.99, 0.18)	−0.04 (− 0.10, 0.02)	0.00%	0.960	Moderate
Ca vs. Ca + Calcitonin	2 (60)	−0.04 (− 0.55, 0.47)	−0.01 (− 0.07, 0.06)	0.00%	0.874	Moderate
Ca + Vit D vs. Ca + Calcitonin	–	–	0.04 (−0.04, 0.12)	–	–	Very low
Percent BMD change at the lumbar spine (466)						
Bis+Ca vs. Bis+Ca + Vit D	–	–	−3.27 (−7.87, 0.84)	–	–	Very low
Bis+Ca vs. Ca	4 (152)	**1.17 (0.80, 1.54)**	**7.24 (3.73, 10.69)**	91.70%	0.000	Moderate
Bis+Ca vs. Ca + Vit D	2 (46)	**1.53 (0.79, 2.27)**	2.22 (−1.44, 5.73)	94.10%	0.000	Low
Bis+Ca vs. Ca + Calcitonin	1 (31)	–	3.13 (−2.51, 8.51)	–	–	Low
Bis+Ca + Vit D vs. Ca	–	–	**10.50 (5.92, 15.34)**	–	–	Very low
Bis+Ca + Vit D vs. Ca + Vit D	3 (145)	**1.32 (1.02, 1.62)**	**5.48 (2.57, 8.42)**	98.30%	0.000	Moderate
Bis+Ca + Vit D vs. Ca + Calcitonin	–	–	**6.39 (0.55, 12.89)**	–	–	Low

Table 2 Summary effect size of pairwise and network meta-analysis *(Continued)*

Comparisons	No. of directed trials (participants)	Pairwise meta-analysis mean differences (95% CI)	Network meta-analysis mean differences (95% CrI)	Heterogeneity I²	P-Value	Quality of evidence
Ca vs. Ca + Vit D	2 (51)	**−2.73 (−3.51, −1.95)**	**−5.02 (−8.84, − 1.20)**	0.00%	0.373	Moderate
Ca vs. Ca + Calcitonin	1 (30)	–	−4.11 (−9.01, 0.72)	–	–	Low
Ca + Vit D vs. Ca + Calcitonin	–	–	0.91 (−4.38, 6.44)	–	–	Very low

Bis = bisphosphonate, Ca = calcium, Vit D = Vitamin D analogs, 95% CI = 95% Confidence Intervals, 95% CrI = 95% Credible Intervals. The mean difference with 95% CI or 95% CrI was used for continuous outcomes. Significant results are in bold. The Grading of Recommendations Assessment, Development and Evaluation (GRADE) approach specific to NMA served to assess the certainty in the evidence (quality of evidence) associated with specific comparisons, including direct, indirect, and final network meta-analysis estimates. The confidence assessment addressed the risk of bias (in individual studies), imprecision, inconsistency (heterogeneity in estimates of effect across studies), indirectness, and publication bias

95% CrI, 5.92 to 15.34; MD, 5.48; 95% CrI, 2.57 to 8.42; MD, 6.39; 95% CrI, 0.55 to 12.89). Both bisphosphonate and vitamin D analogs combined with calcium displayed a notable improvement compared to calcium alone (MD, 7.24; 95% CrI, 3.73 to 10.69; MD, 5.02; 95% CrI, 1.20 to 8.84). As expected, bisphosphonate combined with calcium and vitamin D analogs had the highest SUCRA value (Fig. 3d 99%), followed by bisphosphonate with calcium (63%), calcium with vitamin D analogs (57%), calcitonin with calcium (29%), and calcium only (2%).

Secondary outcomes

We did not observe a significant difference in the incidence of fractures from the direct comparisons and it could not connect to draw network geometries. All treatments have uncertain effects on all-cause mortality and graft loss metrics. Similarly, there were no statistical

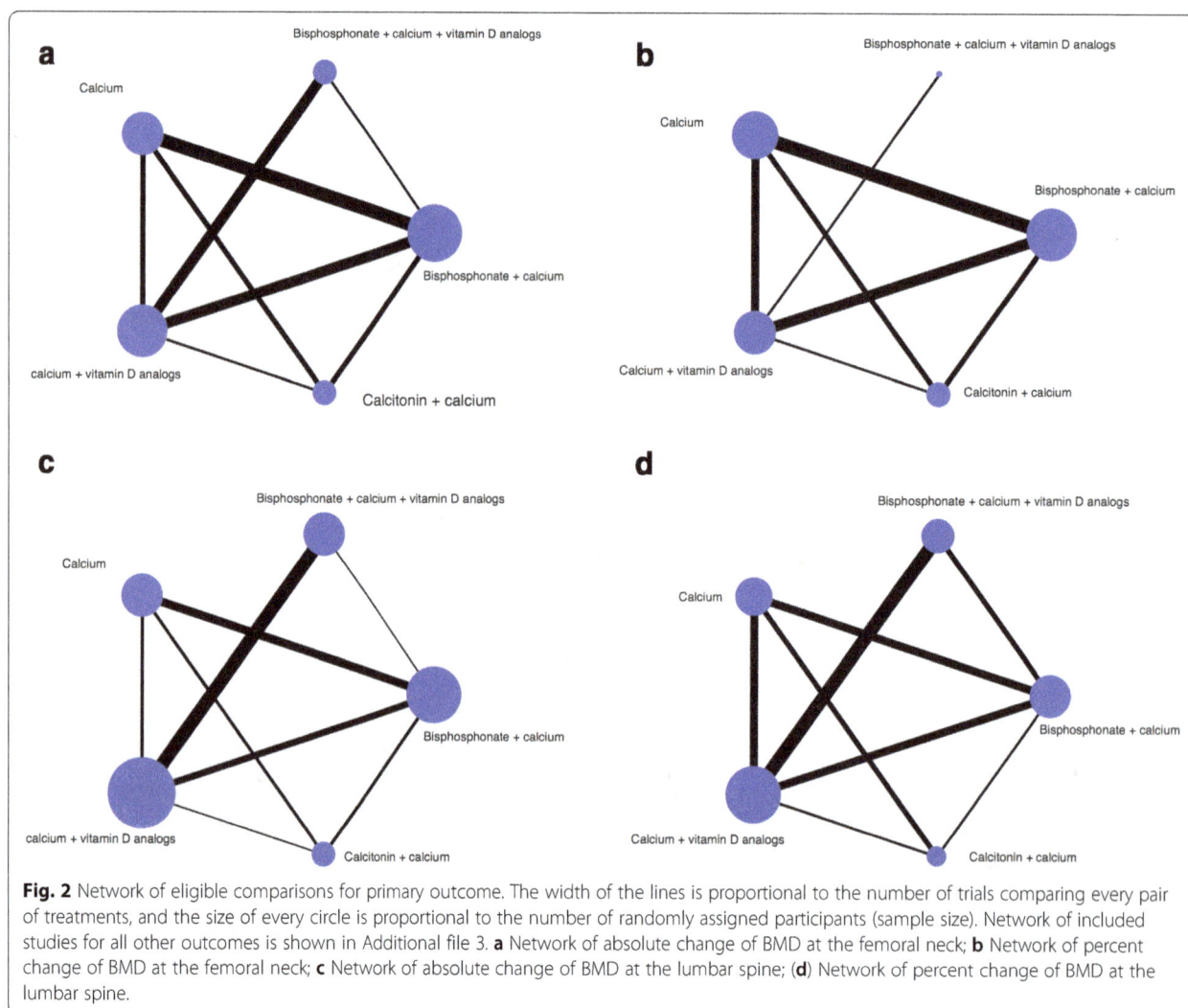

Fig. 2 Network of eligible comparisons for primary outcome. The width of the lines is proportional to the number of trials comparing every pair of treatments, and the size of every circle is proportional to the number of randomly assigned participants (sample size). Network of included studies for all other outcomes is shown in Additional file 3. **a** Network of absolute change of BMD at the femoral neck; **b** Network of percent change of BMD at the femoral neck; **c** Network of absolute change of BMD at the lumbar spine; (**d**) Network of percent change of BMD at the lumbar spine.

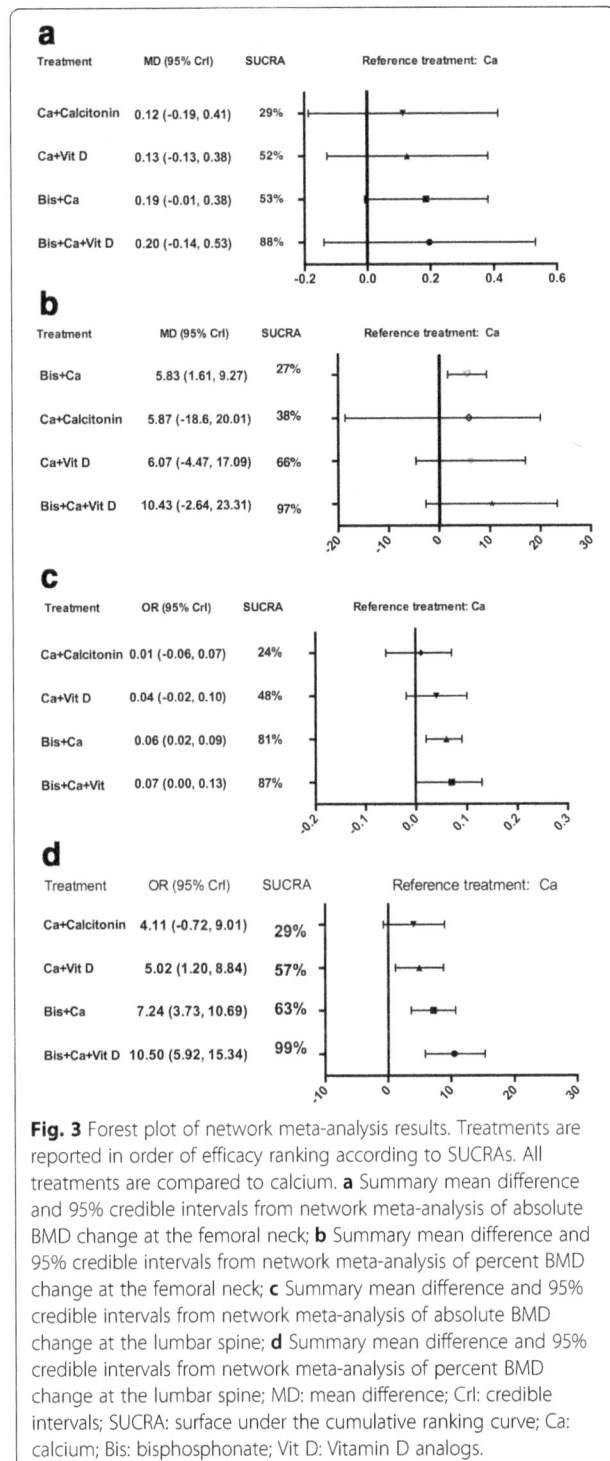

Fig. 3 Forest plot of network meta-analysis results. Treatments are reported in order of efficacy ranking according to SUCRAs. All treatments are compared to calcium. **a** Summary mean difference and 95% credible intervals from network meta-analysis of absolute BMD change at the femoral neck; **b** Summary mean difference and 95% credible intervals from network meta-analysis of percent BMD change at the femoral neck; **c** Summary mean difference and 95% credible intervals from network meta-analysis of absolute BMD change at the lumbar spine; **d** Summary mean difference and 95% credible intervals from network meta-analysis of percent BMD change at the lumbar spine; MD: mean difference; CrI: credible intervals; SUCRA: surface under the cumulative ranking curve; Ca: calcium; Bis: bisphosphonate; Vit D: Vitamin D analogs.

Network consistency

No evidence of small study effects based on funnel plot asymmetry was observed, but the number of studies included in each comparison was small. There was no evidence of inconsistency in the NMA when we applied the node-splitting approach. The total residual deviance for the outcomes of percent change (23.73, pD = 22) and absolute change (43.86, pD = 45) of BMD at the lumbar spine implied a good model fit, as well as percent change (25.22, pD = 26) and absolute change (24.36, pD = 24) at the femoral neck.

Sensitivity analysis

For the sensitivity analyses, we used the full network for the primary outcome. In the first analysis, we investigated the different assumptions regarding the potential relationship between time and treatment effect, Bayesian NMA were repeated using the absolute change of BMD at the twelve-month follow-up period. We observed comparable results at the lumbar spine, adding bisphosphonate showed significant improvement than calcium alone or calcium with vitamin D analogs (Additional file 5: MD, 0.06; 95% CrI, 0.01 to 0.10; MD, 0.03; 95% CrI, 0.00 to 0.07). We also observed that bisphosphonate with calcium and vitamin D analogs outperformed calcium solely (MD, 0.07; 95% CrI, 0.01 to 0.15). At the femoral neck, bisphosphonate with calcium showed a significant preference than calcium alone (Additional file 5; MD, 0.23; 95% CrI, 0.02 to 0.46). The parameter estimates were consistent with the main analysis. We carried out separate meta-regressions to test the effect of length of trial, publication date and modes of administration. No evidence exists for an interaction between any of the trial characteristics assessed and the treatment effect.

Quality of evidence

In general, there was no serious risk of bias, indirectness, inconsistency, or publication bias for any of the direct comparisons. In several comparisons, there was serious imprecision in summary estimate because the 95% credible interval crossed unity. The GRADE quality of evidence supporting the use of each treatment for the primary outcome was outlined in Table 2. According to GRADE, we had moderate confidence in estimates supporting the combination use of bisphosphonate or vitamin D analogs with calcium for improving BMD at the lumbar spine. We detected using bisphosphonate combined with vitamin D analogs and calcium considering BMD change at the lumbar spine with low quality evidence. There was very confidence in estimates supporting using calcitonin with calcium both at the lumbar spine and the femoral neck. Conceptually, there was no significant intransitivity.

differences in the number of biopsy-proven acute rejections as well as adverse events among treatment groups. However, we found more adverse events happened in bisphosphonate and calcium than in calcium alone (OR, 5.41; 95% CrI, 1.15 to 25.49) from pairwise meta-analysis. Further details of the secondary outcome analyses are presented in Additional files 3 and 4.

Discussion

This NMA was aimed to investigate the comparable efficacy and safety of bisphosphonate and its co-interventions for the post-transplantation bone disease. We found the combination of bisphosphonate, calcium and vitamin D analogs was the most effective to prevent bone and restore or improve BMD. However, the effects on fracture risk, adverse events, death, acute renal rejection and graft loss were still uncertain because of insufficient data and short follow-up time.

The current study revealed that only calcium prescription could not benefit KTRs from bone loss. We may suggest KTRs take calcium and vitamin D analogs orally because this NMA showed combination therapy of calcium and vitamin D analogs could improve BMD than calcium alone with moderate quality evidence. The result was supported by previous studies [37, 38]. Our work displayed that calcitonin with calcium seemed only better than calcium alone with low strength of evidence. Two RCTs [26, 33] involving 31 patients allocated to receive calcitonin, and incidence of hypocalcemia was reported so that we did not suggest giving calcitonin for KTRs. In our study, additional use of bisphosphonate could improve BMD changes at the lumbar spine and femoral neck. It was in accordance with previous analyses [9, 39], though they did not examine the effect of calcium and vitamin D analogs supplementation. Importantly, the validity and robustness of NMA depends not only on the heterogeneity in case of standard pairwise meta-analysis, but also on the inconsistency between direct and indirect contrast estimates. No evidence of inconsistency was found in this NMA. Bisphosphonate plus calcium revealed a significant gain in percent BMD change than calcium alone. The heterogeneity was calculated from the pairwise meta-analysis with four RCTs [31–33, 35]. The sample size, races and bisphosphonates which included ibandronate [31], pamidronate [32], clodronate [33], alendronate [35] were different. These resulted in high heterogeneity which would reduce the quality of evidence. Adding bisphosphonates also showed significant improvement than combination of calcium and vitamin D analogs in both absolute and percent BMD change at the lumbar with high heterogeneity. The heterogeneity was associated with characteristics of samples, different inclusion and exclusion criterion. The quality of evidence downgraded because of high heterogeneity. At this stage, limited information made it difficult to perform further analysis. Thus, we could not ignore the impact of heterogeneity when draw the conclusion. Although bisphosphonate with calcium and vitamin D analogs ranked the best, we did not detect any significant differences between combination use of bisphosphonate and calcium with or without vitamin D analogs from the indirect comparisons. Moreover, indirect comparisons would lead to very low quality of evidence. Only RCT conducted by Fan SL et al. [40, 41] compared bisphosphonate alone with placebo. They found that only two intravenous doses of pamidronate can protect the skeleton from bone loss even 4 years later after transplantation. We could not specify the influence of bisphosphonate monotherapy and access the situation of KTRs with no treatment due to lack of relevant studies.

Included RCTs used BMD as a surrogate marker and did not provide sufficient data to make a polygonal network configuration about the fracture. Also, the association between BMD metrics and fracture risk in KTRs is still controversial. West SL et al. [42] indicated that low BMD was a risk factor for subsequent fracture in patients with pre-dialysis CKD, but data for KTRs are scant. According to KDIGO guideline [7], bone biopsy is reasonable to guide treatment in the first twelve-months after transplantation. However, it is an invasive procedure and most centers lack the expertise to properly process and analyze bone biopsy specimens. Recently, the Fracture Risk Assessment Tool (FRAX) [43] and the spine Trabecular bone score (TBS) [44] were detected as new measurements for KTRs to predict fracture risk. Consequently, surrogate outcomes poorly reflect pathological bone changes. Future trials need to find more specific measurements for detecting mineral and bone disorders in KTRs.

Evidence on other secondary outcomes was limited. There was an unexpected finding from previous reviews [9, 45] that bisphosphonate reduced acute graft rejection moderately. Bisphosphonates could suppress cytokine releasing from activated macrophages to inhibit T-cell function. Its immunomodulatory and anti-inflammatory properties may explain this finding. However, the confidence intervals were wide and ignored the influence of co-interventions. The use of bisphosphonate was limited on account of its nephrotoxicity and development of the adynamic bone disease. We did not find additional bisphosphonate use would increase the occurrence of graft loss and adverse events. Apart from mild gastrointestinal side effects, include RCTs did not report or systematically study serious adverse events. Perazella MA et al. [46] summarized that bisphosphonate nephrotoxicity is infusion time-dependent and dose-dependent. Increasing the time interval between doses can limit its nephrotoxicity. On the current situation, bisphosphonate therapy was well tolerated whereas controversial data on its potency in preventing fracture limited its widespread.

Our analysis updated the previous meta-analysis and conducted a comprehensive search with broad inclusion criteria to maximize available data in this field. Only RCTs that supplied BMD results with g/cm^2 were included to standardize each comparison, while some studies used different units such as Z-score or T-score. Furthermore, we used GRADE approach to measure the quality of evidence

Outcomes of bisphosphonate and its supplements for bone loss in kidney transplant...

25

and also performed sensitivity analyses to demonstrate the robustness of estimates. In addition, only adult KTRs were included to offer more reliable evidence and minimize potential bias. To our knowledge, this is the first NMA that took co-intervention (calcium, vitamin D analogs) into account when examining the effect of bisphosphonates and expands on previous meta-analyses as well [9, 45].

However, this NMA still has several limitations including the omission of important methodological details in RCTs and the possibility of reporting biases. Most included studies had a high risk of bias and their impact on results is uncertain. Moreover, some studies only included cadaveric allograft, while some studies excluded patients with diabetes or postmenopausal women. These were risk factors for fracture. Preexisting CKD-MBD, immunosuppression therapy including steroid dosage, CNIs type could also cause bone disease after KT. Because of insufficient information, we could not perform further analysis to identify the influence of relevant factors. These would result in high heterogeneity which may downgrade the quality of evidence as well. Aside from different basic characteristic of the participant, it is unknown if within the drug class of bisphosphonates certain drugs are more favorable than others, and the bisphosphonates regimen (dosage, route, timing, and administration duration) differ among the included studies. We grouped vitamin D, calcitriol, alfacalcidol together as vitamin D analogs and did not distinguish their efficacy. These factors may potentially influence the calculation of BMD between RCTs.

More high-quality RCT is required to determine the optimal therapy for KTRs to prevent fractures with minimal risk for side effects. We also need to find a more correlative measurement than BMD to reflect pathological bone changes in KTRs. Future studies should be powered to show the fracture risk with sufficient follow-up time (≥3 years) and adequate sample sizes, while providing methodological details.

Conclusion

At this stage, we suggested the additional use of bisphosphonate was well-tolerated and more favorable in KTRs to improve BMD at the lumbar spine and femoral neck. However, evidence to reduce fracture risk is insufficient. Clinicians should take all known safety information and compliance of patients into account when using bisphosphonates. Further studies are needed to support our findings and find optimal treatment option for KTRs.

Acknowledgments

The authors would like to acknowledge Ian Charles Tobias for reviewing the manuscript.

Funding

This study was supported by the National Natural Science Foundation of China (Grant No.81570668).

Authors' contributions

PF and QW were responsible for the conception and design of the study. YY, SQ did the analysis and interpreted the analysis in collaboration with XRL and LHD. YY, SQ were responsible for the acquisition of data. YY, SQ wrote the first draft of the manuscript. YY, XT interpreted the data and wrote the final version. All authors critically revised the Article for important intellectual content and approved the final version. PF and QW obtained public funding.

Competing interests

The author declare that they have no competing interests.

Author details

[1]Kidney Research Laboratory, Division of Nephrology, National Clinical Research Center for Geriatrics, West China Hospital, Sichuan University, No. 37, Guoxue Alley, Chengdu, Sichuan, People's Republic of China610041. [2]Department of Nephrology, The First People's Hospital of Changzhou, The Third Affiliated Hospital of Soochow University, Changzhou, Jiangsu, People's Republic of China213000. [3]Department of Urology, Institute of Urology, West China Hospital, Sichuan University, Chengdu, Sichuan, People's Republic of China. [4]Stroke Clinical Research Unit, Department of Neurology, West China Hospital, Sichuan University, Chengdu, Sichuan, People's Republic of China.

References

1. Mitterbauer C, Oberbauer R. Bone disease after kidney transplantation. Transpl Int. 2008;21(7):615–24.
2. Naylor KL, Li AH, Lam NN, Hodsman AB, Jamal SA, Garg AX. Fracture risk in kidney transplant recipients: a systematic review. Transplantation. 2013; 95(12):1461–70.
3. Weisinger JR, Carlini RG, Rojas E, Bellorin-Font E. Bone disease after renal transplantation. Clin J Am Soc Nephrol. 2006;1(6):1300–13.
4. Bouquegneau A, Salam S, Delanaye P, Eastell R, Khwaja A. Bone disease after kidney transplantation. Clin J Am Soc Nephrol. 2016;11(7):1282–96.
5. Cunningham J. Pathogenesis and prevention of bone loss in patients who have kidney disease and receive long-term immunosuppression. J Am Soc Nephrol. 2007;18(1):223–34.
6. Evenepoel P, Cooper K, Holdaas H, Messa P, Mourad G, Olgaard K, Rutkowski B, Schaefer H, Deng H, Torregrosa JV, Wuthrich RP, Yue S. A randomized study evaluating cinacalcet to treat hypercalcemia in renal transplant recipients with persistent hyperparathyroidism. Am J Transplant. 2014;14(11):2545–55.
7. Ketteler M, Block GA, Evenepoel P, Fukagawa M, Herzog CA, McCann L, Moe SM, Shroff R, Tonelli MA, Toussaint ND, Vervloet MG, Leonard MB. Executive summary of the 2017 KDIGO chronic kidney disease-mineral and bone disorder (CKD-MBD) guideline update: what's changed and why it matters. Kidney Int. 2017;92(1):26–36.
8. Palmer SC, McGregor DO, Strippoli GF. Interventions for preventing bone disease in kidney transplant recipients. Cochrane Database Syst Rev. 2007.
9. Versele EB, Van Laecke S, Dhondt AW, Verbeke F, Vanholder R, Van Biesen W, Nagler EV. Bisphosphonates for preventing bone disease in kidney transplant recipients: a meta-analysis of randomized controlled trials. Transpl Int. 2015;29(2):153–64.
10. Hutton B, Salanti G, Caldwell DM, Chaimani A, Schmid CH, Cameron C, Ioannidis JP, Straus S, Thorlund K, Jansen JP, Mulrow C, Catalá-López F, Gøtzsche PC, Dickersin K, Boutron I, Altman DG, Moher D. The PRISMA extension statement for reporting of systematic reviews incorporating network meta-analyses of health care interventions: checklist and explanations. Ann Intern Med. 2015;162(11):777–84.

11. Higgins G, Green S. Cochrane handbook for systematic reviews of interventions version 5.1.0. Updated march, 2011. London: The Cochrane Collaboration; 2011.

12. DerSimonian R, Laird N. Meta-analysis in clinical trials. Control Clin Trials. 1986;7:177–88.

13. Salanti G, Higgins JP, Ades AE, Ioannidis JP. Evaluation of networks of randomised trials. Stat Methods Med Res. 2008;17(3):279–301.

14. Higgins JP, Jackson D, Barrett JK, Lu G, Ades AE, White IR. Consistency and inconsistency in network meta-analysis: concepts and models for multi-arm studies. Res Synth Methods. 2012;3(2):98–110.

15. Higgins JP, Thompson SG, Deeks JJ, Altman DG. Measuring inconsistency in meta-analyses. BMJ. 2003;327(7414):557–60.

16. Guyatt GH, Oxman AD, Vist GE, Kunz R, Falck-Ytter Y, Alonso-Coello P, Schünemann HJ, GRADE Working Group. GRADE: an emerging consensus on rating quality of evidence and strength of recommendations. BMJ. 2008; 336(7650):924–6.

17. Salanti G, Del Giovane C, Chaimani A, Caldwell DM, Higgins JP. Evaluating the quality of evidence from a network meta-analysis. PLoS One. 2014;9(7):e99682.

18. Smerud KT, Dolgos S, Olsen IC, Åsberg A, Sagedal S, Reisæter AV, Midtvedt K, Pfeffer P, Ueland T, Godang K, Bollerslev J, Hartmann A. A 1-year randomized, double-blind, placebo-controlled study of intravenous ibandronate on bone loss following renal transplantation. Am J Transplant. 2012;12(12):3316–25.

19. Coco M, Pullman J, Cohen HW, Lee S, Shapiro C, Solorzano C, Greenstein S, Glicklich D. Effect of risedronate on bone in renal transplant recipients. J Am Soc Nephrol. 2012;23(8):1426–37.

20. Torregrosa JV, Fuster D, Gentil MA, Marcen R, Guirado L, Zarraga S, Bravo J, Burgos D, Monegal A, Muxí A, García S. Open-label trial: effect of weekly risedronate immediately after transplantation in kidney recipients. Transplantation. 2010;89(12):1476–81.

21. Torregrosa JV, Fuster D, Monegal A, Gentil MA, Bravo J, Guirado L, Muxí A, Cubero J. Efficacy of low doses of pamidronate in osteopenic patients administered in the early post-renal transplant. Osteoporos Int. 2011;22(1):281–7.

22. Walsh SB, Altmann P, Pattison J, Wilkie M, Yaqoob MM, Dudley C, Cockwell P, Sweny P, Banks LM, Hall-Craggs M, Noonan K, Andrews C, Cunningham J. Effect of pamidronate on bone loss after kidney transplantation: a randomized trial. Am J Kidney Dis. 2009;53(5):856–65.

23. Lan G, Peng L, Xie X, Peng F, Wang Y, Yu S. Alendronate is effective to treat bone loss in renal transplantation recipients. Transplant Proc. 2008;40(10):3496–8.

24. Trabulus S, Altiparmak MR, Apaydin S, Serdengecti K, Sariyar M. Treatment of renal transplant recipients with low bone mineral density: a randomized prospective trial of alendronate, alfacalcidol, and alendronate combined with alfacalcidol. Transplant Proc. 2008;40(1):160–6.

25. Nayak B, Guleria S, Varma M, Tandon N, Aggarwal S, Bhowmick D, Agarwal SK, Mahajan S, Gupta S, Tiwari SC. Effect of bisphosphonates on bone mineral density after renal transplantation as assessed by bone mineral densitometry. Transplant Proc. 2007;39(3):750–2.

26. El-Agroudy AE, El-Husseini AA, El-Sayed M, Mohsen T, Ghoneim MA. A prospective randomized study for prevention of postrenal transplantation bone loss. Kidney Int. 2005;67(5):2039–45.

27. Schwarz C, Mitterbauer C, Heinze G, Woloszczuk W, Haas M, Oberbauer R. Nonsustained effect of short-term bisphosphonate therapy on bone turnover three years after renal transplantation. Kidney Int. 2004;65(1):304–9.

28. Jeffery JR, Leslie WD, Karpinski ME, Nickerson PW, Rush DN. Prevalence and treatment of decreased bone density in renal transplant recipients: a randomized prospective trial of calcitriol versus alendronate. Transplantation. 2003;76(10):1498–502.

29. Coco M, Glicklich D, Faugere MC, Burris L, Bognar I, Durkin P, Tellis V, Greenstein S, Schechner R, Figueroa K, McDonough P, Wang G, Malluche H. Prevention of bone loss in renal transplant recipients: a prospective, randomized trial of intravenous pamidronate. J Am Soc Nephrol. 2003; 14(10):2669–76.

30. Haas M, Leko-Mohr Z, Roschger P, Kletzmayr J, Schwarz C, Mitterbauer C, Steininger R, Grampp S, Klaushofer K, Delling G, Oberbauer R. Zoledronic acid to prevent bone loss in the first 6 months after renal transplantation. Kidney Int. 2003;63(3):1130–6.

31. Grotz W, Nagel C, Poeschel D, Cybulla M, Petersen KG, Uhl M, Strey C, Kirste G, Olschewski M, Reichelt A, Rump LC. Effect of Ibandronate on bone loss and renal function after kidney transplantation. J Am Soc Nephrol. 2001; 12(7):1530–7.

32. Nam JH, Moon JI, Chung SS, Kim SI, Park KI, Song YD, Kim KR, Lee HC, Huh K, Lim SK. Pamidronate and calcitriol trial for the prevention of early bone loss after renal transplantation. Transplant Proc. 2000;32(7):1876.

33. Grotz WH, Rump LC, Niessen A, Schmidt-Gayk H, Reichelt A, Kirste G, Olschewski M, Schollmeyer PJ. Treatment of osteopenia and osteoporosis after kidney transplantation. Transplantation. 1998;66(8):1004–8.

34. Giannini S, D'Angelo A, Carraro G, Nobile M, Rigotti P, Bonfante L, Marchini F, Zaninotto M, Dalle Carbonare L, Sartori L, Crepaldi G. Alendronate prevents further bone loss in renal transplant recipients. J Bone Miner Res. 2001;16(11):2111–7.

35. Koc M, Tuglular S, Arikan H, Ozener C, Akoglu E. Alendronate increases bone mineral density in long-term renal transplant recipients. Transplant Proc. 2002;34(6):2111–3.

36. Torregrosa JV, Fuster D, Pedroso S, Diekmann F, Campistol JM, Rubí S, Oppenheimer F. Weekly risedronate in kidney transplant patients with osteopenia. Transpl Int. 2007;20(8):708–11.

37. Elagroudy AE, et al. Preventing bone loss in renal transplant recipients with vitamin D. J Am Soc Nephrol. 2003;14(11):2975–9.

38. Josephson MA, Schumm LP, Chiu MY, Marshall C, Thistlethwaite JR, Sprague SM. Calcium and calcitriol prophylaxis attenuates posttransplant bone loss. Transplantation. 2004;78(8):1233–6.

39. Kan SL, Ning GZ, Chen LX, Zhou Y, Sun JC, Feng SQ. Efficacy and safety of bisphosphonates for low bone mineral density after kidney transplantation: a meta-analysis. Medicine. 2016;95(5):e2679.

40. Fan SL, Almond MK, Ball E, Evans K, Cunningham J. Pamidronate therapy as prevention of bone loss following renal transplantation. Kidney Int. 2000; 57(2):684–90.

41. Fan SL, Kumar S, Cunningham J. Long-term effects on bone mineral density of pamidronate given at the time of renal transplantation. Kidney Int. 2003; 63(6):2275–9.

42. West SL, Lok CE, Langsetmo L, Cheung AM, Szabo E, Pearce D, Fusaro M, Wald R, Weinstein J, Jamal SA. Bone mineral density predicts fractures in chronic kidney disease. J Bone Miner Res. 2015;30(5):913–9.

43. Naylor KL, Leslie WD, Hodsman AB, Rush DN, Garg AX. FRAX predicts fracture risk in kidney transplant recipients. Transplantation. 2014;97(9):940–5.

44. Luckman M, Hans D, Cortez N, Nishiyama KK, Agarwal S, Zhang C, Nikkel L, Iyer S, Fusaro M, Guo EX, McMahon DJ, Shane E, Nickolas TL. Spine trabecular bone score as an Indicator of bone microarchitecture at the peripheral skeleton in kidney transplant recipients. Clin J Am Soc Nephrol. 2017;12(4):644–52.

45. Palmer SC, Mcgregor DO, Strippoli GF. Interventions for preventing bone disease in kidney transplant recipients: a systematic review of randomized controlled trials. Am J Kidney Dis. 2005;45(4):638–49.

46. Perazella MA, Markowitz GS. Bisphosphonate nephrotoxicity. Kidney Int. 2008;74(11):1385–93.

3

Switching iron sucrose to ferric carboxymaltose associates to better control of iron status in hemodialysis patients

Jesse M. G. Hofman[1,6]* [iD], Michele F. Eisenga[1], Adry Diepenbroek[1], Ilja M. Nolte[2], Bastiaan van Dam[3], Ralf Westerhuis[4], Stephan J. L. Bakker[1], Casper F. M. Franssen[1] and Carlo A. J. M. Gaillard[5]

Abstract

Background: Although the efficacy of iron sucrose (IS) and ferric carboxymaltose (FCM) in treating anemia in hemodialysis (HD) patients has been studied individually, a comparison of these two intravenous iron formulations has not yet been performed in HD patients.

Methods: We performed a retrospective audit on records of 221 stable HD patients from different HD centers in the Netherlands, who were switched from IS to FCM on a 1:1 ratio. To assess the effect of the switch on iron status parameters, data from 3 time points before and 3 time points after the switch were analyzed using linear mixed effects models. Subanalyses were done in 2 subgroups of patients anemic or iron deficient at baseline.

Results: Hemoglobin increased in all groups (anemic [1.4 g/dL, $P < 0.001$] iron deficient [0.6 g/dL, $P < 0.001$]), while the weekly iron dose was significantly lower when patients received FCM compared to IS (48 vs 55 mg/week, $P = 0.04$). Furthermore, serum ferritin and transferrin saturation increased in all groups (anemic [64 μg/L, 5.0%, $P < 0.001$] iron deficient [76 μg/L, 3.6%, $P < 0.001$]). Finally, the darbepoetin α dose decreased significantly in all groups (anemic [− 16 μg/wk., $P = 0.01$] iron deficient [− 11 μg/wk., $P < 0.001$]).

Conclusions: In this real-life study in HD patients, a switch from IS to FCM resulted in an improvement of iron status parameters despite a lower weekly dose of FCM. Furthermore, the ESA dose was reduced during FCM, while hemoglobin levels increased.

Keywords: Ferric carboxymaltose, Iron sucrose, Hemodialysis, Iron status, ESA

Background

Anemia is a frequent complication of chronic kidney disease (CKD) [1]. In CKD, the main causes of anemia are deficiency of erythropoietin, iron-restricted erythropoiesis and anemia of the chronic disease (ACD) [2–4]. The latter originates from the chronic inflammation that is a hallmark of CKD patients and has been shown to be associated with adverse outcomes such as cardiovascular events, end-stage renal disease, increased mortality, and decreased quality of life [5]. In ACD, pro-inflammatory cytokines upregulate hepcidin production in the liver which subsequently hampers iron uptake from the gut and iron release from the reticulo-endothelial system [6, 7] which leads to functional iron deficiency that negatively affects erythropoiesis. Furthermore, increased iron utilization due to the use of erythropoiesis stimulating agents (ESA), and iron loss as a result of dialysis-related blood loss contribute to the high prevalence of anemia in patients with CKD [8].

Oral administration of iron has limited efficaciousness and is associated with gastrointestinal side effects. By means of intravenous iron, gastrointestinal absorption is bypassed and incorporated more rapidly [5]. Indeed, it has been established that intravenous iron supplementation as a treatment for iron deficiency anemia is superior

* Correspondence: j.m.g.hofman@umcg.nl
[1]Department of Nephrology, University Medical Center Groningen, University of Groningen, Hanzeplein 1, Groningen 9713GZ, The Netherlands
[6]Department of Internal Medicine, Division of Nephrology, University Medical Center Groningen, Hanzeplein 1, 9713GZ Groningen, The Netherlands
Full list of author information is available at the end of the article

to oral iron supplementation in non-dialysis dependent CKD, hemodialysis (HD) and peritoneal dialysis patients [9–11]. Furthermore, ESA requirements have been shown to be decreased in patients receiving intravenous iron [12].

Nowadays, several intravenous iron supplementations are available, of which iron sucrose (IS) and a more recently introduced intravenous (IV) iron compound, ferric carboxymaltose (FCM) (brand names Venofer and Ferinject, respectively) are frequently used. Although the efficacy of IS and that of FCM for treatment of anemia in CKD patients have been studied individually by comparing the formulations to oral iron supplementation [10, 13], a head to head comparison of these two intravenous formulations has never been performed in HD patients. Therefore, the goal of this audit is to analyze the effects of a switch from IS to equally dosed FCM. Hence, we performed an audit on records of HD patients in three dialysis centers that switched from IS to FCM.

Methods

Study design

We conducted an audit using data retrospectively gathered from HD patients who were switched from IS to FCM because of a change in hospital policies. Patients from four dialysis centers were included (Dialysis Center Groningen, $n = 110$, University Medical Center Groningen, $n = 11$, Dialysis Center "Noord-West Ziekenhuizgroep", $n = 54$, and Dialysis Center Amersfoort, $n = 46$). We analyzed a study period of 15 months in total, during which we studied 6 time points, each 3 months apart, as illustrated in Fig. 1. During the 6 months pre-switch patients received IS, and during the 9 months post switch they received FCM. During both periods, blood was sampled every 3 months as part of the clinical routine, at least one week after administration of IV iron. The baseline time point was one of the three time points before the switch, and was defined for each patient separately when the patient had at that time point

been using maintenance IV iron medication for ≥ 6 months, and the patient had been on HD treatment for at least 3 months. The need for participant consent was waived by the medical ethical committee in the UMCG for the act on Medical Research Involving Human Subjects (in Dutch:WMO).

Study population

The study population consisted of CKD patients who were at least 18 years old, were on uninterrupted HD treatment for a period of at least 3 months before the switch and 3 months after the switch, were using IS at the start of the investigational period, and were subsequently switched from IS to FCM. Patients with any malignancy diagnosed in the five years prior to the investigational period were excluded. In all three cohorts anemia was diagnosed when hemoglobin was < 12 g/dL. Subsequently a diagnostic workup was performed to rule out causes of anemia besides CKD, like bleeding or active infection. If these were ruled out, IV iron therapy was initiated when there was an absolute iron deficiency (transferrin saturation (TSAT) < 20% and ferritin < 100 ng/mL) or when TSAT was ≤20%, or ferritin was ≤200 µg/l, and an increase in hemoglobin concentration was desired without increasing the ESA dose. In this case, the patient received 100 mg of iron per week for 10 weeks. Subsequently, iron medication was ceased, and after 4 weeks the patient's iron stores were assessed by the treating nephrologist, who decided on the treatment plan. If ferritin was < 200 µg/l, or TSAT was < 20%, IV iron was initiated at a dose of 100 mg per week. If ferritin was 200–500 µg/l, and/or TSAT was 20–30%, the dose was 100 mg every two weeks. If ferritin was 500–800 µg/l and/or TSAT was 30–50%, the dose was 100 mg every four weeks. If ferritin was > 800 µg/l and/or TSAT was > 50%, no IV iron was administered. If IV iron alone was not sufficient to improve hemoglobin levels, the treating nephrologist added an ESA to the therapeutic regime. In all cases, the patient was re-evaluated every three months, at least a week after the

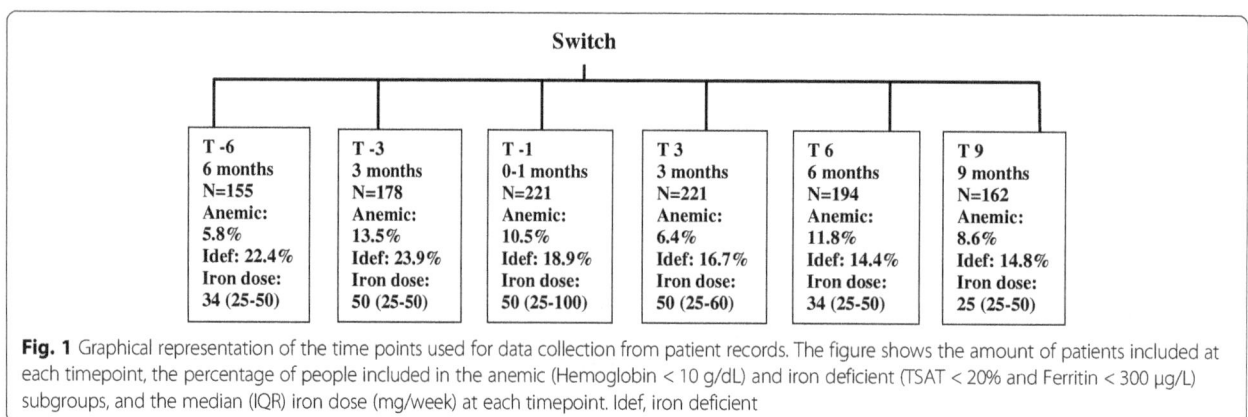

Fig. 1 Graphical representation of the time points used for data collection from patient records. The figure shows the amount of patients included at each timepoint, the percentage of people included in the anemic (Hemoglobin < 10 g/dL) and iron deficient (TSAT < 20% and Ferritin < 300 µg/L) subgroups, and the median (IQR) iron dose (mg/week) at each timepoint. Idef, iron deficient

last administration of IV iron. The goal of this treatment was to prevent hemoglobin from dropping below 10 g/dL, while not routinely exceeding 12 g/dL. Iron was always administered in the final 30 min of the HD session. The protocol did not change after switching from IS to FCM. This is in accordance with the 2015 Dutch National federation for Nephrology guidelines for management of anemia in kidney disease that are based on the most recent KDIGO guidelines and the ERBP position statement on the KDIGO guidelines [14].

After application of the exclusion criteria, data from 221 of the original 280 patients who were switched from IS to FCM were included in the final analyses. Following inclusion of data from the baseline time point, data was included for analysis up until the final time point 9 months after the switch, or until follow-up was censored because the patient died, stopped using FCM, or stopped HD treatment due to any cause. As depicted in Fig. 1, at T-6 data from 155 patients were included, at T-3 data from 178 patients were included, and at T-1, by definition, data from all 221 patients were included. After inclusion, all patients were followed up until T3, the first time point, i.e. 3 months after the switch, 194 patients were followed up until T6, i.e. 6 months after the switch, and 162 until T9, i.e. 9 months after the switch. As a result, we analyzed the data with linear mixed models, which is considered to be robust to missing values and is therefore able to deal with missing data at certain time points. We also assessed the effect of the factor "time" on the period from T-6 to T-1 (patients on IS) and T3 to T9 (patients on FCM).

Audit

The primary objective of this analysis was to determine whether the switch from IS to FCM modulated iron status parameters in relation to iron dose and ESA dose. We used the parameters TSAT and serum ferritin over time to quantify the effect on both absolute and functional iron deficiency, as they have been shown to be key parameters in the diagnosis of iron deficiency anemia (IDA) [15], and hemoglobin over time to determine the effect on the severity of anemia. To further address other effects of the switch on erythropoiesis, iron metabolism and inflammation, we included ESA dose, iron dose, serum iron, mean corpuscular volume (MCV), hematocrit, reticulocyte count, total iron-binding capacity and C-reactive protein (CRP) as secondary objectives. All data was gathered from blood samples that were analyzed at the main laboratory in each hospital.

Statistical analysis

Normally distributed variables are described as mean ± standard deviation (SD), and skewed variables as median and interquartile range (IQR). Categorical variables are expressed as percentage. Linear mixed effects models, which are within-person analyses, were used to assess the effect of the medication switch on iron status and dialysis parameters. Random effects were patient identification number (ID) and an interaction between ID and switch. The most appropriate covariance structure was determined for each outcome variable separately. Fixed effects were switch, factor time classified as three options for the three time moments before and after switch, $time^2$ to account for the possible nonlinear relation between time and the outcome variable, iron deficiency at baseline, anemia at baseline, and interactions between switch and anemia, switch and iron deficiency, switch and time, and switch and $time^2$. The least significant fixed effects were removed in a stepwise manner for each variable, until only effects with a significance of < 0.1 were left in order to achieve a good model fit. Subsequently, the estimated marginal means of parameters before and after the switch were compared to determine the main effect of the switch. Skewed variables were ln-transformed in order to achieve a normal distribution. Subanalyses were performed in a subgroup of iron deficient patients, characterized by TSAT $< 20\%$ and ferritin < 300 µg/L ($n = 55$), and anemic patients, characterized by a hemoglobin of < 10 g/dL in men and women [16], which was the lower end of the hemoglobin target range of 10–12 g/dL ($n = 24$). Data analysis was performed in SPSS statistics version 22.0 (IBM Corporation, Chicago, IL, USA).

Results

We included 221 HD patients (mean age 65 ± 15 years), of whom 24 were anemic at baseline, and 55 iron deficient at baseline. The prevalence of hypertension and diabetes mellitus was 58.6% and 31.8%, respectively. There was no significant correlation between ferritin and CRP at baseline in the entire group ($\beta -0.090$, $P = 0.33$), the anemic group (β 0.286, $P = 0.32$), or the iron deficient group ($\beta -0.128$, $P = 0.64$). Additional baseline characteristics of the entire group, as well as anemic and iron deficient subgroups are shown in Table 1.

Effects of the switch in the entire cohort

The models used to analyze the effect of the switch on each parameter are described in Additional file 1: Table S1. The main effects of the switch from IS to FCM on all parameters are reported in Table 2. The dosage of iron medication decreased significantly after switch from IS to FCM (-7 mg/wk., $P = 0.04$), while hemoglobin (0.64 g/dL, $P < 0.001$) and hematocrit (0.02, $P < 0.001$) increased significantly. Furthermore,

Table 1 Baseline characteristics of patients included in the study

	All patients $n = 221$	Anemic $n = 24$	Iron deficient $n = 55$
Sex (% male)	62.3	45.5	67.3
Age (years)	65 ± 15	62 ± 16	64 ± 18
Diabetes mellitus (%)	31.8	35.0	20.8
Hypertension (%)	58.6	65.0	54.2
BMI (kg/m^2)	24.7 ± 4.1	25.4 ± 4.5	25.0 ± 3.7
Systolic BP pre-HD (mmHg)	140 ± 24	135 ± 26	141 ± 21
Diastolic BP pre-HD (mmHg)	69 ± 14	70 ± 15	69 ± 13
Residual diuresis (%)	47.6	37.5	42.9
Ultrafiltration (L)	2.15 ± 0.96	2.55 ± 0.76	1.98 ± 0.92
Dialysis vintage (months)	22 (11–49)	22 (10–44)	26 (9–55)
Urea pre-HD (mg/dL)	23.2 ± 7.2	21.8 ± 7.8	24.5 ± 6.9
Creatinine pre-HD (µg/dL)	808 ± 250	842 ± 257	870 ± 259
Hb (g/dL)	11.7 ± 1.2	9.4 ± 0.5	11.8 ± 1.3
Ht	0.35 ± 0.03	0.30 ± 0.02	0.36 ± 0.04
Reticulocytes (%)	13.7 (10.3–19.0)	14.0 (12.0–22.3)	14.0 (12.0–18.0)
MCV (fL)	95.4 ± 6.4	96.8 ± 6.9	91.0 ± 5.6
Ferritin (µg/L)	416 (227–625)	514 (297–700)	176 (116–226)
Transferrin (g/L)	1.9 ± 0.3	1.9 ± 0.4	2.1 ± 0.3
TSAT (%)	20.8 (15.0–26.5)	18.5 (14.0–31.3)	14.0 (12.0–16.0)
Serum iron (µg/L)	9.3 (7.0–12.8)	9.0 (7.0–14.0)	7.0 (6.0–8.0)
TIBC (µmol/L)	46.0 ± 9.2	44.3 ± 9.0	49.4 ± 9.6
Iron medication (mg/wk)	50 (25–100)	100 (50–100)	50 (33–100)
Darbepoetin α (µg/wk)	30 (10–50)	40 (50–60)	30 (16–60)
Epoetin β (IE/wk)	8000 (4000–12,000)	8000 (7000–13,500)	8000 (4000–12,000)
CRP (mg/L)[a]	6.2 (2.0–16.0)	13.5 (2.0–40.0)	15.0 (1.5–56.0)
Phosphate (mmol/L)	1.59 (1.29–1.93)	1.73 (1.31–2.16)	1.61 (1.3–2.0)
Potassium (mmol/L)	4.9 (4.5–5.4)	4.8 (4.5–5.6)	5.0 (4.6–5.5)
Sodium (mEq/L)	138.0 ± 3.1	138.7 ± 2.8	137.3 ± 3.3

Normally distributed variables are described as mean ± SD and variables with a skewed distribution as median, IQR. Dialysis duration and frequency are described as mode

BP, blood pressure; HD, hemodialysis; Hb, hemoglobin; Ht, hematocrit; MCV, mean corpuscular volume; TSAT, transferrin saturation; TIBC, total iron binding capacity; CRP, C-reactive protein

[a]Data available in 119 HD patients before the switch

after the switch from IS to FCM, serum ferritin increased significantly (64 µg/L, $P < 0.001$) as well as TSAT (3.4%, $P < 0.001$) (Fig. 2). The proportion of reticulocytes in the blood and serum transferrin decreased significantly (– 0.1 g/L, $P = 0.002$). The factor time was not a significant predictor of TSAT and serum ferritin both before and after the switch; hence the data shown below are fully the result of the switch. The ESA dose was decreased significantly in patients using darbepoetin α, but not in those using epoetin β. MCV showed a slight significant increase. Other parameters did not change significantly as result of the switch of IS to FCM.

Effects of the switch in anemic patients alone

When assessing the same parameters in specifically anemic patients at baseline, hemoglobin (1.4, $P < 0.001$), hematocrit (0.04 $P < 0.001$), TSAT (5.0%, $P < 0.001$), and serum iron (1.9 µmol/L, $P = 0.008$) seemed to increase more as a result of the switch in this subgroup compared to the entire population, while the darbepoetin α dose decreased more (– 16 µg/wk., $P = 0.010$), as shown in Table 2. The models show that having a hemoglobin level of < 10 g/dL at baseline enhances the effect of the switch beyond the effect the switch has in non-anemic individuals on hemoglobin, hematocrit, TSAT, serum iron, and ESA dose. For the other variables, including

Table 2 Main effect of medication switch in the total population and subgroups

	Total population (n = 221)			Anemic at baseline (n = 24)			Iron deficient at baseline (n = 55)		
	Before (SE)	After (SE)	P	Before (SE)	After (SE)	P	Before (SE)	After (SE)	P
Ln Irondose (mg/wk)	4.007 (0.063)	3.880 (0.063)	0.04	4.114 (0.046)	3.987 (0.045)	0.006	4.094 (0.086)	3.967 (0.086)	0.11
Irondose (mg/wk)	55	48		61	54		60	53	
Ln Darbepoetin α (μg/wk)	3.528 (0.122)	3.299 (0.121)	0.001	3.809 (0.230)	3.375 (0.227)	0.01	3.649 (0.155)	3.290 (0.155)	< 0.001
Darbepoetin α (μg/wk)	34	27		45	29		38	27	
Ln Epoetin β (IE/wk)	9.038 (0.099)	8.911 (0.096)	0.06	N/A[a]	N/A[a]	N/A[a]	N/A[a]	N/A[a]	N/A[a]
Epoetin β (IE/wk)	8400	7400		N/A[a]	N/A[a]		N/A[a]	N/A[a]	
Hb (g/dL)	11.00 (0.11)	11.64 (0.10)	< 0.001	10.10(0.196)	11.50 (0.184)	< 0.001	11.21 (0.134)	11.85 (0.130)	< 0.001
Ht	0.338 (0.003)	0.358 (0.003)	< 0.001	0.316 (0.006)	0.358 (0.006)	< 0.001	0.345 (0.004)	0.364 (0.004)	< 0.001
MCV (fL)	94.10 (0.453)	94.92 (0.452)	0.001	94.10 (0.453)	94.92 (0.452)	0.001	91.46 (0.759)	92.28 (0.758)	0.08
Ln Reticulocytes (%)	2.613 (0.036)	2.704 (0.033)	< 0.001	2.613 (0.036)	2.704 (0.033)	0.002	2.613 (0.036)	2.704 (0.033)	0.004
Reticulocytes (%)	13.6	14.9		13.6	14.9		13.6	14.9	
Ln Ferritin (μg/L)	5.659 (0.041)	5.860 (0.055)	< 0.001	5.659 (0.041)	5.860 (0.055)	< 0.001	5.132 (0.071)	5.503 (0.095)	< 0.001
Ferritin (μg/L)	287	351		287	351		169	245	
Ln Transferrin (g/L)	0.640 (0.013)	0.611 (0.014)	0.002	0.640 (0.013)	0.611 (0.014)	0.04	0.702 (0.022)	0.674 (0.023)	0.03
Transferrin (g/L)	1.9	1.8		1.9	1.8		2.0	2.0	
Ln TSAT (%)	2.841 (0.037)	3.019 (0.044)	< 0.001	2.760 (0.067)	3.035 (0.080)	< 0.001	2.609 (0.050)	2.844 (0.062)	< 0.001
TSAT (%)	17.1	20.5		15.8	20.8		13.6	17.2	
TIBC (μmol/L)	47.648 (0.707)	47.225 (0.764)	0.35	47.648 (0.707)	47.225 (0.764)	0.12	50.240 (1.112)	49.818 (1.148)	0.53
Ln Serumiron (μmol/L)	2.13 (0.04)	2.26 (0.04)	0.003	2.08 (0.07)	2.29 (0.08)	0.008	1.96 (0.05)	2.14 (0.06)	0.001
Serumiron (μmol/L)	8.4	9.6		8.0	9.9		7.1	8.5	
Ln CRP (mg/L)	1.999	1.825 (0.092)	0.23	1.999 (0.121)	1.825 (0.092)	0.004	1.999 (0.121)	1.825 (0.092)	0.20
CRP	7.4	6.2		7.4	6.2		7.4	6.2	
Ultrafiltration (L)	2.307 (0.103)	2.214 (0.100)	0.23	2.459 (0.193)	2.235 (0.186)	0.22	2.307 (0.103)	2.214 (0.100)	0.32
Ln Phosphate	0.440 (0.020)	0.416 (0.020)	0.19	0.440 (0.020)	0.416 (0.020)	0.14	0.440 (0.020)	0.416 (0.020)	0.17
Phosphate	1.55	1.52		1.55	1.52		1.55	1.52	

Shown in this table are the marginal estimated means of all data before and after the switch, as calculated with our model. Data is described as mean (SE).
P-values of paired samples t-tests are shown. Ln-transformed variables were transformed back in order to give insight into the effect size
SE, standard error; Hb, hemoglobin; Ht, hematocrit; MCV, mean corpuscular volume; TSAT, transferrin saturation; TIBC, total iron binding capacity; CRP, C-reactive protein
[a]Sample size was too small to draw useful conclusions

ferritin (Fig. 2), results were similar to those described for the entire population.

Effects of the switch in iron deficient patients alone
In this subgroup, the ESA dose decreased more than in the entire population (darbepoetin α: − 11 μg/wk., P < 0.001) (Table 2). Furthermore, it shows that being iron deficient at baseline enhances the effect of the switch on serum ferritin (76 μg/l, P < 0.001). For all the other variables the results were similar to those described for the entire population.

Discussion
In this analysis, we have shown that the switch from IS to FCM in HD patients was associated with a significant improvement of iron status, unrelated to iron dose. After the switch to FCM hemoglobin, hematocrit, serum ferritin, TSAT, and MCV increased, while transferrin levels decreased, reflecting erythropoiesis which is less restricted by iron deficiency [17]. Furthermore, ESA dose decreased after the switch to FCM. This is, to our knowledge, the first investigation to compare the effects on iron status of a switch to FCM from IS in dialysis-dependent CKD patients.

In the subgroup of anemic patients at baseline especially, the effect of the switch on iron status was even more pronounced, despite the fact that these patients were prescribed significantly less iron and a smaller ESA dose after the switch. Switching from IS to FCM resulted in a marked increase in TSAT in both groups, a large increase of MCV in the anemic group, and an increase in serum ferritin in both groups. Although the baseline hemoglobin and iron status in the anemic and iron deficient groups were worse, the large improvement of iron

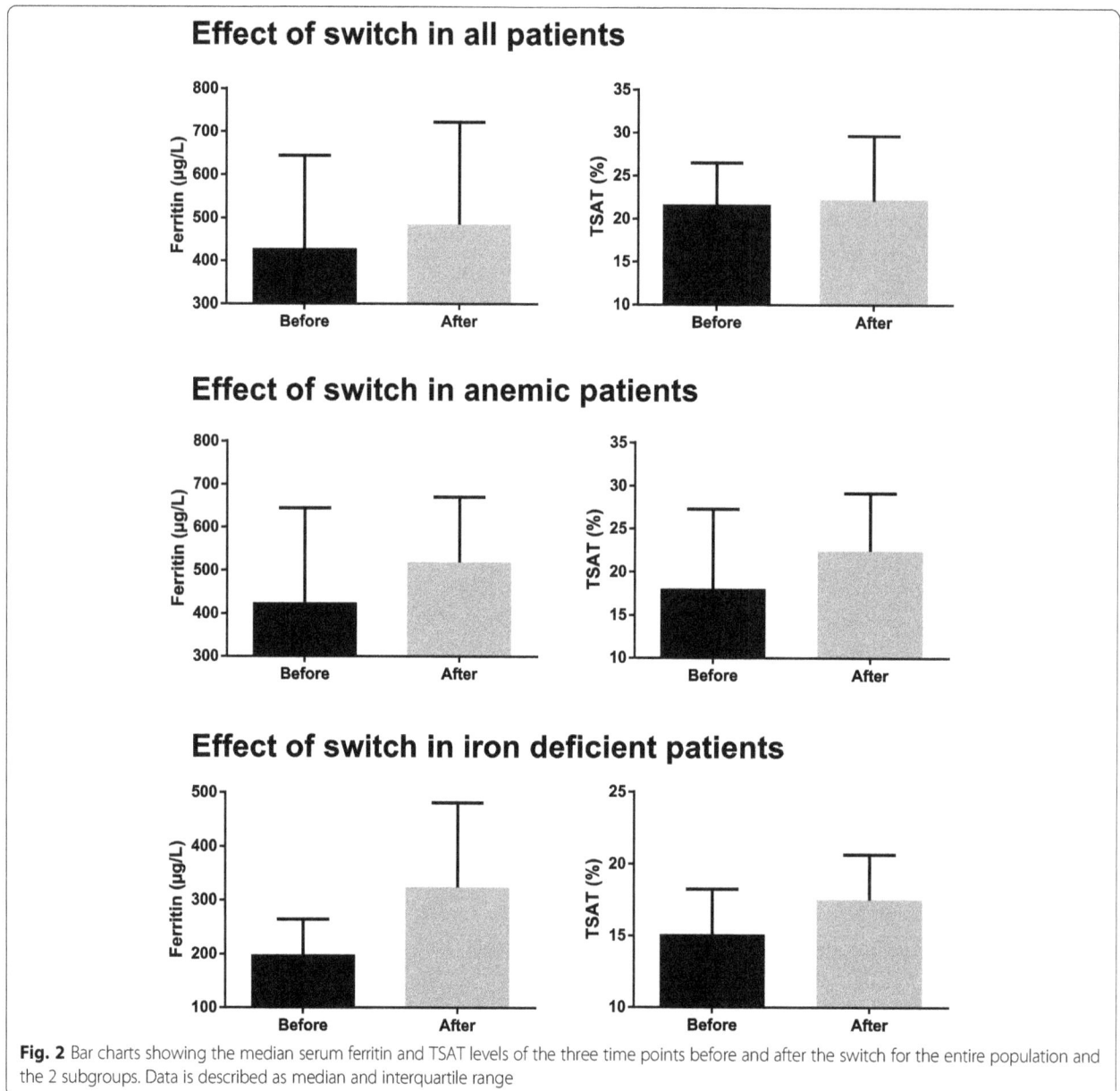

Fig. 2 Bar charts showing the median serum ferritin and TSAT levels of the three time points before and after the switch for the entire population and the 2 subgroups. Data is described as median and interquartile range

status in these groups seems attributable to the effect of switching from IS to FCM since we did not identify a statistically significant general trend based solitarily on the factor time.

These results seem to indicate that switching from IS to similarly dosed FCM causes an increase in ferritin and TSAT in all groups, which is more pronounced in anemic patients. When speculating on possible mechanisms why FCM seems to be more effective than IS in replenishing iron stores, one could put forth the argument that FCM has increased bioavailability of elemental iron compared to IS. FCM and IS are both composed of an iron(III)-hydroxide core, surrounded by a carbohydrate shell (carboxymaltose and sucrose, respectively)

[18]. FCM has a higher molecular weight than IS (150,000 v 43,300 Da) and a longer half-life (7–12 v 5–6 h) which increase the area under the curve, indicating that the bioavailability of FCM is greater than that of IS [18]. A second explanation might be that FCM is much more stable than IS, which prevents release of labile iron into the blood, where it can saturate transferrin and lead to significant amounts of non-transferrin bound iron (NTBI) [19]. This causes not only a less efficient uptake of iron by reticuloendothelial macrophages [18], but the NTBI may also lead to oxidative stress [20]. At this point it should be noted that there is no long-term data available on the pharmacokinetics of both compounds; therefore a direct comparison between the two compounds

cannot be performed. A head to head pharmacokinetic study would be required before conclusions can be drawn.

These results are in accordance with the results of the REPAIR-IDA trial, a randomized controlled trial comparing FCM to IS in a group of 2584 non-renal IDA patients. Onken et al. describe a significant increase in serum ferritin and TSAT in favor of FCM, 56 days after drug administration [21]. We have demonstrated that over a period of 9 months, a significant difference in serum ferritin and TSAT continues to exist due to administration of FCM.

One of the adverse effects of FCM described is hypophosphatemia. We observed a nonsignificant 0.03 mmol/L decrease in serum phosphate levels; hence, hypophosphatemia did not become more prevalent as a result of the switch from IS to FCM. This is in accordance with a clinical trial in inflammatory bowel disease patients, which described a transient decrease of serum phosphate levels in the FCM group which resolved between week 4 and week 12 after the switch [22]. Our results contradict the findings of a study by Hardy et al. specifically assessing the effect of FCM on serum phosphate levels compared to IS in iron deficiency anemia patients. The authors found that FCM caused significantly more hypophosphatemia than IS, which resolved after a mean duration of 6 months [23]. It should be noted, however, that the latter study did not comprise solitarily chronic kidney disease patients. Hence, the diminished renal function and as such the lower risk of developing hypophosphatemia in our study might have resulted in a substantive difference between our identified prevalence and the results as described by Hardy and colleagues.

It is known, at least theoretically, that administration of intravenous iron in CKD patients on the long term might lead to an iron overload, which may produce endothelial dysfunction, cardiovascular disease, and immune dysfunction [24]. It seems plausible, based on our results, that we can correct iron status parameters more efficiently with FCM, at a lower dose, and as such a putative iron overload can be prevented. Furthermore, we can also speculate that FCM administration could be more cost-efficient than IS due to the lower iron and ESA dose, which may lead to financial savings in the long term [25]. A well performed cost-benefit analysis is needed to substantiate this possible advantage of using FCM as compared to IS.

A strength of our investigation is that it comprises a comparison of multiple data points within one patient, meaning that our results correspond better to a real-life situation where a patient is switched from IS to FCM. Moreover, it should be kept in mind that we censored patients who stopped using FCM as data was no longer available, likely contributing to the underestimation of the effect of FCM as these patients will likely have iron status parameters longer in target.

A limitation of our study is the longitudinal study design without randomization, making it difficult to draw firm conclusions. A head-to-head comparison between IS and FCM is needed to confirm our results. Furthermore, we acknowledge as limitation that we did not assess the tolerability or safety of either IV iron preparation even though these factors play an important role when prescribing. Although the safety of FCM has never been compared to IS in the HD population specifically, it has been assessed in other patient groups such as non-dialysis dependent CKD in the REPAIR-IDA trial [21]. In this trial, Onken et al. found no significant difference in the number of patients that reached a primary composite safety endpoint. Hypertensive events immediately following drug administration occurred significantly more in the FCM group than in the IS group, with 7.45% of patients compared to 4.36% experiencing an event, however, hypertensive events occurred on non-dosing days nearly twice as often in the IS group.

Conclusions

In conclusion, the switch from IS to FCM was accompanied by a marked improvement in iron status parameters, despite a lower iron dose. In addition, use of FCM resulted in an increase in hemoglobin levels while ESA dose was decreased. Our results need to be confirmed and delineated in more detail in larger prospective studies.

Abbreviations
ACD: Anemia of chronic disease; CKD: Chronic kidney disease; CRP: C-reactive protein; ESA: Erytrhropoiesis-stimulating agents; FCM: Ferric carboxymaltose; HD: Hemodialysis; ID: Identification number; IDA: Iron deficiency anemia; IQR: Interquartile range; IS: Iron sucrose; IV: Intravenous; MCV: Mean corpuscular volume; NTBI: Non-transferrin bound iron; SD: Standard deviation; TIBC: Total iron binding capacity; TSAT: Transferrin saturation

Funding
This research was supported by a grant from Vifor Pharma (no grant numbers are attributed). All statements in this report, including its findings and conclusions, are solely those of the authors and do not necessarily represent the views or policies of Vifor Pharma.

Authors' contributions
CAJMG, AD, RW, BvD, and SJLB: designed the research; JMGH and MFE: conducted the research; JMGH, MFE, and IMN: analyzed data and performed the statistical analysis; JMGH, MFE, CAJMG, SJLB, and CFMF: wrote the manuscript and had primary responsibility for the final content; and all authors: read and approved the final manuscript.

Competing interests
C.A.J.M.G. received speaking fees and research funding from Vifor Pharma. The other authors have declared that no conflict of interest exists.

Author details

[1]Department of Nephrology, University Medical Center Groningen, University of Groningen, Hanzeplein 1, Groningen 9713GZ, The Netherlands. [2]Department of Epidemiology, University Medical Center Groningen, University of Groningen, Hanzeplein 1, Groningen 9713GZ, The Netherlands. [3]Department of Internal Medicine, Medical Center Alkmaar, Wilhelminalaan 12, 1815JD Alkmaar, The Netherlands. [4]Dialysis Center Groningen, Hanzeplein 1, Groningen 9713GZ, The Netherlands. [5]Department of Internal Medicine and Dermatology, University Medical Center Utrecht, University of Utrecht, Heidelberglaan 100, 3584CX Utrecht, The Netherlands. [6]Department of Internal Medicine, Division of Nephrology, University Medical Center Groningen, Hanzeplein 1, 9713GZ Groningen, The Netherlands.

References

1. Stauffer ME, Fan T. Prevalence of anemia in chronic kidney disease in the United States. PLoS One. 2014;9:e84943. https://doi.org/10.1371/journal.pone.0084943.

2. O'Mara NB. Anemia in patients with chronic kidney disease. Diabetes Spectr. 2010;21:12–9.

3. de Benoist B, McLean E, Egli I, Cogswell M. Worldwide prevalence of anaemia 1993–2005. Geneva: WHO Press, world health organization; 2008. https://doi.org/10.1017/S1368980008002401.

4. Zarychanski R, Houston DS. Anemia of chronic disease: a harmful disorder or an adaptive, beneficial response? CMAJ. 2008;179:333–7. https://doi.org/10.1503/cmaj.071131.

5. Macdougall IC. Iron supplementation in the non-dialysis chronic kidney disease (ND-CKD) patient: oral or intravenous? Curr Med Res Opin. 2010;26:473–82.

6. van der Weerd NC, Grooteman MPC, Nubé MJ, ter Wee PM, Swinkels DW, Gaillard CAJM. Hepcidin in chronic kidney disease: not an anaemia management tool, but promising as a cardiovascular biomarker. Neth J Med. 2015;73:108–18.

7. Nemeth E, Tuttle MS, Powelson J, Vaughn MB, Donovan A, Ward DM, et al. Hepcidin regulates cellular iron efflux by binding to ferroportin and inducing its internalization. Science. 2004;306:2090–3. https://doi.org/10.1126/science.1104742.

8. Fishbane S. Iron Management in Nondialysis-Dependent CKD. Am J Kidney Dis. 2007;49:736–43.

9. Rozen-Zvi B, Gafter-Gvili A, Paul M, Leibovici L, Shpilberg O, Gafter U. Intravenous versus Oral Iron supplementation for the treatment of Anemia in CKD: systematic review and meta-analysis. Am J Kidney Dis. 2008;52:897–906. https://doi.org/10.1053/j.ajkd.2008.05.033.

10. Macdougall IC, Bock AH, Carrera F, Eckardt K-U, Gaillard C, Van Wyck D, et al. FIND-CKD: a randomized trial of intravenous ferric carboxymaltose versus oral iron in patients with chronic kidney disease and iron deficiency anaemia. Nephrol Dial Transplant. 2014;29:2075–84. https://doi.org/10.1093/ndt/gfu201.

11. Shepshelovich D, Rozen-Zvi B, Avni T, Gafter U, Gafter-gvili A. Intravenous versus Oral Iron supplementation for the treatment of Anemia in CKD: an updated systematic review and meta-analysis. Am J Kidney Dis. 2016;68: 677–90. https://doi.org/10.1053/j.ajkd.2016.04.018.

12. Hörl WH. Clinical aspects of iron use in the anemia of kidney disease. J Am Soc Nephrol. 2007;18:382–93. https://doi.org/10.1681/ASN.2006080856.

13. Van Wyck DB, Roppolo M, Martinez CO, Mazey RM, McMurray S. A randomized, controlled trial comparing IV iron sucrose to oral iron in anemic patients with nondialysis-dependent CKD. Kidney Int. 2005;68:2846–56.

14. Smets Y, Gaillard C. Richtlijn Anemie bij Chronische Nierziekte. 1st ed. Amsterdam: Nederlandse federatie voor Nefrologie; 2015.

15. De FL, Iolascon A, Taher A, Domenica M. European journal of internal medicine clinical management of iron de fi ciency anemia in adults : systemic review on advances in diagnosis and treatment. Eur J Intern Med. 2017;42:16–23. https://doi.org/10.1016/j.ejim.2017.04.018.

16. Kidney Disease: Improving global outcomes (KDIGO) Anemia work group. KDIGO clinical practice guideline for Anemia in chronic kidney disease. Kidney Int Suppl. 2012;2:279–335.

17. Brugnara C, Mohandas N. Red cell indices in classification and treatment of anemias: from M.M. Wintrobes's original 1934 classification to the third millennium. Curr Opin Hematol. 2013;20:222–30. https://doi.org/10.1097/MOH.0b013e32835f5933.

18. Geisser P, Burckhardt S. The pharmacokinetics and pharmacodynamics of iron preparations. Pharmaceutics. 2011;3:12–33. https://doi.org/10.3390/pharmaceutics3010012.

19. Danielson BG. Structure, chemistry, and pharmacokinetics of intravenous iron agents. J Am Soc Nephrol. 2004;15(suppl 2):S93–8. https://doi.org/10.1097/01.ASN.0000143814.49713.C5.

20. Evans RW, Rafique R, Zarea A, Rapisarda C, Cammack R, Evans PJ, et al. Nature of non-transferrin-bound iron: studies on iron citrate complexes and thalassemic sera. J Biol Inorg Chem. 2008;13:57–74. https://doi.org/10.1007/s00775-007-0297-8.

21. Onken JE, Bregman DB, Harrington RA, Morris D, Buerkert J, Hamerski D, et al. Ferric carboxymaltose in patients with iron-deficiency anemia and impaired renal function: the REPAIR-IDA trial. Nephrol Dial Transplant. 2014; 29:833–42. https://doi.org/10.1093/ndt/gft251.

22. Evstatiev R, Marteau P, Iqbal T, Khalif IL, Stein J, Bokemeyer B, et al. FERGIcor, a randomized controlled trial on ferric carboxymaltose for iron deficiency anemia in inflammatory bowel disease. Gastroenterology. 2011;141:846–853.e2.

23. Hardy S, Vandemergel X. Intravenous iron administration and hypophosphatemia in clinical practice. Int J Rheumatol. 2015;2015:468675. https://doi.org/10.1155/2015/468675.

24. Van Buren P, Velez RL, Vaziri ND, Zhou XJ. Iron overdose: a contributor to adverse outcomes in randomized trials of anemia correction in CKD. Int Urol Nephrol. 2012;44:499–507. https://doi.org/10.1007/s11255-011-0028-5.

25. Keating GM. Ferric Carboxymaltose: a review of its use in Iron deficiency. Drugs. 2015;75:101–27. https://doi.org/10.1007/s40265-014-0332-3.

4

Home hemodialysis treatment and outcomes: retrospective analysis of the Knowledge to Improve Home Dialysis Network in Europe (KIHDNEy) cohort

Shashidhar Cherukuri[1], Maria Bajo[2], Giacomo Colussi[3], Roberto Corciulo[4], Hafedh Fessi[5], Maxence Ficheux[6], Maria Slon[7], Eric Weinhandl[8,9]* (iD) and Natalie Borman[10]

Abstract

Background: Utilization of home hemodialysis (HHD) is low in Europe. The Knowledge to Improve Home Dialysis Network in Europe (KIHDNEy) is a multi-center study of HHD patients who have used a transportable hemodialysis machine that employs a low volume of lactate-buffered, ultrapure dialysate per session. In this retrospective cohort analysis, we describe patient factors, HHD prescription factors, and biochemistry and medication use during the first 6 months of HHD and rates of clinical outcomes thereafter.

Methods: Using a standardized digital form, we recorded data from 7 centers in 4 Western European countries. We retained patients who completed ≥6 months of HHD. We summarized patient and HHD prescription factors with descriptive statistics and used mixed modeling to assess trends in biochemistry and medication use. We also estimated long-term rates of kidney transplant and death.

Results: We identified 129 HHD patients; 104 (81%) were followed for ≥6 months. Mean age was 49 years and 66% were male. Over 70% of patients were prescribed 6 sessions per week, and the mean treatment duration was 15.0 h per week. Median HHD training duration was 2.5 weeks. Mean standard Kt/V_{urea} was nearly 2.7 at months 3 and 6. Pre-dialysis biochemistry was generally stable. Between baseline and month 6, mean serum bicarbonate increased from 23.1 to 24.1 mmol/L ($P = 0.01$), mean serum albumin increased from 36.8 to 37.8 g/L ($P = 0.03$), mean serum C-reactive protein increased from 7.3 to 12.4 mg/L ($P = 0.05$), and mean serum potassium decreased from 4.80 to 4.59 mmol/L ($P = 0.01$). Regarding medication use, the mean number of antihypertensive medications fell from 1.46 agents per day at HHD initiation to 1.01 agents per day at 6 months ($P < 0.001$), but phosphate binder use and erythropoiesis-stimulating agent dose were stable. Long-term rates of kidney transplant and death were 15.3 and 5.4 events per 100 patient-years, respectively.

Conclusions: Intensive HHD with low-flow dialysate delivers adequate urea clearance and good biochemical outcomes in Western European patients. Intensive HHD coincided with a large decrease in antihypertensive medication use. With relatively rapid training, HHD should be considered in more patients.

Keywords: Adequacy, Antihypertensive medication, Home hemodialysis, Intensive hemodialysis, Kidney transplant, Lactate, Low-flow dialysate, Ultrapure dialysate

* Correspondence: eweinhandl@nxstage.com; wein0205@umn.edu
[8]NxStage Medical, Inc., 350 Merrimack Street, Lawrence, MA 01843, USA
[9]Department of Pharmaceutical Care and Health Systems, University of Minnesota, Minneapolis, MN, USA
Full list of author information is available at the end of the article

Background

The prevalence of chronic kidney disease (CKD) is growing internationally, partly due to the steadily growing prevalence of diabetes. This has led to a rise in need for renal replacement therapy (RRT); the number of patients receiving RRT is expected to double by 2030 [1]. Between 2013 and 2014 alone, the number of adult patients receiving RRT in the United Kingdom rose 4.0% [2]. Although use of hemodialysis outpaces use of peritoneal dialysis in the UK and almost every other country [3], patients on home hemodialysis (HHD) represent only slightly more than 4% of dialysis patients in the UK [2]. Across all of Europe, patients on HHD represent < 2% of dialysis patients [4]. Compared to in-center hemodialysis, HHD is associated with lower risk of cardiovascular death and hospitalization [5, 6]. This association may reflect increased treatment frequency, which has been shown in randomized clinical trials to reduce left ventricular mass, improve blood pressure control, and lower serum phosphorus [7–12]. HHD also permits patients the flexibility to dialyze at times that they choose. On the other hand, HHD is associated with higher risk of infection-related hospitalization, compared to in-center hemodialysis [6]. Increased treatment frequency may increase risk of vascular access complications [13].

Despite the potential benefits of HHD, utilization of the modality is low. Historically, this has been attributed to cost and logistics. In the UK, funding for HHD setup costs are a challenge for most hospitals, as the therapy is not included in the tariff set by the specialist commissioners. The recommendation from the National Institute of Clinical Excellence (NICE) to provide HHD to all suitable patients has encouraged renal units to improve HHD programs [14]. Introduction of more compact and user-friendly dialysis machines has also changed the way that patients are dialyzed at home. The aim of this study is to describe patient and treatment factors, short-term biochemical outcomes, and long-term clinical outcomes in HHD patients at European centers that participate in the Knowledge to Improve Home Dialysis Network in Europe (KIHDNEy). The overarching aim of KIHDNEy is to evaluate an array of outcomes on intensive HHD with low-volume dialysate, a newer modality in Europe than in North America.

Methods

Study cohort

We performed a retrospective cohort study of anonymized data that were voluntarily provided by 7 dialysis centers throughout Europe. Centers were in England (Portsmouth), France (Caen, Paris), Italy (Bari, Niguarda [Milan]), and Spain (Madrid, Navarre). All patients in the KIHDNEy cohort initiated HHD with the NxStage System One (NxStage Medical, Lawrence, Massachusetts, United States), a portable hemodialysis machine that employs a low volume of lactate-buffered, ultrapure dialysate per session and inverts the traditional ratio between dialysate and blood flow rates. Patients used either a set of 5-l bags of sterile, premixed dialysate ("Express System") or fluid that was produced in the home with 5-l bags of dialysate concentrate and purified tap water ("PureFlow SL"), without need for a reverse osmosis system. Preceding initiation of HHD, patients were educated in a health care facility about the practice of HHD (including cannulation) and technical aspects of the machine.

Patient factors

During 2015, centers entered data into a standardized Microsoft Excel worksheet. Data comprised patient characteristics; HHD prescription factors; standard Kt/V_{urea} and ultrafiltration volume after 3 and 6 months of HHD; pre-dialysis biochemical parameters at baseline and after 3 and 6 months of HHD; and medication use at baseline and after 3 and 6 months of HHD. Medications comprised erythropoiesis-stimulating agents, heparin, antihypertensive agents, and phosphate binders; units of darbepoetin alfa were converted to units of epoetin alfa-equivalent by multiplying by 250. We also derived ultrafiltration rate after 3 and 6 months of HHD, but with hemodialysis session duration and weight ascertained at baseline. In addition, centers entered data regarding long-term outcomes, including kidney transplant, return to in-center hemodialysis, and death. Patients were followed until October 31, 2015.

Statistical analysis

Centers were instructed to enter data only for patients who completed ≥ 6 months of HHD. Therefore, we retained patients who initiated HHD no later than April 30, 2015, and excluded any retained patient with < 6 months of follow-up. Furthermore, we excluded patients with missing data regarding HHD prescription factors. We used descriptive analysis to assess patient characteristics and HHD prescription factors. For each clearance and biochemical parameter, we calculated the mean, standard deviation, median, interquartile range, and 10th–90th percentile interval at baseline (as applicable) and months 3 and 6. For each parameter, we assessed statistical significance of the linear trend across measured times; the test was derived from a linear mixed model of the parameter regressed on time, with random effects (intercept and slope) for each patient, but without further covariate adjustment. With long-term follow-up, we estimated the cumulative incidence of kidney transplant, return to in-center hemodialysis, and death, beginning at 6 months after HHD initiation and ending at the earlier of 48 months after HHD initiation or October 31, 2015. All statistical analyses were performed with SAS, version 9.4 (Cary, North Carolina, United States) and R, version 3.2.3 (Vienna, Austria).

Results

We collected data regarding 129 patients in 7 centers. After we excluded patients with missing data regarding the home hemodialysis prescription ($n = 2$), patients who initiated HHD after April 30, 2015 ($n = 14$), and patients with < 6 months of HHD before therapy attrition ($n = 9$), we retained 104 (81%) patients for analysis (Fig. 1). Therapy attrition was attributable to kidney transplant and return to in-center HD; the latter was due to both medical complications and psychosocial issues. Among retained patients, we identified 59 (57%) patients in England, 23 (22%) in France, 10 (10%) in Italy, and 12 (12%) in Spain.

Patient characteristics are displayed in Table 1. Mean age was 49 years (range, 19 to 75 years) and 66% of patients were male. Merely 15% of patients had either diabetes mellitus or hypertensive nephrosclerosis as their primary renal diagnosis. Prevalence of moderate (body mass index, 30–34 kg/m^2), severe (35–39 kg/m^2), and morbid (≥40 kg/m^2) obesity was 13%, 6%, and 3%, respectively. The Charlson comorbidity score was ≤6

points in nearly all patients. Most patients were on conventional hemodialysis before HHD initiation; only 16% of patients were incident cases of end stage renal disease (ESRD).

HHD prescription factors are displayed in Table 2. Over 70% of patients were prescribed 6 sessions per week. Mean (standard deviation) hemodialysis hours per session and per week were 2.6 (0.4) and 15.0 (2.9), respectively, and more than 68% received ≥15 h per week. Dialysate preparation varied by country: in France and Italy, only premixed dialysate was used; in Spain, only dialysate concentrate was used; and in the United Kingdom, both preparations were used, although dialysate concentrate was dominant (86%). Most patients dialyzed with a fistula. Regarding the number of training weeks, mean and median (interquartile range) estimates were 3.8 and 2.5 (3.0), respectively; regarding the number of training sessions, corresponding estimates were 16.8 and 10.0 (16.5) respectively (Fig. 2). Training duration was ≤2 weeks in 50% of all patients and 80% of patients in the United Kingdom.

Details of hemodialytic clearance are displayed in Table 3. With HHD, mean standard Kt/V_{urea} was nearly 2.7 at months 3 and 6 and roughly 90% of patients had standard $Kt/V_{urea} \geq 2.1$. Among the minority of patients with recorded ultrafiltration volume at months 3 and 6, mean ultrafiltration volume was roughly 1 L, mean

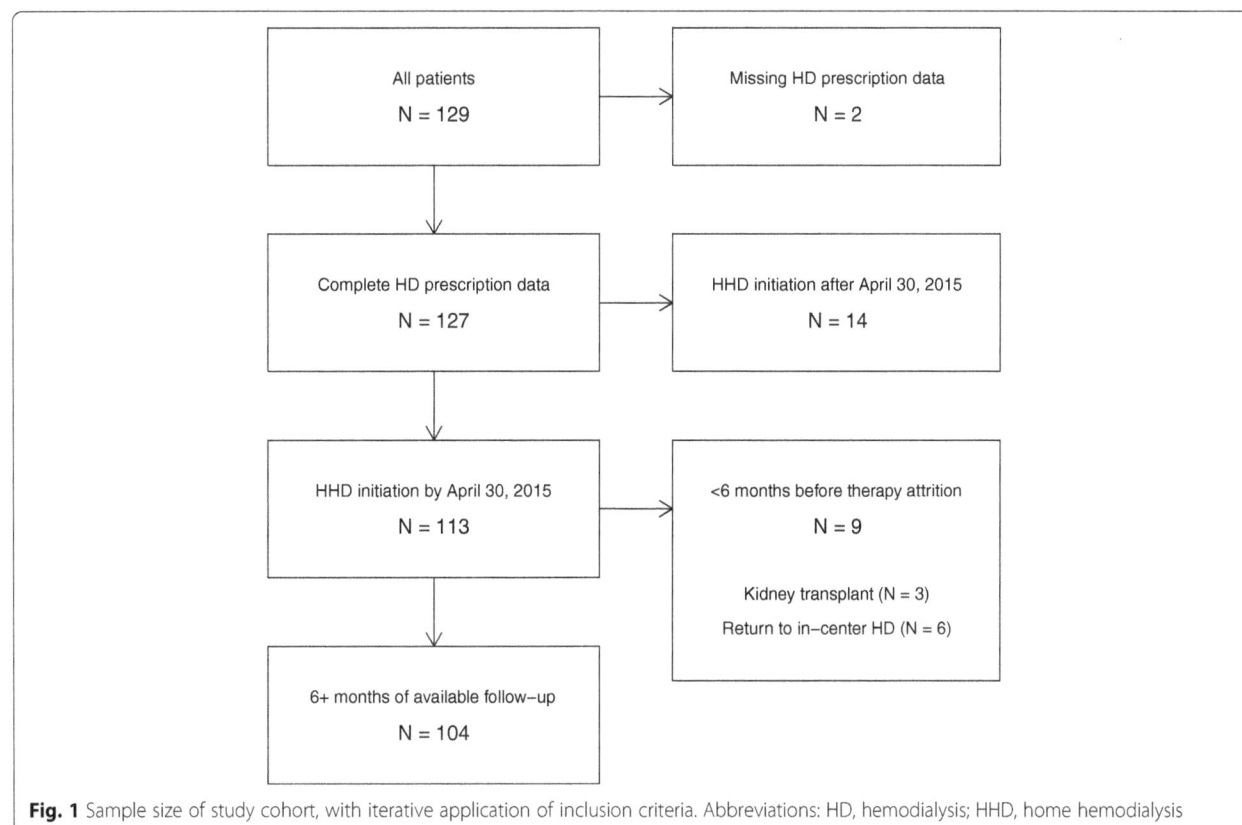

Fig. 1 Sample size of study cohort, with iterative application of inclusion criteria. Abbreviations: HD, hemodialysis; HHD, home hemodialysis

Table 1 Home hemodialysis patient characteristics

	Statistic
Age (years)	
Mean (SD)	49.3 (12.8)
Median (IQR)	49 (19)
10th–90th percentile interval	31.6–65.0
Sex (%)	
Female	33.7
Male	66.3
Primary renal diagnosis (%)	
Diabetes mellitus	9.6
Hypertensive nephrosclerosis	5.8
Glomerulonephritis	29.8
Polycystic kidney disease	10.6
Other diagnosis	44.2
Body mass index (kg/m^2)	
Mean (SD)	26.7 (6.0)
Median (IQR)	25.7 (7.5)
10th–90th percentile interval	20.4–34.3
Charlson comorbidity score (points)	
Mean (SD)	3.7 (2.0)
Median (IQR)	3 (3)
10th–90th percentile interval	2–6
Prior renal replacement modality (%)	
Conventional hemodialysis	70.2
Intensive hemodialysis	3.8
Peritoneal dialysis	6.7
Kidney transplant	2.9
Incident ESRD	16.3
Prior dialysis duration (months)	
Mean (SD)	36.9 (55.2)
Median (IQR)	18 (35)
10th–90th percentile interval	0–127
History of kidney transplant (%)	
No	63.5
Yes	36.5

Abbreviations: *ESRD* end stage renal disease, *IQR* interquartile range, *SD* standard deviation

Table 2 Home hemodialysis prescription factors

	Percentage
Hemodialysis sessions per week (%)	
4	1.9
5	24.0
6	70.2
7	3.8
Hours per hemodialysis session (%)	
2.0–2.4	30.8
2.5–2.9	41.3
3.0–3.4	22.1
≥ 3.5	5.8
Hemodialysis hours per week (%)	
10.0–11.9	7.7
12.0–14.9	24.0
15.0–17.9	47.1
≥ 18.0	21.2
Dialysate preparation (%)	
Premixed dialysate	39.4
Dialysate concentrate	60.6
Dialysate liters per session (%)	
15	2.9
20	39.4
25	31.7
30	25.0
40	1.0
Vascular access modality (%)	
Catheter	17.3
Graft	2.9
Fistula	79.8
Cannulation technique [a] (%)	
Sharp needle	8.4
Buttonhole needle	80.7
Plastic needle	10.8

[a] In patients with a fistula

with serum C-reactive protein > 10 mg/L increased from 22% at baseline to 30% at month 6.

Medication use is displayed in Table 5. The mean number of antihypertensive agents per day fell significantly ($P < 0.001$), from 1.46 at baseline to 1.01 at month 6. The percentage of patients using no antihypertensive agents increased from 31% at baseline to 41% at month 6, while the percentage of patients using > 2 antihypertensive agents per day decreased from 23 to 11%. Phosphate binder pill count and ESA dose were stable. The percentage of patients using no heparin for anticoagulation nearly doubled between baseline and month 6 ($P < 0.001$).

ultrafiltration rate was < 7 mL/hour/kg, and over 80% of patients had ultrafiltration rate < 10 mL/hour/kg.

Biochemical parameters are displayed in Table 4. Mean changes between baseline and months 3 and 6 were modest. Serum bicarbonate increased by 1 mmol/L between baseline and month 6, whereas serum potassium decreased by 0.2 mmol/L. Calcium and phosphorus were stable, while serum albumin and C-reactive protein increased during follow-up. The percentage of patients

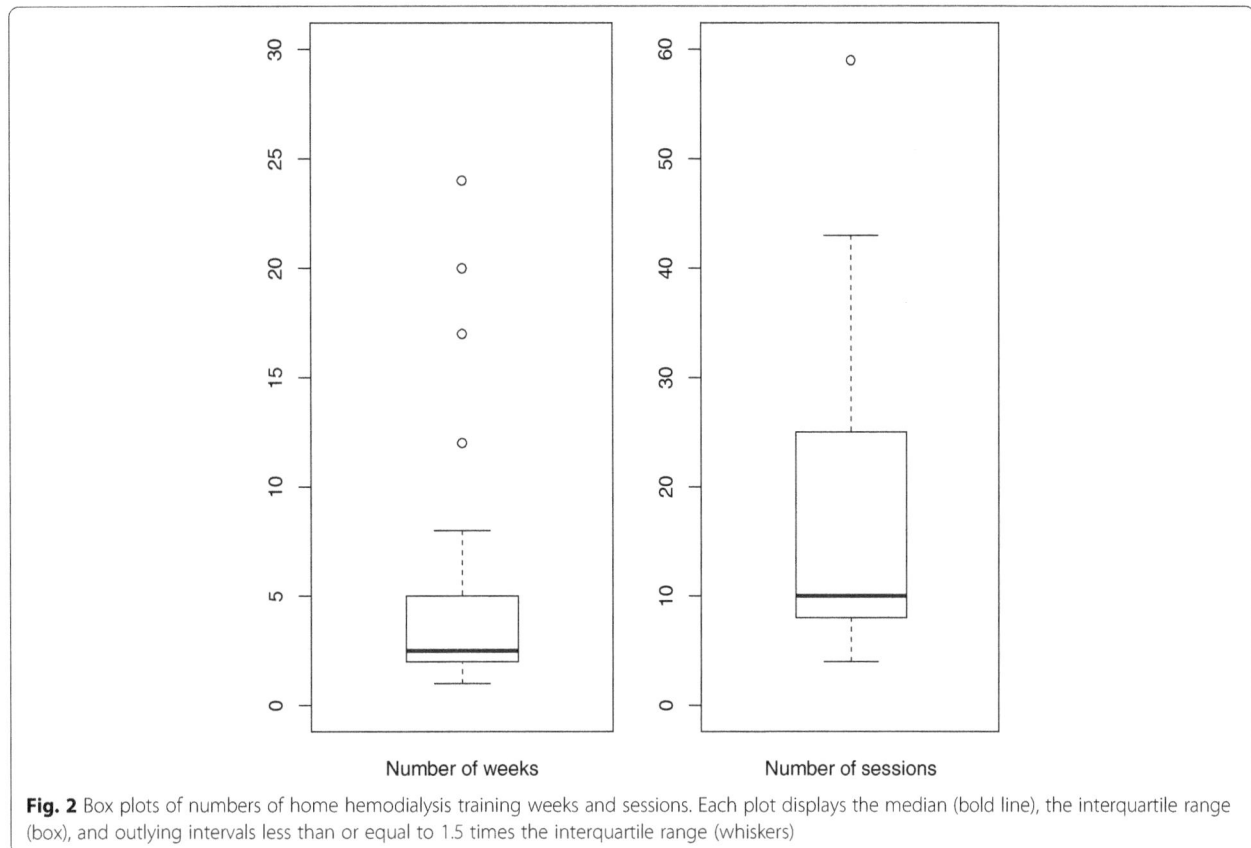

Fig. 2 Box plots of numbers of home hemodialysis training weeks and sessions. Each plot displays the median (bold line), the interquartile range (box), and outlying intervals less than or equal to 1.5 times the interquartile range (whiskers)

Mean follow-up duration was 18.8 months. During follow-up, there were 17 kidney transplants, 8 returns to in-center hemodialysis, and 6 deaths. After the first 6 months of follow-up, transplant and death rates were 15.3 and 5.4 events per 100 patient-years, respectively. At 24 months after HHD initiation, the cumulative incidence of kidney transplant, return to in-center hemodialysis, and death was 20%, 8%, and 6%, respectively. At 48 months after HHD initiation, corresponding estimates of cumulative incidence were 32%, 10%, and 15%. Thus, approximately 43% of patients remained on HHD at 48 months after HHD initiation (Fig. 3). Returns to in-center hemodialysis were due to medical complications in 2 cases and psychosocial problems in 6 cases.

Discussion

HHD continues to have limited penetration in Europe and is not currently offered as an option to all ESRD patients. In the most recent annual report of the European Renal Association-European Dialysis and Transplant Association (ERA-EDTA), the highest percentages of dialysis patients on HHD were in Finland (7.1%), Denmark (5.8%), the Netherlands (4.4%), the UK (4.3%), and Sweden (3.6%); corresponding percentages in all other countries were less than 3% [15]. The reasons for low use of HHD are myriad, but primary reasons include

the relative simplicity of peritoneal dialysis and the shortage of patient-friendly hemodialysis equipment for application in the home setting [16]. In the KIHDNEy cohort, HHD patients used equipment that employs lactate-buffered, ultrapure dialysate, which is either supplied in premixed bags or produced from concentrate and tap water (without a reverse osmosis system). Each treatment consumes 15 to 60 l of dialysate, which flow at a maximum rate of 200 mL/minute. From the patient's perspective, the device presents a relatively simple user interface, is sufficiently small to transport, and requires neither electrical nor plumbing modifications to the home; the costs of those modifications are ordinarily between $1000 and $4000 [17]. In this observational study, we evaluated patient and treatment factors, biochemical outcomes, and clinical outcomes in European patients on intensive HHD with low-volume dialysate. Despite its modest sample size, this study is the largest study of European patients on such treatment.

The mean age of patients in the KIHDNEy cohort was almost 50 years. That is roughly 10 years less than the mean age of prevalent ESRD patients in many European countries [15], but similar to the relative youthfulness of HHD patients in the United States [18, 19]. The majority of patients were male, in concordance with HHD populations in North America, Australia, and New Zealand

Table 3 Urea clearance, ultrafiltration volume, and ultrafiltration rate in home hemodialysis patients

	Month 3	Month 6
Standard Kt/V_{urea}		
Patients (n)	87	87
Mean (SD)	2.67 (0.49)	2.69 (0.55)
Median (IQR)	2.63 (0.46)	2.63 (0.57)
10th–90th percentile interval	2.14–3.30	2.09–3.49
Ultrafiltration volume [a] (L)		
Patients (n)	32	32
Mean (SD)	1.07 (0.84)	1.08 (0.87)
Median (IQR)	1.00 (1.02)	1.00 (0.92)
10th–90th percentile interval	0.20–2.00	0.20–2.00
Ultrafiltration rate (mL/hour/kg)		
Patients (n)	32	32
Mean (SD)	6.54 (4.85)	6.82 (5.61)
Median (IQR)	6.21 (6.35)	6.46 (5.11)
10th–90th percentile interval	1.51–13.95	0.76–11.88

Abbreviations: *IQR* interquartile range, *SD* standard deviation
[a] Per hemodialysis session

Table 4 Biochemical parameters in home hemodialysis patients

	Baseline	Month 3	Month 6	p [a]
Bicarbonate (mmol/L)				
Mean (SD)	23.1 (3.5)	24.1 (2.8)	24.1 (2.9)	0.01
Median (IQR)	23.3 (4.2)	24.0 (4.0)	24.0 (3.5)	
10th–90th percentile interval	18.0–27.3	20.7–27.5	20.0–28.0	
Potassium (mmol/L)				
Mean (SD)	4.80 (0.63)	4.64 (0.71)	4.59 (0.78)	0.01
Median (IQR)	4.80 (0.90)	4.60 (1.10)	4.40 (1.00)	
10th–90th percentile interval	3.9–5.6	3.8–5.5	3.8–5.6	
Calcium (mmol/L)				
Mean (SD)	2.29 (0.19)	2.30 (0.20)	2.28 (0.19)	0.43
Median (IQR)	2.30 (0.24)	2.29 (0.22)	2.30 (0.23)	
10th–90th percentile interval	2.03–2.52	2.06–2.53	2.04–2.49	
Phosphorus (mmol/L)				
Mean (SD)	1.73 (0.49)	1.67 (0.49)	1.68 (0.48)	0.38
Median (IQR)	1.64 (0.72)	1.64 (0.66)	1.62 (0.60)	
10th–90th percentile interval	1.16–2.40	1.10–2.33	1.11–2.28	
Albumin (g/L)				
Mean (SD)	36.8 (5.2)	37.5 (4.0)	37.8 (4.5)	0.03
Median (IQR)	37.0 (5.0)	37.0 (5.0)	38.0 (6.0)	
10th–90th percentile interval	31.0–43.0	32.3–43.0	38.0–50.0	
Hemoglobin (g/dL)				
Mean (SD)	11.4 (1.5)	11.1 (1.6)	11.2 (1.4)	0.25
Median (IQR)	11.5 (1.7)	11.1 (1.9)	11.1 (2.0)	
10th–90th percentile interval	9.2–13.5	9.2–13.0	9.5–13.1	
Beta-2-microglobulin (mg/L)				
Mean (SD)	23.6 (9.7)	26.8 (12.5)	25.4 (10.8)	0.64
Median (IQR)	22.0 (14.7)	25.3 (15.1)	24.0 (14.2)	
10th–90th percentile interval	10.3–36.3	14.4–42.7	13.7–42.0	
C-reactive protein (mg/L)				
Mean (SD)	7.3 (8.9)	11.4 (16.6)	12.4 (24.8)	0.05
Median (IQR)	4.4 (7.2)	5.0 (12.3)	5.0 (12.0)	
10th–90th percentile interval	1.0–18.0	0.7–31.0	0.9–30.0	

Abbreviations: *IQR* interquartile range, *SD* standard deviation
[a] From test of linear trend across displayed times

[18, 20, 21]. Furthermore, the prevalence of diabetes as the primary etiology of ESRD was low. However, characterization of the KIHDNEy cohort as a collection of young, healthy men is inaccurate. Age ranged from 19 to 75 years and the Charlson comorbidity score ranged from 2 to 10 points. Notably, body mass index ranged from 13 (underweight) to 51 (obese). Thus, HHD appears to be a viable dialytic modality across a wide array of patients, including patients in poorer health. This observation contradicts the assumption that HHD is feasible exclusively in younger patients with limited comorbidity. In the KIHDNEy cohort, more than 70% of patients converted from in-center hemodialysis to HHD, and mean dialysis duration at HHD initiation was more than 3 years. In the United States, HHD is also commonly prescribed subsequently to in-center hemodialysis [18].

Almost all patients in the KIHDNEy cohort were prescribed either 5 or 6 treatments per week. Because treatment duration was typically between 2.0 and 3.5 h, over 70% of patients accumulated at least 15 treatment hours per week. By comparison, large majorities of in-center hemodialysis patients in France, Italy, Spain, and the UK accumulate no more than 12 treatment hours per week [22]. The ease of delivering more treatment hours per week in the home setting is one of the primary advantages of HHD. The most commonly prescribed dialysate volume was 20 l per session and most patients dialyzed against 20 to 30 l per session. The majority of patients used a fistula and cannulated with a buttonhole needle. Buttonhole cannulation may be associated with increased risks of local and systemic infection, although mupirocin prophylaxis may greatly reduce risk [23, 24]. Slightly more than 17% of patients in the KIHDNEy cohort used a catheter. Catheters are widely used by HHD patients in Canada [21] and do not constitute an absolute contraindication to HHD.

HHD training, which is more complex than peritoneal dialysis training, is an obstacle to the growth of HHD. Needed nursing labor and corresponding costs may be substantial. In the Frequent Hemodialysis Network (FHN) Nocturnal Trial, patients required an average of 27.7 training sessions, which spanned between 11 and 59 days [17]. However, patients in that trial used

Table 5 Medication use in home hemodialysis patients

	Baseline	Month 3	Month 6	p [a]
Antihypertensive medication use (agents/day)				
Mean (SD)	1.46 (1.49)	1.10 (1.29)	1.01 (1.11)	< 0.001
Median (IQR)	1 (2)	1 (1)	1 (1)	
10th–90th percentile interval	0–4	0–3	0–3	
Phosphate binder use (pills/day)				
Mean (SD)	3.25 (2.91)	3.13 (2.66)	3.21 (2.84)	0.83
Median (IQR)	3 (4)	3 (3)	3 (5)	
10th–90th percentile interval	0–6	0–6	0–6	
ESA dose (EPO-equivalent IU/week)				
Mean (SD)	8792 (6936)	8211 (6654)	8551 (7086)	0.57
Median (IQR)	8000 (6000)	7750 (6000)	8000 (8000)	
10th–90th percentile interval	2000–17,000	1250–16,000	0–16,125	
Anticoagulant use [b] (%)				
No	21.4	NR	40.2	< 0.001
Yes	78.6	NR	59.8	

Abbreviations: *EPO* epoetin alfa, *ESA* erythropoiesis-stimulating agent, *IQR* interquartile range, *IU* international units, *NR* not recorded, *SD* standard deviation
[a] From test of linear trend across displayed times
[b] Heparin use during hemodialysis session

traditional hemodialysis equipment in the home setting. Patients in the KIHDNEy cohort required an average of 16.8 training sessions. This apparent reduction in training intensity may reflect the simple user interface of the equipment. On the other hand, this reduction may reflect that some patients were familiar with self-cannulation before commencing HHD training. More research about the nature of HHD training is needed. Ultimately, equipment that permits more rapid training can improve the economic feasibility of HHD. Despite the rapid pace of training in the KIHDNEy cohort, we observed good patient retention after the first 6 months of HHD. The rate of death was relatively low, whereas the rate of kidney transplant was relatively high. However, the magnitude of the transplant rate may primarily reflect the age distribution of the KIHDNEy cohort, as nearly all patients were non-elderly; whether HHD directly influences the likelihood of transplant is unknown. We also observed that most returns to in-center hemodialysis occurred in the first 12 months of follow-up and were attributable to psychosocial problems. High incidence of technique failure during the first year of HHD has been observed in the United States [19], and in the FHN Nocturnal Trial, HHD increased perceived caregiver burden [25].

Although intensive HHD with low-flow dialysate is widely used in the United States and is associated with lower risk of death and similar risk of hospitalization, relative to thrice-weekly in-center hemodialysis [5, 6], very little data about solute clearance and biochemistry

with this therapeutic approach have been published. Kraus et al. reported that mean standard Kt/V_{urea} was nearly 2.3 in patients who were prescribed 6 sessions per week [26]. In the KIHDNEy cohort, mean standard Kt/V_{urea} was nearly 2.7 at both 3 and 6 months after HHD initiation. Furthermore, roughly 90% of patients achieved standard Kt/V_{urea} of ≥2.1, even without accounting for residual function. Adequate small solute clearance with low-volume dialysate is achievable because the dialysate is highly saturated when the blood flow rate is high and the dialysate flow rate is low. On average, ultrafiltration intensity was low. Multiple studies correlate lower ultrafiltration rate with improved survival and shorter post-dialysis recovery time [27–29]. Changes in biochemistry were generally modest. Serum concentrations of calcium, phosphorus, hemoglobin, and beta-2-microglobulin did not change significantly. The absence of a significant decline in serum phosphorus contrasts with the effect of intensive hemodialysis in the FHN Daily Trial [30]. It is possible that while dialytic clearance of phosphorus increased after HHD initiation [31], dietary intake of phosphorus also increased; to that point, serum albumin increased significantly. Mean serum potassium declined after initiation of HHD, although the 10th–90th percentile range was unchanged. The decline probably reflects the effect of shortening the usual interdialytic interval. Finally, serum C-reactive protein (CRP) increased. Serum CRP > 10 mg/L most often reflects acute or chronic inflammation [32]. Infection may have contributed to the increase, as infection – specifically, vascular access infection – has been reported to be a challenge with HHD [33]. We did not collect data regarding vascular access complications, so the incidence of access infection in the KIHDNEy cohort is unknown. However, serum CRP data suggest that dialysis centers should closely monitor signs of infection on HHD, including tenderness and localized redness at the buttonhole site [34].

Regarding medication use, there were no significant changes in either phosphate binder use or erythropoiesis-stimulating agent dose. There was a significant decline in antihypertensive medication use between baseline and follow-up; the same change was observed in the Following Rehabilitation, Economics and Everyday-Dialysis Outcome Measurements (FREEDOM) Study of short daily HHD [35]. Intensive hemodialysis reduces pre-dialysis systolic blood pressure and the need for antihypertensive medications [11, 36]. We did not collect longitudinal data about blood pressure, but the significant decline in medication use is compatible with a reduction in systolic blood pressure. The percentage of patients who did not require heparin administration nearly doubled after 6 months of HHD. Less need for anticoagulation may have been due to the absence of an air-blood interface in the disposable cartridge in the hemodialysis machine, lower session duration, and possibly, better volume control.

The primary limitations of this study are the small sample size and the brief follow-up interval. Many trends in the KIHDNEy cohort suggest hypotheses that require confirmation in prospective studies with larger sample size and longer follow-up. Nevertheless, this study is one of the largest analyses of biochemistry in patients on intensive HHD with low-flow dialysate. A secondary limitation of this study is the absence of controls, with respect to either hemodialysis setting, frequency, or equipment. Trends in the KIHDNEy cohort cannot be attributed directly to the home setting, intensive hemodialysis, or equipment. In addition, all patients in the KIHDNEy cohort were prescribed diurnal HHD; these data offer no insight into biochemical and clinical outcomes on nocturnal HHD with low-volume dialysate.

Conclusions

HHD is a unique modality, insofar as it offers the opportunity to individualize treatment and specifically, to increase treatment intensity beyond what is typically feasible in the center setting. For HHD to be attractive to both physicians and patients, HHD equipment must maintain provide good clinical outcomes and be sufficiently easy for patients to use. Preliminary data in the KIHDNEy cohort suggest that transportable equipment

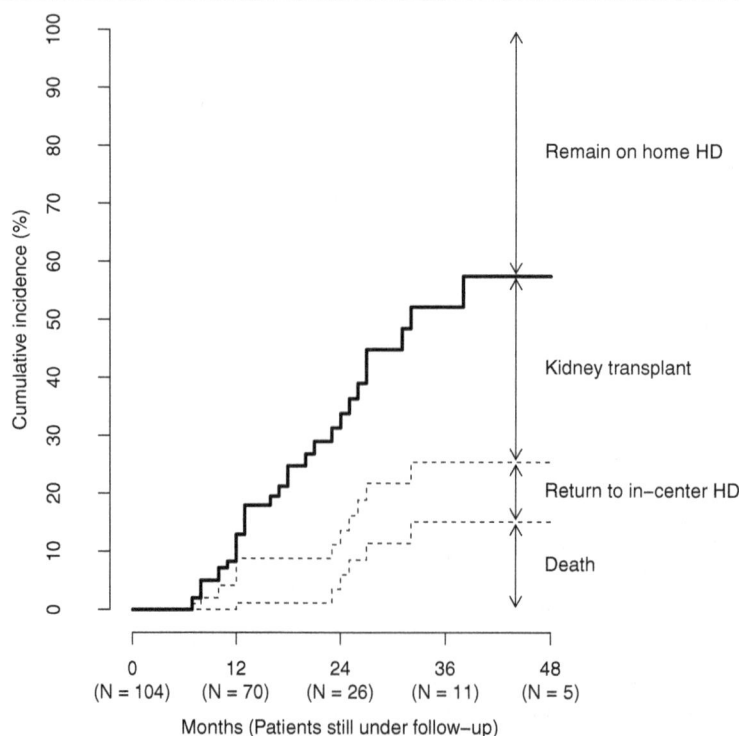

Fig. 3 Cumulative incidence of home hemodialysis cessation due to kidney transplant, return to in-center hemodialysis, and death. Abbreviations: HD, hemodialysis

that employs low-flow dialysate achieves these objectives when patients are prescribed > 3 sessions per week. However, infection may pose a risk in HHD patients. Ultimately, larger studies of European patients are needed to better understand clinical outcomes associated with this emerging therapeutic approach.

Abbreviations
CKD: Chronic kidney disease; ERA-EDTA: European Renal Association-European Dialysis and Transplant Association; ESRD: End stage renal disease; FHN: Frequent Hemodialysis Network; FREEDOM Study: Following rehabilitation, economics and everyday-dialysis outcome measurements study; HHD: Home hemodialysis; KIHDNEy: The Knowledge to Improve Home Dialysis Network in Europe; NICE: National Institute of Clinical Excellence; RRT: Renal replacement therapy

Acknowledgements
The authors thank Susan Everson, PhD, for proofreading and organizing references. Dr. Everson is a consultant to NxStage Medical.

Funding
All authors except Dr. Weinhandl collected data in the course of clinical care. Those authors voluntarily entered data in a standardized digital form; NxStage Medical provided no compensation for extraction and recording of data. Dr. Weinhandl, a clinical epidemiologist and biostatistician, coordinated statistical analysis of data.

Authors' contributions
MB, GC, RC, HF, MF, MS, and NB conceived the study and recorded data. EW was primarily responsible for processing and analyzing data. SC, EW, and NB were primarily responsible for data interpretation and initial writing. MB, GC, RC, HF, MF, and MS critically reviewed initial writing and suggested revisions. All authors gave final approval of the submitted manuscript and are accountable for all aspects of the work.

Competing interests
All authors except Dr. Weinhandl are members of the NxStage European Medical Board. Members receive nominal compensation for participation. Dr. Weinhandl is an employee of NxStage Medical.

Author details
[1]Royal Wolverhampton Hospital, Renal Services, Wolverhampton, England. [2]Hospital Universitario La Paz, Servicio de Nefrologia, Madrid, Spain. [3]Niguarda Hospital, Nefrologia – Centro Trapianti Rene, Milan, Italy. [4]Policlinic University, Azienda Ospedaliero-Universitaria Consorziale Policlinico, Bari, Italy. [5]Hôpital Tenon, Service de Néphrologie et Dialyses, Paris, France. [6]CHR Clémenceau, Service Néphrologie-Hémodialyse-Transplantation, Caen, France. [7]Hospital de Navarra, Servicio de Nefrologia, Pamplona, Spain. [8]NxStage Medical, Inc., 350 Merrimack Street, Lawrence, MA 01843, USA. [9]Department of Pharmaceutical Care and Health Systems, University of Minnesota, Minneapolis, MN, USA. [10]Queen Alexandra Hospital, Wessex Kidney Centre, Portsmouth, England.

References
1. Liyanage T, Ninomiya T, Jha V, Neal B, Patrice HM, Okpechi I, Zhao MH, Lv J, Garg AX, Knight J, et al. Worldwide access to treatment for end-stage kidney disease: a systematic review. Lancet (London England). 2015; 385(9981):1975 82.

2. MacNeill SJ, Casula A, Shaw C, Castledine C. UK Renal Registry 18th Annual Report: Chapter 2 UK Renal Replacement Therapy Prevalence in 2014: National and Centre-specific analyses. Nephron. 2016;132(Suppl 1):41–68.
3. Saran R, Robinson B, Abbott KC, Agodoa LY, Ayanian J, Bragg-Gresham J, Balkrishnan R, Chen JL, Cope E, Eggers PW, et al. US renal data system 2016 annual data report: epidemiology of kidney disease in the United States. Am J Kidney Dis. 2017;69(3s1):A7–a8.
4. Pippias M, Kramer A, Noordzij M, Afentakis N, de la Alonso Torre R, Ambuhl PM, Aparicio Madre MI, Arribas Monzon F, Asberg A, Bonthuis M, et al. The European renal association - European Dialysis and transplant association registry annual report 2014: a summary. Clin Kidney J. 2017;10(2):154–69.
5. Weinhandl ED, Liu J, Gilbertson DT, Arneson TJ, Collins AJ. Survival in daily home hemodialysis and matched thrice-weekly in-center hemodialysis patients. J Am Soc Nephrol. 2012;23(5):895–904.
6. Weinhandl ED, Nieman KM, Gilbertson DT, Collins AJ. Hospitalization in daily home hemodialysis and matched thrice-weekly in-center hemodialysis patients. Am J Kidney Dis. 2015;65(1):98–108.
7. Culleton BF, Walsh M, Klarenbach SW, Mortis G, Scott-Douglas N, Quinn RR, Tonelli M, Donnelly S, Friedrich MG, Kumar A, et al. Effect of frequent nocturnal hemodialysis vs conventional hemodialysis on left ventricular mass and quality of life: a randomized controlled trial. Jama. 2007;298(11): 1291–9.
8. Chertow GM, Levin NW, Beck GJ, Depner TA, Eggers PW, Gassman JJ, Gorodetskaya I, Greene T, James S, Larive B, et al. In-center hemodialysis six times per week versus three times per week. N Engl J Med. 2010;363(24): 2287–300.
9. Rocco MV, Lockridge RS Jr, Beck GJ, Eggers PW, Gassman JJ, Greene T, Larive B, Chan CT, Chertow GM, Copland M, et al. The effects of frequent nocturnal home hemodialysis: the frequent hemodialysis network nocturnal trial. Kidney Int. 2011;80(10):1080–91.
10. McCullough PA, Chan CT, Weinhandl ED, Burkart JM, Bakris GL. Intensive hemodialysis, left ventricular hypertrophy, and cardiovascular disease. Am J Kidney Dis. 2016;68(5s1):S5–s14.
11. Bakris GL, Burkart JM, Weinhandl ED, McCullough PA, Kraus MA. Intensive hemodialysis, blood pressure, and antihypertensive medication use. Am J Kidney Dis. 2016;68(5s1):S15–s23.
12. Copland M, Komenda P, Weinhandl ED, McCullough PA, Morfin JA. Intensive hemodialysis, mineral and bone disorder, and phosphate binder use. Am J Kidney Dis. 2016;68(5s1):S24–s32.
13. Suri RS, Larive B, Sherer S, Eggers P, Gassman J, James SH, Lindsay RM, Lockridge RS, Ornt DB, Rocco MV, et al. Risk of vascular access complications with frequent hemodialysis. J Am Soc Nephrol. 2013;24(3):498–505.
14. National Institute for Health and Care Excellence. Renal replacement therapy services for adults. Quality standard [QS72]. 2014; https://www.nice. org.uk/guidance/qs72/chapter/about-this-quality-standard.
15. ERA-EDTA Registry. ERA-EDTA Registry Annual Report 2015. Amsterdam, the Netherlands: Academic Medical Center, Department of Medical Informatics; 2017.
16. Trinh E, Chan CT. The rise, fall, and resurgence of home hemodialysis. Semin Dial. 2017;30(2):174–80.
17. Pipkin M, Eggers PW, Larive B, Rocco MV, Stokes JB, Suri RS, Lockridge RS Jr. Recruitment and training for home hemodialysis: experience and lessons from the nocturnal dialysis trial. Clin J Am Soc Nephrol. 2010;5(9): 1614–20.
18. Weinhandl ED, Gilbertson DT, Collins AJ. Mortality, hospitalization, and technique failure in daily home hemodialysis and matched peritoneal Dialysis patients: a matched cohort study. Am J Kidney Dis. 2016;67(1): 98–110.
19. Seshasai RK, Mitra N, Chaknos CM, Li J, Wirtalla C, Negoianu D, Glickman JD, Dember LM. Factors associated with discontinuation of home hemodialysis. Am J Kidney Dis. 2016;67(4):629–37.
20. Marshall MR, Hawley CM, Kerr PG, Polkinghorne KR, Marshall RJ, Agar JW, McDonald SP. Home hemodialysis and mortality risk in Australian and New Zealand populations. Am J Kidney Dis. 2011;58(5):782–93.
21. Tennankore KK, Na Y, Wald R, Chan CT, Perl J. Short daily-, nocturnal- and conventional-home hemodialysis have similar patient and treatment survival. Kidney Int. 2018;93(1):188–94.
22. Tentori F, Zhang J, Li Y, Karaboyas A, Kerr P, Saran R, Bommer J, Port F, Akiba T, Pisoni R, et al. Longer dialysis session length is associated with better intermediate outcomes and survival among patients on in-center three

times per week hemodialysis: results from the Dialysis outcomes and practice patterns study (DOPPS). Nephrol Dial Transplant. 2012;27(11):4180–8.

23. Wong B, Muneer M, Wiebe N, Storie D, Shurraw S, Pannu N, Klarenbach S, Grudzinski A, Nesrallah G, Pauly RP. Buttonhole versus rope-ladder cannulation of arteriovenous fistulas for hemodialysis: a systematic review. Am J Kidney Dis. 2014;64(6):918–36.

24. Nesrallah GE, Cuerden M, Wong JH, Pierratos A. Staphylococcus aureus bacteremia and buttonhole cannulation: long-term safety and efficacy of mupirocin prophylaxis. Clin J Am Soc Nephrol. 2010;5(6):1047–53.

25. Suri RS, Larive B, Hall Y, Kimmel PL, Kliger AS, Levin N, Tamura MK, Chertow GM. Effects of frequent hemodialysis on perceived caregiver burden in the frequent hemodialysis network trials. Clin J Am Soc Nephrol. 2014;9(5):936–42.

26. Kraus M, Burkart J, Hegeman R, Solomon R, Coplon N, Moran J. A comparison of center-based vs. home-based daily hemodialysis for patients with end-stage renal disease. Hemodial Int. 2007;11(4):468–77.

27. Assimon MM, Wenger JB, Wang L, Flythe JE. Ultrafiltration rate and mortality in maintenance hemodialysis patients. Am J Kidney Dis. 2016;68(6):911–22.

28. Chazot C, Vo-Van C, Lorriaux C, Deleaval P, Mayor B, Hurot JM, Jean G. Even a moderate fluid removal rate during individualised Haemodialysis session times is associated with decreased patient survival. Blood Purif. 2017;44(2): 89–97.

29. Hussein WF, Arramreddy R, Sun SJ, Reiterman M, Schiller B. Higher ultrafiltration rate is associated with longer Dialysis recovery time in patients undergoing conventional hemodialysis. Am J Nephrol. 2017;46(1):3–10.

30. Daugirdas JT, Chertow GM, Larive B, Pierratos A, Greene T, Ayus JC, Kendrick CA, James SH, Miller BW, Schulman G, et al. Effects of frequent hemodialysis on measures of CKD mineral and bone disorder. J Am Soc Nephrol. 2012; 23(4):727–38.

31. Brunati CCM, Gervasi F, Casati C, Querques ML, Montoli A, Colussi G. Phosphate and calcium control in short frequent hemodialysis with the NxStage system one cycler: mass balance studies and comparison with standard thrice-weekly bicarbonate Dialysis. Blood Purif. 2018;45(4):334–42.

32. Beerenhout CH, Kooman JP, van der Sande FM, Hackeng C, Leunissen KM. C-reactive protein levels in dialysis patients are highly variable and strongly related to co-morbidity. Nephrol Dial Transplant. 2003;18(1):221.

33. Poon CK, Chan CT. Home hemodialysis associated infection-the "Achilles' heel" of intensive hemodialysis. Hemodial Int. 2017;21(2):155–60.

34. Christensen LD, Skadborg MB, Mortensen AH, Mortensen C, Moller JK, Lemming L, Hogsberg I, Petersen SE, Buus NH. Bacteriology of the buttonhole cannulation tract in hemodialysis patients: a prospective cohort study. Am J Kidney Dis. 2018;72(2):234–42.

35. Jaber BL, Collins AJ, Finkelstein FO, Glickman JD, Hull AR, Kraus M, McCarthy J, Miller B, Spry L. Daily Hemodialysis (DHD) Reduces the Need for Anti-Hypertensive Medications. In: Renal Week 2009: 2009: J Am Soc Nephrol; 2009. p. 675A.

36. Kotanko P, Garg AX, Depner T, Pierratos A, Chan CT, Levin NW, Greene T, Larive B, Beck GJ, Gassman J, et al. Effects of frequent hemodialysis on blood pressure: results from the randomized frequent hemodialysis network trials. Hemodial Int. 2015;19(3):386–401.

5

Prevalence of chronic kidney disease in South Asia: a systematic review

Mehedi Hasan[1*†] ⓘ, Ipsita Sutradhar[1†], Rajat Das Gupta[1†] and Malabika Sarker[2,3]

Abstract

Background: Chronic kidney disease (CKD) is becoming a major public health problem around the world. But the prevalence has not been reported in South Asian region as a whole. This study aimed to systematically review the existing data from population based studies in this region to bridge this gap.

Methods: Articles published and reported prevalence of CKD according to K/DOQI practice guideline in eight South Asian countries between December 1955 and April 2017 were searched, screened and evaluated from seven electronic databases using the PRISMA checklist. CKD was defined as creatinine clearance (CrCl) or GFR less than 60 ml/min/1.73 m^2.

Results: Sixteen population-based studies were found from four South Asian countries (India, Bangladesh, Pakistan and Nepal) that used eGFR to measure CKD. No study was available from Sri Lanka, Maldives, Bhutan and Afghanistan. Number of participants ranged from 301 in Pakistan to 12,271 in India. Majority of the studies focused solely on urban population. Different studies used different equations for measuring eGFR. The prevalence of CKD ranged from 10.6% in Nepal to 23.3% in Pakistan using MDRD equation. This prevalence was higher among older age group people. Equal number of studies reported high prevalence among male and female each.

Conclusions: This systematic review reported high prevalence of CKD in South Asian countries. The findings of this study will help pertinent stakeholders to prepare suitable policy and effective public health intervention in order to reduce the burden of this deadly disease in the most densely populated share of the globe.

Keywords: Chronic kidney disease, South Asia

Background

Globally, Chronic Kidney Disease (CKD) is one of the leading causes of death and disability. In 1990, CKD was the 27th leading cause of death which rose up and became 18th leading cause of death in 2010 [1]. In 2013, around 1 million people died because of CKD related cause [2]. Despite of being a global concern, CKD disproportionately affects the people from developing countries. A systematic review, conducted in 2015 reported that, 109.9 million people from high-income countries had CKD (men-48.3 million, women-61.7 million) whereas the burden was 387.5 million in lower-middle income countries (men-177.4 million, women- 210.1 million) [3].

CKD is associated with a wide range of life threatening diseases [4]. CKD is considered as one of the major risk factors for developing cardiovascular disease [5]. A study conducted in 2003 reported that patients having Glomerular filtration rate (GFR) between 15 and 59 ml/min/ 1.73 m^2 are at 38% higher risk of development of cardiovascular disease than patients having GFR 90 and 150 ml/ min/1.73m^2 [6]. Along with the impact on individual health, CKD also affects the social life and responsible for loss of productivity [7]. The most common form of social impact due to CKD is financial burden [7]. CKD patients are at higher risk to develop end-stage renal disease (ESRD) which requires costly management like dialysis and kidney transplantation [8]. A study conducted in USA revealed that the treatment cost for CKD and ESRD imposes a huge financial burden to the health care system and the average annual cost for end-stage renal disease without transplantation was near 75 billion US dollar in 2001 [8]. CKD needs to be given priority because it is the

* Correspondence: mehedihasan6376@gmail.com
†Mehedi Hasan, Ipsita Sutradhar and Rajat Das Gupta contributed equally to this work.
1Centre for Non-Communicable Diseases and Nutrition, BRAC James P Grant School of Public Health, BRAC University, 5th Floor (Level-6), icddrb Building, 68 Shahid Tajuddin Ahmed Sarani, Mohakhali, Dhaka 1212, Bangladesh
Full list of author information is available at the end of the article

consequence of uncontrolled diabetes and hypertension that are considered as world wide epidemic now a days.

Despite the acute and chronic harmful consequences, CKD is hardly studied specially in lower and middle income countries of Asia and Africa. Few segregated studies have been conducted in India, Bangladesh, Pakistan, Nepal, and Sri Lanka, however, no systematic review is available in South Asian region portraying the current burden of CKD. Hence, it is difficult for policy makers and public health leaders to get a complete scenario about CKD burden in these countries and formulate relevant policies to overcome CKD related mortality and morbidity. Therefore, we have conducted this systematic review to identify the prevalence of CKD in South Asian countries.

Methods

Search strategy

We conducted a systematic review of relevant existing literatures from South Asian countries using PRISMA guideline [9]. Two researchers separately searched the potential literatures in PubMed, Google Scholar, and POPLINE. In addition, they searched national online journal for India, Pakistan, Bangladesh, Nepal, and Sri Lanka. However, no national online journal was available for Bhutan, Maldives and Afghanistan. During search, medical sub-heading as well as plain text were used for the following keywords: 'epidemiology', 'prevalence', 'chronic renal insufficiency', 'chronic kidney disease', 'India', 'Bangladesh', 'Sri Lanka', 'Nepal', 'Bhutan', 'Maldives', 'Pakistan' and 'Afghanistan'. Using those key terms together with Boolean operators, global search term was developed for potential literature search. We also manually searched the bibliography of all selected studies (snow bowling) to identify more articles.

Inclusion and exclusion criteria

Inclusion criteria for this study were a) study reported data from South Asian countries; b) study published between December 1955 (earliest publication) and 30, April 2017; c) study reported prevalence of CKD; d) study published in English language; and e) study carried out in general population. Exclusion criteria for this study were a) study did not report data from South Asian countries; b) study published in other languages than English; c) conference proceedings, book chapters, editorials, and study published only in abstract form; d) study carried out in high risk group of people (known case of diabetes, hypertension, kidney disease); e) study with a sample size of less than 200 participants; and f) study did not determine CKD based on GFR estimation by serum creatinine-based equations. At first, two researchers (IS and RDG) searched and screened all the articles individually. The third

researcher (MH) critically reviewed the overall search and screening process to ensure the consistency. Finally, the full text of selected publications was assessed for eligibility by all three researchers (MH, RDG, and IS). Any discrepancies were resolved by group (MH, IS, RDG and MS) consensus throughout the whole process.

Quality appraisal

Three researchers (MH, IS and RDG) independently determined risk of bias of included studies. For this purpose, we adopted a quality assessment checklist where eight study characteristics were used to assess the quality of included studies such as selection of representative study participants, sample size, sampling technique, response rate, exclusion rate and method used for determination of CKD. This checklist was prepared based on the criteria used in a systematic review on CKD conducted in Sub-Saharan Africa [10]. If the study participants were representative of the general population, we scored it as "2", however, if the study participants were representative of the population in question, we scored it as "1" otherwise we scored it as "0". If the study participants were not included or excluded on the basis of specific risk factors, sample size was adequate (at least 384 considering 50% prevalence rate), sampling technique was random, response rate was > 40%, exclusion rate was < 10%, methods used to diagnose CKD was mentioned, consistent method for determination of CKD was used, we scored articles as "1", however, if the study participants were included or excluded on the basis of specific risk factors, sample size was not adequate, sampling technique was non-random, response rate was ≤ 40%, exclusion rate was ≥ 10%, methods used to diagnose CKD was not mentioned and consistent method for determination of CKD was not used, we scored articles as "0". Later, the number for each study was added to get the final score. The maximum score was 9. If any study gets 7–9, we considered it as "high quality" study. Score 4, 5 and 6 were considered as "moderate quality" study, and score 0, 1, 2 and 3 were considered as "poor quality" study. All the discrepancies that arouse while quality assessment were solved by consensus.

Definition of CKD

Chronic Kidney Disease (CKD) is defined as the structural/functional abnormalities of kidney or decreased GFR < 60 ml/min/1.73 m^2 for 3 months [11]. We used the definition of CKD from the K/DOQI practice guideline that was published in 2002 by the National Kidney Foundation (NKF). CKD was defined as creatinine clearance (CrCl) or GFR less than 60 ml/min/1.73 m^2 [11, 12]. In the included studies for this review, three equations were used to estimate eGFR: Four-variable MDRD equation [13, 14], CKD-EPI equation [15] and Cockcroft-Gault equation [16].

Data extraction

Two authors (MH and RDG) separately extracted data from the selected articles and for this purpose a data extraction table was developed in excel file. This table included (a) title, (b) journal name, (c) name of authors, (d) publication year, (e) year of data collection, (f) study objective, (g) study setting (urban/rural), (h) study design, (i) sampling strategy (random/non-random), (j) sample size, (k) study population, (l) outcome assessment (objective/subjective), (m) diagnostic criteria for CKD, (n) prevalence (overall), (o) prevalence (gender, age, location specific), and (p) authors' conclusion. After data extraction, a third author (IS) crosschecked both of the tables to ensure consistency. Any dispute that arose during data extraction was resolved by group consensus. Subsequently, data was analyzed using tabulation, grouping and thematic approach.

Result

Search result

The initial search brought up 3906 articles. After removal of duplication, 3031 articles were eligible to be screened by title and abstract. Following title and abstract screening, 79 studies remained for full text assessment. Then 63 studies were excluded after full text review. Finally 16 articles met the eligibility criteria and were reviewed and synthesized (Fig. 1) [17–32]. Articles on CKD were found from India (n = 8), Pakistan (n = 4), Bangladesh (n = 3), and Nepal (n = 1). No study was found from Sri Lanka, Bhutan, Afghanistan and Maldives. Most of the studies were published after 2010 except one Indian and one Pakistani study published in 2009 and 2005 respectively [20, 30]. Numbers of participants ranged from 301 in a study from Pakistan [29] to 12, 271 in an Indian study [17].

Quality of studies and risk of bias

Among the 16 studies included in our systematic review, nine were of high quality [17, 18, 20, 21, 25, 26, 28, 30, 31] and seven were of moderate quality [19, 22–24, 27, 29, 32] based on the preselected criteria described in 'Quality appraisal' section. Detail of the study quality is illustrated in Additional file 1. Closer inspection of the table shows, the study participants were representative of the general population in seven studies [17, 20, 25, 28, 30–32] and representative of the population in question for nine studies [18, 19, 21–24, 26, 27, 29]. No study included or excluded participants on the basis of specific risk factors.

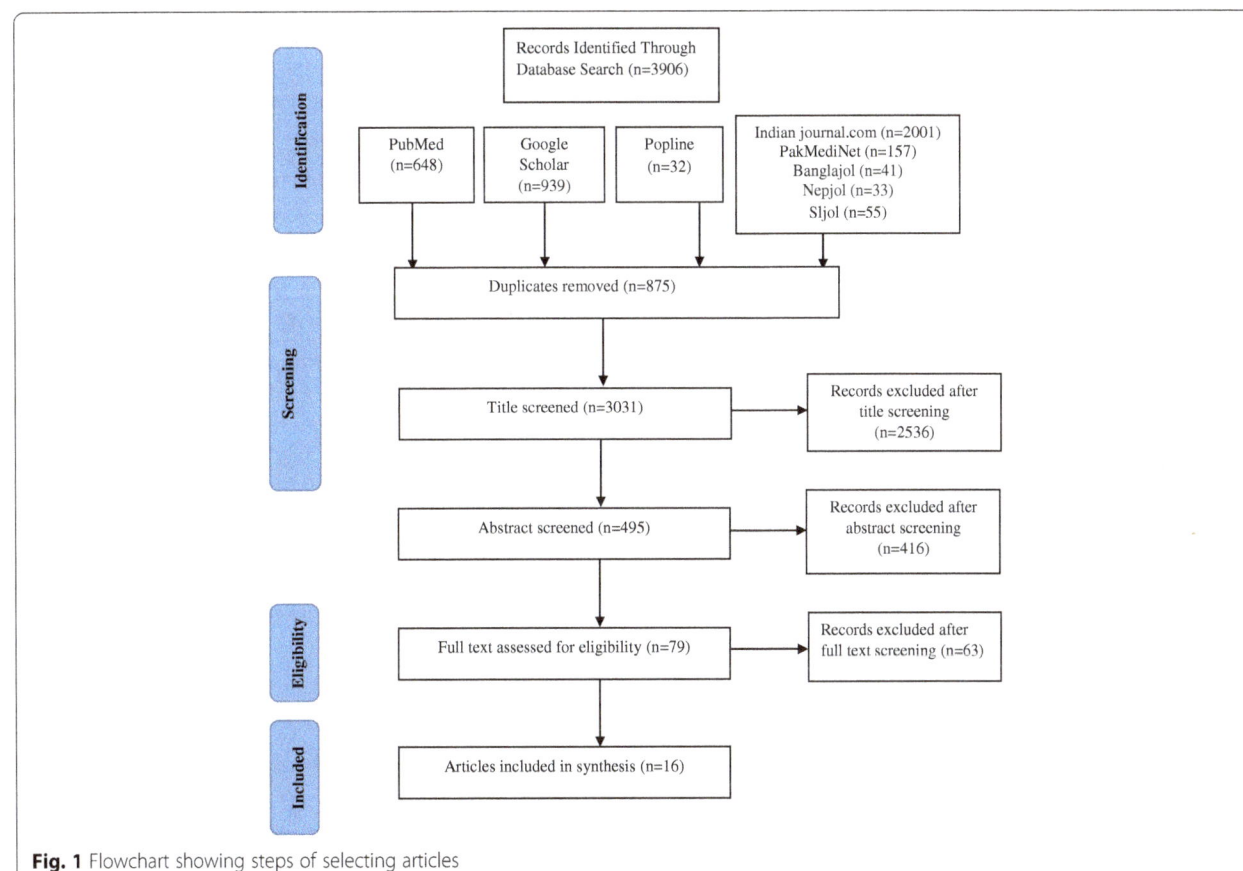

Fig. 1 Flowchart showing steps of selecting articles

Sample size was adequate in 13 studies [17–24, 26, 27, 30–32] and sampling technique was random in eight studies [17, 18, 20, 25, 27, 28, 30, 31]. Twelve studies reported response rate as > 40% [17, 18, 20, 21, 23–26, 28–31] and five studies reported exclusion rate as < 10% [20, 21, 26, 29, 31]. All the 16 studies used a consistent method for determination of CKD and reported the method used [17–32]. Study data were neither sufficient nor homogeneous to allow for meta-analyses.

Description of studies: design, setting and population
India
We found eight studies from India, all of which adopted cross-sectional study design [17–24]. Majority of the studies were done exclusively in urban settings [17, 19, 21, 23, 24], however, only one study was conducted involving participants from both urban, semi urban and rural areas [20]. Three of these studies recruited participants using random sampling technique [17, 18, 20]. Number of respondents in these studies ranged from 1104 to 12,271 and majority of them were adult male (Table 1) [19–23]. The studies measured spot quantitative urine protein and/ or eGFR as biomarker for determination of CKD. Three studies used MDRD equation [19, 21, 22]; one study used CKD-EPI equation [17] and two studies used both [23, 24] to calculate eGFR. Rest of the studies used both CG-BSA and MDRD formula [18, 20].

Bangladesh
Three studies were identified from Bangladesh [25–27], of which all were conducted in Dhaka city (capital of Bangladesh). Two studies performed community based survey [25, 27] of which one targeted slum dwellers [27]. These two studies selected participants using random sampling technique [25, 27]. However, Fatema et al. carried out their study among participants attending a health screening camp and their sampling technique was non-random [26]. The number of participants in Bangladeshi studies ranged from 402 to 1000. Male were predominant in two studies (51.0%, 88.3%) [25, 26]. One study recruited participants from people who were older than 30 years [25]. However, in rest of the two studies, lower age limit was 15 years and 18 years (Table 2) [26, 27].

In these studies, eGFR was measured using MDRD [26, 27], CG [26] and CKD-EPI equation [25].

Pakistan
We found four studies from Pakistan and all of those studies were conducted in urban areas of Karachi [28–31]. Three out of four studies performed community based survey and selected participants using random sampling technique [28, 30, 31]. However, Imran et al., conducted study among volunteers who willingly participated in a health camp and sampling technique of this study was non-random [29]. Amidst three Pakistani studies, lowest

Table 1 Characteristics of the Indian studies

Author [ref.], year	Setting	Study population, study design, sampling strategy	Number of participants, response, age limit and mean age (±S.D.), gender
Anand et al. [17], 2015	Urban	Participants from Delhi and Chennai who took part in Center for Cardio metabolic Risk Reduction in South Asia surveillance, cross sectional, random	12,271, 80%, > 20 years, mean age ± S.D.: 41.4 ± 12.7 years (Chennai), 44.4 ± 13.9 years (Delhi), 43.5% male
Anupama et al. [18], 2014	Rural	Participants from rural Karnataka who took part in a screening survey, cross sectional study, random	2728, 76.6%, ≥18 years, mean age ± S.D.: 39.88 ± 15.87 years, 45.6% male
Mahapatra et al. [19], 2016	Urban	Indian central government Employees in Delhi, cross sectional study, non-random	1104, Not mentioned, > 18 years, Not Mentioned, 61.4% male
Singh et al. [20], 2009	Urban, Semi Urban, Rural	Participants from Delhi and adjoining region, cross sectional, random	5563, 94.4%, ≥ 20 years, Not Mentioned, 60% male
Singh et al. [21], 2013	Urban	Participants attending thirteen academic and private medical centers in India participated in the study under the name of Screening and Early Evaluation of Kidney disease – SEEK, cross sectional study, non-random	6120, 92.3%, ≥18 years, mean age ± S.D.: 45.22 ± 15.2 years, 55.1% male
Trivedi et al. [22], 2016	Semi Urban	Participants attending a health screening camp in six towns of India, cross sectional study, non-random	2350, Not Mentioned, mean age ± S.D.: 48.16 ± 14 years, 61.2% male
Varma et al. [23], 2010	Urban	Indian central government employees in Agra town, cross sectional study, Not Mentioned	3398, 83.9% ≥18 years, mean age ± S.D.: 35.64 ± 8.72 years, 66% male
Varma et al. [24], 2011	Urban	Indian Army personnel in Agra town who were part of 'Comprehensive Health Survey for Detection of Life Style Diseases at the local Military Hospital., cross sectional study, Not Mentioned	1920, 81.9%, > 20 years, mean age ± S.D.: 34.72 ± 7.57 years, gender distribution Not Mentioned

Table 2 Characteristics of the studies from Bangladesh, Pakistan and Nepal

Author [ref.], year	Setting	Study population, study design, sampling strategy	Number of participants, response, age limit and mean age (±S.D.), gender
Bangladesh:			
Anand et al. [25], 2014	Urban	Participants from urban Dhaka, cross sectional study, random	402, 88.8%, > 30 years, mean age ± S.D.: 49.5 ± 12. 7 years, 51% male
Fatema et al. [26], 2013	Urban	Participants attending a health screening camp in urban Dhaka, cross sectional study, non-random	650, 97.5%, 18–70 years, mean age ± S.D.: 37 ± 11 years, 88.3% male
Huda et al. [27], 2012	Urban	Participants from urban slum of Dhaka, cross sectional study, random	1000, not mentioned, 15–65 years, mean age ± S.D.: 34.39 ± 12.70 years, 33% male
Nepal:			
Sharma et al. [32], 2013	Urban	Participants from community-based screening for Chronic Kidney Disease, Hypertension and Diabetes in urban Dharan, cross sectional study, non-random	1000, not mentioned, ≥20 years, not mentioned, 48% male
Pakistan:			
Alam et al. [28], 2014	Urban	Participants from urban Karachi, cross sectional study, random	461, 76%, ≥15 years, not mentioned, 36% male
Imran et al. [29], 2015	Urban	Volunteers who willingly gave their sample in a health camp in urban Karachi, cross sectional study, non-random	301, 97.3%, 30–80 years, not mentioned, 62% male
Jafar et al. [30], 2005	Urban	Participants from urban Karachi, cross sectional study, random	332, 88.9%, > 40 years, mean age ± S.D.: 51.4 ± 9.9 years, 54.2% male
Jessani et al. [31], 2014	Urban	Participants from urban Karachi, cross sectional study, random	3143, 91.4%, ≥ 40 years, not mentioned, 47.8% male

and highest sample size was 301 [29] and 3143 respectively [31]. Minimum age requirement was 15 years [28] to 40 years [31] in these studies. eGFR was measured using MDRD [28, 30], CKD-EPI [29] and CKD-EPI Pakistan equation [31] in Pakistani studies.

Nepal

Only one article was available from Nepal that carried out population based study to identify CKD (according to K/DOQI guideline) prevalence. This study adopted community-based cross sectional survey design and was conducted in urban Dharan [32]. One thousand individuals (male-48%, female-52%) who were at least 20 years old participated in this survey (Table 2) [32]. This study measured eGFR using MDRD equation for diagnosis of CKD [32].

Prevalence of CKD
India

The overall pooled prevalence of CKD among Indian adults was 10.2%. As per high quality studies, highest prevalence was 17.2% found among participants of SEEK (Screening and Early Evaluation of Kidney Disease) study [21] and lowest prevalence was 4.2% found among ≥ 20 years old adult residing in Delhi [20]. Singh et al. (MDRD-17.2%, CKD EPI-16.4%) and Varma et al. (MDRD-15%, CKD EPI-13.1%) found that CKD prevalence was slightly higher while using MDRD equation compared to that found using CKD-EPI equation [21, 23].

Studies that used both MDRD and CG-BSA equations found that the prevalence of CKD was markedly higher using CG-BSA equation than that found using MDRD equation (Anupama et al.: MDRD-6.3%, CG/BSA-16.69%; MDRD-4.2%, CG/BSA-13.3%) (Table 3) [18, 20].

Age-specific prevalence: Three studies from India reported age-specific prevalence of CKD. Two studies reported the age specific prevalence using MDRD equation and the rest one used CKD-EPI equations. All of these studies found that prevalence of CKD rose with increasing age (Table 3) [17, 18, 22].

Gender specific prevalence: Six Indian studies reported gender specific CKD prevalence. Three out of these six studies reported higher prevalence of CKD among men ranged between 8.1% and 21.0% [18, 21, 22]. However, rest three studies reported that the CKD prevalence was higher among female participants ranged between 16.3% and 19.1% than their male counterparts [17, 18, 20, 23] (Table 3).

Bangladesh

The overall pooled prevalence of CKD among Bangladeshi adults was 17.3%. As per high quality studies, in Bangladesh, highest prevalence of CKD was reported as 26.0% [25] whereas Fatema et al. reported the lowest prevalence (12.8%) [26] (Table 4). This discrepancy might be attributable to the age difference of study participants in these two studies. Mean age of study participants were 49.5 years and 37 years in Anand et al. [25] and

Table 3 Prevalence of CKD in India

Author [ref.], year	Assessment of Kidney Function	Prevalence of CKD			
Anand et al. [17], 2015	Spot quantitative urine protein and eGFR (CKD-EPI)	Overall: 7.5% (crude), 8.7% after age standardization	Age and Gender specific prevalence:		
			Chennai:		
			Male: 6.6% Female: 6.5% (crude)		
			Male: 7.5% Female: 7.7% (age standardized)		
			Age in years	Male	Female
			20–44	3.5%	4.6%
			45–64	10.7%	10.5%
			≥65	21.6%	16.7%
			Delhi:		
			Male: 8.1% Female: 9.4% (crude)		
			Male: 9.0% Female: 10.8% (age standardized)		
			Age in years	Male	Female
			20–44	5.1%	6.6%
			45–64	9.5%	12.0%
			≥65	29.4%	28.9%
Anupama et al. [18], 2014	Spot quantitative urine protein, creatinine clearance and eGFR (CG/BSA & MDRD)	Overall: 6.3% (MDRD), 16.69% (CG/BSA)	Age specific prevalence:		
			Age in Years		Prevalence
			18–19		0.8%
			20–29		2.4%
			30–39		3.8%
			40–49		6.4%
			50–59		7.5%
			60–69		16.7%
			≥70		21%
			Gender specific prevalence:		
			Male: 8.1% Female: 4.8% (MDRD)		
Mahapatra et al. [19], 2016	Spot quantitative urine protein and eGFR (MDRD)	Overall: 27.7%	Age specific prevalence: Not Mentioned		
			Gender specific prevalence: Not Mentioned		
Singh et al. [20], 2009	Spot quantitative urine protein and eGFR (MDRD, CG/BSA)	Overall: 13.3% (CG/BSA), 4.2% (MDRD)	Age specific prevalence: Not Mentioned		
			Gender specific prevalence: Male: 11.1% Female: 16.6% (CG/BSA)		
			Male: 2.7% Female: 6.3% (MDRD)		
Singh et al. [21], 2013	Spot quantitative urine protein and eGFR (MDRD)	Overall: 17.2% (MDRD), 16.4% (CKD-EPI)	Age specific prevalence: Not Mentioned		
			Gender specific prevalence: Male: 19% Female: 14.9% (MDRD)		
Trivedi et al. [22], 2016	Spot quantitative urine protein and eGFR (MDRD)	Overall: 20.93%	Age specific prevalence:		
			Age in Years	Prevalence	
			18–30	18.53%	
			31–40	13.74%	
			41–50	20.52%	
			51–60	20.93%	
			61–70	26.77%	

Table 3 Prevalence of CKD in India *(Continued)*

Author [ref.], year	Assessment of Kidney Function	Prevalence of CKD			
		> 70	36.36%		
		Gender specific prevalence: Male: 21% Female: 20.8%			
		Age in Years	Prevalence		
				Male	Female
		18–30		18.5%	18.58%
		31–40		11.63%	16%
		41–50		20.06%	21.13%
		51–60		22.83%	17.62%
		61–70		25.33%	30%
		> 70%		31.48	58.33%
Varma et al. [23], 2010	Spot quantitative urine protein and eGFR (CKD-EPI & MDRD)	Overall: 15% (MDRD), 13.1% (CKD-EPI)	Age specific prevalence: Not Mentioned		
			Gender specific prevalence: Male: 12.62% Female: 14.13% (CKD-EPI)		
			Male: 13.04% Female: 19.13% (MDRD)		
Varma et al. [24], 2011	Spot quantitative urine protein and eGFR (CKD-EPI & MDRD)	Overall: 9.54%	Age specific prevalence: Not Mentioned		
			Gender specific prevalence: Not Mentioned		

Fatema et al. [26] respectively. The only study that focused on urban slum dwellers, CKD prevalence was found as 16.0% using CG/BSA method (Table 5) [27].

Age-specific prevalence: Among the three Bangladeshi studies, only Huda et al. reported age specific prevalence of CKD. According to this study, the prevalence of CKD was higher among elderly people aged more than 40 years (16.5%) than their counterparts whose age was between 25 years and 40 years (10.7%) (Table 5) [27].

Gender specific prevalence: Two studies from Bangladesh reported gender segregated prevalence of CKD [25, 27]. Anand et al. reported that the prevalence of CKD was higher among women (28.0%) than men (24.7%) [25], however, Huda et al. identified more male (14.3%) to suffer from CKD than their female counterparts (12.7%) (Table 5) [27].

Pakistan

The overall CKD prevalence among Pakistani adults was 21.2%. According to high quality studies, highest CKD prevalence in Pakistan was reported as 29.9% [30] and the lowest prevalence was 12.5% [31]. Though both of these studies were conducted among similar age group participants, use of different equations for determining CKD might be attributable to this difference.

Age-specific prevalence: Among the Pakistani studies, only Alam et al. reported age specific prevalence of CKD. The study found highest prevalence of CKD among elderly participants having age more than 50 years

(43.6%) and lowest prevalence among comparatively younger participants aged less than 30 years (10.5%) (Table 5) [28].

Gender specific prevalence: All the four Pakistani studies reported gender specific prevalence of CKD [28–31]. Alam et al. and Imran et al. reported higher CKD prevalence among men [28, 29], however, Jessani et al. and Jafar et al. identified women to suffer from CKD more frequently than men [30, 31]. In the high quality study that used country specific equation for determining CKD, slightly higher proportion of female participants were found to have CKD than their male counterparts (male-11.6%, female-13.3%) (Table 4) [31].

Nepal

Only one Nepalese study met eligibility criteria for this systematic review [32]. This moderated quality study was conducted among ≥20 years old adults residing in urban Dharan and reported CKD prevalence as 10.6%. While segregated by age, CKD prevalence has shown rising trend with increasing age (Table 4). However, gender specific prevalence was not mentioned in this study.

Discussions

To the best of our knowledge, our systematic review is the first of this type that portrayed the prevalence of CKD in South Asian countries. This study will, expectantly, bring attention of international, regional as well as

Table 4 Prevalence of CKD in South Asian countries according to the quality of primary studies

Author [ref.], year	Study quality	Prevalence of CKD	Study site	Required age of study participants	Mean age (± S.D.) of study participants
India:					
Anand et al. [17], 2015	High	8.7%	Urban	> 20 years	41.4 ± 12.7 years (Chennai), 44.4 ± 13.9 years (Delhi)
Anupama et al. [18], 2014	High	6.3% (MDRD), 16.69% (CG/BSA)	Rural	≥ 18 years	39.88 ± 15.87 years
Mahapatra et al. [19], 2016	Moderate	27.7%	Urban	> 18 years	Not Mentioned
Singh et al. [20], 2009	High	4.2% (MDRD), 13.3% (CG/BSA)	Urban, Semi Urban, Rural	≥ 20 years	Not Mentioned
Singh et al. [21], 2013	High	17.2% (MDRD), 16.4% (CKD-EPI)	Urban	≥ 18 years	45.22 ± 15.2 years
Trivedi et al. [22], 2016	Moderate	20.93%	Semi Urban	Not Mentioned	48.16 ± 14 years
Varma et al. [23], 2010	Moderate	15% (MDRD), 13.1% (CKD-EPI)	Urban	≥ 18 years	35.64 ± 8.72 years
Varma et al. [24], 2011	Moderate	9.54%	Urban	> 20 years	34.72 ± 7.57 years
Bangladesh:					
Anand et al. [25], 2014	High	26%	Urban	> 30 years	49.5 ± 12. 7 years
Fatema et al. [26], 2013	High	12.8%	Urban	18–70 years	37 ± 11 years
Huda et al. [27], 2012	Moderate	13.1% (MDRD), 16% (CG/BSA)	Urban	15–65 years	34.39 ± 12.70 years
Nepal:					
Sharma et al. [32], 2013	Moderate	10.6%	Urban	≥ 20 years	Not Mentioned
Pakistan:					
Alam et al. [28], 2014	High	16.6%	Urban	≥ 15 years	Not Mentioned
Imran et al. [29], 2015	Moderate	25.6%	Urban	30–80 years	Not Mentioned
Jafar et al. [30], 2005	High	29.9%	Urban	> 40 years	51.4 ± 9.9 years
Jessani et al. [31], 2014	High	12.5%	Urban	≥ 40 years	Not Mentioned

national stakeholders to the magnitude of CKD and importance of reducing burden of this deadly disease in the most densely populated share of the globe.

It was reveled from our study that there is a scarcity of population based data on CKD in South Asian countries. This finding approves the statement of a previous study that reported that data on non-communicable diseases are rarely available outside developed countries [33]. Ample inconsistencies in characteristics of study population, study design, sampling technique and methods used to determine CKD makes it challenging to depict exact figure of CKD prevalence as well as to offer persuasive comparison of prevalence estimates in these countries.

Nevertheless, according to the existing literature, one to four out of every 10 individuals in South Asia are suffering from CKD. Highest and lowest prevalence of CKD was reported from Pakistan (21.2%) and India (10.2%) respectively. The country specific prevalence of India, Bangladesh and Nepal is similar with the global prevalence of CKD (13.4%) [34] and with the prevalence in some developed countries like the USA and Japan (10%

to 13%) [35, 36]. However, the unusually high prevalence reported in Pakistan might be due to higher minimum age requirement set as eligibility criteria of study participants in Pakistani studies (≥ 40 years). The age specific distribution of CKD unveiled from this systematic review also supports this finding. Studies from four different countries (India, Bangladesh, Pakistan and Nepal) revealed that the prevalence of CKD was higher among elderly people than their younger counterparts. Age is a well-established risk factor for development of CKD [37, 38]. Usually, as a part of the normal physiologic process, renal function (GFR) starts to decline even in a healthy individual after 30 to 40 years of age, which might deteriorate after 50–60 years of age due to structural changes in kidneys [39, 40]. This increased prevalence of CKD among elderly individuals also can be explained by the higher prevalence of diabetes and hypertension among this group of people that are considered as important risk factors for developing CKD [17, 28, 29, 32].

Seven studies included in our review found higher prevalence of CKD among men whereas rest of the studies reported that women suffer from CKD more frequently

Table 5 Prevalence of CKD in Bangladesh, Pakistan and Nepal

Author [ref.], year	Assessment of Kidney Function	Prevalence of CKD	
Bangladesh:			
Anand et al. [25], 2014	Spot quantitative urine protein and eGFR (CKD-EPI)	Overall: 26%	Age specific prevalence: Not Mentioned
			Gender specific prevalence: Male: 24.7% Female: 28%
Fatema et al. [26], 2013	Spot quantitative urine protein and eGFR (MDRD)	Overall: 12.8%	Age specific prevalence:
			Not Mentioned
			Gender specific prevalence:
			Not Mentioned
Huda et al. [27], 2012	Spot quantitative urine protein, creatinine clearance and eGFR (CG/BSA & MDRD)	Overall: 13.1% (MDRD), 16% (CG/BSA)	Age specific prevalence (MDRD):
			25–40 Years: 10.7%
			> 40 Years: 16%
			Gender specific prevalence (MDRD): Male: 14.7% Female: 12.3%
Nepal:			
Sharma et al. [32], 2013	Spot quantitative urine protein and eGFR (MDRD)	Overall: 10.6%	Age specific prevalence:
			Age in years · · · · · · Prevalence
			20–39 · · · · · · 3.4%
			40–59 · · · · · · 11.4%
			≥ 60 · · · · · · 30.5%
			Gender specific prevalence: Not Mentioned
Pakistan:			
Alam et al. [28], 2014	Spot quantitative urine protein and eGFR (MDRD)	Overall: 16.6%	Age specific prevalence:
			Age in Years · · · · · · Prevalence
			< 30 · · · · · · 10.5%
			30–50 · · · · · · 12.7%
			> 50 · · · · · · 43.6%
			Gender specific prevalence: Male: 20.6% Female: 14.2%
Imran et al. [29], 2015	eGFR (CKD-EPI)	Overall: 25.6%	Age specific prevalence: Not Mentioned
			Gender specific prevalence: Male: 26.3% Female: 22.4%
Jafar et al. [30], 2005	Creatinine clearance and eGFR (MDRD)	Overall: 29.9%	Age specific prevalence: Not Mentioned
			Gender specific prevalence: Male: 26.7% Female: 32.5%
Jessani et al. [31], 2014	Spot quantitative urine protein and eGFR (CKD-EPI Pakistan equation)	Overall: 12.5%	Age specific prevalence: Not Mentioned
			Gender specific prevalence: Male: 11.6% Female: 13.3%

than men. This finding is in contrast with the pattern of gender distribution of CKD across the globe. In a recently conducted systematic review on global prevalence of CKD, two-third of included studies identified that CKD was more prevalent in women than in men [34]. A population-based study conducted in Norway reported that female gender was associated with slower decline of GFR with increasing age [41]. Women are also considered protected from CKD to some extent because of their distinctive biological phenomenon (glomerular structure, glomerular hemodynamics systolic blood pressure, hormonal status) and life style related factors (dietary protein and salt intake, smoking and alcohol consumption) [42, 43]. However, further research is needed to identify gender specific prevalence of CKD in South Asian countries.

This systematic review indicates that CKD poses a huge burden on the health system of South Asian countries (India, Bangladesh, Pakistan and Nepal). This is not unusual considering the high prevalence of diabetes and hypertension in this region [44–50]. However, awareness on different non-communicable diseases like diabetes, hypertension and CKD is very little among South Asian people and people usually do not seek health care until any sign or symptom of CKD appears [44, 45, 51]. In addition, people commonly prefer self-treatment or rely on informal and unqualified practitioners [52–54]. Like other LMICs, health system of South Asian countries are not prepared to combat the huge burden of NCDs [55]. Number human resources dedicated for prevention and treatment of kideny dieseases is also less and disproportonate in these countries [55]. Along with these, poor referral system prevailing in South Asian countries makes it difficult to detect CKD cases in early stage [56–58]. It is evident that untreated CKD is a risk factor for developing end stage renal disease (ESRD) and cardiovascular diseases (CVDs) that are leading causes of death in LMICs [59–62]. CKD is also found to be associated with poor health-related quality of life and loss of productivity [63]. To combat the CKD related burden, prevention and early detection of the disease through low-cost community based screening programs is important especially in resource constrain settings of South Asian countries. It is also a timely need for pertinent stakeholders of these countries to perform advocacy in order to offer low cost kidney transplantation and dialysis facility for advanced stage CKD patients. Further research is warranted to identify actual burden of CKD among people of different age group, sex, ethnicity and geographical location as well as among underprivileged group of people residing in slums and rural areas.

This systematic review is not free from limitations. The main limitation of this review was equations used for determining CKD by included studies were not validated amid South Asian population except one study carried out by Jessani et al. [31]. Moreover, studies considered for this review adopted cross-sectional design, though, to be declared as having CKD, one person needs to show abnormal kidney structure or function for more than 3 months, which cannot be captured by cross sectional studies [64].

Conclusions

Chronic Kidney Disease is a major public health con-cern in South Asian countries. Studies reported that one to four out of every ten individuals in these countries are suffering from CKD with variation attributable to discrepancy in research methodology and methods used for determining CKD. Prevalence of CKD rose with increasing age, however issues such as gender and other socio-economic factors have not been explored fully, therefore, further research is warranted. Limited number of population-based studies using cross-sectional design also created the need for further research to identify actual burden of CKD and its distribution in these countries. It is also a timely need for relevant stakeholders of this region to develop suitable policy and effective public health intervention for prevention, control and treatment of CKD in South Asia.

Abbreviations

CKD: Chronic Kidney Disease; CKD-EPI: Chronic Kidney Disease Epidemiology Collaboration; CVDs: Cardiovascular diseases; ESRD: End stage renal disease; MDRD: Modification of Diet in Renal Disease (MDRD); PRISMA: Preferred Reporting Items for Systematic Reviews and Meta-Analyses

Authors' contributions

MH, IS and RDG conceptualized the study, designed the methodology and contributed to searching the literatures and synthesizing the findings as well as preparing the draft manuscript. MS participated in synthesizing the findings and critically reviewing the manuscript. All authors read and approved the final manuscript.

Competing interests

The authors declare that they have no competing interests.

Author details

[1]Centre for Non-Communicable Diseases and Nutrition, BRAC James P Grant School of Public Health, BRAC University, 5th Floor (Level-6), icddrb Building, 68 Shahid Tajuddin Ahmed Sarani, Mohakhali, Dhaka 1212, Bangladesh. [2]Centre for Science of Implementation and Scale-Up, Centre for Non-Communicable Diseases and Nutrition, BRAC James P Grant School of Public Health, BRAC University, Dhaka, Bangladesh. [3]Adjunct Research Faculty, Institute of Public Health, Heidelberg University, Heidelberg, Germany.

References

1. Jha V, Garcia-Garcia G, Iseki K, Li Z, Naicker S, Plattner B, et al. Chronic kidney disease: global dimension and perspectives. Lancet. 2013;382(9888): 260–72. https://doi.org/10.1016/S0140-6736(13)60687-X.
2. Abubakar II, Tillmann T, Banerjee A. Global, regional, and national age-sex specific all-cause and cause-specific mortality for 240 causes of death, 1990-2013: a systematic analysis for the global burden of disease study 2013. Lancet. 2015;385(9963):117–71. https://doi.org/10.1016/S0140-6736(14)61682-2.

3. Mills KT, Xu Y, Zhang W, Bundy JD, Chen CS, Kelly TN, Chen J, He J. A systematic analysis of worldwide population-based data on the global burden of chronic kidney disease in 2010. Kidney Int. 2015;88(5):950–7.

4. Snively CS, Gutierrez C. Chronic kidney disease: prevention and treatment of common complications. Am Fam Physician. 2004;70(10):1921–8.

5. Mann JF, Gerstein HC, Pogue J, Bosch J, Yusuf S. Renal insufficiency as a predictor of cardiovascular outcomes and the impact of ramipril: the HOPE randomized trial. Ann Intern Med. 2001;134(8):629–36.

6. Manjunath G, Tighiouart H, Ibrahim H, MacLeod B, Salem DN, Griffith JL, et al. Level of kidney function as a risk factor for atherosclerotic cardiovascular outcomes in the community. J Am Coll Cardiol. 2003;41(1): 47–55.

7. Weiner DE. Public health consequences of chronic kidney disease. Clin Pharmacol Ther. 2009;86(5):566–9. https://doi.org/10.1038/clpt.2009.137.

8. Lysaght MJ. Maintenance dialysis population dynamics: current trends and long-term implications. J Am Soc Nephrol. 2002;13(Suppl 1):S37–40.

9. Liberati A, Altman DG, Tetzlaff J, Mulrow C, Gøtzsche PC, Ioannidis JPA, et al. The PRISMA statement for reporting systematic reviews and meta-analyses of studies that evaluate health care interventions: explanation and elaboration. PLoS Med. 2009;6(7):e1000100. https://doi.org/10.1371/journal. pmed.1000100.

10. Stanifer JW, Jing B, Tolan S, Helmke N, Mukerjee R, Naicker S, et al. The epidemiology of chronic kidney disease in sub-Saharan Africa: a systematic review and meta-analysis. Lancet Glob Health. 2014;2(3):e174–81. https://doi. org/10.1016/S2214-109X(14)70002-6.

11. National Kidney Foundation. K/DOQI clinical practice guidelines for chronic kidney disease: evaluation, classification, and stratification. Am J Kidney Dis. 2002;39(2 Suppl 1):S1.

12. Levey AS, Coresh J, Balk E, Kausz AT, Levin A, Steffes MW, et al. National Kidney Foundation practice guidelines for chronic kidney disease: evaluation, classification, and stratification. Ann Intern Med. 2003;139(2):137–47.

13. Levey AS. A simplified equation to predict glomerular filtration rate from serum creatinine. J Am Soc Nephrol. 2000;11:A0828.

14. Levey AS, Bosch JP, Lewis JB, Greene T, Rogers N, Roth D. A more accurate method to estimate glomerular filtration rate from serum creatinine: a new prediction equation. Modification of diet in renal disease study group. Ann Intern Med. 1999;130(6):461–70.

15. Levey AS, Stevens LA, Schmid CH, Zhang YL, Castro AF 3rd, Feldman HI, et al. A new equation to estimate glomerular filtration rate. Ann Intern Med. 2009;150(9):604–12.

16. Cockcroft DW, Gault MH. Prediction of creatinine clearance from serum creatinine. Nephron. 1976;16(1):31–41.

17. Anand S, Shivashankar R, Ali MK, Kondal D, Binukumar B, Montez-Rath ME, et al. Prevalence of chronic kidney disease in two major Indian cities and projections for associated cardiovascular disease. Kidney Int. 2015;88(1):178–85. https://doi.org/10.1038/ki.2015.58.

18. Anupama YJ, Uma G. Prevalence of chronic kidney disease among adults in a rural community in South India: results from the kidney disease screening (KIDS) project. Indian J Nephrol. 2014;24(4):214. https://doi.org/10.4103/ 0971-4065.132990.

19. Mahapatra HS, Gupta YP, Sharma N, Buxi G. Identification of high-risk population and prevalence of kidney damage among asymptomatic central government employees in Delhi, India. Saudi J Kidney Dis Transpl. 2016; 27(2):362–70. https://doi.org/10.4103/1319-2442.178564.

20. Singh NP, Ingle GK, Saini VK, Jami A, Beniwal P, Lal M, et al. Prevalence of low glomerular filtration rate, proteinuria and associated risk factors in North India using Cockcroft-gault and modification of diet in renal disease equation: an observational, cross-sectional study. BMC Nephrol. 2009;10:4. https://doi.org/10.1186/1471-2369-10-4.

21. Singh AK, Farag YM, Mittal BV, Subramanian KK, Reddy SR, Acharya VN, et al. Epidemiology and risk factors of chronic kidney disease in India - results from the SEEK (screening and early evaluation of kidney disease) study. BMC Nephrol. 2013;14:114. https://doi.org/10.1186/1471-2369-14-114.

22. Trivedi H, Vanikar A, Patel H, Kanodia K, Kute V, Nigam L, et al. High prevalence of chronic kidney disease in a semi-urban population of Western India. Clin Kidney J. 2016;9(3):438–43. https://doi.org/10.1093/ckj/sfw009.

23. Varma PP, Raman DK, Ramakrishnan TS, Singh P, Varma A. Prevalence of early stages of chronic kidney disease in apparently healthy central government employees in India. Nephrol Dial Transplant. 2010;25(9):3011–7. https://doi.org/10.1093/ndt/gfq131.

24. Varma PP, Raman DK, Ramakrishnan TS, Singh P. Prevalence of early stages of chronic kidney disease in healthy Army personnel. Med J Armed Forces India. 2011;67(1):9–14. https://doi.org/10.1016/S0377-1237(11)80004-3.

25. Anand S, Khanam MA, Saquib J, Saquib N, Ahmed T, Alam DS, et al. High prevalence of chronic kidney disease in a community survey of urban Bangladeshis: a cross-sectional study. Glob Health. 2014;10(1):9. https://doi. org/10.1186/1744-8603-10-9.

26. Fatema K, Abedin Z, Mansur A, Rahman F, Khatun T, Sumi N, et al. Screening for chronic kidney diseases among an adult population. Saudi J Kidney Dis Transpl. 2013;24(3):534.

27. Huda MN, Alam KS, Harun Ur R. Prevalence of chronic kidney disease and its association with risk factors in disadvantageous population. Int J Nephrol. 2012;2012:267329. https://doi.org/10.1155/2012/267329.

28. Alam A, Amanullah F, Baig-Ansari N, Lotia-Farrukh I, Khan FS. Prevalence and risk factors of kidney disease in urban Karachi: baseline findings from a community cohort study. BMC Res Notes. 2014;7(1):179. https://doi.org/10. 1186/1756-0500-7-179.

29. Imran S, Sheikh A, Saeed Z, Khan SA, Malik AO, Patel J, et al. Burden of chronic kidney disease in an urban city of Pakistan, a cross-sectional study. J Pak Med Assoc. 2015;65(4):366.

30. Jafar TH, Schmid CH, Levey AS. Serum creatinine as marker of kidney function in south Asians: a study of reduced GFR in adults in Pakistan. J Am Soc Nephrol. 2005;16(5):1413–9.

31. Jessani S, Bux R, Jafar TH. Prevalence, determinants, and management of chronic kidney disease in Karachi, Pakistan - a community based cross-sectional study. BMC Nephrol. 2014;15:90. https://doi.org/10.1186/1471-2369-15-90.

32. Sharma SK, Dhakal S, Thapa L, Ghimire A, Tamrakar R, Chaudhary S, et al. Community-based screening for chronic kidney disease, hypertension and diabetes in Dharan. JNMA J Nepal Med Assoc. 2013;52(189):205–12.

33. Halbert RJ, Natoli JL, Gano A, Badamgarav E, Buist AS, Mannino DM. Global burden of COPD: systematic review and meta-analysis. Eur Respir J. 2006; 28(3):523–32.

34. Hill NR, Fatoba ST, Oke JL, Hirst JA, O'Callaghan CA, Lasserson DS, et al. Global prevalence of chronic kidney disease–a systematic review and meta-analysis. PLoS One. 2016;11(7):e0158765. https://doi.org/10.1371/journal. pone.0158765.

35. Coresh J, Selvin E, Stevens LA, Manzi J, Kusek JW, Eggers P, et al. Prevalence of chronic kidney disease in the United States. JAMA. 2007;298(17):2038–47. https://doi.org/10.1001/jama.298.17.2038.

36. Imai E, Horio M, Watanabe T, Iseki K, Yamagata K, Hara S, et al. Prevalence of chronic kidney disease in the Japanese general population. Clin Exp Nephrol. 2009;13(6):621–30. https://doi.org/10.1007/s10157-009-0199-x.

37. Anand S, Kondal D, Montez-Rath M, Zheng Y, Shivashankar R, Singh K, et al. Prevalence of chronic kidney disease and risk factors for its progression: a cross-sectional comparison of Indians living in Indian versus US cities. PLoS One. 2017;12(3):e0173554. https://doi.org/10.1371/journal.pone.0173554.

38. Fischbacher CM, Bhopal R, Rutter MK, Unwin NC, Marshall SM, White M, et al. Microalbuminuria is more frequent in south Asian than in European origin populations: a comparative study in Newcastle, UK. Diabet Med. 2003; 20(1):31–6.

39. Glassock RJ, Winearls C. Ageing and the glomerular filtration rate: truths and consequences. Trans Am Clin Climatol Assoc. 2009;120:419–28.

40. Coresh J, Astor BC, Greene T, Eknoyan G, Levey AS. Prevalence of chronic kidney disease and decreased kidney function in the adult US population: third National Health and nutrition examination survey. Am J Kidney Dis. 2003;41(1):1–12. https://doi.org/10.1053/ajkd.2003.50007.

41. Eriksen BO, Ingebretsen OC. The progression of chronic kidney disease: a 10-year population-based study of the effects of gender and age. Kidney Int. 2006;69(2):375–82. https://doi.org/10.1038/sj.ki.5000058.

42. Iseki K. Gender differences in chronic kidney disease. Kidney Int. 2008;74(4): 415–7. https://doi.org/10.1038/ki.2008.261.

43. Halbesma N, Brantsma AH, Bakker SJ, Jansen DF, Stolk RP, De Zeeuw D, et al. Gender differences in predictors of the decline of renal function in the general population. Kidney Int. 2008;74(4):505–12. https://doi.org/10.1038/ ki.2008.200.

44. Roy A, Praveen PA, Amarchand R, Ramakrishnan L, Gupta R, Kondal D, et al. Changes in hypertension prevalence, awareness, treatment and control rates over 20 years in National Capital Region of India: results from a repeat cross-sectional study. BMJ Open. 2017;7(7):e015639. https://doi.org/10.1136/ bmjopen-2016-015639.

45. Shafi ST, Shafi T. A survey of hypertension prevalence, awareness, treatment, and control in health screening camps of rural Central Punjab, Pakistan. J Epidemiol Glob Health. 2017;7(2):135–40. https://doi.org/10.1016/j.jegh.2017.01.001.

46. Saquib N, Saquib J, Ahmed T, Khanam MA, Cullen MR. Cardiovascular diseases and type 2 diabetes in Bangladesh: a systematic review and meta-analysis of studies between 1995 and 2010. BMC Public Health. 2012;12:434. https://doi.org/10.1186/1471-2458-12-434.

47. Gyawali B, Sharma R, Neupane D, Mishra SR, van Teijlingen E, Kallestrup P. Prevalence of type 2 diabetes in Nepal: a systematic review and meta-analysis from 2000 to 2014. Glob Health Action. 2015;8:29088. https://doi.org/10.3402/gha.v8.29088.

48. Chataut J, Khanal K, Manandhar K. Prevalence and Associated factors of hypertension among adults in rural Nepal: a community based study. Kathmandu Univ Med J (KUMJ). 2015;13(52):346–50.

49. Anjana RM, Deepa M, Pradeepa R, Mahanta J, Narain K, Das HK, et al. Prevalence of diabetes and prediabetes in 15 states of India: results from the ICMR-INDIAB population-based cross-sectional study. Lancet Diabetes Endocrinol. 2017;5(8):585–96. https://doi.org/10.1016/S2213-8587(17)30174-2.

50. Meo SA, Zia I, Bukhari IA, Arain SA. Type 2 diabetes mellitus in Pakistan: current prevalence and future forecast. J Pak Med Assoc. 2016;66(12):1637–42.

51. Ene-Iordache B, Perico N, Bikbov B, Carminati S, Remuzzi A, Perna A, Islam N, Bravo RF, Aleckovic-Halilovic M, Zou H, Zhang L. Chronic kidney disease and cardiovascular risk in six regions of the world (ISN-KDDC): a cross-sectional study. Lancet Glob Health. 2016;4(5):e307–19. https://doi.org/10.1016/S2214-109X(16)00071-1.

52. Ahmed SM, Adams AM, Chowdhury M, Bhuiya A. Changing health-seeking behaviour in Matlab, Bangladesh: do development interventions matter? Health Policy Plan. 2003;18(3):306–15.

53. Patle RA, Khakse GM. Health-seeking behaviour of elderly individuals: a community-based cross-sectional study. Natl Med J India. 2015;28(4):181–4.

54. Anwar M, Green J, Norris P. Health-seeking behaviour in Pakistan: a narrative review of the existing literature. Public Health. 2012;126(6):507–17. https://doi.org/10.1016/j.puhe.2012.02.006.

55. Sharif MU, Elsayed ME, Stack AG. The global nephrology workforce: emerging threats and potential solutions! Clin Kidney J. 2016;9(1):11–22. https://doi.org/10.1093/ckj/sfv111.

56. Bhola N, Kumari R, Nidha T. Utilization of the health care delivery system in a district of North India. East Afr J Public Health. 2008;5(3):147–53.

57. Sakhuja V, Sud K. End-stage renal disease in India and Pakistan: burden of disease and management issues. Kidney Int. 2003;63:S115–S8. https://doi.org/10.1046/j.1523-1755.63.s83.24.x.

58. Hada R, Khakurel S, Agrawal RK, Kafle RK, Bajracharya SB, Raut KB. Incidence of end stage renal disease on renal replacement therapy in Nepal. Kathmandu Univ Med J (KUMJ). 2009;7(3):301–5.

59. Levey AS, Coresh J. Chronic kidney disease. Lancet. 2012;379(9811):165–80. https://doi.org/10.1016/S0140-6736(11)60178-5.

60. Sarnak MJ, Levey AS, Schoolwerth AC, Coresh J, Culleton B, Hamm LL, et al. Kidney disease as a risk factor for development of cardiovascular disease: a statement from the American Heart Association councils on kidney in cardiovascular disease, high blood pressure research, clinical cardiology, and epidemiology and prevention. Circulation. 2003;108(17):2154–69. https://doi.org/10.1161/01.cir.0000095676.90936.80.

61. Weiner DE, Tighiouart H, Amin MG, Stark PC, MacLeod B, Griffith JL, et al. Chronic kidney disease as a risk factor for cardiovascular disease and all-cause mortality: a pooled analysis of community-based studies. J Am Soc Nephrol. 2004;15(5):1307–15.

62. Tonelli M, Wiebe N, Culleton B, House A, Rabbat C, Fok M, et al. Chronic kidney disease and mortality risk: a systematic review. J Am Soc Nephrol. 2006;17(7):2034–47. https://doi.org/10.1681/asn.2005101085.

63. Soni RK, Weisbord SD, Unruh ML. Health-related quality of life outcomes in chronic kidney disease. Curr Opin Nephrol Hypertens. 2010;19(2):153. https://doi.org/10.1097/MNH.0b013e328335f939.

64. Levin A, Stevens P, Bilous RW, Coresh J, De Francisco AL, De Jong PE, Griffith KE, Hemmelgarn BR, Iseki K, Lamb EJ, Levey AS. KDIGO clinical practice guideline for the evaluation and management of chronic kidney disease. Chapter 1: definition and classification of CKD. Kidney Inter Suppl. 2013;3:19–62. https://doi.org/10.1038/kisup.2012.64.

6

The effect of sodium nitrite infusion on renal function, brachial and central blood pressure during enzyme inhibition by allopurinol, enalapril or acetazolamide in healthy subjects: a randomized, double-blinded, placebo-controlled, crossover study

Jeppe B. Rosenbaek*[ID], Erling B. Pedersen[ID] and Jesper N. Bech[ID]

Abstract

Background: Sodium nitrite ($NaNO_2$) causes vasodilation, presumably by enzymatic conversion to nitric oxide (NO). Several enzymes with nitrite reducing capabilities have been discovered in vitro, but their relative importance in vivo has not been investigated. We aimed to examine the effects of $NaNO_2$ on blood pressure, fractional sodium excretion (FE_{Na}), free water clearance (C_{H2O}) and GFR, after pre-inhibition of xanthine oxidase, carbonic anhydrase, and angiotensin-converting enzyme. The latter as an approach to upregulate endothelial NO synthase activity.

Methods: In a double-blinded, placebo-controlled, crossover study, 16 healthy subjects were treated, in a randomized order, with placebo, allopurinol 150 mg twice daily (TD), enalapril 5 mg TD, or acetazolamide 250 mg TD. After 4 days of treatment and standardized diet, the subjects were examined at our lab. During intravenous infusion of 240 μg $NaNO_2$/kg/hour for 2 h, we measured changes in brachial and central blood pressure (BP), plasma cyclic guanosine monophosphate (P-cGMP), plasma and urine osmolality, GFR by ^{51}Cr-EDTA clearance, FE_{Na} and urinary excretion rate of cGMP (U-cGMP) and nitrite and nitrate (U-NO_x). Subjects were supine and orally water-loaded throughout the examination day.

Results: Irrespective of pretreatment, we observed an increase in FE_{Na}, heart rate, U-NO_x, and a decrease in C_{H2O} and brachial systolic BP during $NaNO_2$ infusion. P-cGMP and U-cGMP did not change during infusion. We observed a consistent trend towards a reduction in central systolic BP, which was only significant after allopurinol.

Conclusion: This study showed a robust BP lowering, natriuretic and anti-aquaretic effect of intravenous $NaNO_2$ regardless of preceding enzyme inhibition. None of the three enzyme inhibitors used convincingly modified the pharmacological effects of $NaNO_2$. The steady cGMP indicates little or no conversion of nitrite to NO. Thus the effect of $NaNO_2$ may not be mediated by NO generation.

Keywords: Sodium nitrite, Enzyme inhibition, Natriuresis, Aquaresis, Central blood pressure

* Correspondence: jepros@rm.dk
University Clinic in Nephrology and Hypertension, Regional Hospital West
Jutland and Aarhus University, Laegaardvej 12J, DK-7500 Holstebro, Denmark

Background

Sodium nitrite ($NaNO_2$) has a well known vasodilatory effect, which is believed to rely on the enzymatic and non-enzymatic reduction of nitrite to nitric oxide (NO). The generation of NO from endogenous and exogenous nitrite is an alternative and parallel pathway to the classical synthesis of NO from L-arginine by endothelial NO synthase (eNOS). Several enzymes e.g. xanthine oxidase (XO), carbonic anhydrase (CA), and even eNOS, are reported to possess nitrite reducing capabilities, and hence increasing the bioavailability of NO using nitrite as substrate. Reduction of nitrite to NO occurs preferentially during hypoxia and acidosis, but most of the enzymes retain the ability to generate NO at physiological conditions, although at a lower rate and requiring higher concentrations of nitrite [1].

The XO inhibitor allopurinol has repeatedly been shown to attenuate the blood pressure (BP) reduction by $NaNO_2$ in rats [2–4]. The effect of XO inhibition was selective to nitrite, as the vasodepressor effect of sodium nitroprusside, another NO donor, was intact in all three studies. Ghosh et al. found an association between nitrite reductase activity in erythrocytic XO and the efficacy of dietary nitrate to reduce BP in hypertensive patients [4].

Several studies have found favorable changes in NO metabolites during treatment with various inhibitors of angiotensin-converting enzyme (ACE). The mechanism is suggested to be an up-regulation of eNOS, due to an accumulation of bradykinin [5, 6]. It appears to be a class-effect of ACE inhibitors, as Comini et al. found a consistent increase in rat plasma NO_x (combined nitrate and nitrite), eNOS expression and eNOS activity using a range of ACE inhibitors, including enalapril [7]. In clinical trials, long-term treatments with lisinopril [8, 9] and perindopril [10] were found to elevate plasma levels of NO_x in hypertensive patients. Similarly, injection of quinaprilat in healthy subjects [11] and short-term treatment of normotensive type 1 diabetics with enalapril [12], were shown to enhance endothelial function evaluated by flow-mediated vasodilation.

In vitro studies have shown nitrite reducing effects of CA, and suggest a stimulatory effect of acetazolamide on NO generation, despite the inhibition of CO_2 hydration [13, 14]. A recent clinical trial found a positive effect of nitrate intake on the increase in visually stimulated cerebral blood flow when injecting acetazolamide in healthy male subjects [15].

The relative significance of the individual nitrite reductases for the bioactivation of $NaNO_2$ in vivo has yet to be determined. In this randomized, double-blind, 4-way crossover study we aimed to investigate the relative importance of ACE, XO, and CA for the various effects of $NaNO_2$ under physiological conditions. After preceding enzyme modulation with allopurinol, enalapril, or acetazolamide, we measured the effects of $NaNO_2$ infusion on 1) the central and brachial BP, 2) the renin-angiotensin-aldosterone system 3) plasma and urinary NO_x and guanosine $3',5'$-cyclic monophosphate (cGMP), and 4) the renal water and sodium regulation. We hypothesized the following: Pretreatment with allopurinol inhibits the ability of XO to reduce nitrite to bioactive NO and hence attenuates the effects of $NaNO_2$, while enalapril and acetazolamide, on the contrary, stimulate the generation of NO from nitrite through eNOS and CA respectively, augmenting the effects of $NaNO_2$.

Methods

Subjects

Subjects were recruited by advertisement on local educational institutions. Prior to enrollment, all subjects passed an examination including medical history, physical examination, office BP measurement, urine dipstick, electrocardiography, and the following blood samples: P-cholesterol, P-alkaline phosphatase, P-alanine aminotransferase, P-bilirubin, B-glycated hemoglobin (hemoglobin A1c), P-thyroid-stimulating hormone, P-urate, P-total CO_2 in venous blood, P-sodium, P-potassium, P-creatinine, P-albumin, B-platelets, B-leukocytes, B-hemoglobin, and hematocrit.

Inclusion criteria

Both gender, age 18–40 years, BMI 18.5–30.0 kg/m^2.

Exclusion criteria

Alcohol consumption > 14 drinks per week for women and > 21 drinks per week for men, smoking, substance abuse, current use of medicine except contraception, known intolerance to the study drugs, office BP > 140/90, diabetes mellitus, anemia, estimated GFR < 60 ml/min (MDRD), history or signs of clinically relevant kidney, heart, liver, lung, neurological, or endocrine diseases, pregnancy or lactation, and blood donation within 1 month of the first investigation.

Withdrawal criteria

Development of exclusion criteria, serious or unacceptable adverse events, suspicion of poor compliance to study medication, sustained BP < 90/50 or symptoms of low BP during $NaNO_2$ infusion.

Design

The study was conducted as a double-blinded, placebo-controlled, 4-way crossover trial. Subjects received allopurinol, enalapril, acetazolamide, or placebo for 4 days in random order. Each treatment period was followed by an examination day. The examination days were separated by a wash-out period of at least 3 weeks.

Study drugs

Allopurinol (Tablet Allopurinol "DAK", 300 mg) was produced by Takeda Pharma A/S, Taastrup, Denmark. Enalapril (Tablet Enalapril "Actavis", 5 mg) was produced by Actavis Nordic A/S, Gentofte, Denmark. Acetazolamide (Tablet Diamox, 250 mg) was produced by Goldshield Pharmaceuticals Limited, Surrey, United Kingdom. Placebo contained 120 mg of potato starch and 51 mg lactose monohydrate. All tablets were covered in opaque gelatine capsules and were identical in appearance. Sodium nitrite 10 mg/ml (Skanderborg Pharmacy, Denmark) was diluted in isotonic saline immediately before administration according to subject weight.

Randomization

Treatment order was allocated consecutively at the time of inclusion by the principal investigator according to a randomization plan created on randomization.com by the Hospital Pharmacy, Central Denmark Region. Medication was packed, sealed and labeled by the Hospital Pharmacy. Investigators, lab technicians, and subjects were blinded to treatment order for the duration of the trial.

Number of subjects

Using a power of 80% and a significance level of 5% the minimum number of subjects should be 14 when the minimum relevant relative change in fractional sodium excretion (FE_{Na}) is 10%, and the standard deviation is 12%. Due to expected dropouts and incomplete voiding, the minimum number of included subjects was set to 20.

Experimental procedure

Before examination

For 4 days prior to each examination day, subjects ingested a standard diet prepared by the hospital kitchen. One of two diet sizes, 11.000 kJ per day or 15.000 kJ per day, was chosen according to the estimated energy demands for each subject based on weight and physical activity. Regardless of diet size, the nutritional composition was 55% carbohydrates, 30% fat, and 15% protein, sodium content was 135 mmol per day and content of nitrate and nitrite was minimized. Subjects were asked to drink 2.5 L daily, including a maximum of two small cups of coffee or tea. No alcohol or soft drinks were allowed. The subjects were asked to take the study medication twice daily (TD) between 7–8 AM and 6–8 PM, with the last dose on the morning of the examination day. Dosage: Allopurinol: 150 mg TD, enalapril: 5 mg TD, acetazolamide: 250 mg TD.

Examination day

On each examination day, the subjects arrived at the lab at 7.45 AM after an overnight fast, bringing a 24-h urine collection. Two indwelling catheters were placed in antecubital veins, one for sequential blood samples and one in the opposite arm for the administration of chromium-51 labeled ethylenediamine tetra-acetic acid (^{51}Cr-EDTA) and $NaNO_2$. An oral load of 175 ml of tap water every half hour was started at 7.30 AM with the last dose of study medication. The subjects were installed in supine position in a quiet, temperature-controlled (22–25 °C) room throughout the day. Voiding was done sitting or standing. After 90 min of adaptation, blood and urine samples were collected every 30 min from 9.30 AM to 1.30 PM. The first two clearance periods were used as baseline. The baseline periods were followed by four periods from 10.30 AM to 12.30 PM, during which a sustained infusion of 50 ml saline diluted $NaNO_2$, 240 µg/kg/hour (= 3.48 µmol/kg/hour), was administered, and finally two post-infusion periods from 12.30 PM to 1.30 PM. Blood samples were analyzed for ^{51}Cr-EDTA, P-sodium, and P-osmolality (P-Osm). The sample at 1.30 PM was analyzed for combined nitrite and nitrate ($P-NO_x$) and the samples at 10.30 AM, 11.30 AM and 12.30 PM also for plasma concentrations of renin (PRC), arginine vasopressin (P-AVP), angiotensin II (P-ANGII), P-aldosterone, P-cGMP, P-urate and plasma total carbon dioxide in venous blood (P-(vB)-total CO_2). The sample volume was replaced 1:1 with isotonic saline. Urine samples were analyzed for sodium, creatinine, osmolality (U-Osm), ^{51}Cr-EDTA, γ-subunit of the epithelial sodium channel (U-ENaCγ), and aquaporin-2 (U-AQP2). Samples at 10.30 AM, 11.30 AM, 12.30 PM and 1.30 PM were furthermore analyzed for U-cGMP and $U-NO_x$.

Blood pressure measurements

Brachial blood pressure was measured oscillometrically using Omron 705IT (Omron Healthcare Co. Ltd., Kyoto, Japan) every 15 min. Central systolic blood pressure (cSBP) was estimated by tonometric pulse wave analysis HealthSTATS BPro (HealthSTATS International, Singapore). The device was applied and calibrated according to the directions of the manufacturer, using the averaged last three of four consecutive measurements with the Omron 705IT. Sequential measurements were made every 15 min from 9 AM to 1.30 PM.

Renal function

Glomerular filtration rate (GFR) was measured by the constant infusion clearance technique with ^{51}Cr-EDTA as reference substance [16].

Biochemical analyses

Blood samples were drawn from an indwelling catheter, placed in ice water and centrifuged immediately at 2200 G for 10 min at 4 °C. Immediately after voiding, urine was centrifuged at 2200 G for 10 min at 4 °C. Concentrations of sodium, potassium, and creatinine were measured using routine methods at the Department of Clinical Biochemistry, Regional Hospital West Jutland, Denmark. Urine supernatant and plasma were kept frozen in cryotubes at − 80 °C (PRC, P-aldosterone, P-AVP, and combined nitrate and nitrite (P-NO$_x$ and U-NO$_x$)), or at − 20 °C (P-ANGII, P-cGMP, U-cGMP, U-ENaCγ, U-AQP2, P-Osm, and U-Osm) until assayed.

P-AVP and P-ANGII were extracted from plasma with C$_{18}$ Sep-Pak (Waters Corporation, Milford, MA, USA) and determined by radioimmunoassay (RIA) as previously described [16, 17]. The antibodies against AVP were a gift from Professor Jacques Dürr (Miami, FL, USA). Minimal detection level: 0.5 pmol/L. Coefficients of variation: 13% (inter-assay) and 9% (intra-assay). Antibodies against ANGII were obtained from the Department of Clinical Physiology, Glostrup Hospital, Denmark. Minimal detection level: 2 pmol/L. Coefficients of variation: 12% (inter-assay) and 8% (intra-assay).

P-Aldosterone was determined by RIA (Demeditec Diagnostics GmbH, Kiel, Germany). The minimal detection level was 3.99 pmol/L. The coefficients of variations were 17.2% (inter-assay) and 12.6% (intra-assay).

Plasma renin concentration (PRC) was determined by a RIA kit from Cisbio Bioassays, Codolet, France. The minimal detection level: 1 pg/ml. Coefficients of variation in the range 4–263 pg/ml: 3.6–5.0% (interassay) and 0.9–3.6% (intra-assay).

Plasma and urine osmolality was determined by freeze-point depression (A$_2$O Advanced Automated Osmometer, Advanced Instruments, MA, USA).

U-NO$_x$ and P-NO$_x$ were determined by a colorimetric assay (R&D Systems, Minneapolis, MN, USA). Nitrate was reduced to nitrite by nitrate reductase and subsequently converted to a deep purple azo compound by addition of Griess reagent. The concentration was determined by photometric measurement of absorbance at 540 nm. Minimal detection level in urine: 15.6 μmol/L and in plasma: 6.2 μmol/L. The coefficients of variation were 3.9% (inter-assay) and 1.8% (intra-assay).

U-cGMP and P-cGMP were determined by a competitive enzyme immunoassay kit from R&D Systems, Minneapolis, MN, USA. Minimal detection level: 1.14 pmol/L. Coefficients of variation: 6.9% (inter-assay) and 4.9% (intra-assay).

U-AQP2 was determined by RIA as previously described [18, 19]. Rabbit anti-AQP2 antibodies were a gift from Professor Soren Nielsen and Professor Robert Fenton, The Water and Salt Research Center, Aarhus

University, Denmark. Minimal detection level: 32 pg/tube. Coefficients of variation: 11.7% (inter-assay) and 5.9% (intra-assay).

U-ENaCγ was measured by RIA as previously described [20]. ENaCγ was synthesized and purchased by Lofstrand, Gaithersburg, Maryland, USA. The ENaCγ antibodies were a gift from Professor Soren Nielsen and Professor Robert Fenton, The Water and Salt Research Center, Aarhus University. It was raised against a synthetic peptide in rabbits, and affinity purified as previously described [21].

Calculations

FE$_{Na}$ was calculated using the formula (sodium clearance (C$_{Na}$) / ^{51}Cr-EDTA clearance × 100%). C$_{Na}$ was calculated as (U-Na / P-Na x urine output rate (UOR)). Free water clearance (C$_{H2O}$) was calculated as (UOR − osmolar clearance (C$_{osm}$)). C$_{osm}$ was calculated as (U-osmolality / P-osmolality x UOR). Creatinine clearance was calculated for 24-h urine as (urine volume x U-creatinine) / (P-creatinine x urine collection period).

Statistical analysis

Statistical tests were performed in SPSS Statistics ver. 20 (IBM Corp., Armonk, NY, USA). All data was graphically evaluated for normality using Q-Q plots. Where logarithmic transformation could correct skewed data, parametric tests were performed on the transformed data. Statistics were performed using one-way repeated measures (RM) ANOVA for comparing over time within each pretreatment. A two-way RM ANOVA with time and pretreatment as within factors were used to test for interaction between pretreatment and time. Comparisons between placebo and pretreatments at baseline or between baseline and individual time points within groups were performed using paired t-test. When skewed data could not be normalized by log transformation, Friedman test and Wilcoxon signed-rank test were performed instead. Normal distributed data are presented as means with 95% confidence intervals, and non-parametric data as medians with inter-quartile ranges in brackets. Statistical significance was defined as $p < 0.05$. Pairwise comparisons with baseline were Bonferroni corrected.

Results

Demographics

A total of 25 subjects were assessed for eligibility. Four were excluded due to elevated blood pressure (1), microscopic hematuria (1), elevated liver enzymes (1), and withdrawal of consent (1) prior to participation. During the study, five more dropped out, due to dizziness (1), headache (1), inability to void according to schedule (1), trouble placing intravenous catheters (1), and withdrawal of consent due to personal bustle (1) (Fig. 1). The remaining 16 completed the study; characteristics are presented in Table 1. Two was excluded from the urine analyses due to incomplete voiding during examination days.

Effect of pretreatment on baseline characteristics

As shown in Table 2, pretreatment with acetazolamide reduced creatinine clearance, absolute sodium excretion, and P-potassium, and increased fractional excretion of potassium (FE_K) measured in 24-h urine. It decreased plasma total CO_2 in venous blood and marginally increased P-urate. Pretreatment with allopurinol reduced P-urate, and slightly increased 24-h excretion of $ENaC\gamma$, while enalapril marginally increased 24-h excretion of albumin and slightly reduced P-sodium.

Effect of NaNO$_2$ on NO$_x$ and cGMP

We measured a steady increase in P-NO$_x$ and U-NO$_x$ throughout the NaNO$_2$ infusion, regardless of preceding enzyme inhibition. P-cGMP was unchanged during infusion after all pretreatments. U-cGMP did not change during the infusion ($p > 0.05$ vs. baseline) but decreased significantly in the post-infusion period (Table 3).

Effect of NaNO$_2$ on GFR and renal sodium and water excretion

As shown in Table 4, baseline GFR was significantly lower after acetazolamide compared to placebo ($p < 0.001$), while enalapril and allopurinol did not change baseline GFR. Infusion of NaNO$_2$ did not alter GFR besides transient fluctuations after placebo and acetazolamide. The baseline reduction of GFR after acetazolamide was sustained throughout the examination day. None of the pretreatments changed baseline fractional sodium excretion (FE_{Na}) compared to placebo. During NaNO$_2$ infusion, FE_{Na} increased regardless of

Table 1 Clinical and laboratory characteristics of the 16 subjects

Gender (male/female)	5/11
Age (years)	23 [19;27]
BMI (kg/m^2)	23 [20;29]
Systolic blood pressure (mmHg)	121 [111;132]
Diastolic blood pressure (mmHg)	73 [64;87]
P-alanine aminotransferase (U/l)	23 (16;28)
P-bilirubin (µmol/l)	8.0 (6.3;10.0)
P-alkaline phosphatase (U/l)	57 (44;82)
P-cholesterol (mmol/l)	4.2 [3.7;4.8]
B-glycated hemoglobin (mmol/mol)	34 (32;35)
P-thyroid stimulating hormone (mIE/l)	1.17 (0.78;2.05)
P-urate (mmol/l)	26 [22;30]
P-total CO_2 in venous blood (mmol/l)	27 [26;28]
P-sodium (mmol/l)	140 [139;141]
P-potassium (mmol/l)	3.8 [3.7;3.9]
eGFR$_{MDRD}$ (ml/min/1.73m^2)	100 [92;107]
P-albumin (g/l)	42 [40;43]
B-platelets (×10^9/l)	233 [208;259]
B-leukocytes (×10^9/l)	6.3 [5.3;7.3]
B-hemoglobin (mmol/l)	8.6 [8.2;9.0]
Hematocrit	.40 [.42;.44]

Normal distributed data are presented as means with 95% confidence interval in brackets and non-parametric data as medians with 25th and 75th percentiles in parentheses. Estimated glomerular filtration rate (eGFR$_{MDRD}$) is calculated using the Modification of Diet in Renal Disease Study equation

pretreatment. Urinary sodium excretion increased in a similar way as FE_{Na} (data not presented). Excretion rate of $ENaC\gamma$ was significantly higher at baseline and during NaNO$_2$ infusion after acetazolamide, while the median level of excretion rate did not change consistently during infusion after any of the pretreatments.

At baseline, there was no significant difference in C_{H2O}, or urine output (UO, not presented) between the pretreatments. During and after NaNO$_2$ infusion, we observed a decrease in C_{H2O} and UO (not presented), with the maximum effect after 60–90 min. This response was not modified by any of the pretreatments. At baseline, U-AQP2 was significantly higher after allopurinol, while there was no difference in P-AVP regardless of pretreatment. In response to NaNO$_2$, we observed a significant decrease in P-AVP on the placebo day. The reduction was insignificant after allopurinol, enalapril, and acetazolamide. We could not detect significant changes in U-AQP2 in response to NaNO$_2$, neither after placebo nor after preceding enzyme inhibition.

Effect of NaNO$_2$ on blood pressure

As shown in Table 5, brachial systolic BP was decreased, and heart rate increased during NaNO$_2$ infusion

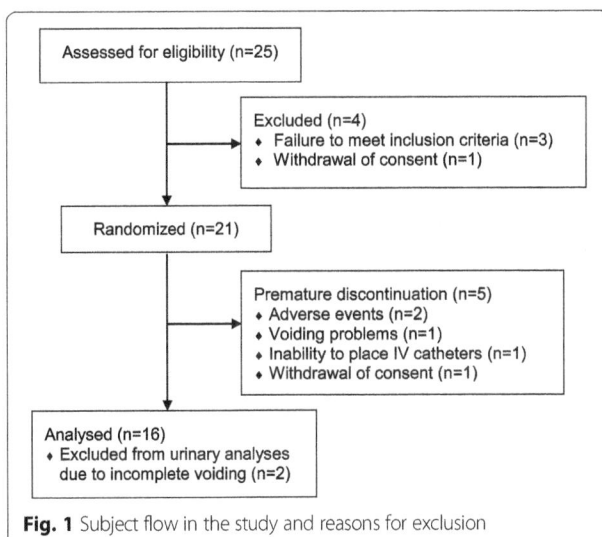

Fig. 1 Subject flow in the study and reasons for exclusion

Table 2 Effect of allopurinol, enalapril and acetazolamide on 24-h urine collection and selected baseline blood samples

	Placebo	Allopurinol	Enalapril	Acetazolamide	$P_{RM\ ANOVA/Friedman}$
CrCl (ml/min/1.73 m^2)	134 [120;148]	137 [124;150]	130 [117;142]	116 [103;130]*	.030
Urine output (ml/min)	1.77 [1.42;2.12]	1.71 [1.38;2.03]	1.58 [1.20;1.96]	1.78 [1.48;2.08]	.411
C_{H2O} (ml/min)	−0.32 [−0.62;-0.01]	−0.43 [− 0.68;-0.17]	−0.36 [− 0.71;0.00]	−0.19 [− 0.49;0.10]	.304
P-sodium (mmol/l)	139 [138;139]	138 [137;139]	137 [137;138]*	138 [137;139]	.025
U-Na (mmol/24 h)	129 [107;151]	135 [115;154]	116 [98;134]	101 [80;122]*	.034
FE$_{Na}$ (%)	0.47 [0.40;0.54]	0.49 [0.39;0.60]	0.45 [0.38;0.52]	0.42 [0.35;0.50]	.412
P-potassium (mmol/l)	4.1 [4.0;4.1]	4.0 [3.9;4.1]	4.1 [4.0;4.2]	3.6 [3.6;3.7]*	<.001
U-K (mmol/24 h)	57.8 [45.9;75.8]	59.2 [41.3;72.1]	51.9 [42.5;83.0]	76.3 [52.7;95.1]	.349
FE$_K$ (%)	7.91 [6.71;9.11]	7.55 [6.17;8.92]	7.67 [6.48;8.85]	11.6 [9.84;13.4]*	<.001
U-albumin (mg/24 h)	2.98 (1.25;4.75)	2.02 (1.00;4.00)	4.50 (1.32;8.25)*	3.00 (2.25;4.75)	.184
U-AQP2 (ng/min)	0.51 [0.41;0.76]	0.64 (0.46;0.83)	0.62 (0.42;0.92)	0.50 (0.38;0.62)	.071
U-ENaCγ (ng/min)	0.23 (0.21;0.31)	0.28 (0.23;0.34)*	0.27 (0.23;0.36)	0.30 (0.24;0.38)	.091
P-urate (mmol/l)	0.29 [0.25;0.33]	0.16 [0.13;0.20]*	0.29 [0.25;0.33]	0.34 [0.30;0.38]*	<.001
P-(vB)-total CO$_2$ (mmol/l)	25.1 [23.9;26.4]	25.0 [24.0;26.0]	24.4 [23.7;25.1]	18.4 [17.4;19.3]*	<.001

Effect of 4 days treatment with allopurinol, enalapril and acetazolamide on 24-h urine collection and selected baseline blood samples in 16 healthy subjects. Creatinine clearance (CrCl), urine output, free water clearance (C_{H2O}), urinary excretion rate of sodium (U-Na) and potassium (U-K) and fractional excretion of sodium (FE$_{Na}$) and potassium (FE$_K$), urinary excretion rate of albumin, aquaporin-2 (U-AQP2), and γ-subunit of the epithelial sodium channel (U-ENaCγ), plasma sodium (P-Na), potassium (P-K), urate, and total carbon dioxide in venous blood (P-(vB)-total CO$_2$). Normal distributed data are presented as means with 95% confidence interval in brackets, and non-parametric data as medians with 25th and 75th percentiles in parentheses. Statistics were performed using one-way repeated measures (RM) ANOVA or Friedman test (U-albumin, U-AQP2, U-ENaCγ). U-K was log transformed before RM ANOVA. Pairwise comparison with placebo was performed using Student's t-test or Wilcoxon signed-rank test (U-albumin, U-AQP2, U-ENaCγ)
Statistically significantly different from placebo: * = p < .05

regardless of pretreatment. The reduction in brachial diastolic BP was only significant after acetazolamide (*p* = 0.035). Brachial mean arterial pressure (MAP) was significantly reduced in response to NaNO$_2$ infusion regardless of pretreatment. There was a trend to a reduction in central systolic BP, which was only significant after allopurinol (*p* = 0.047).

Effect of NaNO$_2$ on the renin-angiotensin-aldosterone system (RAAS)

As depicted in Table 6, PRC was clearly increased at baseline after pretreatment with enalapril, and to a lesser extent after acetazolamide, compared to placebo. In response to NaNO$_2$ infusion, PRC increased further after both enalapril and acetazolamide. Compared to placebo, angiotensin II (AngII) was decreased at baseline after enalapril and allopurinol. In response to NaNO$_2$ infusion, AngII increased marginally only after acetazolamide. Aldosterone was increased at baseline after acetazolamide compared to placebo. The baseline suppression after enalapril was insignificant compared to placebo (*p* = 0.079). NaNO$_2$ infusion did not affect aldosterone levels after any of the pretreatments.

Safety

We observed 26 adverse events, predominantly expected side effects such as paresthesia after acetazolamide (7), gastrointestinal discomfort after enalapril (5), headache (8), and lightheadedness (3) including one event of micturition syncope. None of the adverse events were considered serious.

Discussion

In the present study, our aim was to investigate the impact of preceding short-term modulation of three different enzyme systems on the various acute effects of sodium nitrite infusion. Without active pretreatment, we found that intravenous NaNO$_2$ led to an increased natriuresis, an increase in P-NO$_x$ and U-NO$_x$, a small decrease in AVP, and a systolic BP reduction, along with a decreased aquaresis, an unaffected P-cGMP and even a reduction in U-cGMP in the post-infusion period. Preceding enzyme inhibition did not convincingly modify the effects.

The decrease we observed in brachial BP is in agreement with other studies using comparable doses [22–24]. However, this reduction is smaller than in a recent dose-response study, where our group in addition to a larger decrease in brachial systolic and mean arterial BP found a significant reduction in both the brachial diastolic and the central systolic BP using the same dose of NaNO$_2$ [25]. The reason for this discrepancy might be the different gender ratio in the two studies; the percentage of females was 69% in the present study compared to 42% in the dose-response study. While no gender difference has been reported for NaNO$_2$, Kapil et al. found a substantially greater reduction in both systolic and

Table 3 Effect of intravenous NaNO$_2$ on combined nitrate and nitrite (NOx) and cGMP

| | Baseline | Infusion | | Post-infusion | p_{RM} |
		60 min	120 min	180 min	ANOVA (one-way)
P-NO$_x$ (µmol/l)					
Placebo	17 (13;21)	25 (19;31)*	31 (24;38)*	29 (22;35)*	<.001
Allopurinol	17 (14;23)	24 (19;30)*	32 (26;36)*	30 (26;32)*	<.001
Enalapril	15 (12;19)	24 (21;31)*	29 (26;32)*	27 (24;31)*	<.001
Acetazolamide	17 (13;19)	24 (21;31)*	30 (27;35)*	27 (23;32)*	<.001
$p_{interaction}$ (pretreatment x time)		.742			
U-NO$_x$ (µmol/min)					
Placebo	0.52 (0.37;0.69)	0.72 (0.52;0.79)*	0.94 (0.88;1.09)*	0.95 (0.83;1.21)*	<.001
Allopurinol	0.60 (0.42;0.88)	0.79 (0.65;0.98)*	0.99 (0.87;1.23)*	1.07 (0.90;1.18)*	<.001
Enalapril	0.57 (0.44;0.78)	0.69 (0.59;0.97)*	0.99 (0.87;1.22)*	0.94 (0.80;1.31)*	<.001
Acetazolamide	0.49 (0.45;0.54)	0.63 (0.59;0.67)*	0.98 (0.86;1.05)*	0.94 (0.85;1.06)*	<.001
$p_{interaction}$ (pretreatment x time)		.677			
P-cGMP (pmol/ml)					
Placebo	88 [78;98]	93 [83;104]	87 [78;95]		.310
Allopurinol	91 [83;100]	87 [77;98]	88 [77;98]		.597
Enalapril	82 [71;92]	85 [74;96]	93 [75;110]		.102
Acetazolamide	90 [78;101]	84 [74;93]	84 [74;94]		.088
$p_{interaction}$ (pretreatment x time)		.111			
U-cGMP (pmol/min)					
Placebo	425 (356;530)	426 (371;561)	414 (341;515)	321 (235;343)*	<.001
Allopurinol	487 (388;613)	453 (353;575)	461 (376;570)	367 (287;443)*	<.001
Enalapril	404 (291;527)†	425 (329;552)	409 (309;486)	284 (243;349)*	<.001
Acetazolamide	361 (305;484)†	345 (296;468)	372 (325;470)	269 (236;324)*	<.001
$p_{interaction}$ (pretreatment x time)		.362			

Effect of intravenous NaNO$_2$ on plasma concentrations ($n = 16$) and urinary excretion rates ($n = 14$) of combined nitrate and nitrite (NO$_x$) and guanosine 3',5'-cyclic monophosphate (cGMP) in healthy subjects after 4 days pretreatment with allopurinol, enalapril, acetazolamide, or placebo. Normal distributed data are presented as means with 95% confidence interval in brackets and non-parametric data as medians with 25th and 75th percentiles in parentheses. Statistics were performed using one-way repeated measures (RM) ANOVA for comparing over time and two-way RM ANOVA with time and pretreatment as within factors to test for interaction. Pairwise comparison where performed using Student's t-test. P-NO$_x$, U-NO$_x$ and U-cGMP were log transformed prior to testing
* $p < .05$ within group vs. baseline (Bonferroni), † $p < .05$ vs. placebo at baseline

diastolic brachial BP in males compared to females when ingesting potassium nitrate [26].

We observed an increase in both fractional and absolute sodium excretion during NaNO$_2$ infusion. Although there is not complete agreement on the effects of NO in different nephron segments, a net natriuretic and diuretic effect of NO in vivo is commonly accepted [27]. The natriuretic effect we observed during NaNO$_2$ infusion is in agreement with existing data regarding the overall inhibitory effect of NO on sodium absorption in the nephron. However, we found a reduction in free water clearance and urine output (data not presented), which conflicts with the general notion of NO as a diuretic. A possible explanation could be the reduction in BP. The decrease in P-AVP and steady U-AQP2 suggests that the mechanism is not mediated by AQP2.

Soluble guanylyl cyclase (sGC) releases cGMP to the circulation upon stimulation by NO. Being a renowned second messenger for NO, cGMP is widely used as a surrogate marker of NO activity [28–30]. The lack of increase in P-cGMP and the post-infusion decline in U-cGMP in the present study is puzzling. The findings are nevertheless in agreement with a recent dose-response study from our group [25]. Accordingly, Omar et al. found that an accumulated intra-arterial infusion of approximately 100 mg of NaNO$_2$ did not increase systemic cGMP, measured in the contralateral arm, despite a substantial increase in regional cGMP formation and an 11 mmHg reduction in MAP [31]. In comparison, the accumulated dose used in the present study was approximately 32 mg for the average subject weighing 67 kg.

Table 4 Effect of intravenous NaNO$_2$ on renal sodium and water regulation

	Baseline	Infusion				Post-infusion		p Friedman/ RM ANOVA (one-way)
		30 min	60 min	90 min	120 min	150 min	180 min	
FE$_{Na}$ (%)								
Placebo	1.26 [1.05;1.47]	1.26 [1.09;1.43]	1.43 [1.25;1.62]	1.38 [1.24;1.52]	1.57 [1.36;1.78]	1.53 [1.34;1.73]	1.41 [1.26;1.56]	.001
Allopurinol	1.36 [0.96;1.75]	1.41 [1.05;1.76]	1.52 [1.20;1.83]	1.53 [1.22;1.83]	1.66 [1.32;2.00]*	1.69 [1.40;1.98]*	1.59 [1.33;1.85]	.002
Enalapril	1.15 [0.84;1.46]	1.30 [1.01;1.60]	1.42 [1.15;1.68]*	1.45 [1.20;1.71]*	1.59 [1.34;1.83]*	1.56 [1.32;1.81]*	1.52 [1.29;1.74]*	<.001
Acetazolamide	1.08 [0.86;1.29]	1.25 [1.01;1.49]	1.35 [1.08;1.63]	1.29 [1.07;1.51]	1.42 [1.15;1.69]*	1.44 [1.17;1.71]*	1.28 [1.05;1.52]	.001
$p_{interaction}$ (pretreatment × time)		.535						
GFR (ml/min/1.73 m^2)								
Placebo	98 [90;105]	104 [96;111]	98 [91;105]	105 [97;113]*	101 [92;110]	99 [93;106]	100 [91;109]	.027
Allopurinol	99 [90;108]	102 [93;112]	97 [89;105]	103 [94;112]	98 [88;108]	99 [91;107]	102 [92;111]	.132
Enalapril	101 [92;110]	104 [94;114]	101 [94;108]	104 [96;112]	100 [91;109]	102 [94;109]	102 [94;110]	.568
Acetazolamide	83 [76;89]†	84 [77;92]	77 [70;83]*	83 [75;91]	83 [76;89]	83 [76;89]	85 [78;92]	.012
$p_{interaction}$ (pretreatment × time)		.494						
C$_{H2O}$ (ml/min)								
Placebo	4.58 [3.66;5.50]	2.87 [2.08;3.65]	1.87 [1.36;2.38]*	2.27 [1.46;3.08]*	2.85 [2.11;3.59]	2.64 [2.00;3.28]*	2.85 [2.15;3.55]*	<.001
Allopurinol	4.56 [3.64;5.48]	3.05 [2.02;4.07]	2.54 [1.82;3.27]*	2.04 [0.98;3.10]*	3.00 [2.11;3.90]	3.06 [2.19;3.93]	3.26 [2.40;4.12]	.011
Enalapril	4.82 [3.70;5.94]	3.57 [2.48;4.65]	2.28 [1.26;3.29]*	2.28 [1.48;3.08]*	3.24 [2.59;3.89]	2.23 [1.26;3.21]*	2.67 [1.71;3.63]	.001
Acetazolamide	3.91 [2.80;5.01]	1.99 [1.12;2.87]	1.69 [0.93;2.46]	1.63 [0.87;2.39]*	2.60 [1.78;3.42]	2.67 [1.78;3.55]	2.60 [1.80;3.40]	.004
$p_{interaction}$ (pretreatment × time)		.682						
P-AVP (pg/ml)								
Placebo	0.32 [0.25;0.38]		0.25 [0.20;0.30]*		0.27 [0.21;0.33]*			.012
Allopurinol	0.29 [0.21;0.36]		0.28 [0.22;0.33]		0.25 [0.21;0.29]			.414
Enalapril	0.26 [0.20;0.33]		0.21 [0.17;0.26]		0.23 [0.18;0.28]			.213
Acetazolamide	0.29 [0.22;0.36]		0.27 [0.19;0.35]		0.28 [0.22;0.34]			.770
$p_{interaction}$ (pretreatment × time)		.630						
U-AQP2 (ng/min)								
Placebo	1.26 [1.12;1.41]	1.25 [1.06;1.45]	1.23 [1.10;1.35]	1.18 [1.04;1.33]	1.23 [1.08;1.39]	1.19 [1.06;1.33]	1.13 [1.02;1.23]	.167
Allopurinol	1.45 [1.27;1.63]†	1.37 [1.26;1.48]	1.31 [1.20;1.42]	1.34 [1.21;1.47]	1.33 [1.13;1.54]	1.31 [1.20;1.42]	1.28 [1.17;1.39]	.080
Enalapril	1.29 [1.13;1.44]	1.23 [1.09;1.37]	1.28 [1.14;1.42]	1.26 [1.13;1.40]	1.28 [1.09;1.46]	1.33 [1.18;1.48]	1.18 [1.06;1.31]	.131
Acetazolamide	1.30 [1.15;1.45]	1.26 [1.08;1.44]	1.21 [1.07;1.36]	1.19 [1.04;1.35]	1.25 [1.09;1.41]	1.26 [1.08;1.43]	1.21 [1.06;1.37]	.363
$p_{interaction}$ (pretreatment × time)		.590						
U-ENaCγ (ng/min)								
Placebo	0.44 (0.38;0.51)	0.44 (0.33;0.51)	0.47 (0.35;0.54)	0.45 (0.36;0.59)	0.40 (0.36;0.57)	0.43 (0.36;0.56)	0.43 (0.32;0.46)	.331
Allopurinol	0.43 (0.40;0.65)	0.42 (0.38;0.54)	0.39 (0.34;0.54)	0.47 (0.42;0.61)	0.43 (0.30;0.54)*	0.42 (0.35;0.51)	0.39 (0.34;0.50)	.020
Enalapril	0.44 (0.40;0.64)	0.40 (0.35;0.49)	0.39 (0.34;0.60)	0.45 (0.31;0.53)	0.39 (0.36;0.55)	0.41 (0.33;0.57)	0.45 (0.40;0.53)	.215
Acetazolamide	0.68 (0.48;0.95)†	0.57 (0.42;1.01)	0.59 (0.45;0.94)	0.53 (0.48;0.88)	0.55 (0.45;0.93)	0.71 (0.53;0.94)	0.64 (0.49;0.89)	.561

Effect of intravenous NaNO$_2$ on fractional excretion of sodium (FE$_{Na}$), GFR, free water clearance (C$_{H2O}$), urinary excretion rates of aquaporin-2 (AQP2) and γ-subunit of the epithelial sodium channel (ENaCγ) in 14 healthy subjects and arginine vasopressine (AVP) in 16 healthy subjects after 4 days pretreatment with allopurinol, enalapril, acetazolamide, or placebo. Normal distributed data are presented as means with 95% confidence interval in brackets and non-parametric data as medians with 25th and 75th percentiles in parentheses. Statistics were performed using one-way repeated measures (RM) ANOVA for comparing over time and two-way RM ANOVA with time and pretreatment as within factors to test for interaction. Pairwise comparison where performed using Student's t-test. U-ENaCγ were tested using Friedman test for comparing over time and Wilcoxon's signed rank test for pairwise comparison with placebo or baseline
* $p < .05$ within group vs. baseline (Bonferroni), † $p < .05$ vs. placebo at baseline

Table 5 Effect of intravenous NaNO$_2$ on brachial and central hemodynamics

	Baseline value	Change from baseline to last hour of infusion	$p_{t\text{-test}}$
Brachial systolic BP (mmHg)			
Placebo	115 (111;119)	−2.63 (− 4.41;-0.85)	.007
Allopurinol	115 (111;119)	− 3.07 (−5.12;-1.01)	.006
Enalapril	110 (107;114)[†]	−3.84 (−5.32;-2.35)	<.001
Acetazolamide	114 (111;118)	−3.79 (−5.85;-1.74)	.001
$p_{\text{RM ANOVA}}$		.272	
Brachial diastolic BP (mmHg)			
Placebo	60 (57;62)	−1.50 (−3.28;0.28)	.093
Allopurinol	60 (56;63)	−1.22 (−3.14;0.70)	.196
Enalapril	56 (53;59)[†]	−1.18 (−2.40;0.03)	.054
Acetazolamide	60 (58;63)	−1.58 (−3.04;-0.12)	.035
$p_{\text{RM ANOVA}}$		.923	
Brachial MAP (mmHg)			
Placebo	78 (76;81)	−1.88 (−3.39;-0.37)	.018
Allopurinol	78 (75;81)	−1.84 (−3.63;-0.04)	.046
Enalapril	74 (72;77)[†]	−2.07 (−3.28;-0.86.)	.002
Acetazolamide	78 (76;81)	−2.32 (−3.88;-0.76)	.006
$p_{\text{RM ANOVA}}$		.848	
Heart rate (beats per minute)			
Placebo	55 (52;58)	3.37 (1.95;4.79)	<.001
Allopurinol	55 (52;59)	1.70 (0.12;3.28)[†]	.037
Enalapril	56 (52;60)	2.21 (0.97;3.45)	.002
Acetazolamide	57 (53;61)	1.30 (0.11;2.50)[†]	.035
$p_{\text{RM ANOVA}}$		.050	
Central systolic BP (mmHg)			
Placebo	98 (89;106)	−1.38 (−6.03;3.26)	.528
Allopurinol	99 (91;107)	−4.51 (−8.95;-0.07)	.047
Enalapril	97 (88;106)	−4.04 (−8.13;0.05)	.053
Acetazolamide	101 (90;112)	−2.69 (− 8.30;2.91)	.320
$p_{\text{RM ANOVA}}$		.804	

Effect of intravenous NaNO$_2$ on heart rate, brachial and central blood pressure (BP) in 16 healthy subjects after 4 days pretreatment with allopurinol, enalapril, acetazolamide, or placebo. Data are means with 95% confidence interval in brackets. Baseline values are an average of measurements in the one-hour period prior to infusion. The baseline values were compared to an average of measurements during the last hour of NaNO$_2$ infusion. Pairwise comparisons were performed using Student's t-test. One-way repeated measures (RM) ANOVA was used for comparison of effects between pretreatments
[†]: $p < .05$ vs. placebo

Allopurinol reduced P-urate at baseline, as expected. While NaNO$_2$ infusion lowered the brachial BP without active pretreatment, the reduction in central systolic BP (cSBP) was only significant after pretreatment with allopurinol. The cSBP reduction was not significantly different to the reduction after placebo pretreatment ($p = 0.539$), partly owing to an inherent lesser precision in the tonometry based method [32]. Although the results should be interpreted cautiously, this could indicate a potentiation of the vasodilating effects of NaNO$_2$. The remaining effects of NaNO$_2$ were unaffected by pretreatment with allopurinol. The intact, or even potentiated,

vasodilating effect of NaNO$_2$ after allopurinol is in agreement with the findings by Dejam et al. of an augmented increase in forearm blood flow when NaNO$_2$ and oxypurinol was co-infused [23]. A possible explanation could be a reduced scavenging of NO due to inhibition of xanthine oxidase-generated reactive oxygen species.

We observed an increase in renin concentration during NaNO$_2$ infusion, but only after preceding stimulation of renin secretion by either enalapril or to a lesser extent acetazolamide. The interplay between NO and renin has been studied intensively since the late 1980's. Numerous in vitro studies have shown both inhibitory

Table 6 Effect of intravenous $NaNO_2$ on the renin-angiotensin-aldosteron system

	Baseline	Infusion		p_{RM}
		60 min	120 min	ANOVA (one-way)
PRC (pg/ml)				
Placebo	9 (6;14)	9 (7;16)	9 (8;16)	.262
Allopurinol	9 (5;12)	9 (6;16)*	10 (6;14)	.024
Enalapril	54 (27;89)†	72 (40;93)*	69 (61;95)*	.014
Acetazolamide	15 (9;20)†	16 (12;23)	18 (12;23)*	.008
$p_{interaction}$ (pretreatment x time)		.168		
P-AngII (pg/ml)				
Placebo	16 (12;22)	17 (13;20)	14 (11;23)	.239
Allopurinol	14 (8;19)†	14 (12;21)	13 (10;19)	.175
Enalapril	11 (6;17)†	13 (8;21)	11 (8;21)	.189
Acetazolamide	19 (11;34)	20 (14;34)*	21 (16;35)*	.001
$p_{interaction}$ (pretreatment x time)		.160		
P-Aldo (pmol/l)				
Placebo	128 (98;161)	121 (90;155)	106 (79;155)	.228
Allopurinol	105 (82;158)	98 (64;138)	113 (76;147)	.967
Enalapril	78 (56;106)	77 (54;97)	71 (59;117)	.511
Acetazolamide	184 (132;281)†	178 (125;308)	230 (110;352)	.826
$p_{interaction}$ (pretreatment x time)		.664		

Effect of intravenous $NaNO_2$ on plasma concentrations of renin (PRC), angiotensin II (P-AngII), and aldosterone (P-Aldo) in 16 healthy subjects after 4 days pretreatment with allopurinol, enalapril, acetazolamide, or placebo. Data are medians with 25th and 75th percentiles in parentheses. After log transformation, statistics were performed using one-way repeated measures (RM) ANOVA for comparing over time and two-way RM ANOVA with time and pretreatment as within factors to test for interaction. Pairwise comparison with placebo or baseline where performed using Student's t-test after log transformation
* $p < .05$ within group vs. baseline (Bonferroni), † $p < .05$ vs. placebo at baseline

[33, 34], stimulatory [35, 36] and even biphasic effects [37] of NO or cGMP on renin secretion, while most in vivo studies agree on a stimulatory effect [38–40]. Our findings are in agreement with previous studies from our lab, showing a reduction of renin secretion after systemic NO inhibition in healthy subjects with activated renin system at baseline due to sodium restriction [41] or after angiotensin II receptor blockade [42]. A confounding effect of the BP reduction, being the strongest mediator of renin release, cannot be completely ruled out. However, $NaNO_2$ infusion only increased renin when the basal renin concentration was elevated, after enalapril or acetazolamide, despite a comparable effect on the BP regardless of pretreatment. This pattern corresponds to a previous study by our group, showing no stimulatory effect on the RAAS when infusing BP reducing doses of $NaNO_2$ after moderate sodium intake [25]. Interestingly, the BP lowering effect of $NaNO_2$ was fully preserved after preceding BP reduction with enalapril,

suggesting that the BP reducing mechanism of $NaNO_2$ is independent of ACE activity.

Acetazolamide had a profound effect on multiple baseline values, e.g. 24-h sodium excretion, 24-h creatinine clearance, baseline GFR, and excretion rate of ENaCγ. Previous studies have shown an acute diuretic and natriuretic effect [43, 44] in the proximal tubule, which waned off after a few days of continued treatment [44]. We detected an activation of the RAAS, with significantly elevated levels of renin and aldosterone, most likely caused by a decrease in extracellular volume and pH. Aldosterone, being the primary regulator of ENaC, was most probably responsible for the increase in ENaC and accompanying increase in sodium reabsorption. The decrease in GFR is well known and believed to be mediated by tubuloglomerular feedback [45]. The effects of $NaNO_2$ infusion after acetazolamide did not differ from after placebo pretreatment.

We hypothesized 1) an attenuation of the effects of $NaNO_2$ after inhibition of the nitrite reducing capabilities of XO with allopurinol as shown in rats [2–4], 2) an augmentation of the effects of $NaNO_2$ after enalapril due to accumulation of bradykinin leading to up-regulation of eNOS [5, 6], and 3) an enhanced effect of $NaNO_2$ after acetazolamide due to a stimulated enzymatic conversion of nitrite to NO by carbonic anhydrase [13, 14]. However, apart from a reduction of central systolic BP, which was only significant after allopurinol, we could not detect any consistent differences in the response to $NaNO_2$ between the pretreatments. The results suggest that none of the studied pathways are essential to nitrite bioactivation.

The post-infusion reduction in U-cGMP and steady P-cGMP is consistent with our previous findings [25], but nevertheless puzzling and could indicate that the effects of $NaNO_2$ might not be mediated by the NO-sGC-cGMP pathway. If the actions of $NaNO_2$ under physiologic conditions are independent of NO production, it would explain why modulation of different enzyme systems with suspected nitrite reducing abilities failed to modify the effect. The differences in baseline parameters after each pretreatment were expected and can be ascribed to the fundamental effects of the enzyme inhibitors.

Strengths and limitations

The strengths of the present study lie in the design. It is a rigorously conducted, double-blinded, placebo-controlled, 4-way crossover study. The sodium intake is standardized and controlled. Adherence to the pretreatment was verified by baseline levels of P-renin, P-urate, and P-(vB)-total CO_2 which reflected the pretreatment for all subjects without exception. Previous studies from our laboratory [25, 29, 46, 47] suggest a slightly natriuretic and anti-aquaretic effect of the supine and water loaded model, which might have contributed to the findings in the present study.

The dosage of $NaNO_2$ relies on a previous dose-response study by our group [25]. Evaluated on the effects on $P\text{-}NO_x$, $U\text{-}NO_x$, sodium excretion and BP, we believe to have achieved a relevant increase in nitrite bioavailability.

Conclusion

This study demonstrated a robust BP lowering, natriuretic and anti-aquaretic effect of intravenous $NaNO_2$ regardless of preceding enzyme inhibition. The steady P-cGMP and post-infusion decrease in U-cGMP indicates little or no conversion of nitrite to NO. Thus the effect of $NaNO_2$ may not be mediated by NO generation.

Abbreviations

^{51}Cr-EDTA: Chromium-51 labeled ethylenediamine tetraacetic acid; ACE: Angiotensin-converting enzyme; Aldo: Aldosterone; ANGII: Angiotensin II; AQP2: Aquaporin-2; AVP: Arginine vasopressin; BP: Blood pressure; CA: Carbonic anhydrase; cGMP: Guanosine 3′,5′-cyclic monophosphate; C_{H2O}: Free water clearance; C_{Na}: Sodium clearance; C_{osm}: Osmolar clearance; cSBP: Central systolic blood pressure; ENaCγ: γ-subunit of the epithelial sodium channel; eNOS: Endothelial nitric oxide synthase; FE_K: Fractional excretion of potassium; FE_{Na}: Fractional excretion of sodium; GFR: Glomerular filtration rate; MAP: Mean arterial pressure; $NaNO_2$: Sodium nitrite; NO: Nitric oxide; NO_x: Combined nitrite and nitrate; P-(vB)-total CO_2: Plasma total carbon dioxide in venous blood; PRC: Plasma renin concentration; RIA: Radioimmunoassay; sGC: Soluble guanylyl cyclase; UO: Urine output; UOR: Urine output rate; XO: Xanthine oxidase

Acknowledgements

We thank laboratory technicians Anne Mette Ravn, Kirsten Nygaard and Henriette Vorup Simonsen for skilled assistance in examining the subjects and performing laboratory analyses, Hanne Sahl and the kitchen staff for preparing the diet, and the Department of Clinical Biochemistry, Regional Hospital West Jutland, Denmark for assistance in routine analyses.

Funding

The study was conducted without external grants. All study drugs were paid for by our own lab.

Authors' contributions

JBR, EBP, and JNB designed the project; JBR performed the experiments and analyzed the data; JBR, EBP, and JNB interpreted the results; JBR drafted the manuscript; all authors revised, edited, and approved the manuscript.

Competing interests

The authors declare that they have no competing interests.

References

1. Kim-Shapiro DB, Gladwin MT. Mechanisms of nitrite bioactivation. Tanig Symp Brain Sci. 2014;38:58–68.
2. Casey DB, Badejo AM, Dhaliwal JS, Murthy SN, Hyman AL, Nossaman BD, Kadowitz PJ. Pulmonary vasodilator responses to sodium nitrite are mediated by an allopurinol-sensitive mechanism in the rat. Am J Physiol Heart Circ Physiol. 2009;296(2):H524–33.
3. Golwala NH, Hodenette C, Murthy SN, Nossaman BD, Kadowitz PJ. Vascular responses to nitrite are mediated by xanthine oxidoreductase and mitochondrial aldehyde dehydrogenase in the rat. Can J Physiol Pharmacol. 2009; 87(12):1095–101.
4. Ghosh SM, Kapil V, Fuentes-Calvo I, Bubb KJ, Pearl V, Milsom AB, Khambata R, Maleki-Toyserkani S, Yousuf M, Benjamin N, Webb AJ, Caulfield MJ, Hobbs AJ, Ahluwalia A. Enhanced vasodilator activity of nitrite in hypertension: critical role for erythrocytic xanthine oxidoreductase and translational potential. Hypertension. 2013;61(5):1091–102.
5. Zhao Y, Qiu Q, Mahdi F, Shariat-Madar Z, Rojkjaer R, Schmaier A. Assembly and activation of HK-PK complex on endothelial cells results in bradykinin liberation and NO formation. Am J Physiol Heart Circ Physiol. 2001;280(4): H1821–9.
6. Gauthier KM, Cepura CJ, Campbell WB. Ace inhibition enhances bradykinin relaxations through nitric oxide and b1 receptor activation in bovine coronary arteries. Biol Chem. 2013;394(9):1205–12.
7. Comini L, Bachetti T, Cargnoni A, Bastianon D, Gitti GL, Ceconi C, Ferrari R. Therapeutic modulation of the nitric oxide: all ace inhibitors are not equivalent. Pharmacol Res. 2007;56(1):42–8.
8. Kohno M, Yokokawa K, Minami M, Yasunari K, Maeda K, Kano H, Hanehira T, Yoshikawa J. Plasma levels of nitric oxide and related vasoactive factors following long-term treatment with angiotensin-converting enzyme inhibitor in patients with essential hypertension. Metab Clin Exp. 1999; 48(10):1256–9.
9. Kosenko E, Tikhonova L, Suslikov A, Kaminsky Y. Impacts of Lisinopril and Lisinopril plus simvastatin on erythrocyte and plasma arginase, nitrite, and nitrate in hypertensive patients. J Clin Pharmacol. 2012;52(1):102–9.
10. Kedziora-Kornatowska K, Kornatowski T, Bartosz G, Pawluk H, Czuczejko J, Kedziora J, Szadujkis-Szadurski L. Production of nitric oxide, lipid peroxidation and oxidase activity of ceruloplasmin in blood of elderly patients with primary hypertension. Effects of perindopril treatment. Aging Clin Exp Res. 2016;18(1):1–6.
11. Hornig B, Kohler C, Drexler H. Role of bradykinin in mediating vascular effects of angiotensin-converting enzyme inhibitors in humans. Circulation. 1997;95(5):1115–8.
12. Arcaro G, Zenere BM, Saggiani F, Zenti MG, Monauni T, Lechi A, Muggeo M, Bonadonna RC. ACE inhibitors improve endothelial function in type 1 diabetic patients with normal arterial pressure and microalbuminuria. Diabetes Care. 1999;22(9):1536–42.
13. Kringelholt S, Simonsen U, Bek T. Dorzolamide-induced relaxation of intraocular porcine ciliary arteries in vitro depends on nitric oxide and the vascular endothelium. Curr Eye Res. 2012;37(12):1107–13.
14. Aamand R, Dalsgaard T, Jensen FB, Simonsen U, Roepstorff A, Fago A. Generation of nitric oxide from nitrite by carbonic anhydrase: a possible link between metabolic activity and vasodilation. Am J Physiol Heart Circ Physiol. 2009;297(6):H2068–74.
15. Aamand R, Ho Y, Dalsgaard T, Roepstorff A, Lund TE. Dietary nitrate facilitates an acetazolamide-induced increase in cerebral blood flow during visual stimulation. J Appl Physiol (1985). 2014;116(3):267–73.
16. Pedersen EB, Danielsen H, Spencer ES. Effect of indapamide on renal plasma flow, glomerular filtration rate and arginine vasopressin in plasma in essential hypertension. Eur J Clin Pharmacol. 1984;26(5):543–7.
17. Pedersen EB, Eiskjaer H, Madsen B, Danielsen H, Egeblad M, Nielsen CB. Effect of captopril on renal extraction of renin, angiotensin II, atrial natriuretic peptide and vasopressin, and renal vein renin ratio in patients with arterial hypertension and unilateral renal artery disease. Nephrol Dial Transplant. 1993;8(10):1064–70.
18. Pedersen RS, Bentzen H, Bech JN, Pedersen EB. Effect of water deprivation and hypertonic saline infusion on urinary AQP2 excretion in healthy humans. Am J Physiol Ren Physiol. 2001;280(5):F860–7.
19. Graffe CC, Bech JN, Pedersen EB. Effect of high and low sodium intake on urinary aquaporin-2 excretion in healthy humans. Am J Physiol Ren Physiol. 2012;302(2):F264–75.
20. Al Therwani S, Malmberg MES, Rosenbaek JB, Bech JN, Pedersen EB. Effect of tolvaptan on renal handling of water and sodium, GFR and central hemodynamics in autosomal dominant polycystic kidney disease during inhibition of the nitric oxide system: a randomized, placebo-controlled, double blind, crossover study. BMC Nephrol. 2017;18:268.
21. Hager H, Kwon TH, Vinnikova AK, Masilamani S, Brooks HL, Frokiaer J, Knepper MA, Nielsen S. Immunocytochemical and immunoelectron microscopic localization of alpha-, beta-, and gamma-ENaC in rat kidney. Am J Physiol Ren Physiol. 2001;280(6):F1093–106.

22. Pluta RM, Oldfield EH, Bakhtian KD, Fathi AR, Smith RK, Devroom HL, Nahavandi M, Woo S, Figg WD, Lonser RR. Safety and feasibility of long-term intravenous sodium nitrite infusion in healthy volunteers. PLoS One. 2011;6(1):e14504.

23. Dejam A, Hunter CJ, Tremonti C, Pluta RM, Hon YY, Grimes G, Partovi K, Pelletier MM, Oldfield EH, Cannon RO III, Schechter AN, Gladwin MT. Nitrite infusion in humans and nonhuman primates: endocrine effects, pharmacokinetics, and tolerance formation. Circulation. 2007;116(16):1821–31.

24. Cosby K, Partovi KS, Crawford JH, Patel RP, Reiter CD, Martyr S, Yang BK, Waclawiw MA, Zalos G, Xu X, Huang KT, Shields H, Kim-Shapiro DB, Schechter AN, Cannon RO III, Gladwin MT. Nitrite reduction to nitric oxide by deoxyhemoglobin vasodilates the human circulation. Nat Med. 2003;9(12):1498–505.

25. Rosenbaek JB, Therwani SA, Jensen JM, Mose FH, Wandall-Frostholm C, Pedersen EB, Bech JN. Effect of sodium nitrite on renal function and sodium and water excretion and brachial and central blood pressure in healthy subjects: a dose-response study. Am J Physiol Ren Physiol. 2017;313(2):F378–87.

26. Kapil V, Milsom AB, Okorie M, Maleki-Toyserkani S, Akram F, Rehman F, Arghandawi S, Pearl V, Benjamin N, Loukogeorgakis S, Macallister R, Hobbs AJ, Webb AJ, Ahluwalia A. Inorganic nitrate supplementation lowers blood pressure in humans: role for nitrite-derived NO. Hypertension. 2010;56(2):274–81.

27. Ortiz PA, Garvin JL. Role of nitric oxide in the regulation of nephron transport. Am J Physiol Ren Physiol. 2002;282(5):F777–84.

28. Kanno K, Hirata Y, Emori T, Ohta K, Eguchi S, Imai T, Marumo F. L-arginine infusion induces hypotension and diuresis/natriuresis with concomitant increased urinary excretion of nitrite/nitrate and cyclic GMP in humans. Clin Exp Pharmacol Physiol. 1992;19(9):619–25.

29. Bech JN, Nielsen CB, Pedersen EB. Effects of systemic NO synthesis inhibition on RPF, GFR, UNa, and vasoactive hormones in healthy humans. Am J Phys. 1996;270(5 Pt 2):F845–51.

30. Bode-Boger SM, Boger RH, Galland A, Tsikas D, Frolich JC. L-arginine-induced vasodilation in healthy humans: pharmacokinetic-pharmacodynamic relationship. Br J Clin Pharmacol. 1998;46(5):489–97.

31. Omar SA, Fok H, Tilgner KD, Nair A, Hunt J, Jiang B, Taylor P, Chowienczyk P, Webb AJ. Paradoxical normoxia-dependent selective actions of inorganic nitrite in human muscular conduit arteries and related selective actions on central blood pressures. Circulation. 2015;131(4):381–9.

32. Cheng HM, Lang D, Tufanaru C, Pearson A. Measurement accuracy of non-invasively obtained central blood pressure by applanation tonometry: a systematic review and meta-analysis. Int J Cardiol. 2013;167(5):1867–76.

33. Vidal MJ, Romero JC, Vanhoutte PM. Endothelium-derived relaxing factor inhibits renin release. Eur J Pharmacol. 1988;149(3):401–2.

34. Beierwaltes WH, Carretero OA. Nonprostanoid endothelium-derived factors inhibit renin release. Hypertension. 1992;19(2 Suppl):68–73.

35. Hackenthal E, Taugner R. Hormonal signals and intracellular messengers for renin secretion. Mol Cell Endocrinol. 1986;47(1–2):1–12.

36. Münter K, Hackenthal E. The participation of the endothelium in the control of renin release. J Hypertens. 1991;9(Supplement 6):S238.

37. Schricker K, Kurtz A. Liberators of NO exert a dual effect on renin secretion from isolated mouse renal juxtaglomerular cells. Am J Phys. 1993;265(2 Pt 2):F180–6.

38. Persson PB, Baumann JE, Ehmke H, Hackenthal E, Kirchheim HR, Nafz B. Endothelium-derived NO stimulates pressure-dependent renin release in conscious dogs. Am J Phys. 1993;264(6 Pt 2):F943–7.

39. Johnson RA, Freeman RH. Renin release in rats during blockade of nitric oxide synthesis. Am J Phys. 1994;266(6 Pt 2):R1723–9.

40. Beierwaltes WH. cGMP stimulates renin secretion in vivo by inhibiting phosphodiesterase-3. Am J Physiol Ren Physiol. 2006;290(6):F1376–81.

41. Bech JN, Nielsen CB, Ivarsen P, Jensen KT, Pedersen EB. Dietary sodium affects systemic and renal hemodynamic response to NO inhibition in healthy humans. Am J Physiol Ren Physiol. 1998;274(5 Pt 2):F914–23.

42. Bech JN, Svendsen KB, Nielsen CB, Pedersen EB. The systemic and renal response to NO inhibition is not modified by angiotensin-II-receptor blockade in healthy humans. Nephrol Dial Transplant. 1999;14(3):641–7.

43. Skøtt P, Hommel E, Bruun NE, Arnold-Larsen S, Parving HH. The acute effect of acetazolamide on glomerular filtration rate and proximal tubular reabsorption of sodium and water in normal man. Scand J Clin Lab Invest. 1989;49(6):583 7.

44. Skøtt P, Hommel E, Bruun NE, Arnold-Larsen S, Parving HH. Effects of acetazolamide on kidney function in type 1 (insulin-dependent) diabetic patients with diabetic nephropathy. Diabetologia. 1988;31(11):806–10.

45. Persson A, Wright FS. Evidence for feedback mediated reduction of glomerular filtration rate during infusion of acetazolamide. Acta Physiol Scand. 1982;114(1):1–7.

46. Larsen T, Mose FH, Bech JN, Pedersen EB. Effect of nitric oxide inhibition on blood pressure and renal sodium handling: a dose-response study in healthy man. Clin Exp Hypertens. 2012;34(8):567–74.

47. Lauridsen TG, Vase H, Bech JN, Nielsen S, Pedersen EB. Direct effect of methylprednisolone on renal sodium and water transport via the principal cells in the kidney. Eur J Endocrinol. 2010;162(5):961–9.

7

Incidence and impact on outcomes of acute kidney injury after a stroke: a systematic review and meta-analysis

Julia Arnold[1], Khai Ping Ng[1], Don Sims[2], Paramjit Gill[3,4], Paul Cockwell[1] and Charles Ferro[1]* ⓘD

Abstract

Background: Patients with chronic kidney disease have worse outcomes after stroke. However, the burden of acute kidney injury after stroke has not been extensively investigated.

Methods: We used MEDLINE and Embase to conduct a systematic review and meta-analysis of published studies that provided data on the risk of AKI and outcomes in adults after ischemic and hemorrhagic stroke. Pooled incidence was examined using the Stuart-Ord method in a DerSimonian-Laird model. Pooled Odds Ratios and 95% confidence intervals were calculated for outcomes using a random effects model. This review was registered with PROSPERO (CRD42017064588).

Results: Eight studies were included, five from the United States, representing 99.9% of included patients. Three studies used established acute kidney injury criteria based on creatinine values to define acute kidney injury and five used International Classification of Diseases coding definitions. Overall pooled incidence was 9.61% (95% confidence interval 8.33–10.98). Incidence for studies using creatinine definitions was 19.51% (95% confidence interval 12.75–27.32%) and for studies using coding definitions 4.63% (95% confidence interval 3.65–5.72%). Heterogeneity was high throughout. Mortality in stroke patients who sustained acute kidney injury was increased (Odds Ratio 2.45; 95% confidence interval 1.47–4.10). Three studies reported risk factors for acute kidney injury. There was sparse information on other outcomes.

Conclusions: Mortality in stroke patients who develop acute kidney injury is significantly increased. However the reported incidence of AKI after stroke varies widely and is underestimated using coding definitions. Larger international studies are required to identify potentially preventable factors to reduce acute kidney injury after stroke and improve outcomes.

Keywords: Acute kidney injury, Stroke, Cerebrovascular disease, Meta-analysis, Mortality/survival

Background

Stroke is the leading cause of neurological disability worldwide with huge social and economic impact [1]. In 2015 there were 6.24 million deaths caused by stroke [2]. Chronic kidney disease (CKD) is associated with an increased risk of stroke [3]. Some of this relates to shared traditional risk factors, for example hypertension, hypercholesterolemia, diabetes mellitus and cigarette smoking [4]. However CKD itself has also been recognized as a risk factor for stroke [5, 6]. In a recent systematic review and meta-analysis comprising 83 studies and 30,392 strokes, Masson et al. demonstrated that stroke risk increased by 7% for every 10mls/min/1.73m^2 decline in glomerular filtration rate (GFR) [7].

Acute kidney injury (AKI) is a clinical syndrome defined as an abrupt decrease in kidney function resulting in disturbance of fluid, electrolyte and acid-base homeostasis [8]. AKI is a spectrum, ranging from mild, asymptomatic injury to severe injury requiring renal replacement therapy (RRT) [8, 9]. Over the last decade, with the development and wide adoption of international classification systems [8–10], there has been an increasing amount of research into the incidence of AKI and its influence on adverse outcomes in both high and low income countries [11–14].

After a stroke, neurological deficit leading to dysphagia and physical disability, physiological effects including changes in blood pressure and cerebral salt wasting, as well

* Correspondence: Charles.Ferro@uhb.nhs.uk
[1]Department of Nephrology, University Hospitals Birmingham, Birmingham B15 2WB, UK
Full list of author information is available at the end of the article

as investigations and treatments, can all potentially contribute to the development of AKI. Furthermore, older, comorbid patients are at greatest risk of AKI [14]. Strategies to prevent AKI in stroke patients could therefore be of great importance. Although the association between CKD and stroke outcomes has been the subject of several systematic reviews and meta-analyses [7, 15], the relationship between AKI and stroke is much less clear. We therefore analyzed the reported rates of AKI incidence after a stroke and the associations between AKI and outcomes after a stroke.

Methods

Our systematic review was registered with PROSPERO (CRD42017064588) and we adhered to the PRISMA reporting statement [16]. A literature search of MEDLINE was performed from 1946 through to 30 June 2017 using relevant text words and medical subject headings *acute kidney injury, acute kidney failure, acute renal failure, acute renal insufficiency*, combined with *stroke, cerebrovascular disorders and CVA or TIA*. Embase was searched from 1974 to 30 June 2017, using the same medical subject headings for AKI as for MEDLINE, combined with *cerebrovascular accident, cerebrovascular disease, cerebrovascular disorder, brain hemorrhage; brain infarction* and *stroke* (for a detailed search strategy see Additional file 1). All searches were limited to human studies with no language restrictions. Authors manually reviewed the reference lists of retrieved articles for additional relevant studies.

Study selection

Study eligibility was determined using a standardized form (Additional file 2). Two authors, JA and KN, independently screened the list of studies generated by the search, with disagreements resolved by a third author, CF. Titles and abstracts of all studies were screened before obtaining full text versions of relevant studies. To improve generalizability, studies were included if they were a case control or cohort (prospective or retrospective) study and had a sample size greater than 500 adult subjects hospitalized with either an acute ischemic or hemorrhagic stroke [17]. Included studies had a clear statement regarding the definition of acute kidney injury - creatinine values alone were not sufficient. Subarachnoid hemorrhage was not included in this systematic review in view of the different aetiopathophysiology.

Data collection and analysis

Data was collected using a standardized proforma (Additional file 2) by JA and KN. The following study details were recorded: authors, year of publication, country of publication, type of study, clinical setting, sample size, patient characteristics (age, sex, ethnicity, and comorbidities), definition, type and severity of stroke and definition of AKI. Clinical parameters on admission, including serum creatinine and/or GFR, exposure to radiocontrast media, where

specified and number of patients who developed AKI were recorded. Outcomes including mortality, disability, length of stay, re-stroke or cardiac events were also recorded.

Study quality assessment was performed independently by two authors, JA and CF using the Newcastle-Ottawa scale [18]. A maximum of 9 points can be allocated to a particular study based on quality of selection, comparability and study outcome (including follow up). Scores were defined as poor (0–3), fair (4–6) and good (7–9) [17].

Data synthesis, meta-analysis and statistical analysis were performed using Review Manager v5.3.5 software (The Cochrane Collaboration, UK) and StatsDirect v3.0 (StatsDirect Limited, UK). Meta-analysis of proportions was carried out using the Stuart-Ord (inverse double arcsine square root) method in a DerSimonian-Laird (random effects) model. The Odds Ratio (OR) with accompanying 95% confidence intervals (95% CI) were used to report individual and summary effect measures for dichotomous data. Chi squared tests for heterogeneity were performed to examine if the degrees of freedom were greater than the Cochran Q statistic, with α of below 0.05 considered to be statistically significant. In addition, the I^2 statistic was calculated to provide the estimated percentage of heterogeneity observed. I^2 values of 25%, 50% and 75% correspond to low, medium and high levels of heterogeneity. Any heterogeneity was further explored. A two-sided P value of < 0.05 was considered significant for all analyses.

Results

Study characteristics

A total of 6173 potentially relevant citations were identified (Fig. 1), of which 816 were duplicates. A further 5309 articles were excluded after review of title and abstract and an additional 40 excluded after full text review. The characteristics of the eight included studies are displayed in Table 1 [19–26] with the study outcomes summarized in Table 2. All eight studies were published in the English language between 2007 and 2015. Seven studies were considered to be of good quality and one of fair quality. The eight studies provided data on 12,325,652 patients (range 897 to 7,068,334) from four countries (five from the US [20, 22–24, 26], and one each from China [21], Greece [25] and Romania [19]). The US studies overwhelmingly had the largest sample sizes, with a total of 12,319,724 patients representing 99.9% of all included patients. Three of the US studies used Nationwide Inpatient Sample (NIS) data [23, 24, 26]. Although the same database was used, one study included only patients with ischemic stroke [23], one study included only patients with hemorrhagic stroke [24] and a third included only patients who sustained AKI requiring dialysis treatment (AKI-D) [26]. Therefore it was considered appropriate to include only the first two in the meta-analysis [23, 24]. Five out of eight studies used the International Classification of Diseases-9th or 10th Edition (ICD-9/1CD-10) coding to define AKI [21–24] and AKI-D [26]. Only one of the studies reported data

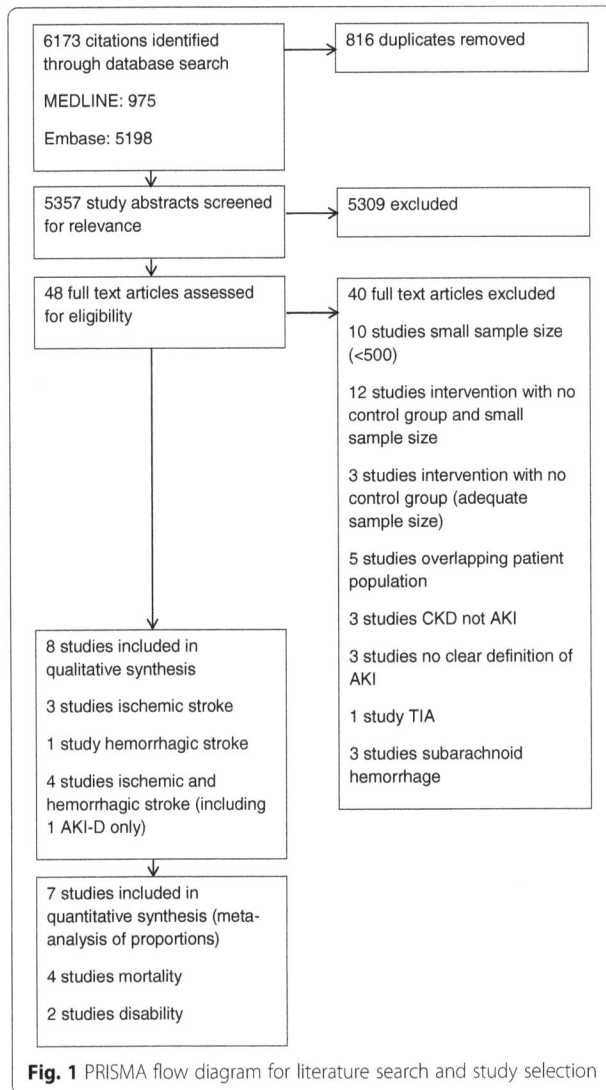

Fig. 1 PRISMA flow diagram for literature search and study selection

on AKI-D in addition to overall AKI incidence [24]. Two studies used the Acute Kidney Injury Network (AKIN) classification [20, 25] and one the Risk/ Injury/ Failure/ Loss/ End-stage (RIFLE) classification [19]. None used urine output criteria. Although there are some differences in the grading of AKI severity between these classifications, both define the absolute incidence of AKI as an increase in serum creatinine > 150%. Stroke was determined using ICD coding in four studies [22–24, 26]. Three studies utilized the World Health Organization (WHO) definition of stroke [27] and extracted clinical data from medical records prospectively [21, 25] or retrospectively [19]. Two studies [21, 25] further subclassified the etiology of ischemic stroke using TOAST criteria [28]. One study utilized stroke registry data as well as clinical records and ICD coding [20].

Five studies followed patients until discharge from hospital [20, 22–24, 26], one for 30 days [19], one from hospitalization up to one year [21] and one from 30 days up to 10 years [25]

(Table 2). Two studies excluded patients with known CKD [23, 24] and two studies excluded patients with end-stage renal disease (ESRD) [20, 26]. Ischemic and hemorrhagic stroke patients were included in four of the studies [19, 20, 25, 26], ischemic stroke alone in three [21–23] and hemorrhagic stroke alone in one study [24] (Table 2).

Pooled incidence of AKI after stroke

Nadkarni et al. reported the incidence of AKI-D only [26]. This was 0.15% in hospitalizations with acute ischemic stroke and 0.35% in intracranial hemorrhage, with an overall incidence of 0.5%. Saeed et al. reported an overall incidence of AKI-D of 1.7% [24].

Using the remaining seven studies, the pooled proportion of AKI as a percentage was 9.61% (95% CI 8.33–10.98) (Fig. 2) with an I^2 statistic of 99.8% indicating high heterogeneity. Excluding Lin et al. [21], which reported a much lower incidence of AKI than any other study (0.82%), made no difference to the heterogeneity (I^2 99.9%).

The pooled incidence of AKI in the studies that utilized ICD coding to define AKI [21–24] was 4.63% (95% CI 3.65–5.72%). Heterogeneity was high (I^2 99.9%). Excluding Lin et al. [21], the pooled incidence of AKI increased to 6.46% (95% CI 5.18–7.86%) and heterogeneity remained high (I^2 99.9%). Further excluding the study of hemorrhagic stroke hospitalizations [24], the pooled incidence of AKI remained similar (6.42%; 95% CI 4.07–9.27%) with high heterogeneity (I^2 90.6%). In comparison, the pooled incidence in studies using creatinine-based AKI definitions [19, 20, 25] was 19.51% (95% CI 12.75–27.32%), again with high heterogeneity (I^2 97.4%).

The pooled incidence of AKI in ischemic stroke [19–23, 25] was 9.62% (95% CI 4.20–16.96%; I^2 statistic 99.5%). Excluding Lin et al. [21], AKI incidence increased to 12.45% (95% CI 4.96–22.70%) and heterogeneity remained high (I^2 99.5%). Using studies with a coding definition for AKI, the pooled incidence was 4.05% (95% CI 1.06–8.86%; I^2 statistic 99.1%). Pooled incidence of AKI in studies utilizing creatinine-based definitions was 17.33% (95% CI 9.42–27.05%) with high heterogeneity (I^2 97.6%).

The pooled incidence of AKI in hemorrhagic stroke [19, 20, 24, 25] was 19.17% (95% CI 7.75–34.15%). Heterogeneity was high (I^2 99.0%). Excluding Saeed et al. 2015 [24], the only study in this group to use a coding definition for AKI, the pooled incidence increased to 24.50% (95% CI 18.03–31.61%). Heterogeneity decreased but remained high (I^2 84.9%).

Risk factors for AKI after stroke

Factors associated with the development of AKI after multivariate analyses are shown in Table 2. Three studies explored risk factors for the development of AKI after stroke [19, 20, 25]. Older age [19], worse renal function on admission [19, 20, 25], ischemic heart disease [19], heart failure

Table 1 Characteristics of the 8 included studies

Author	Type of study/ country	No. of subjects	Age (years) (SD)	Men (%)	Ischemic stroke cases (%)	AKI definition	CKD excluded?	NOS score
Covic et al., 2008 [19]	Observational, retrospective, Romania	1090	66.1 ± 11.5	49.3	932 (85.5%)	Creatinine values; RIFLE	No	7 (3, 2, 2)
Khatri et al., 2014 [20]	Observational, retrospective, United States	1357	64 ± 16	56.0	528 (38.9%)	Creatinine values; AKIN	GFR < 15 ml/min excluded	6 (2, 2, 2)
Lin et al., 2011 [21]	Observational, prospective, China	2683	66.1 ± 13.59 (AF), 63.58 ± 13.64 (no AF)	58.4	2683 (100%)	ICD-10 coding	No	7 (3, 2, 2)
Mohamed et al., 2015 [22]	Observational, retrospective, United States	897	64.4 ± 14.7	44.0	897 (100%)	ICD-9 coding	No	7 (3, 2, 2)
Saeed et al., 2014 [23]	Observational, retrospective, United States (Nationwide Inpatient Sample data)	7,068,334	No AKI 71 ± 31, AKI 74 ± 28	46.1	7,068,334 (100%)	ICD-9 coding	Yes	7 (3, 2, 2)
Saeed et al., 2015 [24]	Observational, retrospective, United States (Nationwide Inpatient Sample data)	614,454	No AKI 69 ± 37, AKI 68 ± 34	52.2	0 (0%) (all cases were hemorrhagic stroke)	ICD-9 coding	Yes	7 (3, 2, 2)
Tsagalis et al., 2008 [25]	Observational, prospective, Greece	2155	70.3 ± 11.9	61.2	1832 (85%)	Creatinine values; AKIN	No	8 (4, 2, 2)
Nadkarni et al., 2015 [26]	Observational, retrospective, United States (Nationwide Inpatient Sample data)	4,634,682	AIS No AKI 73 ± 0.2, AKI 66 ± 0.3 ICH No AKI 69.7 ± 0.13, AKI 65.4 ± 0.21	AIS 50.0 ICH 60.0	3,937,928 (85%)	ICD-9 coding AKI-D only	No	7 (3, 2, 2)

Abbreviations: AIS, acute ischemic stroke; AKI, acute kidney injury; AKI-D, acute kidney injury requiring dialysis; AKIN, Acute Kidney Injury Network; CKD, chronic kidney disease; GFR, estimated glomerular filtration rate; ICD-9/ 10, International Classification of Diseases, 9th/ 10th Revision; ICH, intracranial hemorrhage; mls/ min, milliliters per minute; NOS, Newcastle-Ottawa Scale; RIFLE, Risk, Injury, Failure, Loss, End-Stage Renal Disease

[19, 25] and higher National Institutes of Health Stroke Scale (NIHSS) score on admission [20, 25] were all found to be associated the development of AKI in stroke patients. Use of angiotensin-converting enzyme inhibitors (ACEi) and angiotensin II receptor blockers (ARBs) were only marginally associated with AKI (OR 1.004; 95% CI 0.993–1.058, $P = 0.057$) in one study [19]. One study also tested the association between contrast-enhanced computerized tomography (CT) and AKI and found no relationship [20].

None of the studies presented data on the adjusted rates of AKI associated with cerebral angiography, thrombolysis or any vascular intervention (mechanical thrombectomy, carotid stenting or endarterectomy).

Two studies [19, 25] examined the relationship between stroke type and risk of developing AKI after adjustment for confounders. Covic et al. [19] reported an OR of 2.50 (95% CI 1.42–4.41; $P = 0.001$) in hemorrhagic stroke and Tsagalis et al. [25] an OR of 2.02 (95% CI 1.34–3.04; P = 0.001) with lacunar stroke used as the reference.

AKI and severity of stroke

Two studies found an association between stroke severity (as determined by NIHSS score) and the development of AKI

[20, 25]. In Khatri et al. [20] the adjusted OR per 5 point increase in NIHSS score was 1.13 (95% CI 1.07–1.19; $P < 0.001$). Tsagalis et al. [25] reported an OR of 1.02 (95% CI 1.01–1.03; $P = 0.020$) after adjustment for age, sex, presence of atrial fibrillation (AF), serum glucose, hematocrit and antihypertensive agent use in the first 48 hours of admission.

AKI and degree of disability

Five studies reported disability post stroke with varying definitions. Two studies [21, 22] recorded degree of disability post stroke, as measured by the modified Rankin Scale (mRS). However data from Lin et al. [21] could not be analyzed with respect to AKI. Mohamed et al. [22] found no association between AKI and degree of disability after multiple adjustments. Two studies [23, 24] used coded discharge destination from NIS data as a surrogate marker for disability. Discharge was categorized as none to minimal disability and any other discharge status (home health care, short-term hospital or other facility including intermediate care and skilled nursing home or death) as moderate to severe disability. Both studies found a higher incidence of moderate to severe disability in patients with AKI after adjustment for multiple confounders (Saeed et al. 2014, OR 1.3 (95% CI

Table 2 Incidence of AKI, associated factors, measured outcomes and adjustments in the 8 included studies

Study	Follow up	Factors associated with AKI	Crude Mortality in AKI	AKI an independent risk factor for mortality	Disability and AKI	LOS (days) and AKI	Cost and AKI
Covic et al., 2008 [19]	30 days	Age, renal function on admission, IHD, CHF, hemorrhagic stroke	43.1% vs 12.8% (P = 0.001)	No	Not reported	Not reported	Not reported
Khatri et al., 2014 [20]	Hospital discharge	Admission creatinine, NIHSS score	AIS: 33% vs 10% (P ≤ 0.001) ICH: 40% vs 30% (P = 0.020)	For AIS only OR 3.08 (95% CI 1.49–6.35, P = 0.002) Adjusted for age, sex, race, comorbidities, smoking, CTA, creatinine, NIHSS score	Not reported	Unadjusted AIS: 17.6 vs 8.4 days (P ≤ 0.001) ICH: 13.0 vs 8.0 days (P ≤ 0.001)	Not reported
Lin et al., 2011 [21]	1 year	Not reported	Not reported	Not reported	Not reported	Not reported	Not reported
Mohamed et al., 2015 [22]	Hospital discharge	Not reported	Not reported	Not reported	Not significant after adjustment	OR 2.63, 95% CI 1.51–4.58 Adjusted for comorbidities, complications, NIHSS score	Not reported
Saeed et al., 2014 [23]	Hospital discharge	Not reported	8.4% vs 2.9% (P ≤ 0.001)	OR 2.2 (95% CI 2.0–2.2, P ≤ 0.001) Adjusted for age, sex, race, comorbidities, GI bleeding, sepsis, nicotine dependence	OR for moderate/ severe disability 1.3 (95% CI 1.3–1.4, P ≤ 0.001) Adjusted as for mortality	Unadjusted 6 vs 4 days (P < 0.0001)	Unadjusted USD 38,613 vs 24,474 (P < 0.0001)
Saeed et al., 2015 [24]	Hospital discharge	Not performed	AKI: 28.7% vs 22.4% (P ≤ 0.001) AKI-D vs AKI: 50.2% vs 28.4% (P ≤ 0.001)	OR 1.5 (95% CI 1.4–1.6, P ≤ 0.001) Adjusted for age, sex, race, comorbidities, nicotine dependence, alcohol abuse, hospital bed size, hospital teaching status	OR for moderate/ severe disability 1.2 (95% CI 1.1–1.3, P ≤ 0.001) Adjusted as for mortality	Unadjusted 12 vs 7 days (P < 0.0001)	Unadjusted USD 104,142 vs 54,315 (P < 0.0001)
Tsagalis et al., 2008 [25]	10 years	NIHSS score, CHF, ICH, GFR	30-day mortality 21.8% vs 12.5% (P = 0.001) 10-year mortality 75.9% vs 57.7% (P = 0.001)	10-year HR 1.24 (95% CI 1.07–1.44, P ≤ 0.01), Adjusted for sex, SBP, hematocrit, comorbidities, brain edema, antihypertensives, statin use	Not reported	Not reported	Not reported
Nadkarni et al., 2015 [26] AKI-D only	Hospital discharge	Not performed	AIS: 31.8% vs 5.6% (P ≤ 0.01) ICH: 40.4% vs 28.5% (P ≤ 0.01)	AIS: OR 1.30 (95% CI 1.02–1.48, P ≤ 0.001) ICH: OR 1.95 (95% CI 1.61–2.36, P ≤ 0.01) Adjusted for demographics, hospital characteristics, Charlson comorbidity index and other diagnoses	OR for adverse discharge category AIS: 1.18, 95% CI 1.02–1.37, P ≤ 0.01 ICH: 1.74; 95% CI 1.34–2.24, P ≤ 0.01 Adjusted as for mortality	Unadjusted AIS: 14.1 vs 3.6 days (P ≤ 0.01) ICH: 23.5 vs 5.3 days (P ≤ 0.01)	Unadjusted AIS: USD 32,596 vs 8039 (P ≤ 0.01) ICH: USD 58,111 vs 11,255 (P ≤ 0.01)

Abbreviations: AF, atrial fibrillation; AIS, acute ischemic stroke; AKI, acute kidney injury; AKI-D, acute kidney injury requring dialysis; CHD, coronary heart disease; CHF, congestive heart failure; CT, computerized tomography; CTA, computerized tomography angiography; GFR, glomerular filtration rate; GI, gastrointestinal; ICH, intracranial hemorrhage; IHD, ischemic heart disease; LOS, length of stay; MI, myocardial infarction; mRS, modified Rankin Scale; NIHSS, National Institutes of Health Stroke Scale; OR, Odds Ratio; RIFLE, Risk, Injury, Failure, Loss, End-Stage Renal Disease; SBP, systolic blood pressure; TIA, transient ischemic attack; USD, United States Dollars

1.3–1.4, P < 0.0001); Saeed et al. 2015, OR 1.2 (95% CI 1.1–1.3, P < 0.0001)). A further study [26] utilized an 'adverse discharge' category to classify patients as being discharged to a nursing care facility, hospice or long-term care hospital. Here AKI-D was associated with increased odds of adverse discharge (adjusted OR 1.18, 95% CI 1.02–1.37, P < 0.01 for

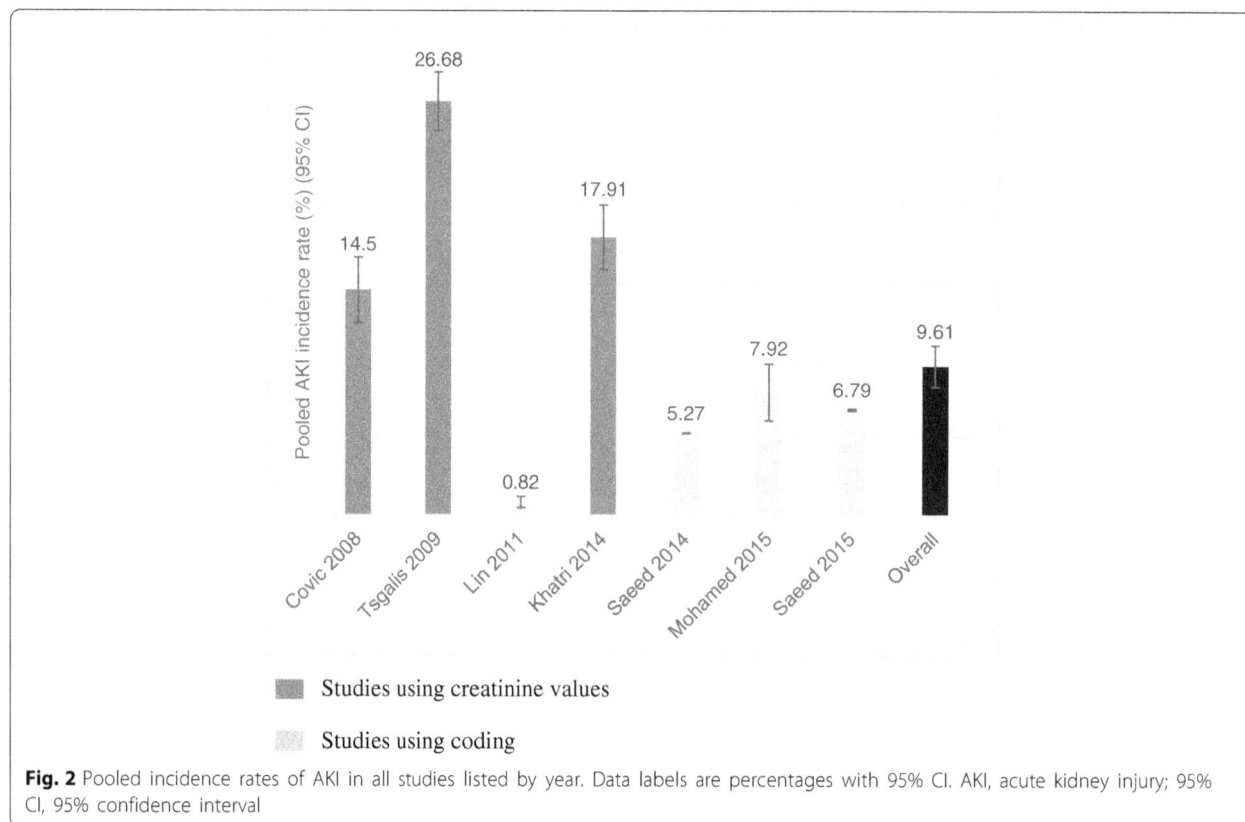

Fig. 2 Pooled incidence rates of AKI in all studies listed by year. Data labels are percentages with 95% CI. AKI, acute kidney injury; 95% CI, 95% confidence interval

ischemic stroke, adjusted OR 1.74; 95% CI, 1.34–2.24; P < 0.01 for ICH) after adjusting for baseline demographics, hospital-level characteristics, Charlson comorbidity index and concurrent diagnoses.

AKI and length of hospital stay and hospitalization costs

Five studies collected data on length of stay (LOS) [20, 22–24, 26]. All studies reported that AKI was associated with an increased length of stay ranging from 2 to 18 extra days spent in hospital (Table 2). In Mohamed et al. [22], this finding persisted after adjustment for age, NIHSS score, previous stroke and insurance status (no OR given, adjusted P < 0.0001).

Three studies analyzed crude inpatient costs using NIS data [23, 24, 26] and all showed AKI was associated with increased inpatients costs ranging from 14,139 to 49,827 US Dollars (Table 2).

AKI and cardiovascular events

One study [25] examined the relationship between AKI after a stroke and long-term cardiovascular events. The probability of having a composite cardiovascular event during the 10-year period was higher in the AKI group than the non-AKI group (cumulative probability 66.8 (95% CI 56.6–76.9) vs 52.7 (95% CI 48.5–56.1); P = 0.001). In a Cox multivariable regression, AKI was an independent predictor of new composite cardiovascular events at 10 years (hazard ratio 1.22; 95% CI 1.01–1.48, P < 0.05)

after adjustment for hypertension, diabetes, stroke subtypes, brain edema on imaging and hematocrit.

AKI and post-thrombolytic ICH

Saeed et al. 2014 [23] found that patients with AKI were more likely to suffer a post-thrombolytic ICH (OR 1.4; 95% CI 1.3–1.6, P < 0.001) after multiple adjustments including age, sex, race/ ethnicity, hypertension, diabetes, AF, dyslipidemia, congestive heart failure, chronic lung disease, myocardial infarction, gastrointestinal bleeding, sepsis and nicotine dependence.

AKI and mortality

Six studies [19, 20, 23–26] compared mortality in AKI versus non-AKI groups with all reporting increased mortality in patients who developed AKI. Two studies reported higher crude mortality rates associated with severity of AKI [19, 20].

Four studies reported in-hospital mortality [20, 23, 24, 26] and two reported 30-day mortality [19, 25]. The OR for all-cause in-hospital mortality in patients with AKI was 2.11 (95% CI 1.09–4.07) with high heterogeneity (I² 100%; Fig. 3). Excluding Saeed et al. 2015, a study of ICH only, the OR increased to 2.67 (95% CI 1.86–3.83) and heterogeneity decreased but remained high (I² 84%). The OR for all-cause 30-day mortality in patients with AKI was 3.13 (95% CI 1.20–8.19), again with high heterogeneity (I² 95%; Fig. 3).

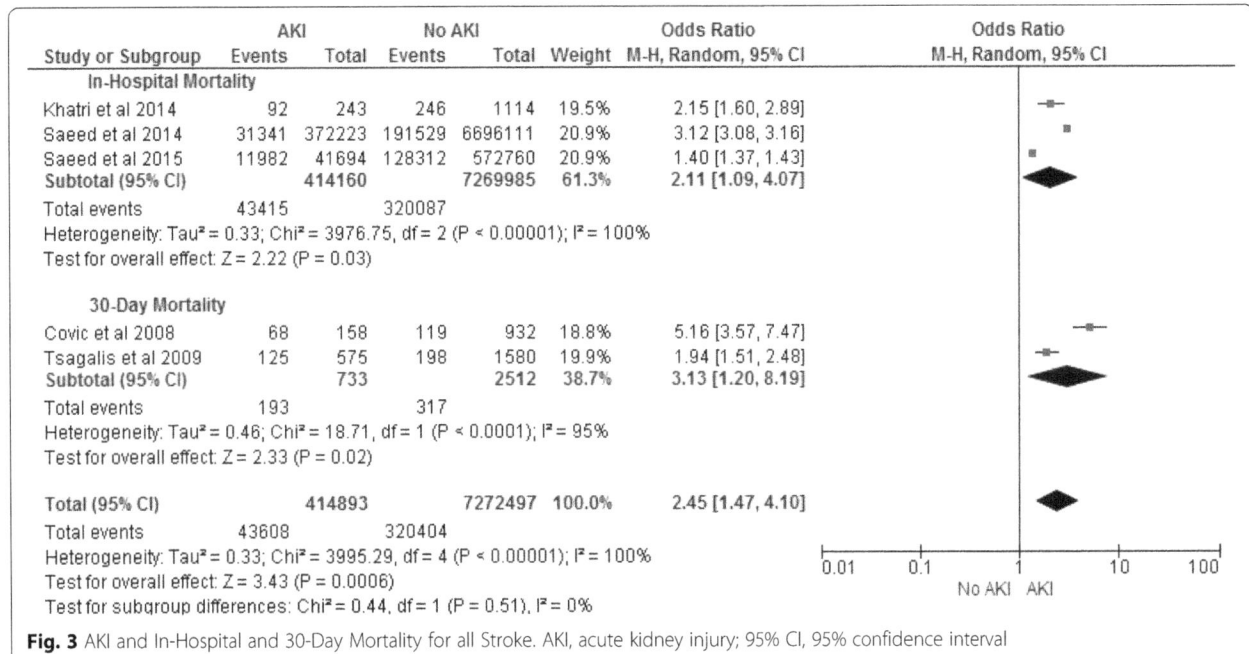

Fig. 3 AKI and In-Hospital and 30-Day Mortality for all Stroke. AKI, acute kidney injury; 95% CI, 95% confidence interval

Two studies [20, 23] provided data on in-hospital mortality after ischemic stroke with a pooled OR of 3.30 (95% CI 2.56–4.26) and low heterogeneity (I² 31%; Fig. 4). Two studies [20, 24] provided data on in-hospital mortality after ICH with a pooled OR of 1.40 (95% CI 1.37–1.43) and low heterogeneity (I² 0%; Fig. 4).

Nadkarni et al. reported an adjusted OR for in-hospital mortality in AKI-D of 1.30 (95% CI 1.12–1.48; $P < 0.001$) in ischemic stroke and 1.95 (95% CI 1.61–2.36; $P < 0.01$) in ICH [26]. Since this study included AKI-D only it was excluded from the meta-analysis. Saeed et al. 2015 reported a higher crude mortality rate in patients with AKI-D than AKI without dialysis (50.2% vs 28.4%, P < 0.001) [24].

Only one study provided long-term mortality data up to 10 years [25], demonstrating higher cumulative mortality in the AKI group at one year (34.6 vs 22.1 in non-AKI group) and 10 years (75.9 vs 57.7; $P = 0.001$). In a Cox proportional hazards model AKI was an independent predictor of 10-year mortality (hazard ratio 1.24; 95% CI 1.07–1.44, P < 0.01) after adjustment for confounders including sex, hypertension, hypercholesterolemia, smoking, systolic blood pressure, brain edema, hematocrit, antihypertensive agent use after the event and ACEi/ARB and statin use on follow-up. The probability of 10-year mortality also increased with severity of AKI.

Discussion

We have shown that reported rates of AKI after stroke vary widely with a range of 0.82% to 26.68%. Increased severity of stroke is related to the risk of AKI. Furthermore, having an episode of AKI after a stroke is associated with worse disability, increased inpatient mortality, LOS and cost, increased risk of future cardiovascular events and longer-term mortality.

There are marked differences in the reported incidence rates depending on the methodology used to identify patients with AKI. Using coding definitions, the pooled incidence of AKI was 4.63%, compared with 19.51% for definitions based on serum creatinine values. ICD coding is known to underestimate the incidence of AKI [29, 30]. Validation of ICD-9 codes for acute renal failure (ARF, which predates present use of the term AKI), used in Saeed et al. 2014 and 2015 are reported to have a sensitivity of 35.4% and a specificity of 97.7%. Thus the low sensitivity for ARF codes may fail to identify patients with mild AKI that is more likely to go unrecognized and uncoded [30]. We know that severe AKI influences a number of outcomes, at high cost to individual patients, the health service and society [14, 31, 32]. Given that milder categories of AKI are much more common they may be even more important to detect and prevent [11, 14, 33]. Furthermore, apart from Nadkarni et al. [26], only one other study reported data on the incidence of AKI-D and outcomes [24]. Since more severe AKI is related to worse outcomes, this is a significant limitation of our meta-analysis. Only three studies reported on the risk factors associated with AKI after stroke [19, 20, 25] and generally confined themselves to reporting on those already known to be associated with AKI. Only two studies reported that stroke severity at presentation was associated with an increased risk of AKI [20, 25]. Two studies reported that hemorrhagic stroke type was associated with the development of AKI [20, 25]. Interestingly, only one study [20] investigated the relationship between radiological contrast exposure and risk of AKI. None of the studies

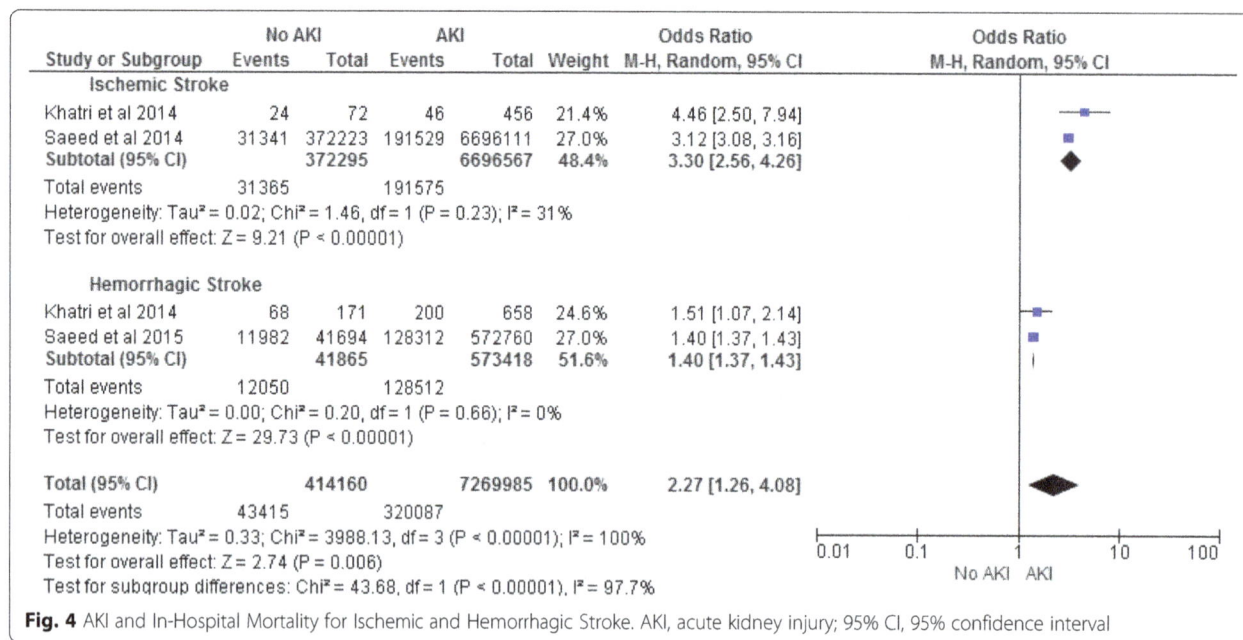

Fig. 4 AKI and In-Hospital Mortality for Ischemic and Hemorrhagic Stroke. AKI, acute kidney injury; 95% CI, 95% confidence interval

presented data on the association between thrombolysis, angiographic procedures or vascular intervention in ischemic stroke and AKI. In light of rapid advances in diagnostic scans and interventional treatments for stroke in recent years, including the use of intra-arterial thrombectomy [3], the incidence of AKI in stroke patients may well increase as these interventions become more widespread [3].

Lower baseline renal function was associated with an increased rate of AKI in three of the studies in this systematic review [19, 20, 25]. Patients with CKD are known to have poorer outcomes after a stroke [34–36]. This leads to the question of whether AKI adds further clinical relevance to what is already known about CKD and stroke. Of the studies that excluded patients with CKD [23, 24], AKI was still a clinically significant determinant of both disability and in-hospital mortality after adjustment for multiple confounding factors. Two further studies found AKI was still associated with worse outcomes after adjustment for baseline renal function or CKD category [20, 25]. This supports the theory that AKI is not merely an extension of the CKD spectrum and represents an important standalone factor that predicts worse outcomes in patients with acute stroke.

Our systematic review demonstrates a clear association between AKI and short-term mortality after stroke. This effect persisted after adjustment for CKD in three studies [19, 22, 26]. A further study [25] also found a relationship between AKI and long-term mortality, up to 10 years post stroke, after adjustment for CKD and post-stroke pharmacological treatments. This is consistent with the effect of AKI on short and long-term mortality in the context of other acute illnesses including myocardial infarction, sepsis and major surgery [37–41]. It is therefore, possible that interventions to prevent AKI may improve outcomes after stroke.

Our study has several strengths in that it encompassed several studies, all within the last decade with a large cumulative sample size and a large number of statistical adjustments. However, there are several significant limitations. Firstly, there was disproportionate representation of US data, accounting for 99.9% of the patient sample, which clearly affects generalizability of the estimates. There may also be significant ascertainment bias in view of the US being a high income country with increased availability of blood test monitoring and other diagnostic tests. Secondly, the number of studies included in the systematic review was small and those included in the meta-analysis smaller still. Despite sensitivity analyses, heterogeneity between studies remained substantial potentially suggesting that these studies should not be combined in a meta-analysis. However, we opted to present the data, warts and all, as this both highlights the need for further research in this area but also gives potential future researchers some idea of the numbers needed for recruitment into studies, as well as the rate and range of AKI to be expected using different definitions.

Conclusions

AKI appears to be a very common complication in hospitalized stroke patients and is associated with increased mortality, disability and healthcare costs. As a potentially preventable condition, further studies are needed in this area to attenuate the effects of AKI, including longer-term morbidity and mortality and the development of CKD. However in the first instance, additional representative studies, ideally using creatinine-based definitions of AKI are required to accurately determine point estimates of AKI post stroke and both short and long-term outcomes.

Abbreviations

ACEi: Angiotensin-converting enzyme inhibitor; AF: Atrial fibrillation; AKI: Acute kidney injury; AKI-D: Acute kidney injury requiring dialysis treatment; AKIN: Acute Kidney Injury Network; ARB: Angiotensin II receptor blocker; ARF: Acute renal failure; CKD: Chronic kidney disease; CT: Computerized tomography; CVA: Cerebrovascular accident; ESRD: End-stage renal disease; GFR: Glomerular filtration rate; ICD-9/10: International Classification of Diseases-9th/10th Edition; ICH: Intracranial hemorrhage; IHD: Ischemic heart disease; mRS: modified Rankin Scale; NIHSS: National Institutes of Health Stroke Scale; NIS: Nationwide Inpatient Sample; OR: Odds ratio; PRISMA: Preferred Reporting Items for Systematic Reviews and Meta-Analyses; PROSPERO: International prospective register of systematic reviews; RIFLE: Risk/ Injury/ Failure/ Loss/ End-stage; RRT: Renal replacement therapy; TIA: Transient ischemic attack; TOAST: Trial of ORG 10172 in Acute Stroke Treatment; WHO: World Health Organization

Acknowledgements

We would like to acknowledge and thank Peter Nightingale of University Hospitals Birmingham NHS Foundation Trust for his statistical expertise and input in analysis for this systematic review.

Authors' contributions

JA and KN devised the search strategy and collected data, overseen by CF. JA and CF carried out quality assessment of the studies, synthesized data and conducted the meta-analysis. KN, DS, PG and PC interpreted the results and contributed to the manuscript. All authors read and approved the final version.

Competing interests

The authors declare that they have no competing interests.

Author details

[1]Department of Nephrology, University Hospitals Birmingham, Birmingham B15 2WB, UK. [2]Department of Stroke, University Hospitals Birmingham, Birmingham, UK. [3]Institute of Applied Health Research, College of Medical and Dental Sciences, University of Birmingham, Birmingham, UK. [4]Warwick Medical School, University of Warwick, Coventry, UK.

References

1. Prabhakaran S, Ruff I, Bernstein RA. Acute stroke intervention: a systematic review. JAMA. 2015;313(14):1451–62.
2. Organisation, W.H. WHO Mortality Database. [cited 9 March 2017; Available from: http://www.who.int/healthinfo/mortality_data/en/.
3. Arnold J, Sims D, Ferro CJ. Modulation of stroke risk in chronic kidney disease. Clin Kidney J. 2016;9(1):29–38.
4. Writing Group Members, et al. Heart disease and stroke Statistics-2016 update: a report from the American Heart Association. Circulation. 2016; 133(4):e38–360.
5. Tomiyama H, Yamashina A. Clinical considerations for the association between vascular damage and chronic kidney disease. Pulse (Basel). 2014; 2(1–4):81–94.
6. Murray AM. The brain and the kidney connection: a model of accelerated vascular cognitive impairment. Neurology. 2009;73(12):916–7.
7. Masson P, et al. Chronic kidney disease and the risk of stroke: a systematic review and meta-analysis. Nephrol Dial Transplant. 2015;30(7):1162–9.
8. KDIGO. Clinical practice guideline for acute kidney injury. Kidney Int Suppl. 2012;2(1):1–138.
9. Mehta RL, et al. Acute kidney injury network: report of an initiative to improve outcomes in acute kidney injury. Crit Care. 2007;11(2):R31.
10. Bellomo R, et al. Acute renal failure - definition, outcome measures, animal models, fluid therapy and information technology needs: the second international consensus conference of the acute Dialysis quality initiative (ADQI) group. Crit Care. 2004;8(4):R204–12.
11. Praught ML, Shlipak MG. Are small changes in serum creatinine an important risk factor? Curr Opin Nephrol Hypertens. 2005;14(3):265–70.
12. Hoste EA, et al. RIFLE criteria for acute kidney injury are associated with hospital mortality in critically ill patients: a cohort analysis. Crit Care. 2006;10(3):R73.
13. Lewington AJ, Cerda J, Mehta RL. Raising awareness of acute kidney injury: a global perspective of a silent killer. Kidney Int. 2013;84(3):457–67.
14. Chertow GM, et al. Acute kidney injury, mortality, length of stay, and costs in hospitalized patients. J Am Soc Nephrol. 2005;16(11):3365–70.
15. Tan J, et al. Warfarin use and stroke, bleeding and mortality risk in patients with end stage renal disease and atrial fibrillation: a systematic review and meta-analysis. BMC Nephrol. 2016;17(1):157.
16. Moher D, et al. Preferred reporting items for systematic reviews and meta-analyses: the PRISMA statement. PLoS Med. 2009;6(7):e1000097.
17. Susantitaphong P, et al. World incidence of AKI: a meta-analysis. Clin J Am Soc Nephrol. 2013;8(9):1482–93.
18. Wells GA, S.B., O'Connell D, Peterson J, Welch V, Losos M, et al. The Newcastle-Ottawa Scale (NOS) for assessing the quality if nonrandomized studies in meta-analyses. [cited 2017 03/03/2017]; Available from: http://www.ohri.ca/programs/clinical_epidemiology/oxford.asp.
19. Covic A, et al. The impact of acute kidney injury on short-term survival in an eastern European population with stroke. Nephrol Dial Transplant. 2008; 23(7):2228–34.
20. Khatri M, et al. Acute kidney injury is associated with increased hospital mortality after stroke. J Stroke Cerebrovasc Dis. 2014;23(1):25–30.
21. Lin S, et al. Characteristics, treatment and outcome of ischemic stroke with atrial fibrillation in a Chinese hospital-based stroke study. Cerebrovasc Dis. 2011;31(5):419–26.
22. Mohamed W, et al. Which comorbidities and complications predict ischemic stroke recovery and length of stay? Neurologist. 2015;20(2):27–32.
23. Saeed F, et al. Acute renal failure is associated with higher death and disability in patients with acute ischemic stroke: analysis of nationwide inpatient sample. Stroke. 2014;45(5):1478–80.
24. Saeed F, et al. Acute renal failure worsens in-hospital outcomes in patients with intracerebral hemorrhage. J Stroke Cerebrovasc Dis. 2015;24(4):789–94.
25. Tsagalis G, et al. Long-term prognosis of acute kidney injury after first acute stroke. Clin J Am Soc Nephrol. 2009;4(3):616–22.
26. Nadkarni GN, et al. Dialysis requiring acute kidney injury in acute cerebrovascular accident hospitalizations. Stroke. 2015;46(11):3226–31.
27. Aho K, et al. Cerebrovascular disease in the community: results of a WHO collaborative study. Bull World Health Organ. 1980;58(1):113–30.
28. Adams HP Jr, et al. Classification of subtype of acute ischemic stroke. Definitions for use in a multicenter clinical trial. TOAST. Trial of org 10172 in acute stroke treatment. Stroke. 1993;24(1):35–41.
29. Waikar SS, et al. Validity of international classification of diseases, ninth revision, clinical modification codes for acute renal failure. J Am Soc Nephrol. 2006;17(6):1688–94.
30. Jannot AS, et al. The diagnosis-wide landscape of hospital-acquired AKI. Clin J Am Soc Nephrol. 2017;12(6):874–84.
31. Silver SA, Chertow GM. The economic consequences of acute kidney injury. Nephron. 2017.
32. Bedford M, et al. What is the real impact of acute kidney injury? BMC Nephrol. 2014;15:95.
33. Lassnigg A, et al. Minimal changes of serum creatinine predict prognosis in patients after cardiothoracic surgery: a prospective cohort study. J Am Soc Nephrol. 2004;15(6):1597–605.
34. Lozano R, et al. Global and regional mortality from 235 causes of death for 20 age groups in 1990 and 2010: a systematic analysis for the global burden of disease study 2010. Lancet. 2012;380(9859):2095–128.
35. Silverwood RJ, et al. Cognitive and kidney function: results from a British birth cohort reaching retirement age. PLoS One. 2014;9(1):e86743.
36. Coresh J, et al. Prevalence of chronic kidney disease in the United States. JAMA. 2007;298(17):2038–47.
37. Levy EM, Viscoli CM, Horwitz RI. The effect of acute renal failure on mortality. A cohort analysis. JAMA. 1996;275(19):1489–94.
38. Wang HE, et al. Acute kidney injury and mortality in hospitalized patients. Am J Nephrol. 2012;35(4):349–55.
39. Coca SG, et al. Long-term risk of mortality and other adverse outcomes after acute kidney injury: a systematic review and meta-analysis. Am J Kidney Dis. 2009;53(6):961–73.
40. Karkouti K, et al. Acute kidney injury after cardiac surgery: focus on modifiable risk factors. Circulation. 2009;119(4):495–502.
41. Bihorac A, et al. Long-term risk of mortality and acute kidney injury during hospitalization after major surgery. Ann Surg. 2009;249(5):851–8.

8

Serum levels of tumor necrosis factor alpha in patients with IgA nephropathy are closely associated with disease severity

Guanhong Li[1], Wei Wu[2], Xinyao Zhang[2], Yuan Huang[2], Yubing Wen[1], Xuemei Li[1] and Ruitong Gao[1*]

Abstract

Background: Tumor necrosis factor alpha (TNF-α) is considered to play an important role in the pathogenesis in IgA nephropathy (IgAN). The correlations between serum TNF-α and disease severity in patients with IgAN remain controversial.

Methods: Concentrations of serum TNF-α of 147 patients with IgAN and 126 healthy subjects were measured by chemiluminescence immunoassay. Correlations with clinicopathological features of patients with IgAN were evaluated.

Results: Serum levels of TNF-α [9.20 (7.70–10.60) pg/mL vs. 6.04 (5.11–7.23) pg/mL, $P < 0.0001$] were higher in patients with IgAN than that in healthy subjects. Receiver operating characteristic curve analysis revealed that TNF-α had better discrimination between patients with IgAN and healthy controls than estimated glomerular filtration rate [TNF-α: (AUC, 0.87; 95% CI, 0.83–0.91; $P < 0.0001$) vs. estimated glomerular filtration rate: (AUC, 0.76; 95% CI, 0.71–0.82; $P < 0.0001$), $P = 0.007$]. Multivariate linear regression analyses showed that serum levels of TNF-α were positively correlated with 24-h urine protein excretion ($r = 0.33$, $P = 0.04$), urinary protein to serum creatinine ratio ($r = 0.33$, $P = 0.03$), serum creatinine ($r = 0.46$, $P < 0.0001$) and Cystatin C ($r = 0.59$, $P < 0.0001$) in IgAN and negatively correlated with estimated glomerular filtration rate ($r = -0.49$, $P < 0.0001$) after adjustment for sex, systolic blood pressure and diastolic blood pressure. Patients with higher mesangial hypercellularity or tubular atrophy/interstitial fibrosis score according to Oxford classification showed higher serum levels of TNF-α.

Conclusions: Our data showed that serum levels of TNF-α detected by chemiluminescence immunoassay was a potential biomarker for evaluating the disease severity in IgAN.

Keywords: Biomarkers, Cytokines, Tumor necrosis factor alpha, IgA nephropathy

Background

IgA nephropathy (IgAN) is the most common cause of primary glomerulonephritis [1]. IgAN is associated with a poor prognosis, about 20–40% of patients with IgAN progress slowly to end-stage renal failure 20–25 years after diagnosis [2, 3]. Heavy proteinuria, hypertension, renal dysfunction, and histological features recently updated Oxford classification have been identified as clinicopathological markers for disease severity and poor prognosis of IgAN [4, 5]. However, these factors are numerous and controversial, and do not always have the specificity to

identify an individual prognosis [2, 4]. Recently, several biomarkers such as serum galactose-deficient IgA1 and the corresponding autoantibodies [6, 7], soluble CD89 levels [8], urinary soluble transferrin receptor [9], urinary interleukin-6/epidermal growth factor (IL-6/EGF) [10] and other serum and urine biomarkers are associated with histological findings of severity and poor outcomes in IgAN. However, the utility of these biomarkers is not yet well defined.

It is considered that cytokines such as tumor necrosis factor-α (TNF-α) play an important role in aberrant mucosal immune response in the early phase of the pathogenesis in IgAN [11, 12], and mesangial cell proliferation, hyperproduction of extracellular matrices, podocyte injury and glomerulosclerosis in the second phase [13].

* Correspondence: gaoruitong@gmail.com
[1]Division of Nephrology, Department of Internal Medicine, Peking Union Medical College Hospital, Chinese Academy of Medical Sciences & Peking Union Medical College, NO.1, Shuaifuyuan, Dongcheng District, Beijing 100730, China
Full list of author information is available at the end of the article

Furthermore, our recent study showed that hydroxychloroquine (HCQ) targeting cytokines including TNF-α was effective in ameliorating proteinuria [14]. Therefore, serum TNF-α may be a potential biomarker for severity in IgAN.

However, the studies concerning serum levels of TNF-α as a biomarker in IgAN were inadequate. The relationship between serum TNF-α levels and clinical parameters, pathological features had not been fully established in IgAN [15, 16].

Concerning the detection method of TNF-α, enzyme linked immunosorbent assay (ELISA) is still recommended. Recently, because of the high sensitivity, rapidity of reaction, simple instrumentation, and wide dynamic range, fully automated chemiluminescence immunoassay (CLIA) has been used as an attractive method in different fields, such as biotechnology, pharmacology, molecular biology [17, 18]. And CLIA has also been used to detect TNF-α in the clinical laboratory of our hospital.

Therefore, in this study, we investigated the value of serum levels of TNF-α in a large sample of patients, detected by CLIA with higher sensitivity and better stability, aiming to explore the role of TNF-α in evaluating disease severity in IgAN.

Methods

Patients

Serum samples were collected from 147 patients with biopsy-proven primary IgAN between July 2016 and April 2017. The patients accepted renal biopsy between November 1999 and December 2016. In addition, 126 serum samples were collected from healthy volunteers who had no known kidney diseases between August 2015 and February 2016. Clinical and laboratory data were collected at the time of cytokines measurement in the clinical laboratory of Peking Union Medical College Hospital. Patients with lupus nephritis, Henoch–Schönlein purpura, liver cirrhosis and other secondary causes of IgAN were excluded from the study. Patients with concomitant systemic disease, autoimmune diseases, neoplastic diseases and infection which might cause abnormal elevation of serum TNF-α or IL-6 were also excluded. All patients gave written informed consent to the study, which had received Local Ethical Committee approval.

Clinical and pathological features

Full medical histories and physical findings were documented. The demographic and the clinical parameters of patients including age, gender, blood pressure (BP), urinary red blood cells count, urine protein/creatinine ratio, 24-h urine protein excretion were recorded. Blood chemistry tests included serum creatinine, Cystatin C and IgA. Estimated glomerular filtration rate (eGFR) was calculated using the Chronic Kidney Disease Epidemiology

Collaboration (CKD-EPI) equation [19]. Chronic Kidney Disease (CKD) stages 1–5 were divided by eGFR≥90 (G1), 60–89 (G2), 45–59 (G3a), 30–44 (G3b), 15–29 (G4), and < 15 (G5) mL/min/1.73 m^2, respectively, according to the new KDIGO (Kidney Disease: Improving Global Outcomes) classification [20]. Histologically, the updated Oxford classification was used for evaluating the pathological lesion [5].

Medication history, including the usage of cortisone, immunosuppressant and renin-angiotensin system blockers such as angiotensin-converting enzymes inhibitors (ACE-Is) and angiotensin II receptor blockers (ARBs) was also recorded.

Measuring serum TNF-α

Blood samples were obtained from each patient after an overnight fast upon admission. The blood samples were allowed to clot at room temperature for 30 mins and centrifuged for 10 minutes at 3000 rpm. The serum samples were separated as soon as possible from the clot of red cells after centrifugation to avoid TNF-α production by blood cells that falsely could increase its values. Separated sera were measured immediately. Levels of serum TNF-α were measured in the clinical laboratory at Peking Union Medical College Hospital using Tumor necrosis factor-alpha Assay Kit (chemiluminescent assay) through IMMULITE® 1000 system (Siemens Healthcare Diagnostics Inc., United Kingdom) according to the manufacturers' instructions. Detection limit of the kits was obtained from the manufacturers, as follows: TNF-α (detection limit 1.7–1000 pg/mL). The recommended reference range was as follows: TNF-α (≤ 8.1 pg/mL).

Statistical analysis

Statistical calculations were performed using SPSS software for Windows, version 20.0 (SPSS Inc., Chicago, IL) and Graph Pad Prism 5.0 (Graph Pad Software Inc., San Diego, CA). Data are presented as medians (interquartile range) or frequency in percent according to the types of variables. The Mann–Whitney U-test was used for statistical comparisons between two groups, and the Kruskal-Wallis Test was used for statistical comparisons among more than two groups. Categorical variables were compared using chi-squared test. To set the cut-off values between IgAN patients and healthy controls (HC), we used the receiver operating characteristic (ROC) curve analyses to find the best compromise value between sensitivity and specificity; we also calculated area under the curve (AUC) with 95% confidence interval (CI) and P values. Serum levels of TNF-α were subjected to logarithmic transformation before correlation analyses. Bivariate correlation analyses were performed using Spearman's correlation analysis. Multivariate linear regression analyses adjusted for sex, systolic BP and dia-stolic BP were performed to examine the correlations between serum levels of TNF-α and clinical parameters. All tests were two-sided and a P-value < 0.05 was considered statistically significant.

Results

Demographic and clinical features in the IgAN patients and healthy subjects

In our study, 147 patients with IgAN [mean age, 35 (29–45) years; male/female ratio, 71/76] and 126 healthy subjects [mean age, 40 (30–49) years; male/female ratio, 61/65] were involved. The main demographic, clinical and the pathological features of patients with IgAN were summarized in Table 1. The average levels of BP, 24-h urine protein excretion, and eGFR were 120 (110–130) / 75 (70–80) mmHg, 0.82 (0.38–1.55) g/24 h, 79.29 (60.00–104.29) mL/min•1.73m^2, respectively. In this study, 35 (23.8%) IgAN patients were untreated, 99 (67.3%) were treated with ACE-Is/ARBs, 71 (48.3%) were treated with oral corticosteroids, and 76 (51.7%) were treated with other immunosuppressive agents at the time of sample collection. The detailed demographic and clinical data of healthy subjects were showed in Additional file 1.

Serum levels of TNF-α in patients with IgAN and controls

As showed in Fig. 1, serum levels of TNF-α [9.20 (7.70–10.60) pg/mL vs. 6.04 (5.11–7.23) pg/mL, P < 0.0001] were significantly higher in IgAN group than that in HC group.

Prediction values of TNF-α in patients with IgAN

ROC analysis confirmed that TNF-α had better discrimination between patients with IgAN and healthy controls (HC) than eGFR [TNF-α: (AUC, 0.87; 95% CI, 0.83–0.91; P < 0.0001) vs. eGFR: (AUC, 0.76; 95% CI, 0.71–0.82; P < 0.0001), P = 0.007] (Fig. 2a and Fig. 2b). The respective optimal derived cut-off values were 7.79 pg/mL (Sensitivity: 74.8%; Specificity: 86.5%) for TNF-α, 80.36 mL/min•1.73m^2 (Sensitivity: 96.8%; Specificity: 52.4%) for eGFR.

Comparison of clinical and pathological features between patients with and without elevated serum TNF-α

We divided the patients into two subgroups based on the reference range of TNF-α which was established by the clinical laboratory in our hospital. The recommended reference range of serum TNF-α was from non-detectable to 8.1 pg/mL. Among 147 patients with IgAN, 98 patients were with elevated serum TNF-α and 49 patients were without elevated serum TNF-α. As showed in Table 2, compared with patients without elevated serum levels of TNF-α, patients with elevated serum levels of TNF-α had older age (P = 0.03) and

higher proportion of male patients (P = 0.047). Significantly higher levels of systolic BP (P = 0.001), diastolic BP (P = 0.02), mean arterial pressure (P = 0.003), 24-h urine protein excretion (P = 0.03), urinary protein to serum creatinine ratio (P = 0.009), serum creatinine (P < 0.0001), Cystatin C (P < 0.0001) and lower levels of eGFR (P < 0.0001) were showed in patients with elevated serum levels of TNF-α. Proportions of mesangial hypercellularity (P = 0.04), segmental glomerulosclerosis (P = 0.02) and tubular atrophy/interstitial fibrosis grade (P = 0.008) were significantly higher in patients with elevated TNF-α than that in patients without elevated TNF-α.

Correlations between serum levels of TNF-α and clinical features of patients with IgAN

Significant higher serum levels of TNF-α were observed in male patients with IgAN than that in female patients [9.70 (8.10–11.10) pg/mL vs. 8.50 (7.20–10.38) pg/mL, P = 0.02]. Serum levels of TNF-α were significantly positively correlated with systolic BP (r = 0.30, P < 0.0001), diastolic BP (r = 0.19, P = 0.02), 24-h urine protein excretion (r = 0.22, P = 0.007), urinary protein to serum creatinine ratio (r = 0.26, P = 0.002), serum creatinine (r = 0.49, P < 0.0001) and Cystatin C (r = 0.51, P < 0.0001) in IgAN. And serum levels of TNF-α were negatively correlated with eGFR (r = – 0.47, P < 0.0001) in bivariate correlation analysis (Table 3). Serum levels of TNF-α was not significantly correlated with age, serum IgA levels or urinary red blood cells count. Multivariate linear regression analyses showed that serum levels of TNF-α were positively correlated with 24-h urine protein excretion (r = 0.33, P = 0.04), urinary protein to serum creatinine ratio (r = 0.33, P = 0.03), serum creatinine (r = 0.46, P < 0.0001) and Cystatin C (r = 0.59, P < 0.0001) in IgAN and negatively correlated with eGFR (r = – 0.49, P < 0.0001) after adjustment for sex, systolic BP and diastolic BP (Table 3).

Correlations between serum levels of TNF-α, and pathological features of patients with IgAN

As showed in Fig. 3, IgAN patients with higher scores in the variable mesangial hypercellularity showed significant higher serum levels of TNF-α [M1: 9.30 (7.90–10.60) pg/mL vs. M0: 6.70 (6.00–10.58) pg/mL, P = 0.03]. Patients with higher scores in the variable tubular atrophy/interstitial fibrosis grade showed higher serum levels of TNF-α [T2:10.60 (8.25–12.85) pg/mL vs. T1: 9.20 (8.00–10.20) pg/mL vs. T0: 8.20 (6.70–10.05) pg/mL, overall P = 0.001]. Serum levels of TNF-α in patients with tubular atrophy/interstitial fibrosis grade T2 were significantly higher than that in grade T0 [T2:10.60 (8.25–12.85) pg/mL vs. T0: 6.70 (6.00–10.58) pg/mL, P = 0.0005] and T1 [T2: 10.60 (8.25–12.85) pg/mL vs. T1: 9.20 (8.00–10.20) pg/mL,

Table 1 Demographic, clinical and pathological features of patients with IgA nephropathy

Characteristics	Values
Patients numbers	147
Cytokines–biopsy time interval[a] (months)	27.93 (6.17–63.37)
Mean age (yr)	35 (29–45)
Male, n (%)	71 (48.3)
Systolic BP (mmHg)	120 (110–130)
Diastolic BP (mmHg)	75 (70–80)
Mean arterial pressure (mmHg)	90 (83–97)
Urinary red blood cell (/μL)	29 (7–79)
Urinary protein to serum creatinine ratio (mg/g Cr)	595 (244–1305)
24-h urine protein excretion (g/24 h)	0.82 (0.38–1.55)
< 0.3	27 (18.4%)
0.3–0.99	59 (40.1%)
1.0–2.99	46 (31.3%)
≥ 3	15 (10.2%)
Serum creatinine (mg/dL)	1.07 (0.84–1.39)
Serum IgA (g/L)	2.22 (1.82–3.22)
Cystatin C (mg/dL)	1.06 (0.93–1.57)
eGFR (mL/min·1.73m^2)[b]	79.29 (60.00–104.29)
CKD Stages[c], n (%)	
1	57 (38.8)
2	49 (33.3)
3a	22 (15.0)
3b	8 (5.4)
4	5 (3.4)
5	6 (4.1)
Oxford classification[d], n (%)	
M0/ M1	16(10.9), 131(89.1)
E0/E1	113(76.9), 34(23.1)
S0/S1	24(16.3), 123(83.7)
T0/T1/T2	45(30.6), 65(44.2), 37(44.2)
C0/C1/C2	66(44.9), 66(44.9), 15(10.2)
Medical treatments, n (%)	
Untreated	35 (23.8)
Corticosteroids	71 (48.3)
Immunosuppressants	76 (51.7)
ACE-Is/ARBs	99 (67.3)

Data are presented as median (interquartile range) or frequency in percent

BP: blood pressure; 1 mmHg = 0.133Kpa; eGFR: estimated glomerular filtration rate; ACE-Is: angiotensin converting enzyme inhibitors; ARBs: angiotensin II receptor blockers. M: mesangial hypercellularity score < 0.5 (M0) or > 0.5 (M1); E: endocapillary hypercellularity absent (E0) or present (E1); S: segmental glomerulosclerosis absent (S0) or present (S1), presence or absence of podocyte hypertrophy/tip lesions in biopsy specimens with S1; T: tubular atrophy/interstitial fibrosis < 25% (T0), 26–50% (T1), or > 50% (T2); C: cellular/fibrocellular crescents absent (C0), present in at least 1 glomerulus (C1), in > 25% of glomeruli (C2)

[a]Time interval between renal biopsy of patients with IgA nephropathy and sample collection

[b]eGFR was calculated according to the Chronic Kidney Disease Epidemiology Collaboration (CKD-EPI) equation [19]

[c]CKD stages 1–5 were divided by eGFR≥90 (G1), 60–89 (G2), 45–59 (G3a), 30–44 (G3b), 15–29 (G4), and < 15 (G5) mL/min/1.73 m^2, respectively, according to the new KDIGO (Kidney Disease: Improving Global Outcomes) classification [20]

[d]Determined in accordance with the Oxford classification [5]

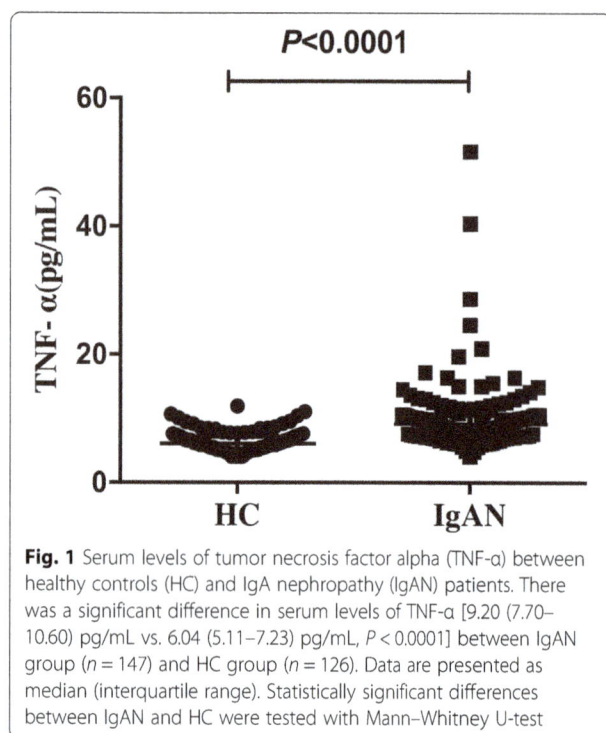

Fig. 1 Serum levels of tumor necrosis factor alpha (TNF-α) between healthy controls (HC) and IgA nephropathy (IgAN) patients. There was a significant difference in serum levels of TNF-α [9.20 (7.70–10.60) pg/mL vs. 6.04 (5.11–7.23) pg/mL, $P < 0.0001$] between IgAN group ($n = 147$) and HC group ($n = 126$). Data are presented as median (interquartile range). Statistically significant differences between IgAN and HC were tested with Mann–Whitney U-test

$P = 0.02$]; But there was no difference between patients with grade T1 and T0 ($P = 0.05$). However, serum levels of TNF-α in patients with different scores of endocapillary hypercellularity, segmental glomerulosclerosis and cellular/fibrocellular crescents show no significant difference ($P > 0.05$).

Discussion

TNF-α is a kind of proinflammatory cytokines that has been involved in certain forms of immune-mediated renal injury, including IgAN [21]. In the present research, we enrolled 147 IgAN patients and investigated the correlations between the serum levels of TNF-α detected by CLIA and the clinicopathological features. Results showed serum levels of TNF-α were significantly higher in patients with IgAN than in healthy subjects. The ROC analysis revealed that the optimal cut-off value of serum TNF-α had better discrimination between IgAN patients and healthy subjects than eGFR. In addition, serum TNF-α significantly correlated with urine protein, and renal function on both bivariate and multivariate linear regression analysis. And serum TNF-α also correlated with mesangial hypercellularity and tubular atrophy/interstitial fibrosis according to Oxford classification in IgAN.

D'Amico G has come the concordance that severe proteinuria, arterial hypertension and impairment of renal function were the strongest and most reliable clinical predictors for an unfavorable prognosis after critical

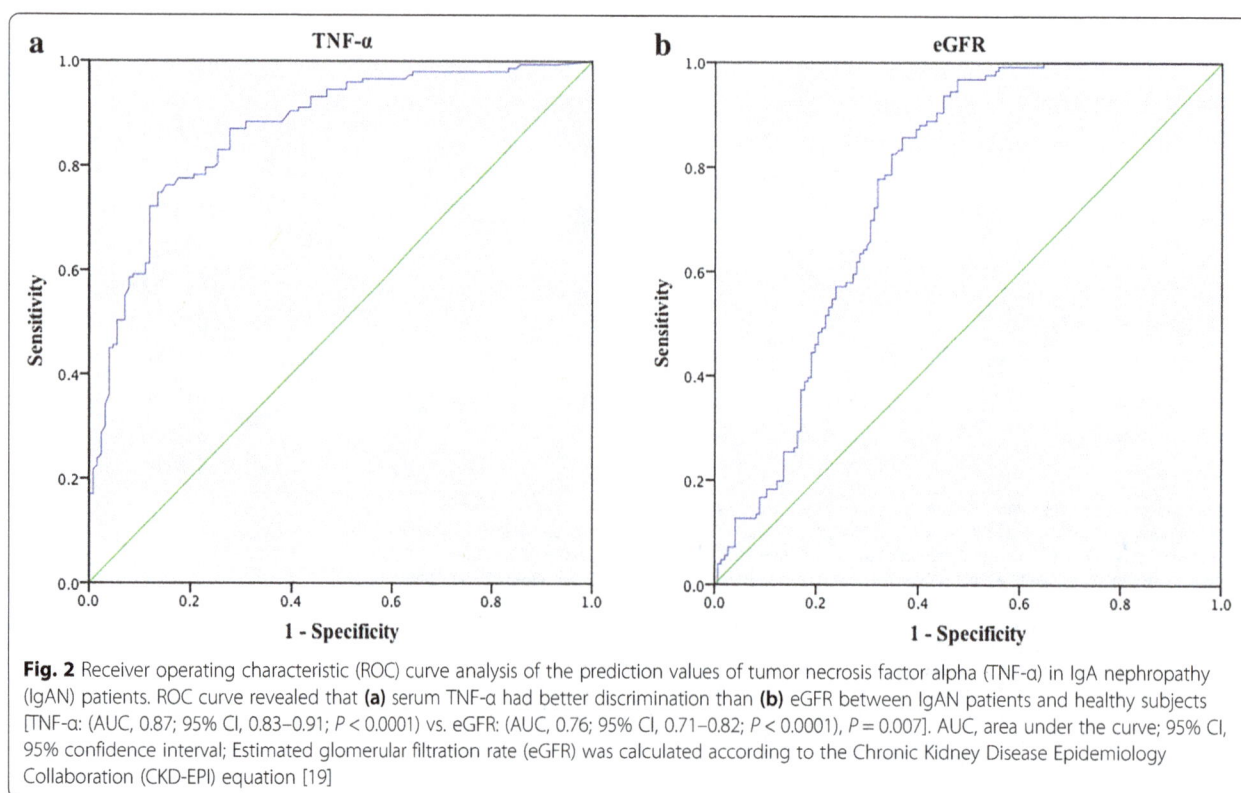

Fig. 2 Receiver operating characteristic (ROC) curve analysis of the prediction values of tumor necrosis factor alpha (TNF-α) in IgA nephropathy (IgAN) patients. ROC curve revealed that (a) serum TNF-α had better discrimination than (b) eGFR between IgAN patients and healthy subjects [TNF-α: (AUC, 0.87; 95% CI, 0.83–0.91; $P < 0.0001$) vs. eGFR: (AUC, 0.76; 95% CI, 0.71–0.82; $P < 0.0001$), $P = 0.007$]. AUC, area under the curve; 95% CI, 95% confidence interval; Estimated glomerular filtration rate (eGFR) was calculated according to the Chronic Kidney Disease Epidemiology Collaboration (CKD-EPI) equation [19]

Table 2 Demographic, clinical and pathological features of patients with and without elevated serum TNF-α

Characteristics	Subgroups		P Value
	TNF-α ≤ 8.1 pg/mL	TNF-α > 8.1 pg/mL	
Patients numbers	49	98	
Cytokines–biopsy time interval[a] (months)	25.93 (5.27–55.90)	28.55 (7.14–67.47)	0.63
Mean age (yr)	33 (28–41)	40 (29–47)	0.03
Male, n (%)	18 (36.7)	53 (54.1)	0.047
Systolic BP (mmHg)	120 (110–120)	120 (118–130)	0.001
Diastolic BP (mmHg)	70 (60–80)	80 (70–80)	0.02
Mean arterial pressure (mmHg)	87 (78–93)	93 (87–97)	0.003
Urinary red blood cell (/μL)	34 (7–131)	22 (7–67)	0.13
Urinary protein to serum creatinine ratio (mg/g Cr)	486 (159–881)	756 (335–1596)	0.009
24-h urine protein excretion (g/24 h)	0.68 (0.30–1.09)	0.99 (0.40–1.70)	0.03
< 0.3	12 (24.5%)	15 (15.3%)	0.009
0.3–0.99	23 (46.9%)	36 (36.7%)	
1.0–2.99	13 (26.5%)	33 (33.7%)	
≥ 3	1 (2.0%)	14 (14.3%)	
Serum creatinine (mg/dL)	0.89 (0.72–1.07)	1.19 (0.92–1.52)	< 0.0001
Cystatin C (mg/dL)	0.98 (0.79–1.12)	1.22 (1.00–2.00)	< 0.0001
eGFR (mL/min·1.73m^2)[b]	92.95 (73.96–118.78)	70.94 (52.26–91.57)	< 0.0001
CKD Stages[c], n (%)			< 0.0001
1	30 (61.2)	27 (27.6)	
2	15 (30.6)	34 (34.7)	
3a	2 (4.1)	20 (20.4)	
3b	1 (2.0)	7 (7.1)	
4	1 (2.0)	4 (4.1)	
5	0 (0.0)	6 (6.1)	
Oxford classification[d], n (%)			
M0/ M1	9 (18.4), 40 (81.6)	7 (7.1),91 (92.9)	0.04
E0/E1	38 (77.6), 11 (22.4)	75 (76.5), 23 (23.5)	0.89
S0/S1	13 (26.5), 36 (73.5)	11 (11.2), 87 (88.8)	0.02
T0/T1/T2	22 (44.9), 19 (38.8), 8 (16.3)	23 (23.5), 46 (46.9), 29 (29.6)	0.008
C0/C1/C2	22 (44.9), 23 (46.9), 4 (8.2)	44 (44.9), 43 (43.9), 11 (11.2)	0.79
Medical treatments, n (%)			
Untreated	10 (20.4)	25 (25.5)	0.49
Corticosteroids	22 (44.9)	49 (50.0)	0.56
Immunosuppressants	26 (53.1)	50 (51.0)	0.82
ACE-Is/ARBs	34 (69.4)	65 (66.3)	0.71

Data are presented as median (interquartile range) or frequency in percent

BP: blood pressure; 1 mmHg = 0.133Kpa; eGFR: estimated glomerular filtration rate; M: mesangial hypercellularity score < 0.5 (M0) or > 0.5 (M1); E: endocapillary hypercellularity absent (E0) or present (E1); S: segmental glomerulosclerosis absent (S0) or present (S1), presence or absence of podocyte hypertrophy/tip lesions in biopsy specimens with S1; T: tubular atrophy/interstitial fibrosis < 25% (T0), 26–50% (T1), or > 50% (T2); C: cellular/fibrocellular crescents absent (C0), present in at least 1 glomerulus (C1), in > 25% of glomeruli (C2)

[a]Time interval between renal biopsy of patients with IgA nephropathy and sample collection

[b]eGFR was calculated according to the Chronic Kidney Disease Epidemiology Collaboration (CKD-EPI) equation [19]

[c]CKD stages 1–5 were divided by eGFR≥90 (G1), 60–89 (G2), 45–59 (G3a), 30–44 (G3b), 15–29 (G4), and < 15 (G5) mL/min/1.73 m^2, respectively, according to the new KDIGO (Kidney Disease: Improving Global Outcomes) classification [20]

[d]Determined in accordance with the Oxford classification [5]

Table 3 Correlation between serum TNF-α and clinical parameters of patients with IgA nephropathy

Variable	Bivariate Regression Coefficient	Bivariate P Value [a]	Multivariate Regression Coefficient	Multivariate P Value [b]
Sex		0.02 [c]		
Systolic BP	0.30	< 0.0001		
Diastolic BP	0.19	0.02		
24-h urine protein excretion	0.22	0.007	0.33	0.04
Urinary protein to serum creatinine ratio	0.26	0.002	0.33	0.03
Serum creatinine	0.49	< 0.0001	0.46	< 0.0001
Cystatin C	0.51	< 0.0001	0.59	< 0.0001
eGFR [d]	−0.47	< 0.0001	0.49	< 0.0001

BP: blood pressure; 1 mmHg = 0.133Kpa; *eGFR*: estimated glomerular filtration rate
[a]Spearman's correlation analysis unless otherwise specified
[b]Multiple linear regression adjusted for sex, Systolic BP and Diastolic BP
[c]Mann–Whitney U-test
[d]eGFR was calculated according to the Chronic Kidney Disease Epidemiology Collaboration (CKD-EPI) equation [19]

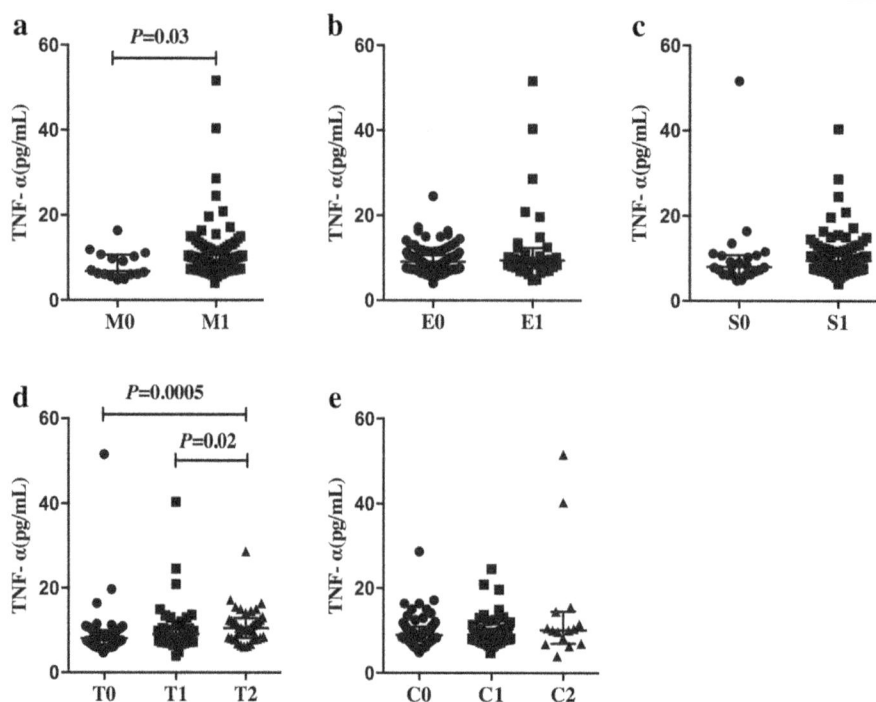

Fig. 3 Correlations between serum levels of tumor necrosis factor alpha (TNF-α) and different grade according to Oxford Classification [a]. (**a**) Serum levels of TNF-α were significantly higher in patients with mesangial hypercellularity grade M1 than that in patients with grade M0 [M1: 9.30 (7.90–10.60) pg/mL vs. M0: 6.70 (6.00–10.58) pg/mL, P = 0.03]. (**d**) Serum levels of TNF-α in patients with tubular atrophy/interstitial fibrosis grade T2 were significantly higher than that in grade T0 [T2: 10.60 (8.25–12.85) pg/mL vs. T0: 6.70 (6.00–10.58) pg/mL, P = 0.0005] and T1 [T2: 10.60 (8.25–12.85) pg/mL vs. T1: 9.20 (8.00–10.20) pg/mL, P = 0.02]; But there was no difference between patients with grade T1 and T0 (P = 0.05). (**b, c** and **e**) Serum levels of TNF-α in patients with different grades of endocapillary hypercellularity [E1: 9.35 (7.53–12.35) pg/mL vs. E0: 9.00 (7.75–10.60) pg/mL, P = 0.66], segmental glomerulosclerosis [S1: 9.40 (7.90–10.60) pg/mL vs. S0: 7.90 (6.20–10.68) pg/mL, P = 0.06] and cellular/fibrocellular crescents [C2:10.20 (7.00–14.50) pg/mL vs. C0: 9.00 (7.53–11.03) pg/mL, P = 0.22; C2: 10.20 (7.00–14.50) pg/mL vs. C1: 9.15 (7.80–10.50) pg/mL, P = 0.26; C1: 9.15 (7.80–10.50) pg/mL vs. C0: 9.00 (7.53–11.03) pg/mL, P = 0.81] did not show any significant difference. Statistically significant differences were tested with Mann–Whitney U-test. [a] Determined in accordance with the Oxford classification [5]

analysis of results of 23 studies [4]. Mesangial hypercellularity and tubular atrophy/interstitial fibrosis lesion judged by updated Oxford classification are also independent predictors of long-term renal outcome [5]. Since serum levels of TNF-α were closely correlated with these three clinical risk factors and pathological features in the study, the results indicated serum levels of TNF-α was a biomarker for disease severity in IgAN.

Human recombinant TNF-α administered intravenously to rabbits induces endothelial damage, and leucocyte and fibrin accumulation in the glomerular capillary lumen [22]. In vitro, TNF-α stimulates the growth of epithelial glomerular cells in culture [23]. However, serum levels of TNF-α were not associated with endocapillary hypercellularity, segmental glomerulosclerosis and cellular/fibrocellular crescents in this study. Since nearly a half of our patients were treated with immunosuppressive therapy in this research, which possibly suppressed the production of cytokines, might interfere with the results. The damage of TNF-α in glomerular endothelial and epithelial cells except that in mesangial cells in IgAN should be determined [11, 12, 24].

Matsumoto K et al. had showed a large proportion of serum TNF originates from serum mononuclear cells, which synthesize increased amounts of TNF-α in IgAN [25]. Since exposure of microbial pathogens triggers the production of TNF-α by Toll-like receptors / myeloid differentiation primary response gene 88 pathways in IgAN [12, 26], TNF-α overproduction in mucosa may be a resource of serum TNF-α. As significantly higher serum levels of TNF-α indicated more severe clinicopathological manifestations and three IgAN patients not involved in this research with the levels of TNF-α higher than 80 pg/mL suffered macroscopic hematuria only hours after respiratory tract infection, we supposed that a direct mucosa-kidney talk that was mediated at least in part by TNF-α may exist [27, 28]. Later researches focusing the mucosa-kidney talk are needed.

To our acknowledgement, this is the first study measuring the serum levels of TNF-α by CLIA in patients with IgAN. Tumor necrosis factor – alpha Assay Kit (chemiluminescence) using in the present study to detect serum TNF-α is a novel and reliable method. The method comparison result shows that the linear relationship between CLIA and ELISA assay is 0.97 for measuring TNF-α. The most importantly, CLIA as a quantitative method which has higher sensitivity than semi-quantitative ELISA, and better stability and wider dynamic range for detecting TNF-α [18, 29]. Furthermore, CLIA is a fully automated technique which can save time, reduce intra- and inter-laboratory variability and improve the reproducibility of the results [18, 29]. Therefore, monitoring serum levels of TNF-α in patients with IgAN will be easy in clinical practice.

There were some limitations in our research. First, a well-designed study with appropriate follow-up period is needed to assess the correlation between serum levels of TNF-α and the renal outcomes in patient with IgAN. Second, variable time differences between renal biopsy and sample collection of the patients might affect the correlations between TNF-α and clinicopathological features. Different treatment regimens in the research might interfere with the results of cytokines. Although it may be tempting to speculate that the serum levels of TNF-α is a prognostic biomarker in IgAN patients, the cross-sectional nature of the study did not allow us to draw a definitive conclusion. This hypothesis may be tested in prospective investigations. Our 10-year cohort study determining whether serum levels of TNF-α is an independent prognostic factor recently approved by Ethics Committee and our randomized controlled study focusing on the therapeutic response of cytokines including TNF-α treated with HCQ in IgAN (ClinicalTrials.gov number, NCT02765594) are both in progress.

Conclusions

We reported that the serum levels of TNF-α, detected by CLIA, were closely associated with disease severity in IgAN. Serum TNF-α was a potential biomarker for severity of patients with IgAN.

Abbreviations

95% CI: 95% Confidence interval; ACE-Is: Angiotensin-converting enzymes inhibitors; ARBs: Angiotensin II receptor blockers; AUC: Area under the curve; BP: Blood pressure; C: Cellular/fibrocellular crescents; CKD: Chronic kidney disease; CKD-EPI: Chronic Kidney Disease Epidemiology Collaboration; CLIA: Chemiluminescence immunoassay; E: Endocapillary hypercellularity; EGF: Epidermal growth factor; eGFR: Estimated glomerular filtration rate; ELISA: Enzyme linked immunosorbent assay; HC: Healthy controls; HCQ: Hydroxychloroquine; IgAN: IgA nephropathy; IL-6: Interleukin-6; LN: Lupus nephritis; M: Mesangial hypercellularity; MCD: Minimal change disease; MN: Membranous nephropathy; ROC: Receiver operating characteristic; S: Segmental glomerulosclerosis; T: Tubular atrophy/interstitial fibrosis; TNF-α: Tumor necrosis factor alpha

Funding

This work was funded by Wu Jieping Medical Foundation of China (No.320.6750.16023). The sponsor of this study is a public organization that supports science in general; it had no role in gathering, analyzing, or interpreting the data.

Authors' contributions

LGH carried out data collection, cytokines measurement, statistical analysis, interpretation of results and wrote the manuscript. WW and ZXY participated in cytokines measurement. HY reviewed medical records. WYB and LXM made the pathological confirmations of IgAN. GRT participated in the study design and coordination, and managing the research project. All authors read and approved the final version prior to submission.

Competing interests

The authors declare that they have no competing interests.

Author details

[1]Division of Nephrology, Department of Internal Medicine, Peking Union Medical College Hospital, Chinese Academy of Medical Sciences & Peking Union Medical College, NO.1, Shuaifuyuan, Dongcheng District, Beijing 100730, China. [2]Department of Clinical Laboratory, Peking Union Medical College Hospital, Chinese Academy of Medical Sciences & Peking Union Medical College, Beijing, China.

References

1. Donadio JV, Grande JP. IgA nephropathy. N Engl J Med. 2002;347(10):738–48.
2. Droz D, Kramar A, Nawar T, Noel LH. Primary IgA nephropathy: prognostic factors. Contrib Nephrol. 1984;40:202–7.
3. Barratt J, Feehally J. IgA nephropathy. J Am Soc Nephrol. 2005;16(7):2088–97.
4. D'Amico G. Natural history of idiopathic IgA nephropathy and factors predictive of disease outcome. Semin Nephrol. 2004;24(3):179–96.
5. Trimarchi H, Barratt J, Cattran DC, Cook HT, Coppo R, Haas M, et al. Oxford classification of IgA nephropathy 2016: an update from the IgA nephropathy classification working group. Kidney Int. 2017;91(5):1014–21.
6. Zhao N, Hou P, Lv J, Moldoveanu Z, Li Y, Kiryluk K, et al. The level of galactose-deficient IgA1 in the sera of patients with IgA nephropathy is associated with disease progression. Kidney Int. 2012;82(7):790–6.
7. Hastings MC, Moldoveanu Z, Suzuki H, Berthoux F, Julian BA, Sanders JT, et al. Biomarkers in IgA nephropathy: relationship to pathogenetic hits. Expert Opin Med Diagn. 2013;7(6):615–27.
8. Vuong MT, Hahn-Zoric M, Lundberg S, Gunnarsson I, van Kooten C, Wramner L, et al. Association of soluble CD89 levels with disease progression but not susceptibility in IgA nephropathy. Kidney Int. 2010;78(12):1281–7.
9. Delanghe SE, Speeckaert MM, Segers H, Desmet K, Vande Walle J, Laecke SV, et al. Soluble transferrin receptor in urine, a new biomarker for IgA nephropathy and Henoch-Schonlein purpura nephritis. Clin Biochem. 2013; 46(7–8):591–7.
10. Ranieri E, Gesualdo L, Petrarulo F, Schena FP. Urinary IL-6/EGF ratio: a useful prognostic marker for the progression of renal damage in IgA nephropathy. Kidney Int. 1996;50(6):1990–2001.
11. Fagarasan S, Kawamoto S, Kanagawa O, Suzuki K. Adaptive immune regulation in the gut: T cell-dependent and T cell-independent IgA synthesis. Annu Rev Immunol. 2010;28:243–73.
12. Tezuka H, Abe Y, Iwata M, Takeuchi H, Ishikawa H, Matsushita M, et al. Regulation of IgA production by naturally occurring TNF/iNOS-producing dendritic cells. Nature. 2007;448(7156):929–33.
13. Lai KN, Leung JC, Chan LY, Saleem MA, Mathieson PW, Lai FM, et al. Activation of podocytes by mesangial-derived TNF-alpha: glomerulo-podocytic communication in IgA nephropathy. Am J Physiol Renal Physiol. 2008;294(4):F945–55.
14. Gao R, Wu W, Wen Y, Li X. Hydroxychloroquine alleviates persistent proteinuria in IgA nephropathy. Int Urol Nephrol. 2017;49(7):1233–41.
15. Rostoker G, Rymer JC, Bagnard G, Petit-Phar M, Griuncelli M, Pilatte Y. Imbalances in serum proinflammatory cytokines and their soluble receptors: a putative role in the progression of idiopathic IgA nephropathy (IgAN) and Henoch-Schonlein purpura nephritis, and a potential target of immunoglobulin therapy? Clin Exp Immunol. 1998;114(3):468–76.
16. Wu TH, Wu SC, Huang TP, Yu CL, Tsai CY. Increased excretion of tumor necrosis factor alpha and interleukin 1 beta in urine from patients with IgA nephropathy and Schonlein-Henoch purpura. Nephron. 1996;74(1):79–88.
17. Meneghel L, Ruffatti A, Gavasso S, Tonello M, Mattia E, Spiezia L, et al. The clinical performance of a chemiluminescent immunoassay in detecting anti-cardiolipin and anti-beta2 glycoprotein I antibodies. A comparison with a homemade ELISA method. Clin Chem Lab Med. 2015;53(7):1083–9.
18. Wang C, Wu J, Zong C, Xu J, Ju H-X. Chemiluminescent immunoassay and its applications. Chin J Anal Chem. 2012;40(1):3–9.
19. Stevens LA, Claybon MA, Schmid CH, Chen J, Horio M, Imai E, et al. Evaluation of the chronic kidney disease epidemiology collaboration equation for estimating the glomerular filtration rate in multiple ethnicities. Kidney Int. 2011;79(5):555–62.
20. Chapter 2: Definition, identification, and prediction of CKD progression. Kidney Int Suppl. 2013;3(1):63–72.
21. Abboud HE. Growth factors in glomerulonephritis. Kidney Int. 1993;43(1): 252–67.
22. Bertani T, Abbate M, Zoja C, Corna D, Perico N, Ghezzi P, et al. Tumor necrosis factor induces glomerular damage in the rabbit. Am J Pathol. 1989; 134(2):419–30.
23. Yanagisawa M, Imai H, Fukushima Y, Yasuda T, Miura AB, Nakamoto Y. Effects of tumour necrosis factor alpha and interleukin 1 beta on the proliferation of cultured glomerular epithelial cells. Virchows Arch. 1994; 424(6):581–6.
24. Kiryluk K, Novak J. The genetics and immunobiology of IgA nephropathy. J Clin Invest. 2014;124(6):2325–32.
25. Matsumoto K. Increased release of tumor necrosis factor-alpha by monocytes from patients with glomerulonephritis. Clin Nephrol. 1993;40(3): 148–54.
26. Yu HH, Chu KH, Yang YH, Lee JH, Wang LC, Lin YT, et al. Genetics and immunopathogenesis of IgA nephropathy. Clin Rev Allergy Immunol. 2011; 41(2):198–213.
27. Floege J, Feehally J. The mucosa-kidney axis in IgA nephropathy. Nat Rev Nephrol. 2016;12(3):147–56.
28. Han L, Fang X, He Y, Ruan XZ. ISN forefronts symposium 2015: IgA nephropathy, the gut microbiota, and gut–kidney crosstalk. Kidney Int Rep. 2016;1(3):189–96.
29. Zhao L, Sun L, Chu X. Chemiluminescence immunoassay. TrAC Trends Anal Chem. 2009;28(4):404–15.

9

Perceptions about the dialysis modality decision process among peritoneal dialysis and in-center hemodialysis patients

Jarcy Zee[1*], Junhui Zhao[1], Lalita Subramanian[1], Erica Perry[2], Nicole Bryant[3], Margie McCall[3], Yanko Restovic[3], Delma Torres[3], Bruce M. Robinson[1], Ronald L. Pisoni[1] and Francesca Tentori[1,4]

Abstract

Background: Patients reaching end-stage renal disease must make a difficult decision regarding renal replacement therapy (RRT) options. Because the choice between dialysis modalities should include patient preferences, it is critical that patients are engaged in the dialysis modality decision. As part of the Empowering Patients on Choices for RRT (EPOCH-RRT) study, we assessed dialysis patients' perceptions of their dialysis modality decision-making process and the impact of their chosen modality on their lives.

Methods: A 39-question survey was developed in collaboration with a multi-stakeholder advisory panel to assess perceptions of patients on either peritoneal dialysis (PD) or in-center hemodialysis (HD). The survey was disseminated to participants in the large US cohorts of the Dialysis Outcomes and Practice Patterns Study (DOPPS) and the Peritoneal DOPPS (PDOPPS). Survey responses were compared between PD and in-center HD patients using descriptive statistics, adjusted logistic generalized estimating equation models, and linear mixed regression models.

Results: Six hundred fourteen PD and 1346 in-center HD participants responded. Compared with in-center HD participants, PD participants more frequently reported that they were engaged in the decision-making process, were provided enough information, understood differences between dialysis modalities, and felt satisfied with their modality choice. PD participants also reported more frequently than in-center HD participants that partners or spouses (79% vs. 70%), physician assistants (80% vs. 66%), and nursing staff (78% vs. 60%) had at least some involvement in the dialysis modality decision. Over 35% of PD and in-center HD participants did not know another dialysis patient at the time of their modality decision and over 60% did not know the disadvantages of their modality type. Participants using either dialysis modality perceived a moderate to high impact of dialysis on their lives.

Conclusions: PD participants were more engaged in the modality decision process compared to in-center HD participants. For both modalities, there is room for improvement in patient education and other support for patients choosing a dialysis modality.

Keywords: End-stage renal disease, Dialysis modality, Hemodialysis, Peritoneal dialysis, Renal replacement therapy

* Correspondence: Jarcy.Zee@ArborResearch.org
[1]Arbor Research Collaborative for Health, 340 E. Huron Street Suite 300, Ann Arbor, MI 48104, USA
Full list of author information is available at the end of the article

Background

Over 120,000 patients reaching end-stage renal disease (ESRD) every year in the United States (US) are faced with a complex and difficult decision regarding renal replacement therapy (RRT) modality options [1]. Although kidney transplant results in the best clinical outcomes, 97% of ESRD patients will require dialysis, most frequently peritoneal dialysis (PD) or in-center hemodialysis (HD) [1]. Although clinical contraindications restrict modality choice in occasional cases, most patients are candidates for both PD and HD [2]. Either dialysis modality may be a better fit for a specific patient based on dialysis treatment characteristics and their impact on daily life. Thus, the choice between modalities should center on patient preferences, and it is critical that patients are included and engaged in the dialysis modality decision [3, 4]. This is supported by increasing evidence that aligning treatment with patient preferences may improve adherence to therapy, quality of life, and ultimately better medical outcomes [5–8].

Clinical practice guidelines support the role of patients and their caregivers in the dialysis modality decision-making process [5, 9–11]. Unfortunately, interviews with dialysis patients show that many did not feel they were given an active choice of modality [3, 12–14], despite wanting to be involved in decision-making [3, 15]. To do so effectively, patients and their caregivers must have a comprehensive understanding of the differences between dialysis modalities and their impacts on daily life [16, 17]. However, previous studies have shown many patients felt unprepared and ill-informed about starting dialysis and about different dialysis modalities [13, 18]. Dialysis education can prepare patients for shared decision-making, and may ultimately lead to better outcomes through more active engagement in care [16, 19–22].

The Empowering Patients on Choices for Renal Replacement Therapy (EPOCH-RRT) study, supported by the Patient-Centered Outcomes Research Institute (PCORI), sought to develop a decision aid (http://choosingdialysis.org) to help patients choose a dialysis modality. To determine factors that are most important to patients when considering dialysis, the EPOCH-RRT study first conducted semi-structured interviews of patients with chronic kidney disease (CKD) and patients undergoing PD or in-center HD. Some of the factors participants identified were independence, flexibility in daily lives, concerns about looks, and quality and quantity of life [14]. For this part of the EPOCH-RRT study, we developed a survey partly based on the information gained from interviews, and we administered the survey to the large, national US samples of participants in the Dialysis Outcomes and Practice Patterns Study (DOPPS) and the Peritoneal DOPPS (PDOPPS). Our aim was to assess participants' perceptions of the dialysis modality decision-making process and compare the impact of their chosen modality on their lives with the goal to inform efforts to increase patient engagement and ultimately contribute to improving patient-centered outcomes.

Methods

Survey design

A 39-question survey (Additional file 1: Figure S1) to assess participants' experiences with the dialysis modality decision and factors that participants had previously identified as important ("patient-centered outcomes") was developed in collaboration with a multi-stakeholder advisory panel and partly based on the analysis of qualitative data collected from 180 advanced CKD participants [14]. The advisory panel included dialysis patients, caregivers (e.g., dialysis patients' family members), and patient advocates (e.g., social workers), who provided perspectives on experiences with CKD and ESRD. The advisory panel informed the development of the survey, tested the survey for readability and comprehension, and helped to review and finalize survey questions. Given the panel members' expertise with the target study population and their personal experience as either patients or caregivers, they were able to assess face validity, interpretability, relevance, and comprehensiveness of questionnaire items. Questionnaires for PD vs. in-center HD patients were identical except for the exchange of the words "peritoneal dialysis" vs. "hemodialysis." The survey was designed for both paper and electronic (tablet) formats, with substantial advisory panel input on layout and design of the electronic survey. The survey was professionally translated from English to Spanish and reviewed by Spanish-speaking members of the institutional review boards, then made available to study participants in either English or Spanish.

Participants were asked whether they were told they had a choice between PD and HD when starting dialysis and to indicate if their involvement in this decision was more, less, or just what they wanted. The survey proceeded with three sets of questions: (1) Participants ranked the degree to which 10 groups of family members, peers, and clinical staff were involved in their dialysis modality decision, as suggested by the Decisional Needs Assessment in Populations [23]. A Cronbach's alpha estimate of 0.89 indicated good reliability of these questions to measure involvement of others in the decision process. (2) Participants rated their level of agreement with nine statements focused on their recollection of their experiences and satisfaction with their dialysis modality decision. This set of questions was adapted for the current study population from the COMRADE scale [24] and Decision Regret Scale [25] and had a Cronbach's alpha estimate of 0.86. Additionally, participants were asked whether the information they had received before starting dialysis was more, less, or just the amount that they had wanted and if they and their doctor had agreed on the type of dialysis that was best for them. (3) Participants ranked the degree to which dialysis affected 16 factors compared with before starting dialysis. These factors were chosen directly based on previous research of the themes most often reported as important to patients when choosing a dialysis modality [14]. Cronbach's alpha for this set of items was 0.93.

Participant enrollment

The DOPPS and PDOPPS are ongoing, international prospective cohort studies of dialysis facility practices and patient outcomes for adult in-center HD and PD participants, respectively [26–28]. DOPPS and PDOPPS participants are selected randomly from a national sample of dialysis facilities. All consented participants in the US DOPPS and PDOPPS studies were eligible for the EPOCH-RRT study. Study coordinators targeted as many eligible participants as possible between February 2015 and August 2015 to participate in the EPOCH-RRT survey (Fig. 1). Some participants departed the dialysis facility before study coordinators could approach them with the survey or were unable to participate due to other reasons, such as cognitive, physical, language, or social impediments. Others were approached for participation but unwilling to complete the EPOCH-RRT survey. Facilities were randomly assigned to receive the survey on either paper or tablet platforms. Local institutional review boards (Ethical and Independent Review Services #13016, Henry Ford Health Systems #8144, University of Michigan HUM00073058) approved all study procedures.

Statistical analysis

For questions on the level of involvement of clinical staff, families, and peers in the dialysis modality selection, we treated the responses as continuous outcomes. Each degree of involvement (i.e., not at all, somewhat, moderately, very much, or extremely) was assigned an integer value from 1 to 5 such that the difference between two adjacent levels represented a 1-unit change. For outcomes on experiences and satisfaction with the dialysis modality decision, responses were dichotomized into agreement (agree or strongly agree) vs. non-agreement (strongly disagree, disagree, or neither agree or disagree) for better model fit and ease of interpretation. For outcomes on factors important to patients, responses were also dichotomized into a large impact (very much or extremely) vs. not large impact (not at all, somewhat, or moderately). Participants who reported not applicable were excluded from analyses of each corresponding question. Missing responses for each question were excluded.

For dichotomized outcomes (experiences and satisfaction with the dialysis modality decision and factors important to patients), logistic generalized estimating equation (GEE) regression models were used to compare outcomes between PD and in-center HD participants. An exchangeable working correlation matrix was used to account for participant clustering within facility. For continuous outcomes (involvement of clinical staff, families, and peers), linear mixed regression models were used to compare dialysis modality, accounting for clustering by including a random intercept for each facility. The primary predictor in all models was dialysis

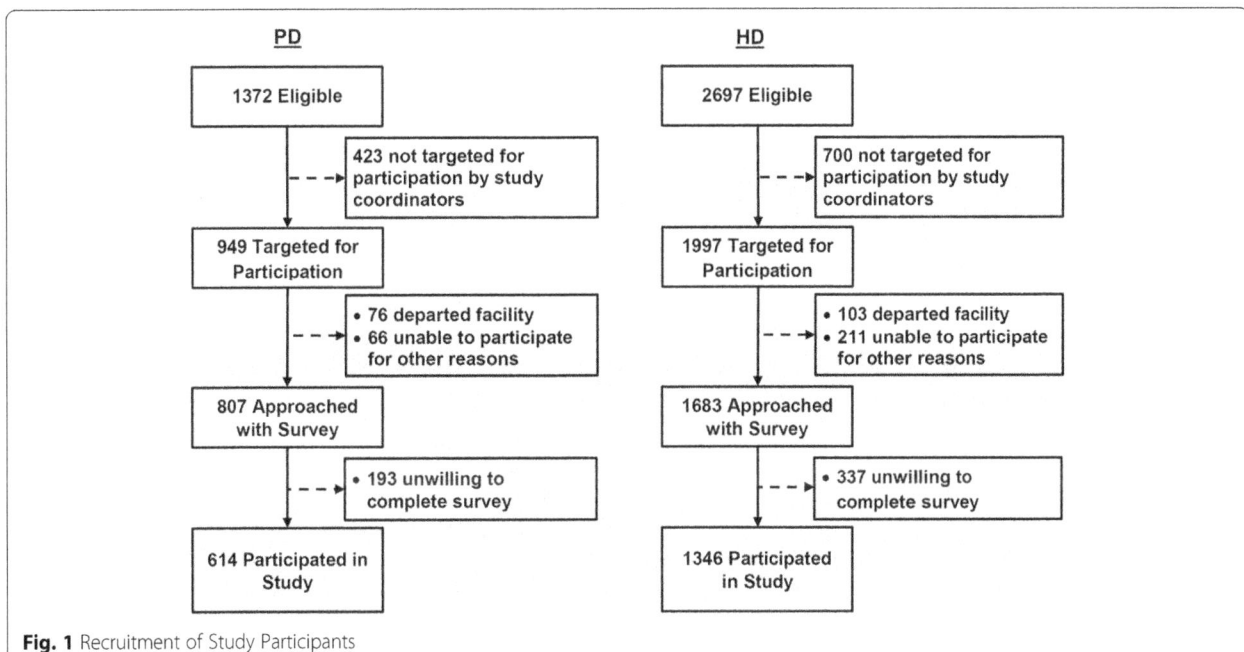

Fig. 1 Recruitment of Study Participants

modality, and all models were adjusted for age, sex, black race, time on dialysis (vintage), and diabetes. Adjusted differences in probabilities or levels of each outcome between PD and in-center HD, along with 95% confidence intervals (CI), were estimated using model parameter estimates. Predicted probabilities from logistic regression models were estimated using means for continuous adjustment covariates and most frequent categories for categorical adjustment covariates.

We tested for an interaction between modality and time on dialysis (< 1 year vs. ≥1 year and < 3 years vs. ≥3 years) in each model to assess whether dialysis vintage modified differences in modality. Similarly, among the subgroup of patients with such information, we tested for an interaction between modality and having prior RRT experience (i.e., in-center HD patients with prior PD experience, PD patients with prior in-center HD experience, and in-center HD or PD patients with prior transplant). Because each interaction analysis involved 38 different hypothesis tests, we applied the Benjamini-Hochberg correction for multiple comparisons to control for false discovery rate [29]. We also conducted two sets of sensitivity analyses: 1) we added paper or tablet platform as an additional adjustment factor and tested for dialysis modality effect modification by platform; 2) for dichotomized outcomes, we treated them as continuous variables using linear models and treated them as ordinal using proportional odds models. All analyses were conducted using SAS, Version 9.4 (SAS Institute Inc., 2013, Cary, NC) or Stata, Version 13.1 (StataCorp, 2013, College Station, TX).

Results
Study participants
Out of 807 PD and 1683 in-center HD participants approached for participation, 614 (76.1%) PD participants from 55 facilities and 1346 (80.0%) HD participants from 80 facilities responded to at least one question in the survey (Fig. 1). Participant characteristics are shown in Table 1. Compared to in-center HD participants, PD participants were younger and were less likely to be black, on average. PD participants also had shorter dialysis vintage, with 46% having started dialysis less than 2 years ago compared to 32% for in-center HD participants. Age, sex, and race distributions of our study sample were similar to those of the US dialysis population, while participants in our study had shorter time on dialysis, on average, than point prevalent dialysis patients in the US in 2013 when these data were collected [1].

Survey completion
Out of 39 total questions, the median (interquartile range) number of questions answered was 36 (33–38) among PD participants and 35 (32–37) among in-center

Table 1 Patient characteristics, by dialysis modality

Variable	PD (n = 614)[a]	HD (n = 1346)[a]
Patient age, mean (SD) years	59.9 (15.0)	63.0 (14.5)
Male	53.9%	57.4%
Race		
White	70.2%	59.5%
Black	23.0%	35.8%
Other	6.8%	4.7%
Time on dialysis		
0 to < 6 months	5.6%	6.2%
6 to < 12 months	11.4%	8.6%
12 to < 36 months	46.1%	31.1%
36+ months	30.6%	54.1%
Diabetes	41%	43.3%

[a]One PD patient and 9 HD patients were missing demographic data

HD participants. The amount of missingness for each question ranged from 3 to 7%, with the exception of question two, regarding the amount of patient involvement in the dialysis modality decision compared to what the participant wanted. This question was left unanswered by 11% of PD participants and 36% of in-center HD participants. In addition, there was a technical error with the question, "I know the disadvantages of hemodialysis compared to peritoneal dialysis" on some of the tablet questionnaires disseminated to in-center HD participants. Therefore, responses to these questions among tablet users (43%) were suppressed and only responses from paper users were used for analyses.

Survey implementation platform
Among participants < 65 years old, response rates across platform (i.e., paper vs. tablet) were similar among both PD (63.2% paper vs. 66.1% tablet) and in-center HD (68.4% paper and 71.9% tablet) participants. However, participants older than 65 who were offered tablets had lower response rates than those offered paper surveys for PD (72.5% paper vs. 55.7% tablet) and in-center HD (69.4% paper vs. 59.7% tablet).

Experience regarding dialysis modality choice
PD participants reported that they were more frequently (93%) told that they had a choice between dialysis modalities than were in-center HD participants (66%). 10% of PD participants and 20% of HD participants felt their involvement in the type of dialysis they would start on was either more than or less than they wanted, rather than just what they wanted.

Involvement of clinical staff, family, and peers
Clinical staff members, especially nephrologists, were most frequently involved in the dialysis modality decision

overall (Fig. 2). Compared to in-center HD, fewer PD participants reported involvement of primary care doctors (60% vs. 70%). Greater differences were observed in the two modalities when it came to involvement of other clinical staff, with for example, 22% of PD participants and 40% of in-center HD participants reporting no involvement at all of nursing staff in the dialysis decision. In adjusted models, the mean [95% CI] level of involvement of physician assistants was 0.4 [0.2,0.6] higher for PD patients and of nursing staff was 0.7 [0.5,0.9] higher for PD patients compared to in-center HD patients. Less than 65% of all participants reported knowing someone on dialysis at the time of their modality decision; among them, over 50% recalled no peer involvement. Also, more PD participants than in-center HD participants reported at least some involvement of partners/spouses (PD 79%, with 55% reporting very much or extremely; in-center HD 70%, with 46% reporting very much or extremely; adjusted mean [95% CI] difference of 0.3 [0.1,0.4] between PD and HD). For both PD and in-center HD participants,

involvement of other family and friends was low to moderate (32–60%).

Experiences and satisfaction with dialysis modality decision

In-center HD participants felt less informed and less confident than PD participants at the time of the dialysis modality decision and were less satisfied with their modality choice (Fig. 3). PD participants more often felt the information they were given was enough and easy to understand, with adjusted differences [95% CI] between PD and HD in the probability of agreement of 0.10 [0.07,0.13] and 0.08 [0.05,0.12], respectively. PD participants more frequently agreed that dialysis choices were explained (0.13 [0.09,0.16]), they understood the advantages (0.22 [0.17,0.26]) and disadvantages (0.15 [0.09,0.22]) of their dialysis modality type, and they were happy with their type of dialysis (0.14 [0.10,0.18]). Almost all PD participants felt their dialysis choices had been explained in a way that was easily understandable,

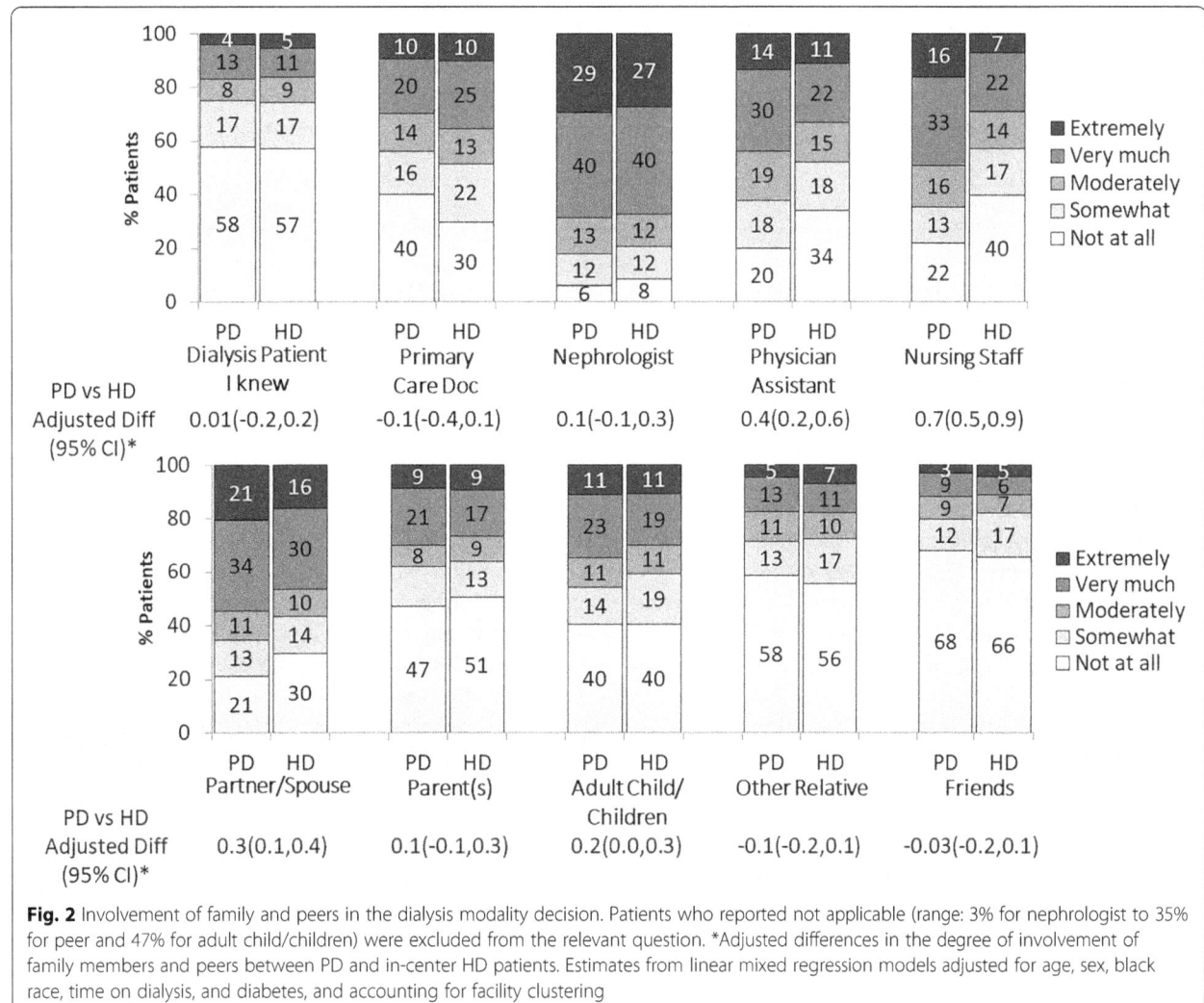

Fig. 2 Involvement of family and peers in the dialysis modality decision. Patients who reported not applicable (range: 3% for nephrologist to 35% for peer and 47% for adult child/children) were excluded from the relevant question. *Adjusted differences in the degree of involvement of family members and peers between PD and in-center HD patients. Estimates from linear mixed regression models adjusted for age, sex, black race, time on dialysis, and diabetes, and accounting for facility clustering

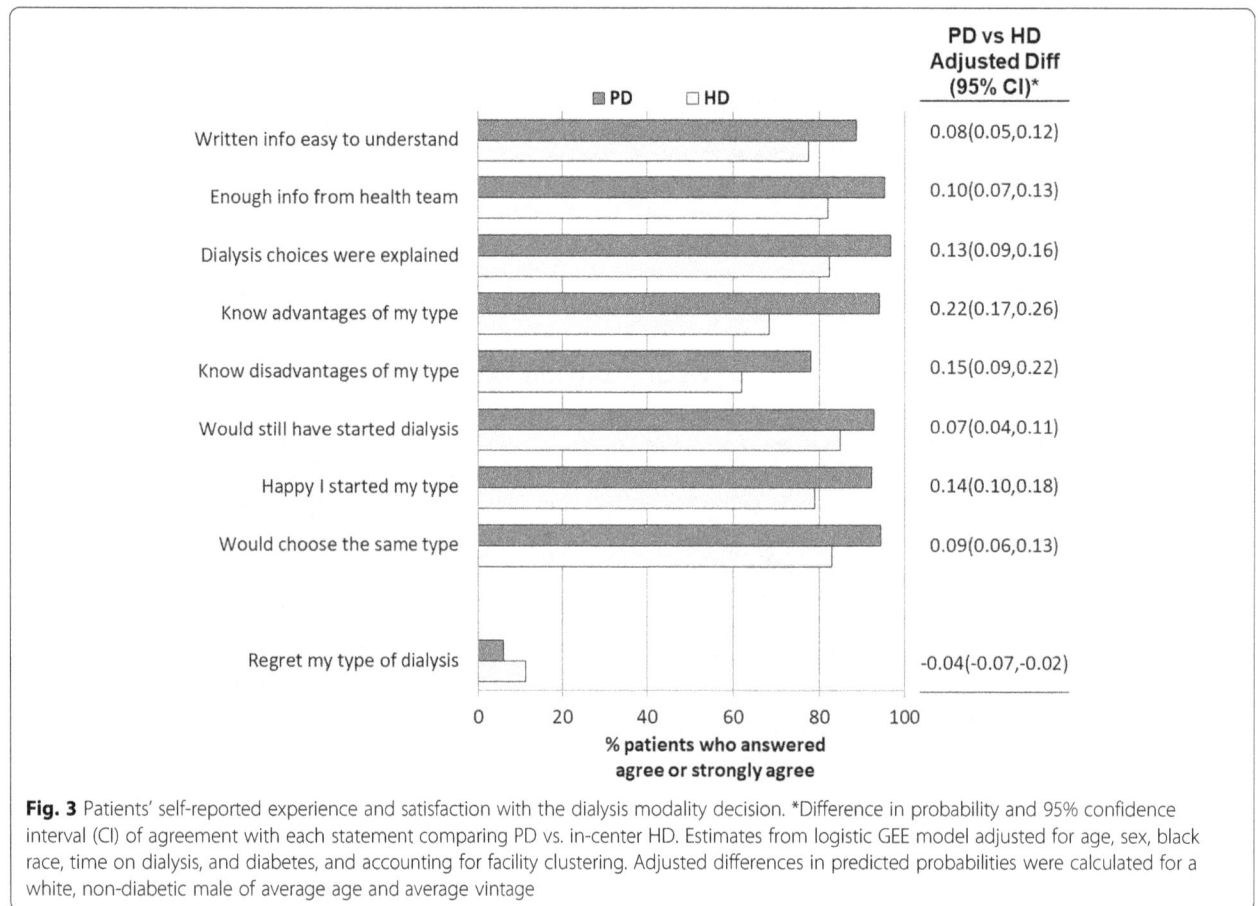

Fig. 3 Patients' self-reported experience and satisfaction with the dialysis modality decision. *Difference in probability and 95% confidence interval (CI) of agreement with each statement comparing PD vs. in-center HD. Estimates from logistic GEE model adjusted for age, sex, black race, time on dialysis, and diabetes, and accounting for facility clustering. Adjusted differences in predicted probabilities were calculated for a white, non-diabetic male of average age and average vintage

whereas close to 20% of in-center HD participants did not. Only 6% of PD participants regretted their choice of dialysis modality, compared with 11% of in-center HD participants (adjusted difference between PD and HD of − 0.04 [− 0.07,-0.02]). While 26% of PD participants reported that the information they had before starting dialysis was either more (9%) or less (17%) than they wanted, rather than just what they wanted, 36% of in-center HD participants reported they had either more or less information (11% and 25%, respectively) (p = 0.178). 95% of PD participants and 84% of in-center HD participants reported that they and their doctor agreed about the type of dialysis that was best for them (p < 0.05).

Impact of dialysis on patients' lives
A sizable number of participants on both in-center HD and PD reported that dialysis had a large impact on all factors assessed (range 17–46%, Fig. 4). In-center HD participants were more affected than PD participants for 15 of 16 factors, but the differences were generally small. PD participants felt their dialysis modality affected reliance on themselves slightly more than HD participants, with an adjusted difference in probability of agreement

of 0.05 [− 0.01,0.10] between PD and HD. The largest differences between PD and in-center HD participants were observed for the factors: doing what I want in my free time (− 0.08 [− 0.13,-0.02]), doing activities I am interested in (hobbies) (− 0.07 [− 0.12,-0.02]), drinking as much water as I want (− 0.20 [− 0.25,-0.15]), and eating what I like (− 0.14 [− 0.19,-0.08]).

Effect modification and sensitivity analyses
The interaction between modality and time on dialysis (using 1 year or 3 years as a cut-point) was not statistically significant in any model. The interaction between modality and prior RRT experience was also not statistically significant in any model among the N = 140 patients with prior RRT experience and N = 1159 patients without prior RRT experience. Therefore, we did not find evidence that time on dialysis or prior RRT experience modified the differences in outcomes between PD and in-center HD. For all outcomes, similar results were obtained after adjusting additionally for platform (tablet vs. paper). In analyses testing for interactions between modality (PD vs. in-center HD) and questionnaire platform (tablet vs. paper), we found little effect modification. In sensitivity analyses treating dichotomized outcomes as continuous or ordinal,

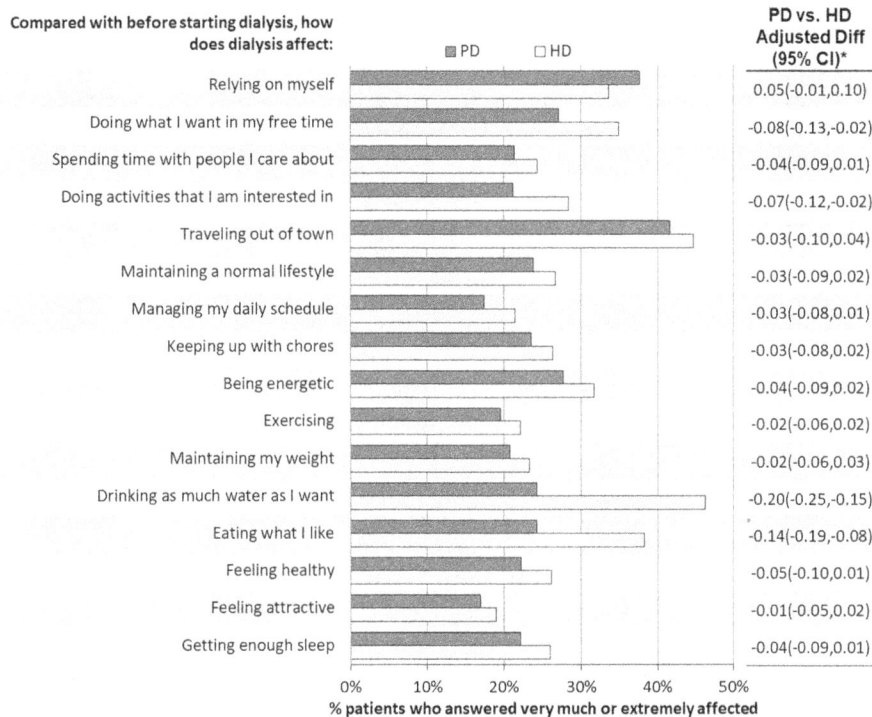

Fig. 4 Effect of dialysis on patient-centered outcomes. Patients who reported not applicable (range: 1% to 9%) were excluded from the relevant question. * Difference in probability and 95% confidence interval (CI) of a large impact of dialysis on each factor comparing PD vs. in-center HD. Estimates from logistic GEE model adjusted for age, sex, black race, time on dialysis, and diabetes, and accounting for facility clustering. Adjusted differences in predicted probabilities were calculated for a white, non-diabetic male of average age and average vintage

results were similar but model assumptions (i.e., normality or proportional odds) were sometimes violated. Thus, we concluded that logistic regressions were most appropriate for these outcomes.

Discussion

By collaborating with an advisory panel and using analyses from qualitative data collected from EPOCH-RRT participant interviews, we developed a survey specifically designed to focus on patient-centered outcomes. This approach was consistent with PCORI goals for multi-stakeholder engagement in research and was invaluable for informing the survey content and interpretation of results. Our survey results showed that that participants who were on PD were more informed and engaged in dialysis modality decision-making compared with in-center HD participants overall. This may be expected, given that PD participants undergo intense training coordinated by clinical staff and that this dialysis technique has an impact on an entire household's quality of life [30]. Therefore, those who choose PD may already be more involved in their own care and likely more receptive to education they receive. Nonetheless, the low involvement of several groups in the dialysis modality decision for both PD and in-center HD participants demonstrates an opportunity to increase family and peer engagement to promote shared

decision-making. Such engagement may result in a better fit of the dialysis modality with each patient's life, as well as improved experience for their families and other caregivers [31–33]. The large number of dialysis participants who did not know someone else on dialysis highlights a potentially useful but underutilized resource, for example. Beyond having support of peers, peer mentoring programs have been successful in different clinical conditions [34–37], and anecdotal evidence indicates that existing peer support programs in dialysis are highly valued by patients and their caregivers [38, 39]. By improving awareness of and access to peers and peer mentors, patients new to dialysis may benefit from increased practical information about dialysis, empathy and understanding, advice on coping strategies, and a greater sense of empowerment and agency [39].

PD participants were much more likely than in-center HD participants to report greater involvement in the dialysis modality decision. Previous studies have found that deficiencies in awareness of options are a barrier to choosing PD and that educational interventions can increase PD use [40–42]. Thus, health care providers may offer PD as an option more often to patients with higher health literacy or better self-care abilities. PD participants also more frequently indicated they were happy with the modality they chose compared to in-center HD participants. This result may reflect a more deliberate and informed decision-making process among PD participants and/or greater involvement in the dialysis modality decision. It may also reflect a more positive perception of the dialysis experience specifically due to self-reinforcement from feeling involved in the modality decision process. Still, many PD participants did not know the disadvantages of their modality and did not feel they had written information that was easy to understand. In both PD and HD groups, such a lack of information and regret in the dialysis modality choice points to opportunities to improve ESRD education for advanced CKD patients. Increased education could then lead to increased understanding of dialysis modalities and satisfaction with treatment, especially among those who ultimately choose in-center HD [19, 20].

Several impactful factors were more frequently identified by in-center HD participants compared to PD participants. Some of these differences may be explained not only by the differences in modality technique but also the location and medical environment where dialysis is performed. For example, clinical characteristics (e.g., lack of residual urine output) of HD patients may require more restrictive diets and fluid intake, while technical aspects of in-center HD (e.g., intermittent dialysis in a facility setting) often limit the time in-center HD patients have for their own interests like travel [43]. Some in-center HD patients have also reported that dialyzing in a clinical setting and being surrounded by other patients makes them feel less healthy, although this opportunity to interact with other patients in the in-center setting was not always perceived as a negative aspect of in-center HD [3].

Overall, the proportion of participants who skipped each question was low, supporting the fact that the survey questions were appropriate and easily interpretable by most dialysis participants. This likely reflected the high engagement of the advisory panel in the development of the survey and reviews of survey questions. There was a higher amount of missingness for one question about the amount of the participant's involvement in the dialysis modality decision. The reasons for which participants did not answer this question could include not having preconceived desires about involvement in the dialysis modality decision and/or unwillingness to admit low involvement. Both suggest that more effort should be made to give participants adequate choice and involvement in their dialysis modality decision process and to monitor patient involvement during that process [44].

There are a few limitations of our study worth noting. First, survey questions asked the extent to which participants felt affected by dialysis, but did not ask whether participants perceived the effects to be positive or negative. Therefore, the direction of impact can only be speculated based on what is known about the different modalities until it can be elucidated by future research. Second,

patients' perceptions of others' involvement in PD training may have inflated their perceptions of involvement in the dialysis modality decision process. While it is plausible that those who must later be involved in training also have some involvement in the decision process, we cannot separate the two periods of involvement in our data. Third, surveys were administered to both incident and prevalent dialysis participants, so the time between dialysis initiation and survey was variable and experiences reflect those of survivors. Particularly for participants who had longer dialysis vintage, recall bias may have affected survey responses related to the dialysis modality decision. However, we have no reason to believe that the recall bias would be different across PD and in-center HD participants, indicating that comparisons between modalities may still have little bias. We also adjusted for vintage in models and found no evidence of modality effect modification by vintage. Fourth, we did not have information on whether participants in the study had contraindications to either dialysis modality, which also may have affected survey responses. For example, some in-center HD participants may not have had PD available if starting dialysis acutely (information not available in our data), which limited their exposure to PD information. Still, these patients should be empowered with information to decide whether to stay on in-center HD or switch to PD when available. Finally, comparisons between PD and in-center HD participants may have been confounded by factors like frailty, comorbid diseases, educational background, social support, and dialysis modality history. Although these variables were not available for analysis, we did control for the most common comorbidity of diabetes and age which is likely to be correlated with frailty.

Conclusions

Our study has several strengths and important implications for ESRD patients and their families as well as for health care providers. By comparing the experiences of PD and in-center HD patients, we identified important differences between these modalities. We found several aspects of the dialysis modality decision that require improvement for both PD and in-center HD patients, including patient education, access to peers, and other support. Increased efforts are needed to encourage a holistic approach to care that involves multiple stakeholders and provides resources such as decision aids for patients facing the choice between dialysis modalities. It is our hope that a focus on education and multi-stakeholder engagement in the dialysis modality decision will empower patients, their caregivers, and health care professionals to collaboratively choose a dialysis modality that best fits the individual patient, with the goals of ultimately improving satisfaction and health outcomes.

Abbreviations

CKD: Chronic kidney disease; DOPPS: Dialysis Outcomes and Practice Patterns Study; EPOCH-RRT: Empowering Patients on Choices for RRT; ESRD: End-stage renal disease; GEE: Generalized estimating equation; HD: Hemodialysis; PCORI: Patient-Centered Outcomes Research Institute; PD: Peritoneal dialysis; PDOPPS: Peritoneal DOPPS; RRT: Renal replacement therapy

Acknowledgements

This work would not have been possible without the contributions of all study participants involved in EPOCH-RRT. Of particular note is the successful collaboration, active engagement, and participation of the advisory panel. In addition, patients and staff at dialysis units participating in the DOPPS and the PDOPPS were invaluable to the current study. Shauna Leighton, BA, Medical Editor at Arbor Research Collaborative for Health, provided editorial assistance on this manuscript.

Funding

Research reported in this article was partially funded through a Patient-Centered Outcomes Research Institute (PCORI) Award (1109). The views presented are solely the responsibility of the author(s) and do not necessarily represent the views of the Patient-Centered Outcomes Research Institute (PCORI), its Board of Governors or Methodology Committee. The Patient-Centered Outcomes Research Institute (PCORI) is an independent, nonprofit organization authorized by Congress in 2010. Its mission is to fund research that will provide patients, their caregivers, and clinicians with the evidence-based information needed to make better-informed health care decisions. PCORI is committed to continually seeking input from a broad range of stakeholders to guide its work. FT is supported in part by NIDDK grant K01DK087762.

Authors' contributions

Research idea and study design: LS, EP, NB, MM, YR, DT, BMR, RLP, FT; Data acquisition: LS, BMR, RLP, FT; Data analysis/interpretation: JZ1 (Zee), JZ2 (Zhao), LS, FT; Statistical analysis: JZ1, JZ2; Supervision or mentorship: JZ1, LS, BMR, RLP, FT. Each author contributed to the manuscript drafting or revision and accepts accountability for the overall work. All authors have read and approved the final version of the manuscript.

Competing interests

FT has received consulting fees from MedScape and is an employee at DaVita HealthCare Partners, Inc. but was not employed there at the time of study conduct. The other authors have nothing to disclose.

Author details

[1]Arbor Research Collaborative for Health, 340 E. Huron Street Suite 300, Ann Arbor, MI 48104, USA. [2]University of Michigan Health System, Ann Arbor, MI, USA. [3]Advisory panel, Ann Arbor, MI, USA. [4]Vanderbilt University Medical Center, Nashville, TN, USA.

References

1. United States Renal Data System (USRDS). Annual Data Report: Atlas of chronic kidney disease and end-stage renal disease in the United States. Bethesda: National Institutes of Health, National Institute of Diabetes and Digestive and Kidney Diseases; 2015.
2. Lameire N, Van Biesen W. Epidemiology of peritoneal dialysis: a story of believers and nonbelievers. Nat Rev Nephrol. 2010;6:75–82.
3. Lee A, Gudex C, Povlsen JV, Bonnevie B, Nielsen CP. Patients' views regarding choice of dialysis modality. Nephrol Dial Transplant. 2008;23: 3953–9.
4. Segall L, Nistor I, Van Biesen W, et al. Dialysis modality choice in elderly patients with end-stage renal disease: a narrative review of the available evidence. Nephrol Dial Transplant. 2017;32:41–9.
5. O'hare AM, Armistead N, Funk Schrag WL, Diamond L, Moss AH. Patient-centered care: an opportunity to accomplish the "three aims" of the national quality strategy in the Medicare ESRD program. Clin J Am Soc Nephrol. 2017;9:2189–94.
6. Kimmel PL, Peterson RA. Depression in end-stage renal disease patients treated with hemodialysis: tools, correlates, outcomes, and needs. Semin Dial. 2005;18:91–7.
7. Mapes DL, Lopes AA, Satayathum S, et al. Health-related quality of life as a predictor of mortality and hospitalization: the Dialysis outcomes and practice patterns study (DOPPS). Kidney Int. 2003;64:339–49.
8. Lopes AA, Bragg J, Young E, et al. Depression as a predictor of mortality and hospitalization among hemodialysis patients in the United States and Europe. Kidney Int. 2002;62:199–207.
9. KDOQI. Clinical Practice Guidelines and Clinical Practice Recommendations for 2006 Updates: Hemodialysis Adequacy, Peritoneal Dialysis Adequacy and Vascular Access Guideline 1. Initiation of dialysis. 1.1 Preparation for kidney failure. Am J Kidney Dis. 2006;48:S1–S322.
10. Renal Physicians Association. Shared Decision-making in the Appropriate Initiation of and Withdrawal from Dialysis. Clinical Practice Guideline. 2nd ed. Rockville: Renal Physicians Association; 2010.
11. Williams AW, Dwyer AC, Eddy AA, et al. Critical and honest conversations: the evidence behind the "choosing wisely" campaign recommendations by the American Society of Nephrology. Clin J Am Soc Nephrol. 2012;7:1664–72.
12. Winterbottom A, Bekker HL, Conner M, Mooney A. Choosing dialysis modality: decision-making in a chronic illness context. Health Expect. 2012; 17:710–23.
13. Song M, Lin F, Gilet CA, Arnold RM, Bridgman JC, Ward SE. Patient perspectives on informed decision-making surrounding dialysis initiation. Nephrol Dial Transplant. 2013;28:2815–23.
14. Dahlerus C, Quinn M, Messersmith E, et al. Patient perspectives on the choice of Dialysis modality: results from the empowering patients on choices for renal replacement therapy (EPOCH-RRT) study. Am J Kidney Dis. 2016;68:901–10.
15. Deber RB, Kraetschmer N, Irvine J. What role do patients wish to play in treatment decision-making? Arch Intern Med. 1996;156:1414–20.
16. Covic A, Bammens B, Lobbedez T, et al. Educating end-stage renal disease patients on dialysis modality selection: clinical advice from the European renal best practice (ERBP) advisory board. Nephrol Dial Transplant. 2010;25: 1757–9.
17. Robinski M, Mau W, Wienke A, Girndt M. Shared decision-making in chronic kidney disease: a retrospection of recently initiated dialysis patients in Germany. Patient Educ Couns. 2016;99:562–70.
18. Whittaker AA, Albee BJ. Factors influencing patient selection of dialysis treatment modality. ANNA J. 1996;23:369–75 Discussion 376-7.
19. Klang B, Björvell H, Clyne N. Predialysis education helps patients choose dialysis modality and increases disease-specific knowledge. J Adv Nurs. 1999;29:869–76.
20. King K. Patients' perspective of factors affecting modality selection: a National Kidney Foundation patient survey. Adv Ren Replace Ther. 2000;7: 261–8.
21. Mehrotra R, Marsh D, Vonesh E, Peters V, Nissenson A. Patient education and access of ESRD patients to renal replacement therapies beyond in-center hemodialysis. Kidney Int. 2005;68:378–90.
22. Golper T. Patient education: can it maximize the success of therapy? Nephrol Dial Transplant. 2001;16(Suppl 7):20–4.
23. Jacobsen MJ, O'Connor AM, Stacey D. Decisional Needs Assessment in Populations: A workbook for assessing patients' and practitioners' decision making needs. Ottawa: University of Ottawa; 1999. [Updated 2013]. Available from https://decisionaid.ohri.ca/docs/implement/Population_Needs.pdf
24. Edwards A, Elwyn G, Hood K, et al. The development of COMRADE—a patient-based outcome measure to evaluate the effectiveness of risk communication and treatment decision making in consultations. Patient Educ Couns. 2003;50:311–22.
25. O'Connor AM. User Manual – Decision Regret Scale. Ottawa: Ottawa Hospital Research Institute; 1996. p. 3. [modified 2004]. Available from http://decisionaid.ohri.ca/docs/develop/User_Manuals/UM_Regret_Scale.pdf
26. Young EW, Goodkin DA, Mapes DL, et al. The Dialysis outcomes and practice patterns study (DOPPS): an international hemodialysis study. Kidney Int. 2000;57:S74–81.
27. Pisoni RL, Gillespie BW, Dickinson DM, Chen K, Kutner MH, Wolfe RA. The Dialysis outcomes and practice patterns study (DOPPS): design, data elements, and methodology. Am J Kidney Dis. 2004;44 Suppl 2:7–15.

28. Perl J, Davies SJ, Lambie M, et al. The peritoneal Dialysis outcomes and practice patterns study (PDOPPS): unifying efforts to inform practice and improve global outcomes in peritoneal Dialysis. Perit Dial Int. 2016; 36:297–307.

29. Benjamini Y, Hochberg Y. Controlling the false discovery rate: a practical and powerful approach to multiple testing. J R Stat Soc Series B Stat Methodol. 1995;57:289–300.

30. Fan SL, Sathick I, McKitty K, Punzalan S. Quality of life of caregivers and patients on peritoneal dialysis. Nephrol Dial Transplant. 2008;23: 1713–9.

31. Huang KB, Weber U, Johnson J, Anderson N, et al. Primary care physician involvement in shared decision making for critically ill patients and family satisfaction with care. J Am Board Fam Med. 2018;31:64–72.

32. Cantekin I, Kavurmaci M, Tan M. An analysis of caregiver burden of patients with hemodialysis and peritoneial dialysis. Hemodial Int. 2016;20:94–7.

33. Sheu J, Ephraim PL, Powe NR, et al. African American and non-African American patients' and families' decision making about renal replacement therapies. Qual Health Res. 2012;22:997–1006.

34. Giese-Davis J, Bliss-Isberg C, Carson K, et al. The effect of peer counseling on quality of life following diagnosis of breast cancer: an observational study. Psycho-Oncology. 2006;15:1014–22.

35. Latimer-Cheung AE, Arbour-Nicitopoulos KP, Brawley LR, et al. Developing physical activity interventions for adults with spinal cord injury. Part 2: motivational counseling and peer-mediated interventions for people intending to be active. Rehabil Psychol. 2013;58:307–15.

36. Ti L, Hayashi K, Kaplan K, et al. Willingness to access peer-delivered HIV testing and counseling among people who inject drugs in Bangkok, Thailand. J Community Health. 2013;38:427–33.

37. Hanks RA, Rapport LJ, Wertheimer J, Koviak C. Randomized controlled trial of peer mentoring for individuals with traumatic brain injury and their significant others. Arch Phys Med Rehabil. 2012;93:1297–304.

38. Perry E, Swartz J, Brown S, Smith D, Kelly G, Swartz R. Peer mentoring: a culturally sensitive approach to end-of-life planning for long-term dialysis patients. Am J Kidney Dis. 2005;46:111–9.

39. Hughes J, Wood E, Smith G. Exploring kidney patients' experiences of receiving individual peer support. Health Expect. 2009;12:396–406.

40. Manns BJ, Taub K, VanderStraeten C, et al. The impact of education on chronic kidney disease patients' plans to initiate dialysis with self-care dialysis: a randomized trial. Kidney Int. 2005;68:1777–83.

41. Devoe DJ, Wong B, James MT, et al. Patient education and peritoneal dialysis modality selection: a systematic review and meta-analysis. Am J Kidney Dis. 2016;68:422–33.

42. McLaughlin K, Manns B, Mortis G, Hons R, Taub K. Why patients with ESRD do not select self-care Dialysis as a treatment option. Am J Kidney Dis. 2003; 41:380–5.

43. Wu AW, Fink NE, Marsh-Manzi JVR, et al. Changes in quality of life during hemodialysis and peritoneal Dialysis treatment: generic and disease specific measures. JASN. 2004;15:743–53.

44. Durand M, Bekker HL, Casula A, et al. Can we routinely measure patient involvement in treatment decision-making in chronic kidney care? A service evaluation in 27 renal units in the UK. Clin Kidney J. 2016;9:252–9.

10

Factors associated with anaemia in kidney transplant recipients in the first year after transplantation: a cross-sectional study

Andy K.H. Lim[1,2]* (iD), Arushi Kansal[1] and John Kanellis[1,2]

Abstract

Background: Anaemia after kidney transplantation may reduce quality of life, graft or patient survival. We aimed to determine the prevalence and risk factors for anaemia in the initial 12 months after transplantation.

Methods: We conducted a cross-sectional study at 6 and 12 months after transplantation. Anaemia was defined by World Health Organization criteria taking into consideration erythropoietin use. Logistic regression was used to determine the association between demographic, clinical and pharmacological risk factors for the main outcome of moderate-severe anaemia.

Results: A total of 336 transplant recipients were included and the prevalence of moderate-severe anaemia was 27.4% at 6 months and 15.2% at 12 months. Lower kidney function, female gender, transferrin saturation below 10% and proteinuria were associated with moderate-severe anaemia at both time points. Recent intravenous immunoglobulin treatment was associated with anaemia at 6 months. Recent infection and acute rejection were also associated with anaemia 12 months. Around 20% of patients had at least one blood transfusion but they were uncommon beyond 3 months.

Conclusions: Anaemia remains highly prevalent requiring treatment with erythropoietin and transfusions. Most identifiable risk factors relate to clinical problems rather than pharmacological management, while markers of iron-deficiency remain difficult to interpret in this setting.

Keywords: Anaemia, Kidney transplantation, Haemoglobin, Iron-deficiency, Haematinics, Blood transfusion

Background

Post-transplant anaemia affects 10–40% of kidney transplant recipients in the first 12 months. The prevalence partly depends on the definition of anaemia and timing post-transplant [1]. Transplant patients have more anaemia than the GFR-matched general population, suggesting that the transplantation process itself may contribute to anaemia [2].

Anaemia requiring transfusions is a risk factor for immunological sensitisation, which may affect future re-transplantation. Post-transplant anaemia is also associated with left ventricular hypertrophy, reduced systolic function and long-term mortality [3, 4]. In the French DIVAT study, anaemia at 12 months based on World Health Organization (WHO) criteria was associated with reduced patient survival in those with chronic kidney disease (CKD) stages 1–3 [5]. Anaemia may also reduce graft survival [6–9], quality of life and affect mental health [10, 11].

Early anaemia is often due to surgical factors, haemodilution and withdrawal of previous erythropoiesis-stimulating agents (ESA). Most anaemia resolves by 3–6 months with restoration of erythropoietin levels. Anaemia after this time frame is particularly relevant as the potential causes are less obvious. The prevalence of anaemia has also changed with the evolving immunosuppressive practices and use of co-administered medications (era-effect). Thus, evaluation of anaemia requires consideration of both clinical and pharmacological factors, and extrapolating from the general CKD population is not necessarily valid.

We aimed to determine the prevalence of anaemia and haematinic deficiency at 6 and 12 months in a

* Correspondence: andy.lim@monash.edu
[1]Department of Nephrology, Monash Health, Clayton, Victoria 3168, Australia
[2]Department of Medicine, Monash University, Clayton, Victoria 3168, Australia

contemporary kidney transplant cohort, and to determine the risk factors associated with anaemia. We focussed on moderate-severe anaemia, as patients with mild anaemia are not likely to be candidates for ESA intervention and the long-term consequences of mild anaemia may be less significant.

Methods

Study design and patients

This was a cross-sectional study of all adult (> 18 years) kidney transplant recipients including combined kidney-pancreas transplants from a single centre (Monash Health). The time points examined were at 6 and 12 months post-transplantation. The study period included transplants performed from 1 Jan 2011 to 31 Dec 2015. Patients were excluded from the study if they were deceased or returned to dialysis within 12 months post-transplantation. Patients with inadequate clinical data were also excluded.

Data collection

Clinical information was obtained from electronic medical records, including demographics (age, sex, diabetes, polycystic kidney disease [PKD], vasculitis and gastrointestinal bleeding risk) and transplantation details (donor type, delayed graft function, combined pancreas-kidney).

Information on clinical progress recorded included: *Recent (within the last 3 months)* episode of recognised bleeding, acute rejection, cytomegalovirus viraemia or nephropathy, BK virus viraemia or nephropathy. *Recent (within the last 4 weeks)* clinically evident systemic infection determined by history, examination and/or laboratory or imaging tests; for example, urinary or respiratory infections. We did not collect qualitative data on symptoms related to anaemia.

Information on medications (immunosuppressant, ESA, proton-pump inhibitors, anticoagulants, antiplatelets, renin-angiotensin system inhibitor, valganciclovir, trimethoprim-sulfamethoxazole, iron supplementation or infusion, vitamin supplementation or injections), treatments for rejection (plasma exchange, intravenous immunoglobulin [IVIG]) and episodes of blood transfusions were also extracted.

Laboratory data was obtained from routine follow up tests per transplant protocols. This included haematinics, parathyroid hormone (PTH) and urinary protein excretion at 6 and 12 months post-transplantation. Laboratory results up to 6 weeks before or after the study time points were considered acceptable for this cross-sectional design. Therefore, missing laboratory data could be due to true missing results or tests performed outside the accepted time frame.

The transplant physicians used their discretion to investigate potential causes of anaemia. They may have organised endoscopy or specialist haematological assessment. We did not collect data on any additional anaemia work-up beyond that routinely collected per protocol.

Definitions

Anaemia was defined by gender-specific WHO criteria: mild anaemia in male 110–129 g/L, female 110–119 g/L; moderate anaemia < 110 g/L, severe anaemia < 80 g/L. A haemoglobin of < 110 g/L defines moderate-severe anaemia for both genders. Patients requiring ESAs to maintain their haemoglobin levels were considered to have moderate-severe anaemia as these patients had a haemoglobin level < 100 g/L to qualify for ESA treatment.

B12 deficiency was defined as a serum level < 140 pmol/L or receiving B12 injections initiated within the last 3 months due to a documented deficiency. Low ferritin was defined as a level < 20 µg/L. Low transferrin saturation was defined as < 15%. Folate deficiency was defined as a serum folate < 10 nmol/L or red cell folate < 800 nmol/L. Serum PTH level is normally between 1.0 and 7.0 pmol/L. We analysed proteinuria as a categorical variable because a 24-h urine collection result was not available for all patients. We defined a 24-h urine protein excretion greater than 0.1 g/day or a spot urine protein-creatinine ratio greater than 0.03 g/mmol, as a positive result. Urine protein-creatinine ratios were also grouped into three ordinal levels: (1) ≤0.03 g/mmol, (2) > 0.03 to ≤0.1 g/mmol, (3) > 0.1 g/mmol.

Statistical analysis

All analyses were performed with STATA, version 15 (StataCorp, TX USA). To compare continuous variables at 6 and 12 months, a paired t-test or Wilcoxon signed-rank test was used depending on the distribution of the variables. To compare paired proportions for dichotomous variables, Mc Nemar's test was used. Logistic regression was used to analyse the association between the clinical and pharmacological predictors and the main binary outcome of anaemia for each time point. Variables with $P < 0.10$ in univariable analysis were included in a baseline multivariable model and a backward-elimination method was used to determine a final multivariable model. In the final model, multiple imputation was performed for missing transferrin saturation data, using a linear regression imputation method (imputed datasets, m = 50). The variables used in the imputation model were: age, gender, haemoglobin, haematocrit, mean corpuscular volume, white cell count, recent infection, recent rejection and proteinuria. We used orthogonal polynomial contrasts of the marginal predictions from the multivariable models to test for trend in the association between urine protein-creatine ratio levels and anaemia. The test for trend was conducted on five individual imputed datasets at both 6 and 12 months, and the conservative P-values were reported. A P-value less than 0.05 was considered statistically significant (or $P < 0.01$ when testing for interaction).

Results

Patient demographics

A total of 413 patients were in the database from 1 Jan 2011 to 31 Dec 2015. Of these, 336 patients were suitable for analysis (Fig. 1) and the demographics of the included patients are shown in Table 1. Most of exclusions were due to the lack of follow-up data. There was a slight preponderance of males. There were only 63/336 (18.8%) cardiac death donors but these accounted for 68.3% of all cases of delayed graft function (post-transplant dialysis). There were 32.7% pre-existing diabetics and 5.1% newly diagnosed post-transplant. Known upper gastrointestinal disorders were more common than lower gastrointestinal disorders as risk factors for gastrointestinal bleeding.

Clinical characteristics

Recognised bleeding (within prior 3 months) was infrequent at both 6 and 12 months (5.1 and 3.3%, respectively). Episodes of biopsy proven rejection (within prior 3 months) were common (14.0% at 6 months, 11.3% at 12 months). Isolated cellular rejection was less common (< 2%), with

the majority of biopsies showing some element of antibody-mediated rejection. The proportion of patients with a recent infection (within prior 4 weeks) was higher at 6 months (20.8%) than 12 months (13.7%), which was statistically significant (difference 7.1%, 95%CI 1.5–13.8%; X^2 = 6.70, df = 1, $P = 0.010$). A recent cytomegalovirus viraemia or infection (within prior 3 months) was uncommon at both time points (3.9%). BK viraemia or infection (within prior 3 months) was more common (15.2% at 6 months, 14.3% at 12 months).

Immunosuppression and medications

A comparison of immunosuppression and medication use for both time points is shown in Table 2. At 12 months, patients were generally on lower mycophenolate mofetil (MMF) doses and lower average prednisolone use compared to 6 months. Calcineurin-inhibitor use was no different with most patients on tacrolimus. As calcineurin-inhibitor doses were targeted to levels, the actual dosage carries little meaning and was not examined. Plasma exchange and IVIG use were less frequent at 12 months compared to 6 months. Our centre does not use anti-thymocyte globulin or rituximab for induction therapy. We use an interleukin-2 receptor antibody (basiliximab) for induction in high

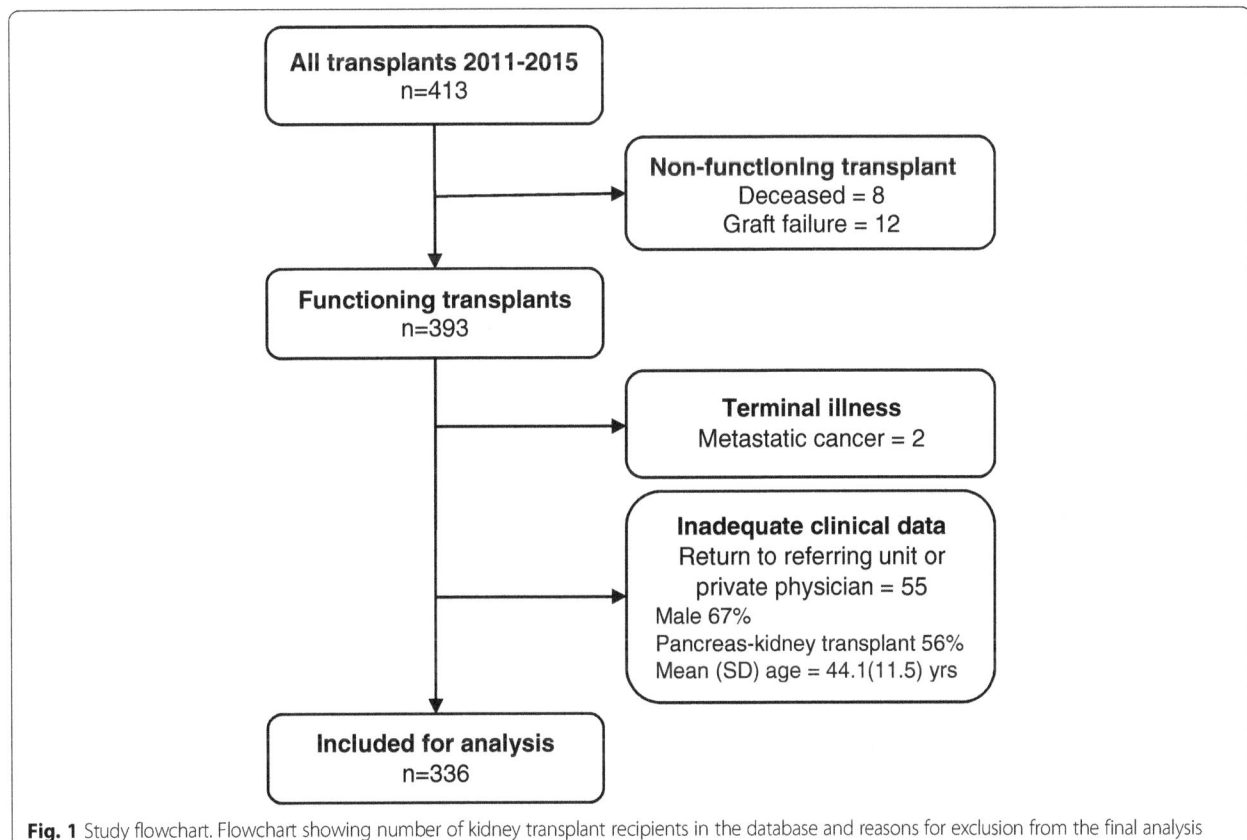

Fig. 1 Study flowchart. Flowchart showing number of kidney transplant recipients in the database and reasons for exclusion from the final analysis

Table 1 Characteristics of included patients (n = 336)

Characteristic	n (%)
Mean (± s.d.) age *years*[a]	51.3 ± 12.9
Male sex	218 (64.9)
Donor type:	
Brain death	176 (52.4)
Cardiac death	63 (18.7)
Living	82 (24.4)
ABO incompatible	15 (4.5)
Delayed graft function[b]	83 (24.7)
Pancreas-kidney transplant	23 (6.9)
Polycystic kidney disease	37 (11.0)
Diabetes:	
Type 1	39 (11.6)
Type 2	71 (21.1)
New-onset after transplant	17 (5.1)
Gastrointestinal bleeding risk:	
Upper gastrointestinal[c]	38 (11.3)
Lower gastrointestinal[d]	21 (6.3)
Vasculitis	11 (3.3)

[a]age at 6-month follow-up
[b]needed at least one dialysis treatment
[c]gastro-oesophageal reflux, oesophagitis, gastritis or ulceration
[d]polyps, angiodysplasia, diverticular disease or haemorrhoidal

Table 2 Medications and immunosuppression (n = 336)

Medication/immunosuppression	6 months n (%)	12 months n (%)	P value
Mycophenolate dose < 1.5 g/day	70 (20.8)	107 (31.8)	< 0.001
Calcineurin inhibitor:			
Tacrolimus	329 (97.9)	325 (96.7)	0.13[b]
Cyclosporine	4 (1.2)	8 (2.4)	
None	3 (0.9)	3 (0.9)	
Sirolimus/everolimus	11 (3.3)	7 (2.1)	0.13[b]
Prednisolone[a]	6.9 (2.6)	5.3 (1.5)	< 0.001
Plasma exchange	18 (5.4)	8 (2.4)	0.041
Intravenous immunoglobulin	49 (14.6)	28 (8.3)	0.006
Proton pump inhibitor	301 (89.6)	287 (85.4)	0.006
Trimethoprim-sulfamethoxazole	301 (89.6)	256 (76.2)	< 0.001
Valganciclovir	180 (53.4)	51 (15.2)	< 0.001
Renin-angiotensin inhibitor	49 (14.6)	60 (17.9)	0.055
Anticoagulation			
None	239 (71.1)	238 (70.8)	1.00[b]
Aspirin	82 (24.4)	78 (23.2)	
Clopidogrel	2 (0.6)	2 (0.6)	
Dual antiplatelets	1 (0.3)	2 (0.6)	
Warfarin	8 (2.4)	10 (3.0)	
Novel anticoagulants	4 (1.2)	6 (1.8)	
Iron supplementation			
None	321 (95.5)	322 (95.8)	1.00[b]
Oral	7 (2.1)	8 (2.4)	
Intravenous	8 (2.4)	6 (1.8)	
Erythropoiesis-stimulating agent	58 (17.3)	28 (8.3)	< 0.001
B12 injections	7 (2.1)	6 (1.8)	0.77[b]

[a]mean (s.d.)
[b]McNemar's exact test due to low frequency of discordant pairs

immunological risk patients. Basiliximab effects are not expected to last 6 months.

Use of prophylactic medications (proton pump inhibitor, trimethoprim-sulfamethoxazole and valganciclovir) reduced from 6 to 12 months, consistent with practice guidelines. Use of renin-angiotensin system inhibitors increased slightly at 12 months but remained < 20% overall. A quarter of patients received antiplatelet agents, mostly with aspirin as a single agent. Less than 5% were on anticoagulants, which were similar at both times. There was low use of supplemental iron and B12 injections were limited to those with documented low B12.

Laboratory characteristics

Results are summarised in Table 3. Haemoglobin and haematocrit were higher at 12 months than 6 months. This was associated with a small reduction in mean corpuscular volume associated with a lower ferritin level, on average. Serum iron, iron binding capacity and transferrin saturation were similar at both time points. However, the proportion of patients with actual laboratory defined low ferritin levels was not different. On the other hand, there was a smaller proportion of patients with transferrin saturation < 10% at 12 months compared to 6 months.

Overall, B12 levels were lower at 12 months than 6 months but the proportion with actual deficiency was similar. Folate deficiency was rare. Overall, kidney

function remained stable between 6 and 12 months with a mean eGFR of 56 ml/min/m^2. PTH levels were lower at 12 months but there was a similar proportion with PTH levels greater than 3 times the upper limit of normal. The proportion of patients with proteinuria was similar at both time points.

Moderate-severe anaemia and ESA use

We confirmed that all patients receiving ESA had a haemoglobin less than 100 g/L at initiation. The proportion of patients using ESAs dropped from 17.3% at 6 months to 8.3% at 12 months. This difference of 8.9% (95% CI: 4.5–13.4%) was statistically significant ($X^2 = 16.67$, df = 1, $P < 0.001$). The prevalence of anaemia based on WHO criteria is shown in Table 4. There is very strong evidence that the proportion of patients with moderate-severe anaemia or ESA use was lower at 12 months than at 6 months ($X^2 = 23.68$, df = 1, P < 0.001). The difference in

Table 3 Comparison of laboratory parameters at 6 and 12 months

Parameter	6 months (n)	12 months (n)	P value[b] (n)
Haemoglobin (g/L)	127 ± 18 (336)	133 ± 18 (336)	< 0.001 (336)
Haematocrit (%)	39.2 ± 0.1 (336)	40.7 ± 0.1 (336)	< 0.001 (336)
Percentage with haematocrit > 0.51	1.5 (336)	3.0 (336)	0.10 (336)
Mean cell volume(fL)	89 ± 7 (336)	87 ± 7 (336)	< 0.001 (336)
White cell count ($\times\ 10^9$/L)	6.9 ± 2.8 (336)	7.4 ± 2.6 (336)	0.002 (336)
[a]Serum iron (µmol/L)	13 (9–18) (248)	13 (10–17) (295)	0.44[c] (225)
Iron binding capacity (µmol/L)	60.5 ± 10.6 (229)	62.1 ± 11.1 (274)	0.06 (209)
[a]Transferrin saturation (%)	23 (15–30) (248)	22 (16–30) (292)	0.48[c] (225)
Percentage with TSAT < 20%	40.7 (248)	37.7 (292)	0.32[d] (225)
Percentage with TSAT < 10%	12.9 (248)	7.9 (292)	0.02[d] (225)
[a]Ferritin (µg/L)	95 (37–269) (248)	75 (31–193) (294)	< 0.001[c] (227)
Percentage with ferritin < 20 µg/L	12.5 (248)	13.6 (294)	0.37[d] (227)
Transferrin (g/L)	2.43 ± 0.43 (247)	2.48 ± 0.46 (291)	0.11 (225)
[a]Serum B_{12} (pmol/L)	299 (217–442) (222)	268 (199–380) (284)	0.002[c] (197)
Percentage with B_{12} < 140 pmol/L	7.7 (222)	6.7 (284)	0.56[d] (197)
Percentage with serum folate < 10 or red cell folate < 800 nmol/L	2.3 (222)	2.2 (278)	0.41[d] (193)
Creatinine (µmol/L)	125 ± 44 (336)	126 ± 52 (336)	0.29 (336)
CKD-EPI eGFR (ml/min/m^2)	56.1 ± 18.5 (336)	56.3 ± 19.0 (336)	0.77 (336)
[a]PTH (pmol/L)	9.8 (6.9–15.5) (244)	9.5 (6.6–15.1) (299)	0.022[c] (232)
Percentage with PTH > 20 pmol/L	16.4 (244)	14.4 (299)	0.13 (232)
Proteinuria (%)	23.8 (336)	26.2 (336)	0.22[d] (336)

Results are mean ± s.d. or [a]median (interquartile range). [b]Significance test is based on paired data, which is paired t-test unless specified as [c]Wilcoxon signed rank test or [d]McNemar's test

the proportion of anaemic patients was 12.2% (95% CI: 7.2–17.2%).

Factors associated with moderate-severe anaemia

The results of univariate analysis are shown in Additional file 1: Table S1. In multivariable logistic regression analysis, the significant factors associated with moderate-severe anaemia at 6 months were: female gender, allograft function, transferrin saturation < 10%, recent treatment with IVIG and proteinuria (Table 5). Every 5 ml/min/m^2 increase in eGFR was associated with 19% lower odds of having moderate-severe anaemia at 6 months. The c-statistic for this model was 0.79.

The significant factors associated with moderate-severe anaemia at 12 months were: female gender, allograft function, recent rejection, recent infection, transferrin

Table 4 Prevalence of anaemia at 6 and 12 months (n = 336)

	6 months	12 months
Original WHO categories		
No anaemia	54.4%	67.3%
Mild anaemia	28.0%	22.9%
Moderate-severe anaemia	17.6%	9.8%
Study categories (inclusive of ESA use)		
No/mild anaemia	72.6%	84.8%
Moderate-severe anaemia	27.4%	15.2%

WHO criteria (mild anaemia males: 110–129 g/L, females: 110–119; moderate: < 110, severe: < 80)

Table 6 Logistic regression showing association of different levels of proteinuria with moderate-severe anaemia (n = 336)

Urine protein/creatinine (g/mmol)	Odds ratio	95% C.I.	P value
6 months[a]			
≤ 0.03	1.00	reference	0.052
> 0.03 to ≤ 0.1	1.69	0.88–3.26	
> 0.1	4.00	1.09–14.6	
12 months[b]			
≤ 0.03	1.00	reference	0.023
> 0.03 to ≤ 0.1	2.43	1.09–5.40	
> 0.1	3.70	1.18–11.6	

Note: The odds ratios and 95% confidence intervals for the covariates were nearly identical to the multivariable models in Table 5 (with proteinuria as a binary variable)
[a]adjusted for eGFR, sex, intravenous immunoglobulin use, transferrin saturation < 10%
[b]adjusted for eGFR, sex, acute rejection, recent infection, transferrin saturation < 10%

saturation < 10% and proteinuria (Table 5). Every 5 ml/min/m^2 increase in eGFR was associated with 20% lower odds of having moderate-severe anaemia at 12 months. The c-statistic for this model was 0.86.

There was a linear trend in the association between urine protein-creatinine ratio and moderate-severe anaemia (Table 6) at 6 months ($X^2 = 4.30$, df = 1, $P = 0.038$) and 12 months ($X^2 = 4.43$, df = 1, $P = 0.035$), after adjusting for the relevant covariates. However, including proteinuria as an ordinal rather than binary variable in the multivariable models resulted in nearly identical coefficients and confidence intervals for the covariates. The c-statistics were also unchanged. Thus, using proteinuria as a binary variable in the multivariable models is parsimonious and did not result in loss of model discrimination.

To determine the impact of including ESA use in the definition of moderate-severe anaemia, we performed a comparison logistic regression analysis with moderate-severe anaemia defined by the original

Table 5 Risk factors for moderate-severe anaemia in multivariable modelling (n = 336)

	Odds ratio	95% C.I.	P value
6 months			
eGFR/5 (ml/min/m^2)	0.81	0.74–0.88	< 0.001
Female sex	4.26	2.41–7.55	< 0.001
Recent intravenous immunoglobulin[a]	2.28	1.12–4.63	0.023
Transferrin saturation < 10%	3.87	1.69–8.90	0.001
Proteinuria	1.95	1.05–3.60	0.035
12 months			
eGFR/5 (ml/min/m^2)	0.80	0.71–0.89	< 0.001
Female sex	3.12	1.46–6.66	0.003
Recent acute rejection[a]	3.09	1.27–7.53	0.013
Recent infection[b]	2.80	1.21–6.51	0.016
Transferrin saturation < 10%	3.45	1.11–10.76	0.033
Proteinuria	2.69	1.29–5.61	0.008

[a]within the last 3 months
[b]within the last 4 weeks

WHO criteria (Additional file 2: Table S2). In this comparison analysis, we excluded patients using ESAs who did not have moderate-severe anaemia (patients included purely on ESA criteria independent of WHO criteria; n = 33 at 6 months, n = 18 at 12 months). In the comparison analysis, recent rejection at 12 months was not significantly associated with the outcome (odds ratio, 1.07 [95% CI: 0.27–4.30], P = 0.92), after allowing for the other covariates. There was also little evidence that proteinuria was associated with the outcome at 6 months (odds ratio, 2.00 [95% CI: 0.97–4.18], P = 0.06). The association of the other factors with moderate-severe anaemia remain significant.

Blood transfusions

A total of 66/336 (19.6%) patients had at least one transfusion episode within 12 months of transplantation, excluding intra-operative transfusions. Of these, 47/66 (71%) had only one transfusion episode. The mean ± s.d. number of transfusions per episode was 1.4 ± 0.7 units (median number of transfusions per episode = 1 unit, interquartile range = 1 unit). The timing of all transfusion episodes in relation to time after transplantation is shown in Fig. 2.

Half of all transfusions occurred in the immediate post-operative period (within 10 days of transplantation) and 75% occurred within 25 days of transplantation. There were 13/336 (3.9%) patients who had at least one transfusion episode after 3 months. Of these 10/13 were already classified as having moderate-severe anaemia at 6 months. There were 4/336 (1.2%) patients with at least one transfusion episode after 9 months. All except one were already classified as having moderate-severe anaemia. A sensitivity analysis was conducted assuming a worst-case scenario that these four patients were

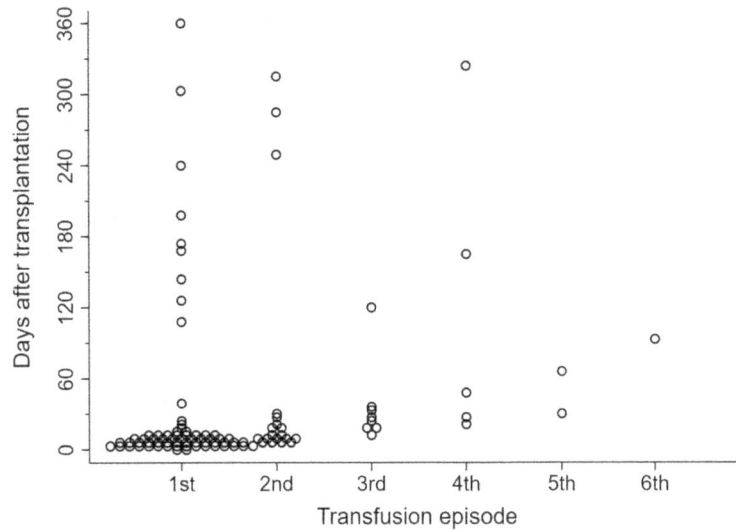

Fig. 2 Plot showing timing of transfusions in 66 patients who received at least one blood transfusion after transplantation. Each circle represents a transfusion episode. Time after transplantation is shown on the y-axis and the transfusion episode number on the x-axis. Most transfusions occurred in the early post-transplant period and the majority of patients only had one or two transfusion episodes

misclassified due to a transfusion within the last 3 months (data not shown). There was no statistically meaningful change in the final multivariable model and the c-statistic remained the same.

Discussion

The prevalence of anaemia in this study of 32.7% at 12 months post-transplant is consistent with estimates reported in the literature. However, a large proportion of these patients only had mild anaemia. For further discussion, we refer to the WHO-defined moderate-severe anaemia (haemoglobin < 110 g/L) in this study simply as "anaemia". We did not examine anaemia risk in the immediate post-surgical period as this is mostly related to surgical issues, transient haemodilution due to fluid loading and the significant volume of early phlebotomies [12]. These risk factors may not necessarily be modifiable so our focus was on anaemia beyond 3 months. We noted that the prevalence of anaemia declined between 6 and 12 months, which is consistent with other studies [8].

There was also a low prevalence of polycythaemia (haematocrit > 0.51) of 1.5% at 6 months and 3.0% at 12 months. These patients were exclusively male. Of these, 2/5 and 3/10 had PKD at 6 and 12 months, respectively. Our prevalence of polycythaemia is relatively low compared to previous data, and may certainly reflect changes in transplantation practice, which was as high as 19% in the mid-1990's and around 8% in the early 2000's [13]. One of these differences may be the proportions of patients with PKD in the transplant cohort, increasing use of renin-angiotensin system inhibitors or impact of MMF use.

Among patient factors, female sex has been associated with moderate-severe anaemia at both time points. This sex association is noted in a number of other studies as well [14–16]. It is postulated that this may partly be due to an increase in irregular menses and menorrhagia after kidney transplantation compared to prior [17]. This abnormal bleeding may be associated with changes to the hormonal profile post-transplantation [18]. However, we did not have data on menopausal status to address this hypothesis. Recipient age showed no association with moderate-severe anaemia even when stratified by sex (data not shown). We found no association between donor type and delayed graft function with anaemia. Diabetic status was associated with anaemia in univariate analysis at 12 months but not multivariate analysis. The highest risk group may be those with new-onset diabetes after transplantation.

Poor graft function is a very consistent correlate with anaemia across many transplant centres and studies [19, 20]. Indeed, this was confirmed in our study as well. A low eGFR (estimated by CKD-EPI equation) was associated with anaemia, even after adjusting for rejection and infection. A similar finding was noted if serum creatinine was used instead of eGFR (data not shown). The increased odds may be related to the inherent quality of the donor kidney and some studies have found an association between donor age and anaemia [20–22]. With the increasing use of extended criteria donors, this may be an area of concern which requires further study. Serum PTH was associated with anaemia in univariate but not multivariate analysis, presumably a reflection of its association with underlying allograft function.

In our study, proteinuria was associated with anaemia even when adjusted for renal function, and the odds of anaemia increases with higher levels of proteinuria, particularly at 12 months. A retrospective study by Bonofiglio et al. noted an association between anaemia at 1 year and 24-h proteinuria at 6 months in their multivariable model [23]. It is unlikely that proteinuria itself causes anaemia but may be a surrogate for other phenomena. There are several postulated mechanisms on how patients with nephrotic syndrome are at increased risk of anaemia. As reviewed by Iorember et al., this may involve increased urinary losses of iron, B12-transcobolamin, caeruloplasmin (secondary copper deficiency) and erythropoietin [24]. However, whether these mechanisms are involved in patients with sub-nephrotic proteinuria or transplantation is unclear.

In our study, we examined the haematinic profile. Although iron deficiency is common, there is much debate surrounding the definitions and whether the parameters used in the general population are applicable in the post-transplant setting. On average, we noted that serum ferritin and B12 levels were lower at 12 months compared to 6 months. However, the prevalence of laboratory defined deficiency based on standard cut-offs were not different. Serum ferritin was unhelpful and paradoxical, with anaemic patients having higher ferritin than non-anaemic patients (316 ± 359 μg/L vs. 125 ± 152 μg/L, $t_{292} = -5.91$, $P < 0.001$). Serum ferritin levels also showed a positive association with anaemia. This may relate to the inflammatory condition and functional iron deficiency. Thus, the ideal level to define deficiency is a little unclear. Similarly, we found that a serum transferrin saturation below 20% as a standard cut-off was not associated with anaemia but a threshold of 10% did in both univariate and multivariate models. It was difficult to analyse folate levels as a continuous variable due to the change in laboratory reporting from red cell folate to serum folate during the study period. Nonetheless, folate deficiency is uncommon (2% prevalence) with no demonstrable association with anaemia.

It has been previously suggested that a poor response to ESAs pre-transplant was a predictor of post-transplant anaemia [25]. However, we did not collect data on pre-transplant haematinic and haematological parameters. Given that ESA and iron supplementation are usually ceased at the time of transplantation, it is unclear how relevant these baseline values are at 6 months. Furthermore, it has been shown that iron deficiency can develop by 6 months in over half of patients who were iron-replete prior to transplantation [26]. There may also be an association between the malnutrition-inflammation score and post-transplant anaemia [19]. These factors could not be assessed in our study.

The use of azathioprine and MMF as anti-proliferative agents has been associated with anaemia. In our centre, MMF use is almost universal within the first 12 months of transplantation so we were unable to compare these two agents. The proportion of patients on daily MMF doses < 1.5 g was higher at 12 months but we could not detect a statistically significant association with the lower dose and anaemia using logistic regression. However, MMF dose could have been transiently reduced on occasions due to incidental leukopaenia and this may have reduced our ability to detect an association between MMF dose and anaemia. The use of mammalian target of rapamycin inhibitors is also associated with anaemia [27, 28]. In our centre, mammalian target of rapamycin inhibitor use was around 3% in the first 12 months and no association with anaemia could be detected.

In the general population, renin-angiotensin system inhibitors are associated with a 50–60% higher risk of anaemia [29]. In our study, there was no obvious effect of renin-angiotensin system inhibitors on anaemia. In the SMAhRT study of telmisartan versus placebo followed for a mean duration of 15 months, use of telmisartan did not worsen anaemia [30]. Nonetheless, it is unclear if the use of renin-angiotensin system inhibitors has contributed to the low prevalence of polycythaemia as previously mentioned. The use of proton-pump inhibitors has also been linked to poor iron absorption, contributing to iron-deficiency in some patients in the general population. Proton-pump inhibitors are routinely prescribed after transplantation but variably maintained and no information is available regarding its impact on iron status in the transplant population. We noted that patients on proton-pump inhibitors had a lower transferrin saturation than those who did not, at 12 months ($27.5\% \pm 12.3\%$ vs. $23.0 \pm 11.0\%$, $t_{290} = 2.32$, $P = 0.021$). There was a suggestion of an association between proton-pump inhibitor use and anaemia on univariate analysis which did not reach statistical significance ($P = 0.07$). If may be useful to explore this potential association in future studies. We did not find an association between trimethoprim-sulfamethoxazole or valganciclovir use with anaemia. Finally, the prevalence of ESA use of 8.1% in this study is comparable to previous reports of 5–11% [14, 20].

Recent rejection was associated with anaemia at 6 and 12 months in univariate analysis. It remained significant at 12 months with multivariate analysis but not in the comparison analysis using WHO criteria for anaemia and excluding ESA-treated, non-anaemic patients. The mechanism of rejection mediated anaemia is likely multifactorial, with both reduced erythropoietin production and inflammation-related erythropoietin resistance at play. However, we also noted that recent IVIG treatment for antibody-mediated rejection was associated with anaemia at 6 months. There is a theoretical risk of high dose (2 g/kg) IVIG precipitating haemolysis in transplant patients [31]. It was proposed that particular blood groups (A, B or AB) and IVIG preparations may be more likely to be associated with haemolysis. In non-transplant patients, data from neurological studies also showed recurrent high-dose IVIG use was associated with reduction in haematocrit or haemoglobin, and that biochemical evidence of haemolysis may be present even if an overt haemolytic syndrome was not evident [32, 33].

In our study, a clinically evident recent infection within the last 4 weeks was associated with anaemia. The majority of these were urinary tract and respiratory infection. Infections possibly cause derangements in iron utilization and erythropoietin resistance. Of further note, opportunistic infections such as cytomegalovirus, Epstein-Barr virus, BK virus and parvovirus B19 can cause direct bone marrow suppression. In our study, cytomegalovirus infection within the last 3 months was associated with anaemia at 6 months in univariate analysis but not in the multivariate model. One possible confounder of the association between anaemia and rejection or infection is the increased burden of diagnostic phlebotomy during acute management. This is difficult to tease out as data on frequency and volume of blood loss was not estimated.

Strengths and limitations

The strengths of this study include the full evaluation of ESA use and consideration of the potential impact of ESA use on prevalence of anaemia. Anaemia prevalence can be underestimated if patients are rescued from anaemia by ESAs. We also incorporated an audit of blood transfusions received by patients to determine transfusion requirements and potential impact of transfusions on anaemia prevalence. This study also evaluated two time points to determine if the factors associated with anaemia evolved over time, rather than assuming that any factors associated with anaemia remain stable between 6 and 12 months.

Including ESA use in the definition of anaemia can also be a limitation by introducing complexity or bias into the analysis. We attempted to address this by performing a comparison analysis using WHO criteria alone to define the outcome. Ultimately, a prospective study collecting incident data would be needed to confirm these associations.

This was a single-centre study and the cross-sectional design means that the results cannot be used for causal inference. A longitudinal study would be useful to confirm the identified factors associated with anaemia as specific risk factors. It was also not designed to look at outcomes such as graft and patient survival.

Data on the use of oral iron supplementation and multivitamins may not be reliable as they were not systematically recorded although data on iron infusions were robust as they were organised through our infusion centre. We also had missing data on haematinics, particularly at 6 months.

As mentioned in the methods section, this may be related to true missing values (test not performed) or related to timing. Although we used multiple imputation, the missing data could introduce some bias into the results if they were not truly *missing at random*.

In terms of generalisability, we would caution against generalising these results to kidney transplant cohorts with significant mammalian target of rapamycin inhibitor use in the first 12 months post-transplantation. Given the significant proportion of pancreas-kidney transplant recipients excluded from the study due to lack of clinical data, a similar caution applies to pancreas-kidney transplant cohorts. Our models should be validated in cohorts with more complete data from such transplant recipients.

Implications for practice

We have learned that anaemia prevalence can be underestimated when ESA use is not considered. Transplant centres monitoring anaemia prevalence should take this into account. The use of IVIG should be considered in the differential diagnosis of anaemia in kidney transplant patients, which may otherwise appear unexplained. A transferrin saturation below 10% should be a prompt to consider iron supplementation even if serum ferritin is within the normal range.

Conclusions

Post-transplant anaemia remains prevalent even in the modern transplant era. Female gender, allograft function, rejection and infection are associated with moderate-severe anaemia. Iron studies are difficult to interpret in the first post-transplant year but a transferrin saturation less than 10% may be a useful marker of increased risk. The role of proton-pump inhibitors, proteinuria and IVIG use in the development of anaemia requires further study. We also recommend that future studies include a quantitative analysis of protein excretion to confirm if there is a linear increase in the risk of anaemia with increasing levels of proteinuria.

Additional files

Additional file 1: Table S1. Univariate logistic regression analysis. The supplementary table shows the results of univariate analysis with the unadjusted odds ratio, 95% confidence intervals and significance values. It also shows the number of observations with the outcome of interest and the total number of observations where data is available.

Additional file 2: Table S2. Factors associated with WHO criteria defined moderate-severe anaemia in multivariable modelling. This analysis excludes patients who only met ESA criteria independent of WHO criteria for the definition of moderate-severe anaemia. It demonstrates that the factor "recent acute rejection" was no longer significantly associated with moderate-severe anaemia after allowing for the other covariates.

Abbreviations

CKD: Chronic kidney disease; eGFR: Estimated glomerular filtration rate using CKD-EPI; ESA: Erythropoiesis-stimulating agent; IVIG: Intravenous immunoglobulin; MMF: Mycophenolate mofetil; PKD: Polycystic kidney disease; PTH: Parathyroid hormone; WHO: World Health Organization

Authors' contributions

AK contributed to the study concept, majority of data collection, and discussion. AKHL contributed to study design, some data collection, data analysis, interpretation, and discussion and drafting article. JK contributed to the interpretation and critical review. All authors have read and approved the final manuscript.

Competing interests

The authors declare that they have no competing interests.

References

1. Reindl-Schwaighofer R, Oberbauer R. Blood disorders after kidney transplantation. Transplant Rev (Orlando). 2014;28(2):63–75.
2. Chadban SJ, Baines L, Polkinghorne K, et al. Anemia after kidney transplantation is not completely explained by reduced kidney function. Am J Kidney Dis. 2007;49(2):301–9.
3. Gurlek Demirci B, Sezer S, Sayin CB, et al. Post-transplantation Anemia predicts cardiovascular morbidity and poor graft function in kidney transplant recipients. Transplant Proc. 2015;47(4):1178–81.
4. Majernikova M, Rosenberger J, Prihodova L, et al. Posttransplant Anemia as a prognostic factor of mortality in kidney-transplant recipients. Biomed Res Int. 2017;2017:6987240.
5. Garrigue V, Szwarc I, Giral M, et al. Influence of anemia on patient and graft survival after renal transplantation: results from the French DIVAT cohort. Transplantation. 2014;97(2):168–75.
6. Kamar N, Rostaing L, Ignace S, Villar E. Impact of post-transplant anemia on patient and graft survival rates after kidney transplantation: a meta-analysis. Clin Transpl. 2012;26(3):461–9.
7. Ichimaru N, Obi Y, Nakazawa S, et al. Post-transplant Anemia has strong influences on renal and patient outcomes in living kidney transplant patients. Transplant Proc. 2016;48(3):878–83.
8. Huang Z, Song T, Fu L, et al. Post-renal transplantation anemia at 12 months: prevalence, risk factors, and impact on clinical outcomes. Int Urol Nephrol. 2015;47(9):1577–85.
9. Winkelmayer WC, Chandraker A, Alan Brookhart M, Kramar R, Sunder-Plassmann G. A prospective study of anaemia and long-term outcomes in kidney transplant recipients. Nephrol Dial Transplant. 2006;21(12):3559–66.
10. Majernikova M, Rosenberger J, Prihodova L, et al. Anemia has a negative impact on self-rated health in kidney transplant recipients with well-functioning grafts: findings from an 8-year follow-up study. Qual Life Res. 2016;25(1):183–92.
11. Abaci SH, Alagoz S, Salihoglu A, et al. Assessment of Anemia and quality of life in patients with renal transplantation. Transplant Proc. 2015;47(10):2875–80.
12. Zheng S, Coyne DW, Joist H, et al. Iron deficiency anemia and iron losses after renal transplantation. Transpl Int. 2009;22(4):434–40.
13. Kiberd BA. Post-transplant erythrocytosis: a disappearing phenomenon? Clin Transpl. 2009;23(6):800–6.
14. Molnar MZ, Mucsi I, Macdougall IC, et al. Prevalence and management of anaemia in renal transplant recipients: data from ten European centres. Nephron Clin Pract. 2011;117(2):c127–34.
15. Jones H, Talwar M, Nogueira JM, et al. Anemia after kidney transplantation; its prevalence, risk factors, and independent association with graft and patient survival: a time-varying analysis. Transplantation. 2012;93(9):923–8.
16. Shibagaki Y, Shetty A. Anaemia is common after kidney transplantation, especially among African Americans. Nephrol Dial Transplant. 2004;19(9):2368–73.
17. Chakhtoura Z, Meunier M, Caby J, et al. Gynecologic follow up of 129 women on dialysis and after kidney transplantation: a retrospective cohort study. Eur J Obstet Gynecol Reprod Biol. 2015;187:1–5.
18. Kim JM, Song RK, Kim MJ, et al. Hormonal differences between female kidney transplant recipients and healthy women with the same gynecologic conditions. Transplant Proc. 2012;44(3):740–3.
19. Molnar MZ, Czira ME, Rudas A, et al. Association between the malnutrition-inflammation score and post-transplant anaemia. Nephrol Dial Transplant. 2011;26(6):2000–6.
20. Vanrenterghem Y, Ponticelli C, Morales JM, et al. Prevalence and management of anemia in renal transplant recipients: a European survey. Am J Transplant. 2003;3(7):835–45.
21. Kamar N, Rostaing L. Negative impact of one-year anemia on long-term patient and graft survival in kidney transplant patients receiving calcineurin inhibitors and mycophenolate mofetil. Transplantation. 2008;85(8):1120–4.
22. Imoagene-Oyedeji AE, Rosas SE, Doyle AM, Goral S, Bloom RD. Posttransplantation anemia at 12 months in kidney recipients treated with mycophenolate mofetil: risk factors and implications for mortality. J Am Soc Nephrol. 2006;17(11):3240–7.
23. Bonofiglio R, Lofaro D, Greco R, Senatore M, Papalia T. Proteinuria is a predictor of posttransplant anemia. Transplant Proc. 2011;43(4):1063–6.
24. Iorember F, Aviles D. Anemia in nephrotic syndrome: approach to evaluation and treatment. Pediatr Nephrol. 2017;32(8):1323–30.
25. Kitamura K, Nakai K, Fujii H, Ishimura T, Fujisawa M, Nishi S. Pre-transplant erythropoiesis-stimulating agent hypo-responsiveness and post-transplant Anemia. Transplant Proc. 2015;47(6):1820–4.
26. Moore LW, Smith SO, Winsett RP, Acchiardo SR, Gaber AO. Factors affecting erythropoietin production and correction of anemia in kidney transplant recipients. Clin Transpl. 1994;8(4):358–64.
27. Chang Y, Shah T, Min DI, Yang JW. Clinical risk factors associated with the post-transplant anemia in kidney transplant patients. Transpl Immunol. 2016;38:50–3.
28. Webster AC, Lee VW, Chapman JR, Craig JC. Target of rapamycin inhibitors (sirolimus and everolimus) for primary immunosuppression of kidney transplant recipients: a systematic review and meta-analysis of randomized trials. Transplantation. 2006;81(9):1234–48.
29. Cheungpasitporn W, Thongprayoon C, Chiasakul T, Korpaisarn S, Erickson SB. Renin-angiotensin system inhibitors linked to anemia: a systematic review and meta-analysis. QJM. 2015;108(11):879–84.
30. Salzberg DJ, Karadsheh FF, Haririan A, Reddivari V, Weir MR. Specific management of anemia and hypertension in renal transplant recipients: influence of renin-angiotensin system blockade. Am J Nephrol. 2014;39(1):1–7.
31. Kahwaji J, Barker E, Pepkowitz S, et al. Acute hemolysis after high-dose intravenous immunoglobulin therapy in highly HLA sensitized patients. Clin J Am Soc Nephrol. 2009;4(12):1993–7.
32. Levine AA, Levine TD, Clarke K, Saperstein D. Renal and hematologic side effects of long-term intravenous immunoglobulin therapy in patients with neurologic disorders. Muscle Nerve. 2017. https://doi.org/10.1002/mus.25693.
33. Markvardsen LH, Christiansen I, Harbo T, Jakobsen J. Hemolytic anemia following high dose intravenous immunoglobulin in patients with chronic neurological disorders. Eur J Neurol. 2014;21(1):147–52.

11

The two isoforms of matrix metalloproteinase-2 have distinct renal spatial and temporal distributions in murine models of types 1 and 2 diabetes mellitus

Il Young Kim[2†], Sang Soo Kim[1†], Hye Won Lee[1], Sun Sik Bae[3], Hong Koo Ha[4], Eun Soon Jung[1], Min Young Lee[1], Miyeun Han[1], Harin Rhee[1], Eun Young Seong[1], Dong Won Lee[2], Soo Bong Lee[2], David H. Lovett[5] and Sang Heon Song[1*]

Abstract

Background: We recently reported on the enhanced tubular expression of two discrete isoforms of the MMP-2 (full length and N-terminal truncated, FL-MMP-2, NTT-MMP-2) in a murine model and human diabetic kidneys. In the present study, we examined in more detail the temporal and spatial distributions of MMP-2 isoform expression in murine models of Type 1 and Type 2 diabetes mellitus.

Methods: Diabetic models were streptozotocin (STZ)-induced diabetes (Type 1 diabetes mellitus) and db/db mice (Type 2 diabetes mellitus). We quantified the abundance of two isoforms of MMP-2 transcripts by qPCR. A spatial distribution of two isoforms of MMP-2 was analyzed semi-quantitatively according to time after injection of STZ and with increasing age of db/db mice. Furthermore, immunohistochemistry for nitrotyrosine was performed to examine a potential association between oxidative stress and MMP-2 isoform expression.

Results: Both isoforms of MMP-2 were upregulated in whole kidneys from STZ and db/db mice. In the case of FL-MMP-2, mRNA levels significantly increased at 12 and 24 weeks in STZ mice, while the isoform expression was significantly increased only at 16 weeks, in the db/db mice. FL-MMP-2 protein levels increased in the cortices and outer medullae of both STZ and db/db mice as a function of the duration of diabetes. For NTT-MMP-2, mRNA levels increased earlier at 4 weeks in STZ mice and at 10 weeks of age in db/db mice. The expression of NTT-MMP-2 also increased, primarily in the cortices of STZ and db/db mice, as a function of the duration of diabetes. Quantitatively, these findings were consistent with the qPCR results in the case of NTT-MMP-2, respectively (STZ 24 weeks, 3.24 ± 3.70 fold; 16 weeks db/db, 4.49 ± 0.55 fold). In addition, nitrotyrosine was expressed primarily in cortex as compared to medulla as a function of the duration of diabetes similar to NTT-MMP-2 expression.

Conclusions: Two isoforms of MMP-2 are highly inducible in two diabetic murine models and become more abundant as a function of time. As the expression patterns were not the same in the two isoforms of MMP-2, it is possible that each isoform has a discrete role in the development of diabetic renal injury.

Keywords: Diabetes mellitus, Hyperglycemia, Matrix metalloproteinase-2, Oxidative stress

* Correspondence: shsong0209@gmail.com
This study was presented as a poster in 2017 ERA-EDTA 54th Congress.
†Il Young Kim and Sang Soo Kim contributed equally to this work.
[1]Biomedical Research Institute and Department of Internal Medicine, Pusan National University Hospital, Gudeok-ro 179 Seo-gu, Busan 49241, Republic of Korea
Full list of author information is available at the end of the article

Background

Diabetes mellitus (DM) is the most common lifestyle-related disease and a heavy public health burden. In addition, the prevalence of DM is increasing very rapidly worldwide [1]. More than 2.7 million Koreans aged 30 years or older have Type 2 DM and the prevalence of an elevated fasting glucose was approximately 25.0% in 2013 [2]. Moreover, diabetes mellitus is the most common etiology of end-stage renal disease (ESRD) and accounts for 48.4% of new ESRD patients in 2015 Korean Registry [3]. Diabetic nephropathy is the most representative renal complication and related to injury to renal tubular cells and various cells of glomeruli. Given the prevalence and the extent of progression to ESRD, further elucidation of core pathophysiologic mechanisms of diabetic nephropathy is an important research goal.

Our laboratories have identified matrix metalloproteinase-2 (MMP-2) as a central mediator of acute and chronic renal injury in both experimental and human clinical settings [4–7]. Transgenic renal tubular epithelial cell expression of the full length, secreted isoform of MMP-2 (FL-MMP-2) results in loss of tubular basement membrane integrity, with resultant tubular atrophy, interstitial fibrosis and inflammation [6]. More recently, we have identified a novel intracellular isoform of MMP-2, called N-terminal truncated isoform of MMP-2 (NTT-MMP-2) [8]. The NTT-MMP-2 isoform lacks a secretory sequence and the inhibitory propeptide and remains intracellular in association with mitochondria in an enzymatically active form [7, 8]. NTT-MMP-2 isoform activation contributed to tubular epithelial cell regulated necrosis, which induced by the mitochondrial permeability transition and enhancement of sensitivity to ischemia/reperfusion injury [5]. Moreover, we tried to explore the expression of two isoforms of MMP-2 in diabetic kidney and firstly reported on the enhanced tubular epithelial cell expression of the FL-MMP-2 and NTT-MMP-2 isoforms in the murine streptozotocin model of Type 1 diabetes mellitus and in archival renal biopsies from patients with diabetic nephropathy [9]. So, we hypothesized that two isoforms of MMP2 can be important mediators in diabetic injury and the current study was designed to expand on these initial observations and to determine if differences exist between the spatial and temporal patterns of MMP-2 isoform expression in murine models of Type 1 (streptozotocin) and Type 2 (db/db mice) diabetic nephropathy. The findings of this study will provide a solid foundation for future studies to uncover mechanisms related to diabetic renal injury.

Methods

Murine models of diabetic nephropathy

The animal protocol (2014–069, 2016–102) used in this study was reviewed and approved by the Pusan National University–Institutional Animal Care and Use Committee (PNU-IACUC) regarding their ethical procedures and scientific care. Mice were randomized into control and diabetic groups. The first diabetic murine model was induced by five daily intraperitoneal injections of streptozotocin (STZ, 40 mg/kg in citrate buffer, pH 4.5, Sigma-Aldrich) in 8 week-old C57/BL6 male mice as described in the previous report [9]. This murine model is representative of Type 1 diabetes mellitus. The control mice received citrate buffer alone. STZ-induced diabetic mice were euthanized under isoflurane anesthesia at 4, 8, 12 and 24 weeks after the completion of STZ injection. Control mice were euthanized by same method at 12 weeks after the completion of citrate buffer without STZ. Each group was comprised of eight mice and was evaluated at 4, 8, 12 and 24 weeks following STZ treatment.

Male db/db mice (BKS.Cg-*m+/+Leprdb*/BomTac, Samtakobiokorea, South Korea) were used as a model of Type 2 diabetes mellitus. Control and db/m (heterozygote) male mice were obtained at the same time from the same company. The three study groups were euthanized under isoflurane anesthesia at 10 and 16 weeks of age. All kidneys were perfused with 4 °C phosphate-buffered saline (PBS) and then excised. Half of the kidney was fixed in 10% neutralized formalin for immunohistochemistry and the remaining portions were used for quantitative polymerase chain reaction (qPCR) analyses as detailed below. Table 1 summarized the characteristics of both diabetic mice model including body weight, kidney weight and albuminuria.

Quantitative polymerase chain reaction (PCR) analysis

The FL-MMP-2 and NTT-MMP-2 mRNA expression levels were measured by quantitative RT-PCR (qPCR). The procedures were described in the previous report in detail [9]. β-actin as the housekeeping internal control was quantified in parallel with the target genes and all products were verified by melting curve analysis (95 °C 15 s, 60 °C 15 s, 95 °C 15 s). Normalization and the fold-changes for each of the genes were calculated using the $2^{-\Delta\Delta CT}$ method. The primers used for qPCR are summarized in Table 2.

Microscopic analysis/immunohistochemistry

The tissues were fixed in 10% formalin immediately after collection. Subsequently, the tissues were paraffin-processed and embedded. The periodic acid-Schiff (PAS) stain and Masson's trichrome (MT) stain were performed to analyze any diabetic tissue injury and fibrosis. In addition, immunohistochemistry was performed on formalin-fixed 3 μm thick paraffin embedded sections. All of the procedures were conducted in the same way as the previous paper [9]. An isoform-specific antibody for NTT-MMP-2 targets the S1' substrate binding loop as reported in detail [5] and antibody to FL-MMP-2 was purchased from Abcam (ab3158, Abcam, Cambridge, UK). Simultaneouly, immunostaining using negative control omitting the primary antibody was

Table 1 Charateristics of diabetic mice models

DM	variables		control (12wks)	STZ 4wks	STZ 8wks	STZ 12wks	STZ 24wks	p-value
Type 1	BW (gm)	Initial	23(23–23.8)	23.5(23–24)	23.5(22.8–24)	23(23–23)	23(23–24)	0.684
		Last	31(29.2–32.8)	27(26.3–27.3)	26(25–28.5)	26(25–27.8)	29(27–32)	0.001
	KW/BW (mg/mg)		0.005 (0.005–0.006)	0.008 (0.007–0.010)	0.008 (0.008–0.008)	0.008 (0.007–0.008)	0.009 (0.008–0.011)	< 0.001
	ACR (µg/mg)		48.0 (31.6–58.9)			90.6 (78.5–97.5)	70.3 (39.0–101.5)	0.002
DM	variables		control	db/db	db/db			p-value
			(db/m 10wks)	(10wks)	(16wks)			
Type 2	BW	Initial	24(24–26)	45(45–46)	45.5(43.5–47.5)			0.043
		Last	25(25–28)	48(45–49)	55(50.5–58.8)			0.001
	KW/BW (mg/mg)		0.006 (0.005–0.008)	0.004 (0.004–0.004)	0.004 (0.004–0.005)			0.045
	ACR (µg/mg)		77.5 (75.9–84.2)	1000 (702.5–2274.0)	1333 (975.3–3755.0)			0.05

Abbreviations: *DM* diabetes mellitus; *STZ* streptozotocin; *BW* body weight; *KW/BW* kidney weight/body weight; *ACR* albumin creatinine ratio

conducted to ensure the specificity of the immunodetection. The semi-quantitative staining grade was measured as follows: grade 0, negative staining; grade 1, weak patchy staining; grade 2, weak diffuse or dense patchy staining; and grade 3, dense diffuse staining. For the assessment of oxidative stress in the diabetic kidneys, immunostaining for the marker of oxidative stress, nitrotyrosine was performed with mouse monoclonal antibody [EM-30] to nitrotyrosine (ab125106, Abcam, Cambridge, UK). We conducted correlation analysis between NTT-MMP-2 transcript abundance and nitrotyrosin IHC staining score. For two isoforms of MMP-2 transcript abundance, we used the $2^{-\Delta CT}$ method of analysis. Nitrotyrosin IHC scoring was performed as follows: 0, negative staining; 1, weak patch staining; 2, weak diffuse staining or dense patch staining; 3, dense diffuse staining.

Statistical analysis

All statistical analyses were performed using GraphPad Prism 6.0 (GraphPad Software). The Kruskal-Wallis test with Dunn's multiple comparison test or Mann Whitney U test were used to compare the experimental groups where appropriate. The spearman correlation analysis was conducted to prove the correlation between nitrotyrosine score and transcripts of both isoforms of MMP-2. A p-value of less than 0.05 was considered significant. The results are presented as the median (interquartile range) for all experiments.

Results

Streptozotocin model of type 1diabetes mellitus

Quantitative PCR showed that the FL-MMP-2 and NTT-MMP-2 transcripts were increased as compared to the non-diabetic control mice as function of the duration of diabetes (Fig. 1-a, b). In the case of FL-MMP-2, transcript abundance measured by quantitative PCR was significantly increased by 18.2 (14.0–21.7) fold and 13.1 (1.6–17.7) fold at 12 weeks and 24 weeks, respectively (p < 0.01). In the case of NTT-MMP-2, the transcripts were significantly increased 3.0 (2.3–4.9) fold at 4 weeks after the last STZ injection. NTT-MMP-2 transcript abundance was increased 2.5 (1.5–8.3) fold and 2.5 (2.1–5.5) fold at 12 and 24 weeks, respectively, p = 0.017. These experiments indicate that expression of the FL-MMP-2 and NTT-MMP-2 isoform transcripts have distinct temporal patterns in the STZ model of Type 1 diabetes mellitus, with NTT-MMP-2 isoform expression occurring significantly earlier than that of FL-MMP-2.

Figure 2 summarizes the results for IHC staining of renal cross sections for the FL-MMP-2 and NTT-MMP-2 isoforms in the STZ model. As shown in Fig. 2, panel I, there is low, but detectable expression of the FL-MMP-2 isoform in the renal cortex of control kidneys. In parallel with the qPCR studies of FL-MMP-2 transcript abundance, there no significant increase in IHC staining at 4 and 8 weeks. Prominent IHC staining for the FL-MMP-2 isoform was evident at 12 and 24 weeks in both the cortex and medulla. At both time points, cortical staining was comparable with medullary staining. Panel II, A and B, summarize semi-quantitative scoring of IHC staining for the FL-MMP-2 isoform.

In contrast to the FL-MMP-2 isoform, NTT-MMP-2 was not detectable by IHC in the either the cortex or medulla of control kidneys. At 4 weeks following STZ injection, NTT-MMP-2 signal was present primarily in the renal cortex and the intensity increased at 8 weeks and was

Table 2 Quantitative polymerase chain reaction primer sequences

Genes	Forward (5'→3')	Reverse (5'→3')
Full length MMP-2 (mouse)	GACCTCTGCGGGTTCTCTGC	TTGCAACTCTCCTTGGGGCAGC
N-terminal truncated MMP-2 (mouse)	GTGAATCACCCCACTGGTGGGTG	TTGCAACTCTCCTTGGGGCAGC
β-actin (mouse control)	CTCTCTTCCAGCCTTCCTTCC	CTCCTTCTGCATCCTGTCAGC

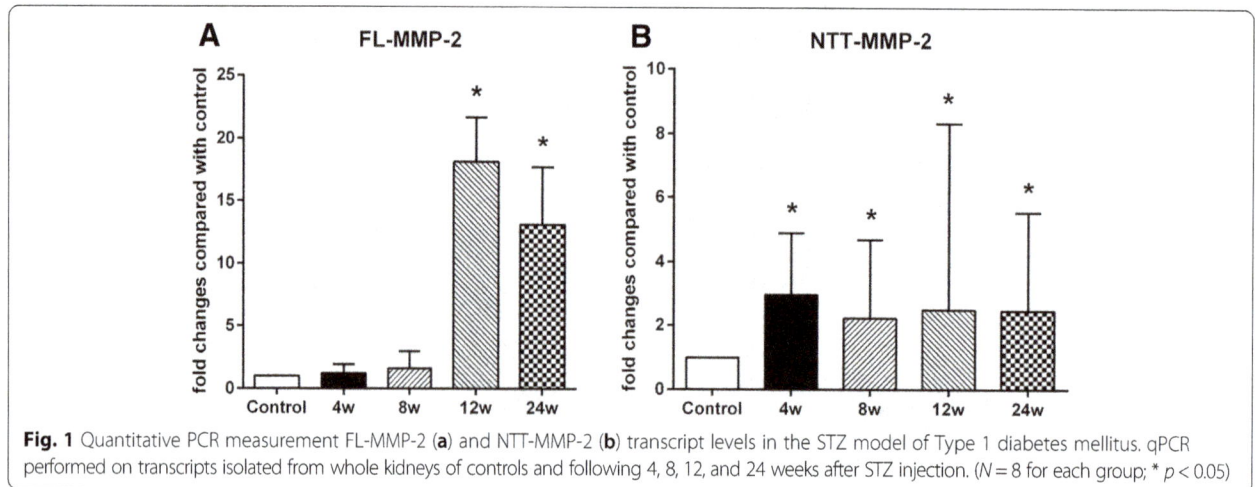

Fig. 1 Quantitative PCR measurement FL-MMP-2 (**a**) and NTT-MMP-2 (**b**) transcript levels in the STZ model of Type 1 diabetes mellitus. qPCR performed on transcripts isolated from whole kidneys of controls and following 4, 8, 12, and 24 weeks after STZ injection. ($N = 8$ for each group; * $p < 0.05$)

primarily limited to the cortex. Panel II, C and D summarize semi-quantitative IHC scoring for the NTT-MMP-2 isoform.

Db/db model of type 2 diabetes mellitus

Quantitative PCR results for expression of the two MMP-2 isoforms in the kidney using the db/db model of Type 2 diabetes mellitus are summarized in Fig. 3. Expression of the FL-MMP-2 transcript in kidneys was not significantly

increased until 10 weeks of age, and was only significantly increased at 16 weeks of age by approximately three-fold as compared to controls. In contrast, NTT-MMP-2 transcript abundance was increased nearly 6-fold by 10 weeks of age. Figure 4 summarizes the results for IHC staining for the MMP-2 isoforms in the db/db model kidneys. The FL-MMP-2 isoform was detected in both the cortex and medulla at 10 and 16 weeks of age, in each case expression of

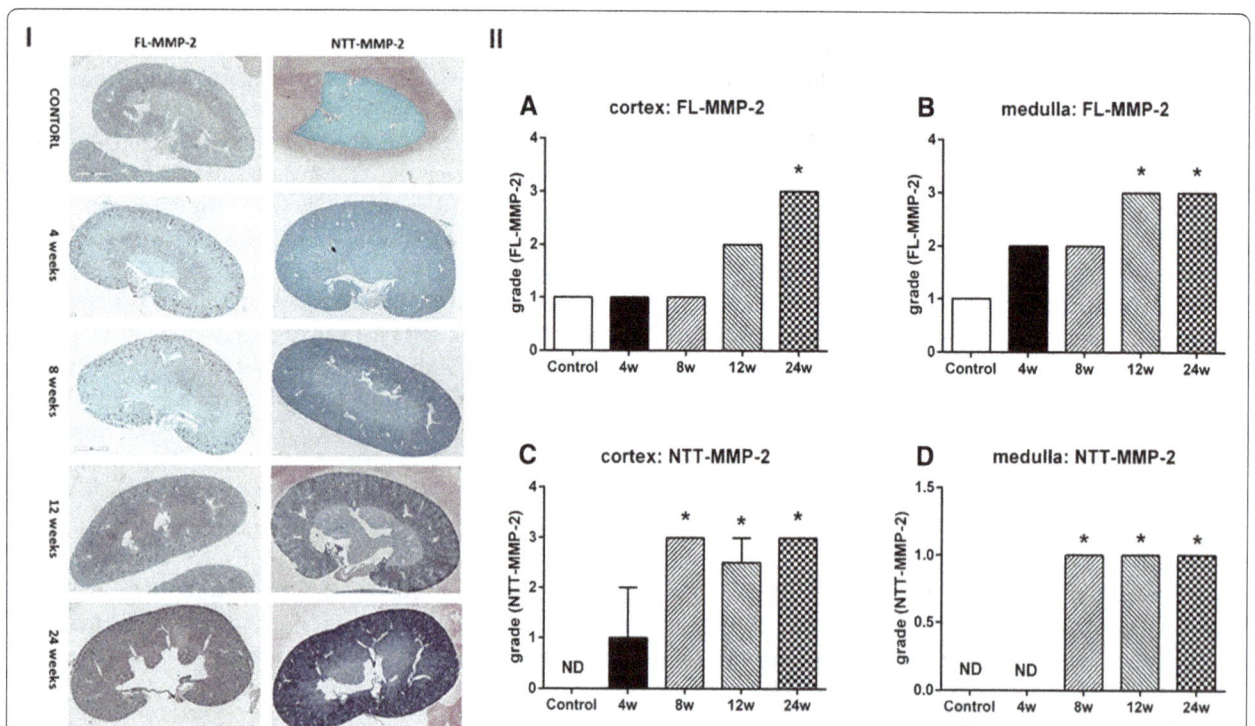

Fig. 2 Immunohistochemical staining of kidneys for FL-MMP-2 and NTT-MMP-2 in the STZ model of Type 1 diabetes mellitus. MMP-2 isoform specific IHC was performed as detailed in Methods. Panel **I**: IHC staining for FL-MMP-2 and NTT-MMP-2 for controls and at 4, 8, 12 and 24 weeks following STZ treatment. There is low basal staining for the FL-MMP-2 isoform in the cortex of control kidneys, while NTT-MMP-2 is not detected. IHC staining for both isoforms progressively increases as a function of time and staining is most prominent in the renal cortex. Panel **II**: Semi-quantitative scoring of IHC staining. ($N = 8$ for each group; * $p < 0.05$; X10))

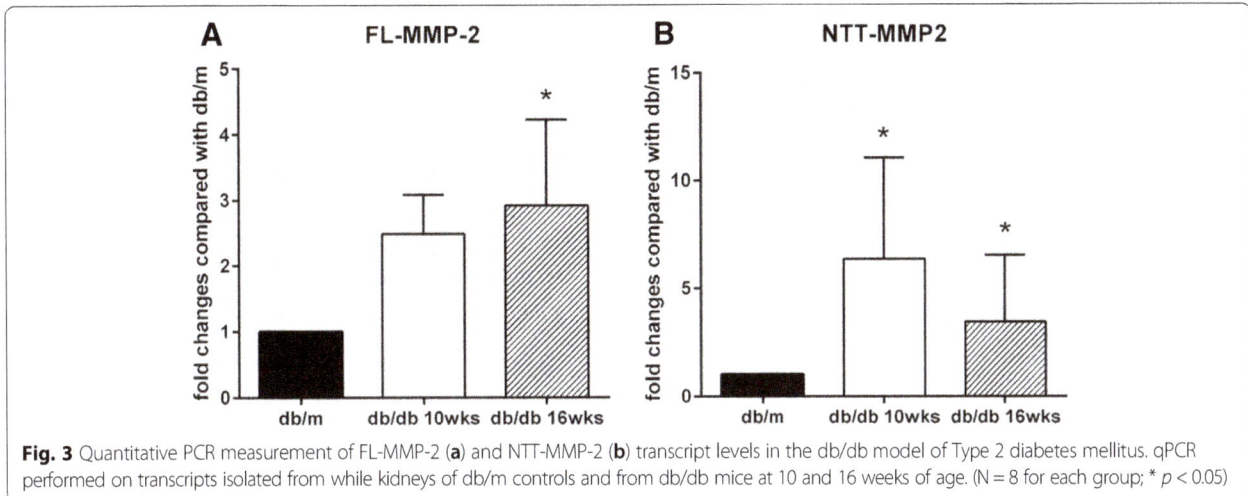

Fig. 3 Quantitative PCR measurement of FL-MMP-2 (**a**) and NTT-MMP-2 (**b**) transcript levels in the db/db model of Type 2 diabetes mellitus. qPCR performed on transcripts isolated from while kidneys of db/m controls and from db/db mice at 10 and 16 weeks of age. (N = 8 for each group; * $p < 0.05$)

the FL-MMP-2 in the cortex was comparable with the medulla. Panel II, A and B summarize the semi-quantitative IHC staining for the FL-MMP-2 isoform. The NTT-MMP-2 isoform was detected mainly in the renal cortex, but not prominent in the medulla of db/db kidneys. Panel II, C and D summarize the semi-quantitative IHC staining for the NTT-MMP-2 isoform.

We performed PAS and Masson trichrome staining on the kidneys from STZ-treated and db/db mice to determine if a correlation exists between the timing of MMP-2 isoform expression and tubular injury and fibrosis. Representative PAS-stained sections for the STZ-treated mice are shown in

Fig. 5, Panel I. Masson trichrome-stained sections are shown in Fig. 5, Panel II. At four weeks following STZ treatment the PAS and Masson trichrome sections are histologically normal. At 8 weeks following STZ treatment, a time at which NTT-MMP-2, but not FL-MMP-2 was upregulated (Figs. 1, 2) there was evidence for cytoplasmic vacuolization of the proximal tubule epithelial cells; however, there was no evidence for fibrosis as determined by Masson trichrome staining. By 24 weeks following STZ treatment when both the FL-MMP-2 and NTT-MMP-2 isoforms are upregulated, there was evidence for widespread proximal tubular epithelial cell necrosis with tubular lumens filled with necrotic cells

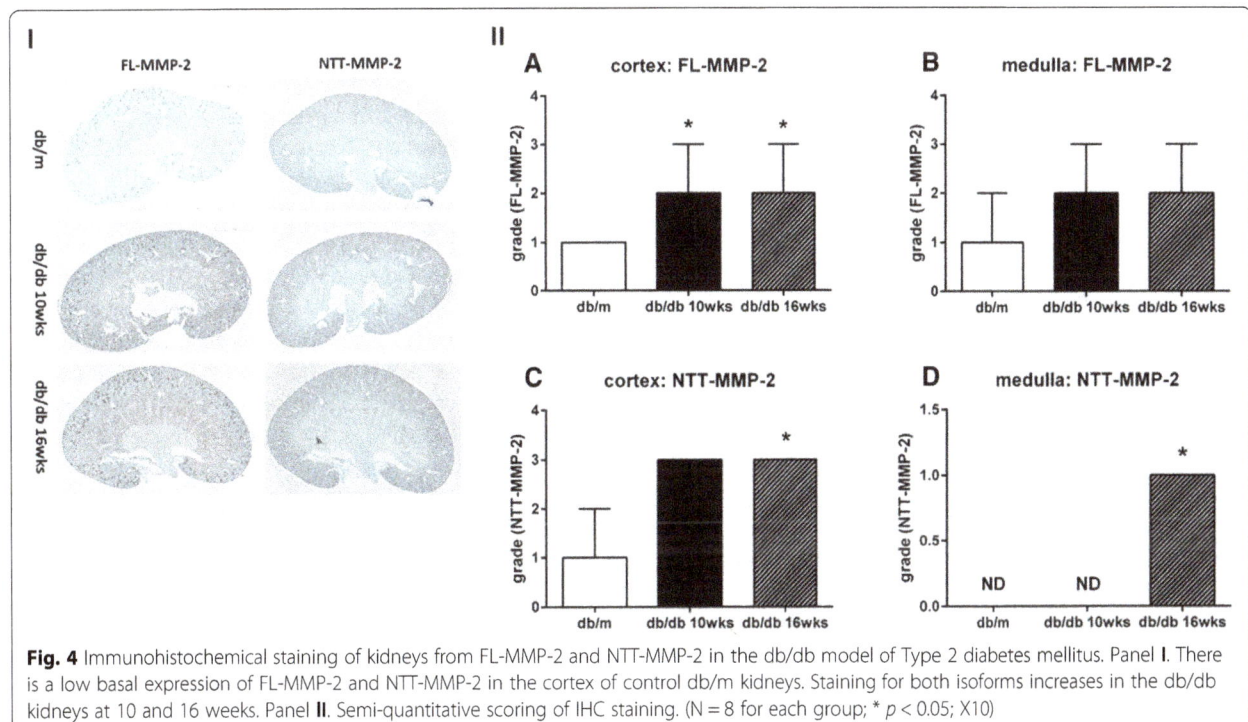

Fig. 4 Immunohistochemical staining of kidneys from FL-MMP-2 and NTT-MMP-2 in the db/db model of Type 2 diabetes mellitus. Panel **I**. There is a low basal expression of FL-MMP-2 and NTT-MMP-2 in the cortex of control db/m kidneys. Staining for both isoforms increases in the db/db kidneys at 10 and 16 weeks. Panel **II**. Semi-quantitative scoring of IHC staining. (N = 8 for each group; * $p < 0.05$; X10)

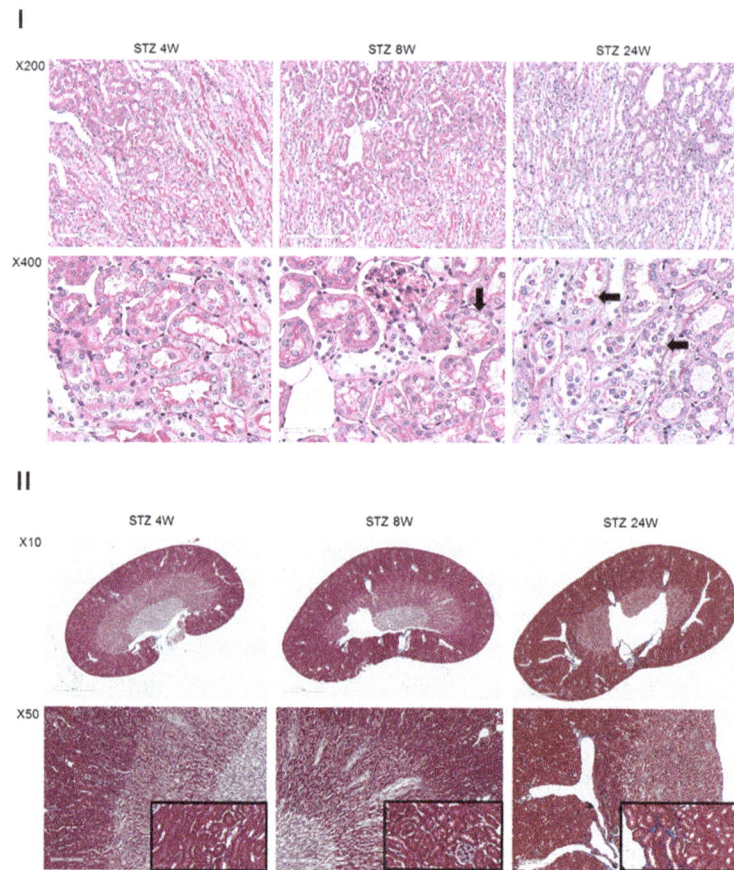

Fig. 5 PAS and Masson trichrome staining of kidneys from the STZ model of Type 1 diabetes mellitus. Panel I: PAS staining of renal cortex at 4, 8 and 24 weeks after STZ treatment. PAS staining is normal in the 4 week STZ group, while vacuolization of tubular epithelial cells is present at 8 weeks (arrow). By 24 weeks there is widespread tubular epithelial cell necrosis with cellular debris in the tubular lumens (arrows). Panel II: Masson trichrome staining of kidneys at 4, 8 and 24 weeks following STZ treatment. There is no detectable fibrosis at 4 and 8 weeks, while there are small foci of fibrosis (blue staining) in the cortex of kidneys at 24 weeks (inset X400)

in PAS-stained renal sections. In contrast to the widespread tubular epithelial cell necrosis at 24 weeks, there were only rare small foci of fibrosis.

We performed similar analyses with PAS and Masson trichrome staining on the db/db mice at 10 and 16 weeks of age. Representative results of these studies are shown in Fig. 6, Panels I and II. Proximal tubular epithelial cell vacuolization was present in the 10 week old db/db kidneys and by 16 weeks there was evidence for tubular epithelial cell necrosis with tubular dilation. Masson trichrome staining revealed only occasional patchy foci of fibrosis in the 16 week old db/db mice, which were not present in the 10 week old db/db mice.

We have recently reported that transgenic expression of the NTT-MMP-2 isoform in renal proximal tubular epithelial cells induces oxidative stress mediated by initiation of the mitochondrial permeability transition [5]. We used IHC staining for nitrotyrosine as a marker of oxidative stress and representative results of these studies are presented in Fig. 7. As compared to controls, there was no increase in nitrotyrosine IHC staining at 4 weeks following STZ treatment; however,

there was prominent staining for nitrotyrosine at 12 weeks following STZ treatment. Notably, nitrotyrosine staining was considerably stronger in the cortex as opposed to the medulla. Nitrotyrosine staining was not detectable in the kidneys of 10 weeks old db/m kidneys, but was readily detected in kidneys of 16 week old db/db mice (Fig. 7-I, II). As with the STZ-treated mice, nitrotyrosine staining was much more abundant in the cortex as compared to the medulla. The temporal patterns and expression levels of nitrotyrosine expression, a marker of oxidative stress, correlated with qPCR determination of MMP-2 isoform expression (Fig. 7-III).

Discussion

The principal findings of this study are that two discrete MMP-2 isoforms are induced in kidneys of murine models representative of Type 1 and Type 2 diabetes. In particular, the expression patterns of FL-MMP-2 and NTT-MMP-2 differed according to the anatomical location and the length of time with hyperglycemia. In the context of the time of a diabetic milieu, NTT-MMP-2 was more significantly

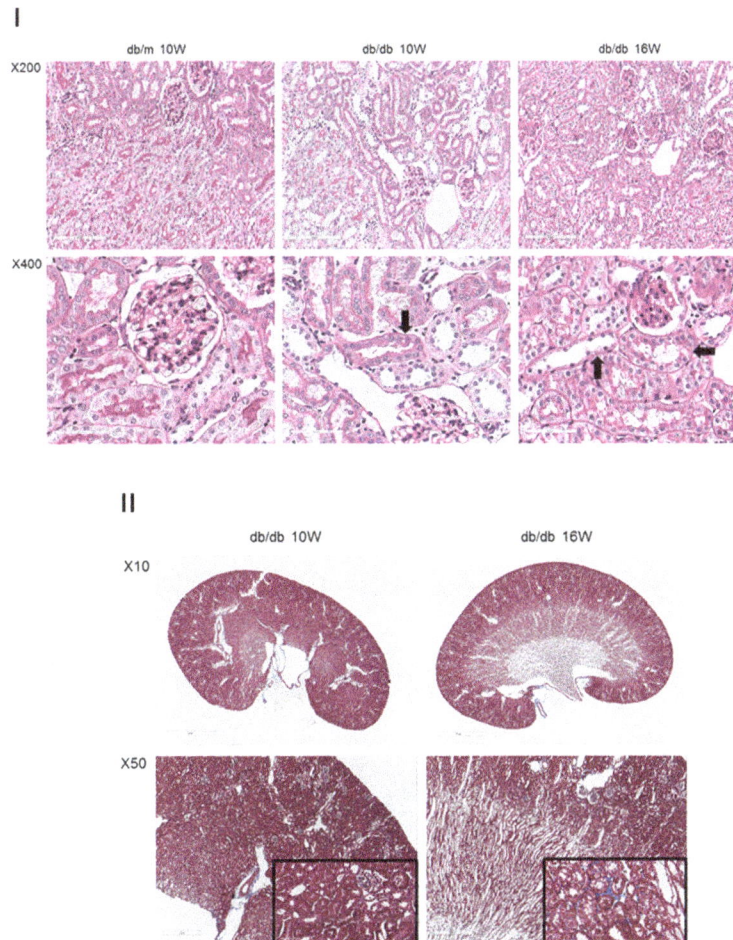

Fig. 6 PAS and Masson trichrome staining of kidneys from the db/db model of Type 2 diabetes mellitus. Panel I: PAS staining of control db/m kidneys is normal. At 10 weeks of age kidneys of db/db mice show occasional tubular epithelial cell vacuolization (arrow), which is much more extensive at 16 weeks of age (arrows). Panel II. Masson trichrome staining of control db/db kidneys at 10 and 16 weeks of age. There are rare, scattered foci of fibrosis (blue) in the deep cortex at 16 weeks, but not at 10 weeks of age (inset X400)

induced earlier in both murine diabetic models as compared to FL-MMP-2. In the context of the anatomical location, although the two isoforms of MMP-2 were expressed gradually in the renal cortical tubular segment according to the time of the two different diabetic milieu, the expression FL-MMP-2 in the outer medulla was more prominent as compared to NTT-MMP-2. Interestingly, NTT-MMP-2 was not expressed in whole kidney of normoglycemic control mice, while low cortical levels of FL-MMP-2 were detected by IHC in normoglycemic kidneys. In addition, although IHC staining for NTT-MMP-2 revealed low, detectable levels in the cortex of the db/m mice, the degree was faint and its expression was not evident in the outer medulla of db/m mice. In the later stage of the STZ induced diabetic model, NTT-MMP-2 was upregulated strongly in the cortex compared to the medulla. In the db/db mice, the two isoforms of MMP-2 were more significantly upregulated in cortex as compared with medulla. Based on these findings and previous data, the abundance

of FL-MMP-2 and NTT-MMP-2 in the two diabetic nephropathy models may be dependent on the degree of hyperglycemia and the degree of associated oxidative stress. Importantly, we showed that the upregulation of NTT-MMP-2 preceded evidence for the tubular injury pattern as previously reported in our transgenic model expressing NTT-MMP-2 in the renal proximal tubule [6].

To date, studies have provided conflcting data about the roles of matrix metalloproteinases in both experimental and clinical diabetic nephropathy [10]. MMP-2 can be expressed in the whole segments anatomically in the animal kidney, even though those kidneys were obtained from the rabbit, rats, and monkeys [11]. The present study is valuable because it defines the anatomical location (cortex vs. medulla) and the time of induction of MMP-2 isoform induction by hyperglycemia in both type 1 and type 2 murine diabetic models.

The NTT-MMP-2 isoform was initially characterized in isolated mitochondria from a murine model of systolic heart failure and accelerated atherogenesis and was

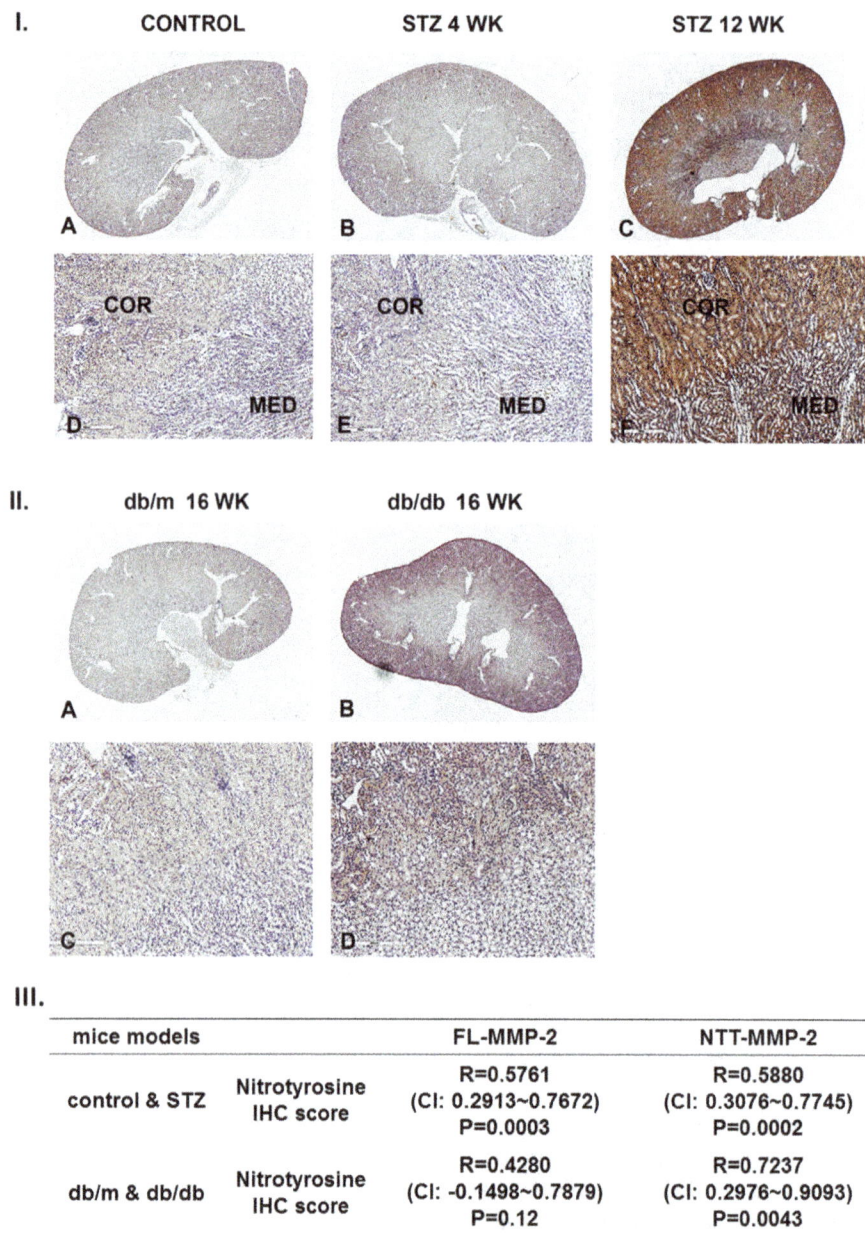

Fig. 7 Nitrotyrosine IHC of kidneys from STZ-treated and db/db mice. Panel **I**: Nitrotyrosine IHC from control kidneys (*a, d*) and at 4 weeks (b, e)and 12 weeks (*c, e*) following STZ treatment. IHC staining for nitrotyrosine is absent in the controls but is detectable at 4 weeks and further increased at 12 weeks. Nitrotyrosine IHC staining is most prominent within the cortex as compared to the medulla. (*a-c* X10; D-F X100). Panel **II**: Nitrotyrosine IHC of kidneys from control db/m (*a, c*) and with 16 week old db/db kidneys (b, d). Nitrotyrosine IHC staining is concentrated in the cortex of the 16 week old db/db kidneys and is not detected in the age-matched db/m controls. (*a, b* X 10; C,D X100). Panel **III**: Nitrotyrosin IHC score is correlated with two isoforms of MMP-2 in STZ and control kidneys. In db/m and db/db kidneys, NTT-MMP-2 is only correlated with nitrotyrosine ICH score. (R, correlation coefficient; CI, 95% confidence interval; ICH, immunohistochemistry)

also detected in the cardiac mitochondrial fraction of aged mice [8]. Subsequently, the NTT-MMP-2 isoform expression significantly correlated with tubular epithelial cell necrosis in human renal transplant delayed graft function [7]. Hyperglycemia- induced oxidative stress is considered as a major driver in diabetic nephropathy [12–14]. We have demonstrated that oxidative stress induces NTT-MMP-2 synthesis via activation of an alternate promoter located in the first intron of the MMP-2 gene [8]. Further, NTT-MMP-2, per se, induces further oxidative stress via induction of the mitochondrial permeability transition, with resultant tubular epithelial cell regulated necrosis [5]. The present study shows that the nitrotyrosine expression in the kidney is associated with the two isoforms of MMP-2, especially NTT-MMP-2. In addition, the hyperglycemia and mitochondrial pathway of regulated necrosis can be related to the increased susceptibility of rodent models and human with diabetes to ischemia-reperfusion injury [15].

Conclusions

Two isoforms of MMP-2 are consistently highly inducible in murine models representative of type 1 and type 2 diabetes and gradually become abundant over time of the diabetic milieu. As the expression patterns were not the same in the two isoforms of MMP-2, it is possible that these isoforms have a respective role in diabetic renal injury.

Abbreviations

DM: Diabetes mellitus; ESRD: End-stage renal disease; FL-MMP-2: The full length matrix metalloproteinase-2; MMP-2: Matrix metalloproteinase-2; MT: Masson's trichrome; NTT-MMP-2: N-terminal truncated isoform; PAS: Periodic acid-Schiff; qPCR: Quantitative polymerase chain reaction; STZ: Streptozotocin

Acknowledgements

SHS was supported by the National Research Foundation of Korea (NRF) grant funded by the Korea government (MSIP) (2016R1A2B4008243). DHL was supported by Department of Veterans Affairs Merit Review Award 1-BX000593 and National Institute of Diabetes, Digestive and Kidney Disease grant RO1DK39776. DHL's contributions are the result of work supported with the resources and the use of facilities at the San Francisco VA Medical Center.

Funding

This study was supported by the National Research Foundation of Korea (NRF) grant funded by the Korea government (MSIP) (2016R1A2B4008243) and fund had roles in the design, experiments, collection, analysis and interpretation of this study.

Authors' contributions

conceptualization: SHS, DHL / study design and coordination: SHS, EYS, DWL, SBL, SSB, DHL / data acquisition and modulation: SHS, IYK, SSK, ESJ, MYL, MH, HR / data analysis: SHS, IYK, SSK, MH, HR, SSB, DHL / investigation: SHS, IYK, SSK, HWL, HKH, ESJ, MYL, DHL / writing and editing of manuscript: SHS, IYK, SSK, DHL. All authors read and approved the final manuscript.

Competing interests

The authors declare that they have no competing interests.

Author details

[1]Biomedical Research Institute and Department of Internal Medicine, Pusan National University Hospital, Gudeok-ro 179 Seo-gu, Busan 49241, Republic of Korea. [2]Research Institute for Convergence of Biomedical Science and Technology and Department of Internal Medicine, Pusan National University Yangsan Hospital, Yangsan, Gyeongsangnamdo, Republic of Korea. [3]MRC for Ischemic Tissue Regeneration, Medical Research Institute, and Department of Pharmacology, Pusan National University School of Medicine, Yangsan, Republic of Korea. [4]Biomedical Research Institute and Department of Urology, Pusan National University Hospital, Busan, Republic of Korea. [5]The Department of Medicine, San Francisco Department of Veterans Affairs Medical Center, University of California San Francisco, California, USA.

References

1. International Diabetes Federation. IDF diabetes atlas. 6th ed. Brussels: International Diabetes Federation; 2013.
2. Noh J. The diabetes epidemic in Korea. Endocrinol Metab (Seoul). 2016;31: 349–53.
3. Jin DC, Yun SR, Lee SW, Han SW, Kim W, Park J. Current characteristics of dialysis therapy in Korea: 2015 registry data focusing on elderly patients. Kidney Res Clin Pract. 2016;35:204–11.
4. Cheng S, Lovett DH. Gelatinase a (MMP-2) is necessary and sufficient for renal tubular cell epithelial-mesenchymal transformation. Am J Pathol. 2003; 162:1937–49.
5. Ceron CS, Baligand C, Joshi S, Wanga S, Cowley PM, Walker JP, et al. An intracellular matrix metalloproteinase-2 isoform induces tubular regulated necrosis: implications for acute kidney injury. Am J Physiol Renal Physiol. 2017;312:F1166–83.
6. Cheng S, Pollock AS, Mahimkar R, Olson JL, Lovett DH. Matrix metalloproteinase 2 and basement membrane integrity: a unifying mechanism for progressive renal injury. The FASEB J. 2006;20:E1248–56.
7. Wanga S, Ceron CS, Delgado C, Joshi SK, Spaulding K, Walker JP, et al. Two distinct isoforms of matrix metalloproteinase-2 are associated with human delayed kidney graft function. PLoS One. 2015;10:e0136276.
8. Lovett DH, Mahimkar R, Raffai RL, Cape L, Maklashina E, Cecchini G, et al. A novel intracellular isoform of matrix metalloproteinase-2 induced by oxidative stress activates innate immunity. PLoS One. 2012;7:e34177.
9. Kim SS, Shin N, Bae SS, Lee MY, Rhee H, Kim IY, et al. Enhanced expression of two discrete isoforms of matrix metalloproteinase-2 in experimental and human diabetic nephropathy. PLoS One. 2017;12:e0171625.
10. Xu X, Xiao L, Xiao P, Yang S, Chen G, Liu F, et al. A glimpse of matrix metalloproteinases in diabetic nephropathy. Curr Med Chem. 2014;21:3244–60.
11. Catania JM, Chen G, Parrish AR. Role of matrix metalloproteinases in renal pathophysiologies. Am J Physiol Renal Physiol. 2007;292(3):F905–11.
12. Lovett DH, Chu C, Wang G, Ratcliffe MB, Baker AJ. A N-terminal truncated intracellular isoform of matrix metalloproteinase-2 impairs contractility of mouse myocardium. Front Physiol. 2014;5:363.
13. Lovett DH, Mahimkar R, Raffai RL, Cape L, Zhu BQ, Jin ZQ, et al. N-terminal truncated intracellular matrix metalloproteinase-2 induces cardiomyocyte hypertrophy, inflammation and systolic heart failure. PLoS One. 2013;8:e68154.
14. Dejonckheere E, Vandenbroucke RE, Libert C. Matrix metalloproteinases as drug targets in ischemia/reperfusion injury. Drug Discov Today. 2011;16:762–78.
15. Peng J, Li X, Zhang D, JK C, Y S, Smith SB, et al. Hyperglycemia, p53, and mitochondrial pathway of apoptosis are involved in the susceptibility of diabetic models to ischemic acute kidney injury. Kidney Int. 2015;87:137–50.

12

Influence of arteriovenous fistula on daily living behaviors involving the upper limbs in hemodialysis patients: a cross-sectional questionnaire study

Yuuta Hara[†], Kosuke Sonoda[†], Koji Hashimoto[†], Kazuaki Fuji, Yosuke Yamada[*] ⓘ and Yuji Kamijo[*]

Abstract

Background: Arteriovenous fistulae can restrict daily living behaviors involving the upper limbs in hemodialysis patients, but no studies have investigated the detailed effects of an arteriovenous fistula on routine life activities. Accordingly, many medical caregivers are unable to explain the effects of an arteriovenous fistula on daily life, particularly during non-dialysis periods, because they cannot observe them directly.

Methods: Thirty outpatients undergoing hemodialysis at 2 facilities scored the difficulty due to an arteriovenous fistula in performing 48 living behaviors during non-dialysis and 10 behaviors during dialysis into 5 grades in a comprehensive questionnaire survey. These behaviors were selected based on an open-answer pre-questionnaire administered to the 30 patients beforehand. The scores were also compared between dominant arm and non-dominant arm arteriovenous fistula groups.

Results: During non-dialysis, the difficulty scores of behaviors restricted out of concern for arteriovenous fistula obstruction (wear a wristwatch, hang a bag on the arm, carry a baby or a dog in the arms, wear a short-sleeved shirt, etc.) increased. The difficulties of "wear a wristwatch" and "hang a bag on the arm" were significantly higher in the non-dominant arm arteriovenous fistula group (both $P < 0.05$). In contrast, scores related to motor function (write, eat or drink, scratch an itch, etc.) increased remarkably during dialysis because of connection of the arteriovenous fistula to the dialysis machine. The difficulties of "write" and "eat or drink" were significantly higher in the dominant arm arteriovenous fistula group (both $P < 0.05$).

Conclusions: Several key daily living behaviors restricted by an arteriovenous fistula were identified in this questionnaire survey. These results will be useful for pre-operative explanation of arteriovenous fistula surgery and arm selection in end-stage renal disease patients.

Keywords: Arteriovenous fistula, Dialysis, Dominant arm, Living behavior, Motor function

---

* Correspondence: yosukeyama@shinshu-u.ac.jp; yujibeat@shinshu-u.ac.jp
[†]Yuuta Hara, Kosuke Sonoda and Koji Hashimoto contributed equally to this work.
Department of Nephrology, Shinshu University School of Medicine, 3-1-1 Asahi, Matsumoto, Nagano 390-8621, Japan

Background

The number of chronic kidney disease patients has been increasing due to lifestyle diseases and an aging population, with those reaching end-stage renal disease requiring the induction of hemodialysis. At that time, many patients require the creation of an arteriovenous fistula (AVF) on either forearm [1, 2].

Once an AVF is made, many patients experience difficulties in using their upper limbs [3] and suffer a decline in quality of life [4], firstly since they must constantly protect the AVF even during non-dialysis [1, 2], secondly because of decreased cosmesis due to vasodilation [5], thirdly as the range of upper-limb motion may become limited from the dilated blood vessel and modification of blood flow [6], and fourthly because moving the arm during dialysis becomes impaired by connection to the dialysis machine. The above issues represent a severe problem for many individuals, who understandably feel uneasy at pre-AVF consultation [7]. However, there are currently no studies investigating precisely how an AVF affects living behaviors. For that reason, many medical providers are unable to give detailed explanations on the influence of AVFs on lifestyle, particularly during non-dialysis, because they cannot observe them. This may fuel patient anxiety when deciding on AVF creation. Qin et al. described that professional strategies of internal fistulae could prolong service time, decrease complications, and increase quality of life [8]. We therefore devised a comprehensive questionnaire to identify which living behaviors were affected most by AVFs in hemodialysis patients. Moreover, we statistically investigated for differences in having the AVF in the dominant or non-dominant arm, a question often discussed at AVF consultations.

Methods

Study design

This was a cross-sectional questionnaire study.

Study patients

Forty-two Japanese patients over the age of 20 years and undergoing outpatient maintenance hemodialysis at either of 2 dialysis clinics (Kanno Dialysis and Vascular Access Clinic or Jishukai Ueda Kidney Clinic) who fulfilled the eligibility criteria below were approached. The inclusion criteria were: 1) currently receiving hemodialysis via an AVF, 2) performance status (PS) [9] of 0 or 1, and 3) having received at least 1 month of regular dialysis. The exclusion criteria were: 1) currently receiving hemodialysis via a non-AVF site, such as an arteriovenous graft, subcutaneously fixed superficial artery, or permanent vascular catheter, 2) having functional AVFs on both arms, 3) having impaired upper limb function due to problems other than AVF, such as hemiplegia, carpal-tunnel syndrome, or traumatic injury, 4) questionnaire response was difficult owing to dementia or a psychiatric disorder, and 5) ambidexterity. Twelve patients who did not provide consent to participate were excluded. The remaining 30 subjects were enrolled for this questionnaire study.

The subjects were analyzed for age, dialysis duration, gender, PS, dominant arm, number of AVF creations, occupation, cause of kidney disease, anastomotic site, AVF vessel size category (0, obscure; 1, thinner than the digitus minimus; 2, thicker than the digitus minimus but thinner than the thumb; 3, thicker than the thumb), and AVF after-effects such as steal syndrome and/or sore finger syndrome. The above information was collected from medical records or direct interviews with the patient.

Method for producing the questionnaire

The living behaviors evaluated in the questionnaire were selected to include activities indispensable in daily life that were affected by the presence of an AVF. To identify such behaviors, a preliminary, open-answer questionnaire (see Additional file 1) was administered to all 30 patients, asking: "Please list as many living behaviors outside of dialysis room as possible that are restricted by your AVF" and "Please list as many living behaviors as possible that are restricted due to your AVF being connected to the dialysis machine during treatment". Based on these results, 19 living behaviors during non-dialysis were identified: wear a wristwatch, carry a heavy object (over 5 kg), wear a short-sleeved shirt, drive a car, hang a bag on the arm, wear wrist-constricting clothes, bend the arm for an extended time, sleep in an unrestricted position, hold a handle strongly, enter a hot spring or public bath, carry a baby or dog in the arms, receive an arm massage, *care not to rub the arm strongly, *care not to hit the arm, *concern the AVF is obstructed due to dehydration, *care to avoid insect bites on the arm, *puncture site itchiness, *listlessness in the shoulder after dialysis, and *care to protect the arm from becoming cold. Five living behaviors during dialysis (eat or drink, operate a TV remote controller, sleep in an unrestricted position, read a book, and write) were listed as well.

To ensure an exhaustive list of living behaviors indispensable in daily life, 26 behaviors were selected according to the Disability of the Arm, Shoulder, and Hand (DASH) score [10], a general upper limb function evaluation tool used in the orthopedic field. As behaviors during non-dialysis, the following items were added: open a tight or new jar, write, turn a key, prepare a meal, push open a heavy door, place an object on a shelf above your head, do heavy household chores, garden or do yard work, make the bed, carry a shopping bag or briefcase, change a light-bulb overhead, wash or blow dry your hair, wash your back, put on a pullover sweater, use a knife to cut food, do recreational activities which require little effort (ex., playing cards, knitting, playing Japanese board games), do recreational activities in which you take some force or impact through your arm, shoulder, or hand (ex., golfing, playing tennis, playing catch ball, using a hammer), do recreational activities in which you move your arm freely (ex., throwing a flying disc, playing badminton), manage transportation needs, and engage in sexual activities. We also asked about *pain in the arm, shoulder, or hand at rest apparently caused by the AVF, *difficulty sleeping due to pain in the arm, shoulder, or hand apparently caused by the AVF, *pain in the arm, shoulder, or hand while performing any specific activity apparently caused by the AVF, *weakness in the arm, shoulder, or hand apparently caused by the AVF, *stiffness in the arm, shoulder, or hand apparently caused by the AVF, and *feel less capable, confident, or useful because of the AVF.

Five doctors in the dialysis field added 3 behaviors during non-dialysis (hold a pot, perform a blood pressure check, and do self-hemostasis of the AVF) and 5 behaviors during dialysis (operate a mobile phone or smart phone, communicate with staff or other patients, remove something from your bag, take medicine, and scratch an itch). Ultimately, these 48 items during non-dialysis and 10 items during dialysis were included in the final questionnaire (see Additional file 2).

The 48 items during non-dialysis were subdivided into 35 items related to activities and 13 items related to symptoms and feelings (indicated above by an asterisk). For the items related to activities, the questionnaire stated "Please rate how much the AVF disturbed the following activities in the past week. If you did not have the opportunity to perform an activity in the past week, please give your best estimate on which response would be the most accurate. It does not matter which hand or arm you used to perform the activity; please answer based on your ability regardless of how well you performed the task. For example, if you wrote with the right hand before having your AVF but are currently writing with the left hand because of the AVF, answer on the ability of writing with the left hand." The patients answered the questionnaire using 5 grades: 1) no difference with the AVF, 2) mild difficulty due to the AVF, 3) moderate difficulty due to the AVF, 4) severe difficulty due to the AVF, and 5) not possible due to the AVF. For the items related to symptoms and feelings, the questionnaire stated: "Please rate the severity of the following symptoms and feelings in the past week." The patients answered the questionnaire using 5 grades: 1) none, 2) mild, 3) moderate, 4) severe, and 5) extreme so I could do nothing.

All 10 items during dialysis were related to activities. The questionnaire stated: "Please rate how much the AVF disturbed the following activities during dialysis in the past week. In this part, AVF means AVF connected to the dialysis machine. If you did not have the opportunity to perform an activity in the past week, please

give your best estimate on which response would be the most accurate. It does not matter which hand or arm you used to perform the activity; please answer based on your ability regardless of how well you performed the task." The grading was identical to that for the non-dialysis activities.

Method for completing the questionnaires

A written questionnaire was given to all of the subjects, who completed it by themselves during or after dialysis. Since the outcomes contained subjective evaluation, there was a possibility of result bias, particularly when a researcher could easily identify a specific individual. Therefore, the surveys were recorded by means of an anonymous identification number for each respondent.

Statistical analysis

For patient characteristics, qualitative data are expressed as the number (percentage) and quantitative data are presented as the median (range). Regarding questionnaire scores, the average of all scores was calculated for each item. Missing data were excluded from the analysis. Response rates (RR) were calculated and shown. Additional comparison between the dominant-arm AVF group (DA-group) and non-dominant arm AVF group (nDA-group) were performed using the chi-square test for qualitative data and the Mann-Whitney U test for quantitative data. Statistical significance was defined as $P < 0.05$ as calculated by IBM SPSS statistics version 20 software (IBM Co., New York, USA).

Results

Table 1 summarizes the patient characteristics. There were 30 patients in total (15 each in the DA-group and nDA-group) with a variety of occupations, age range of 40 to 83 years, and dialysis duration range of 1 to 403 months. No patient had steal syndrome or sore finger syndrome. There were no significant differences between the test groups.

The overall results for living behaviors during non-dialysis and dialysis ranked according to average score value are presented in Figs. 1, 2 and 3. In items related to activity during non-dialysis (median RR: 97% [range: 73 to 100%]) (Fig. 1), the difficulty scores of items that could compress the AVF, such as "wear a wristwatch", "hang a bag on the arm", "bend the arm for an extended time", "wear wrist-constricting clothes", "receive an arm massage", "carry a baby or a dog in the arms", "perform a blood pressure check" and "wear a short-sleeved shirt" were relatively higher. Lower scores were seen for items that did not risk compression of the AVF, such as "write", "prepare a meal", "make the bed", "wash or blow dry your hair", "use a knife to cut food", "turn a key", "put on a pullover sweater", "use a knife to

Table 1 Characteristics of the study patients

	All patients N = 30	Dominant-arm AVF group N = 15	Non-dominant arm AVF group N = 15	P-value
Age (years)	63.5 (48–83)	63.0 (48–81)	64.0 (47–83)	0.65
Dialysis duration (months)	48.5 (1–403)	31.0 (1–331)	51.0 (5–403)	0.33
Gender (male)	22 (73%)	11 (73%)	11 (73%)	1.00
Performance status (0: 1)	26: 4 (87%: 13%)	13: 2 (87%: 13%)	13: 2 (87%: 13%)	1.00
Dominant arm (right)	29 (97%)	15 (100%)	14 (93%)	1.00
Number of AVF creations	1 (1–3)	1 (1–3)	1 (1–2)	0.49
Occupation				
Blue-collar worker	7 (23%)	4 (27%)	3 (20%)	1.00
White-collar worker	5 (17%)	2 (13%)	3 (20%)	1.00
Unemployed	18 (60%)	9 (60%)	9 (60%)	1.00
Cause of kidney disease				
Diabetes mellitus	13 (43%)	7 (47%)	6 (40%)	1.00
Chronic glomerular nephritis	13 (43%)	7 (47%)	6 (40%)	1.00
Other	4 (14%)	1 (6%)	3 (20%)	0.60
Anastomotic site				
Anatomical snuffbox	5 (17%)	2 (13%)	3 (20%)	1.00
Distal forearm	21 (70%)	11 (74%)	10 (67%)	1.00
Middle forearm	4 (13%)	2 (13%)	2 (13%)	1.00
Proximal forearm	0 (0%)	0 (0%)	0 (0%)	–
Vessel size category of AVF[a]				
Distal forearm	1 (0–3)	1 (0–2)	1 (0–3)	0.17
Middle forearm	1 (0–3)	0 (0–3)	1 (0–3)	0.15
Proximal forearm	1 (0–3)	1 (0–3)	1 (0–2)	0.33
After-effect of AVF creation				
Steal syndrome	0 (0%)	0 (0%)	0 (0%)	–
Sore finger syndrome	0 (0%)	0 (0%)	0 (0%)	–
Other	0 (0%)	0 (0%)	0 (0%)	–

AVF arteriovenous fistula. Data are presented as the number (percentage) or median (range).
[a]: 0) obscure, 1) thinner than the digitus minimus, 2) thicker than the digitus minimus but thinner than the thumb, 3) thicker than the thumb

cut food", "do recreational activities which require little effort", and "manage transportation needs". Regarding items related to symptoms and feelings during non-dialysis (median RR: 90% [range: 87 to 100%]) (Fig. 2), the scores of those related to AVF protection, such as "care not to hit the arm", "care not to rub the arm strongly", and "concern the AVF is obstructed due to dehydration", were highest. Scores were lowest for items unrelated to protecting the AVF, such as "listlessness in the shoulder after dialysis", "difficulty sleeping because of pain in the arm, shoulder, or hand apparently caused by the AVF", and "pain in the arm, shoulder, or hand apparently caused by the AVF while performing any specific activity". Among the items related to behaviors during dialysis (median RR: 97%

[range: 94 to 100%]) (Fig. 3), the scores for "write", "eat or drink", and "scratch an itch" were highest, while that for "communicate with staff or patients" was lowest.

The items with an average score of 2 (mild difficulty due to the AVF/mild) or more were next compared between the DA-group and nDA-group (Fig. 4). Concerning the items related to activity during non-dialysis, the scores for "wear a wristwatch" and "hang a bag on the arm" were significantly higher in the nDA-group (both $P < 0.05$). No significant differences were noted between the groups for symptoms and feelings during non-dialysis. Among the items related to activity during dialysis, the scores for "write" and "eat or drink" were significantly higher in the DA-group (both $P < 0.05$).

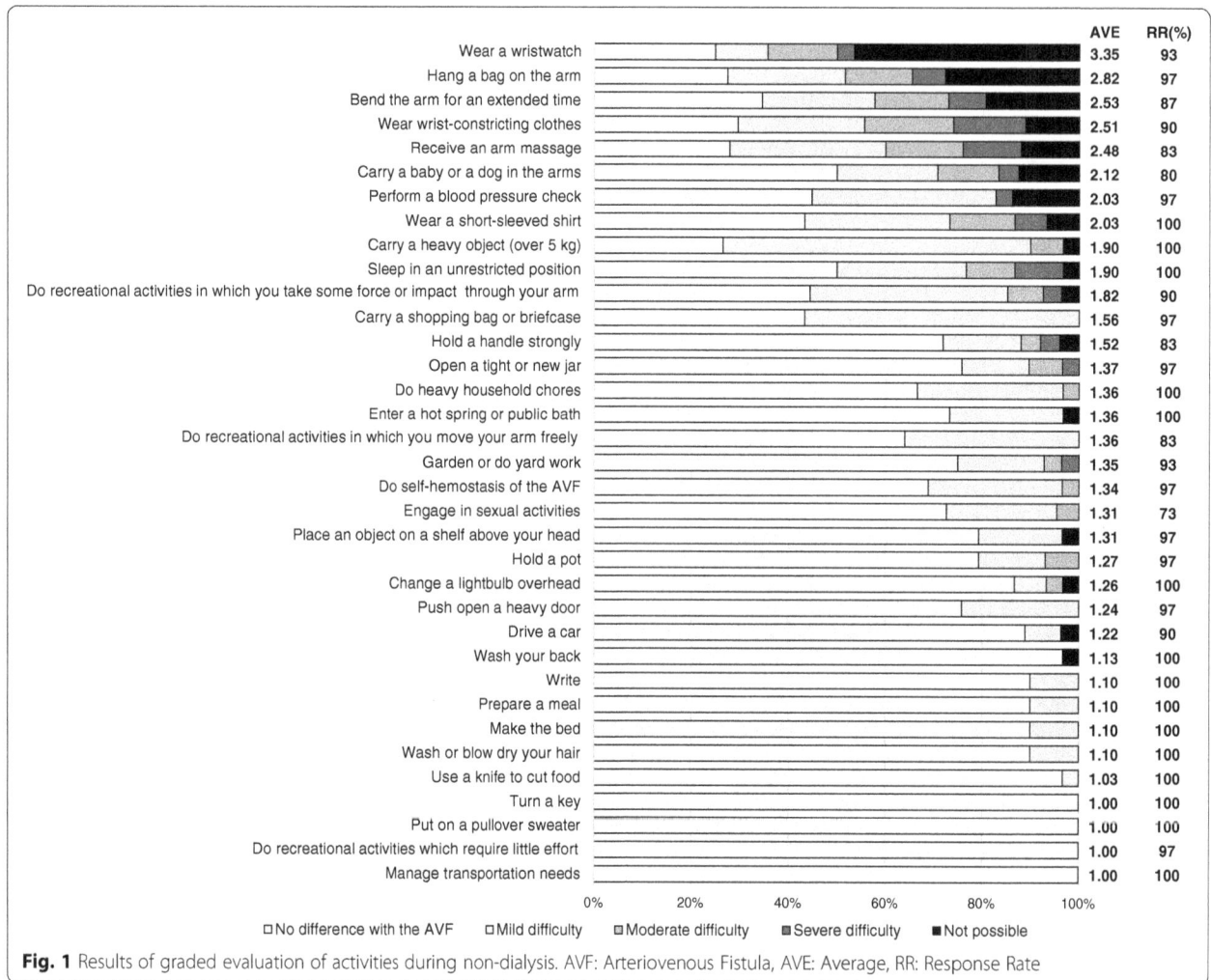

Fig. 1 Results of graded evaluation of activities during non-dialysis. AVF: Arteriovenous Fistula, AVE: Average, RR: Response Rate

Discussion

There have been no studies directly assessing the influence of AVFs on daily living behaviors involving the arms, which can be a serious problem for some hemodialysis patients. The present questionnaire survey revealed the most frequent difficulties among dialysis (activity-related) and non-dialysis (AVF compression avoidance-related) behaviors and clarified the possible differences in having an AVF in the dominant or non-dominant arm. Since AVF is the most often used type of vascular access [11, 12], this information will be very helpful for caregivers to better advise end-stage renal disease patients before and after the AVF procedure.

Based on our findings, it appeared possible to classify all tested items into 4 categories: 1) those that do not compress the arm but become restricted when motor function of the arm declines, 2) those related to physical appearance, 3) those that can compress and/or damage the arm, causing restriction out of worry for AVF obstruction, and 4) those related to unusual sensation (Fig. 5). In this context, the presence of an AVF had little influence on motor function itself during non-dialysis, with many living behaviors instead being restricted due to care for protecting the AVF. Indeed, protection of the AVF is essential for dialysis patients. Compressing the AVF vessel can cause obstruction [1] and wounds on the operated arm may lead to critical bleeding [13] .Additionally, since infection of the AVF site can sometimes be severe, patients need to keep the arm clean [14, 15]. Medical staff accordingly instruct patients to protect the AVF [1, 2], which seems to have the greatest influence on daily life. On the other hand, with little impact on the muscles and nerves, the AVF did not remarkably affect motor function among the respondents.

In the clinical context, patients scheduled to receive an AVF surgery will be better able to visualize post-operative life using the results of this study, which may reduce anxiety prior to surgery. Also, for individuals nervous about AVF protection, advocating long sleeves

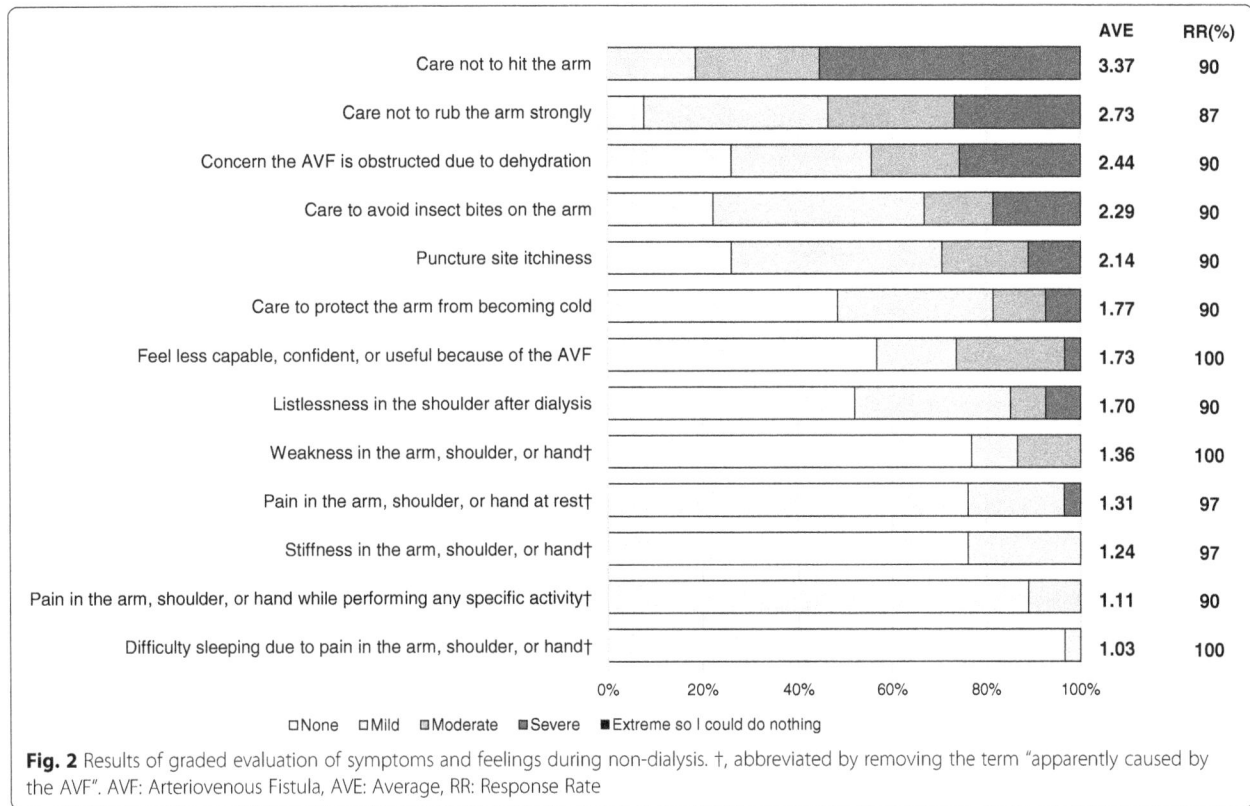

Fig. 2 Results of graded evaluation of symptoms and feelings during non-dialysis. †, abbreviated by removing the term "apparently caused by the AVF". AVF: Arteriovenous Fistula, AVE: Average, RR: Response Rate

that do not constrict the AVF arm and/or an arm cover during non-dialysis periods may provide comfort. In contrast, motor function is more predominantly limited during dialysis because the arm is connected to the dialysis machine. Medical staff should therefore arrange the dialysis room environment such that patients can be entertained and perform behaviors not requiring specific work with their AVF arm during dialysis.

This is a novel study that highlights the influence of AVFs on the daily living behaviors of dialysis patients during non-dialysis, which is normally difficult for medical providers to observe in detail. In addition to

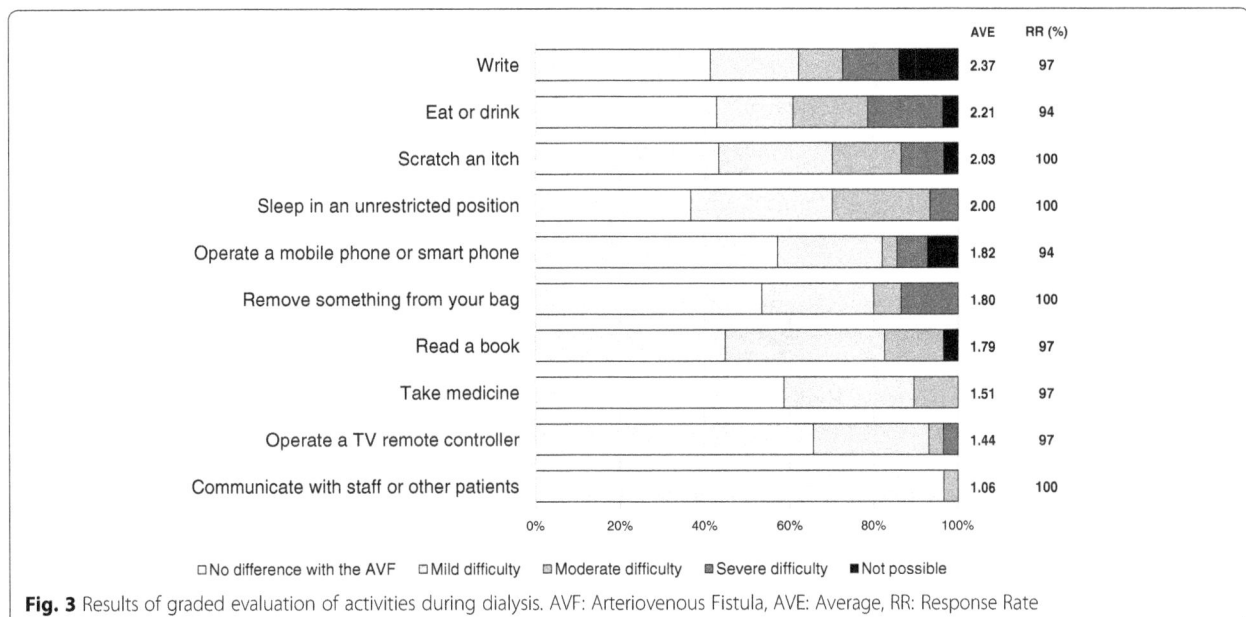

Fig. 3 Results of graded evaluation of activities during dialysis. AVF: Arteriovenous Fistula, AVE: Average, RR: Response Rate

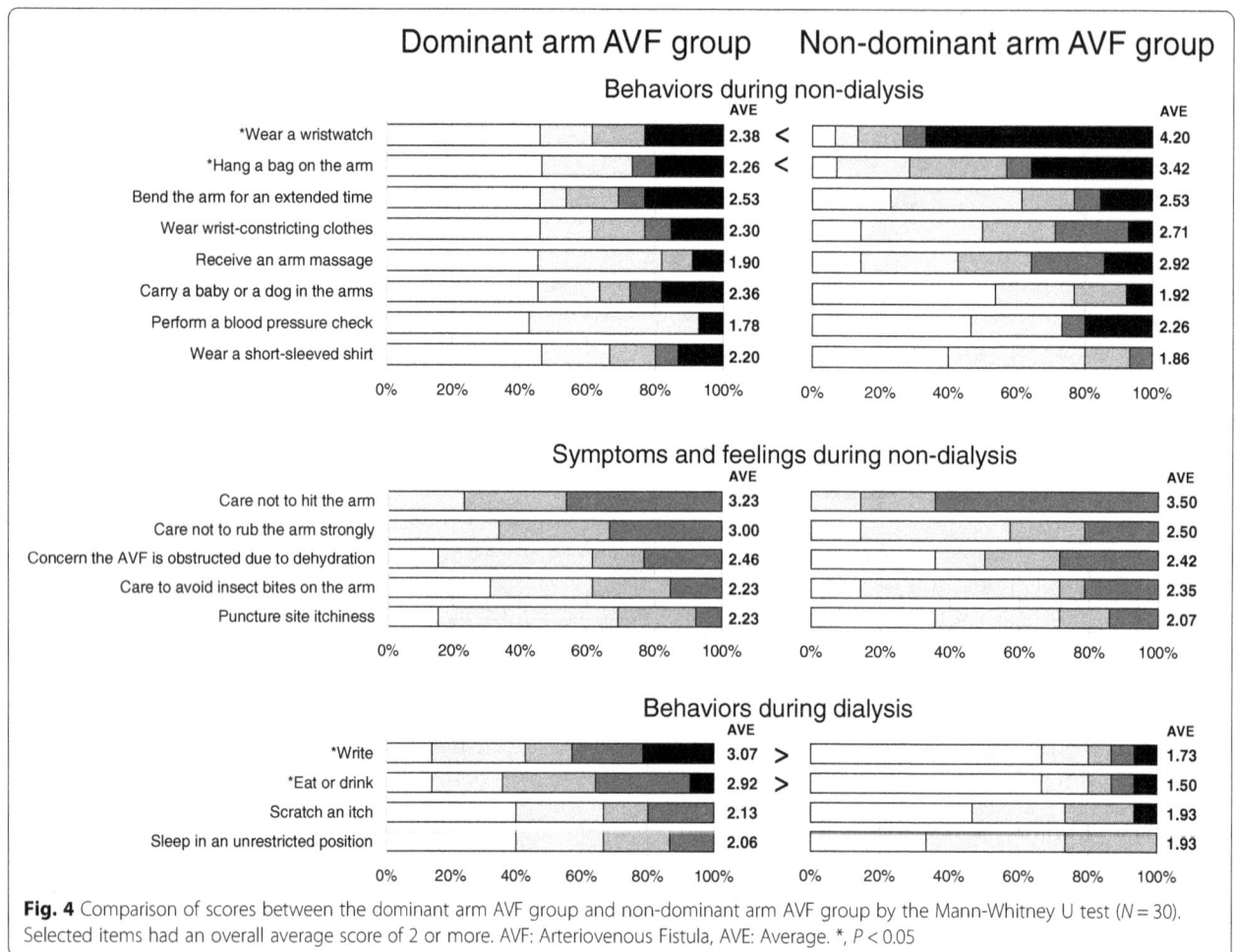

Fig. 4 Comparison of scores between the dominant arm AVF group and non-dominant arm AVF group by the Mann-Whitney U test (N = 30). Selected items had an overall average score of 2 or more. AVF: Arteriovenous Fistula, AVE: Average. *, P < 0.05

increased scores for conventional items said to be avoided during AVF education, such as "hang a bag on the arm", "wear a wristwatch", "bend the arm for an extended time", and "wear wrist-constricted clothes" [1], scores for many items important for communication and physical contact with family and friends, such as "carry a baby or a dog in the arms", "receive an arm massage", "wear a short-sleeved shirt", and "do recreational activities in which you take some force or impact through your arm" were higher as well. Moreover, in items regarding symptoms and feelings during non-dialysis, nearly half of the cohort scored "feel less capable, confident, or useful because of the AVF" as 2 or more. The prevalence of depression is high in dialysis patients [16, 17], and worsened psychological status and quality of life have been associated with mortality [16–18] and the development of itchiness [19]. The presence of an AVF may make dialysis patients reluctant to communicate with others and represents a contributing factor to diminished psychological status, lower quality of life, and higher mortality. Careful monitoring for mental health is therefore advised.

In comparisons between the DA-group and nDA-group, the DA-group tended to have more difficulty with activities during dialysis while the nDA-group appeared to have more trouble with activities during non-dialysis. The dominant arm is generally used in a major role for exercise and fine work [20] and the non-dominant arm often plays a supplementary role, such as to wrap or hang an object on the arm or to immobilize objects [21]. As shown in Fig. 5, the AVF was connected to the dialysis machine during dialysis, thereby strongly affecting motor function. In contrast, it was difficult to perform behaviors such as wrapping or hanging objects on the arm during non-dialysis because of concern for AVF blockage. These findings may be beneficial when consulting patients on which arm is more suitable for an AVF; if the dominant arm that is responsible for primary motor function is selected, the difficulty scores during dialysis will tend to rise, while if the non-dominant arm that is responsible for supplementary roles is chosen, the scores during non-dialysis will likely increase. It is generally considered that the AVF should be made in the non-dominant arm considering behaviors

	DURING NON-DIALYSIS	DURING DIALYSIS
Motor function	Carry a shopping bag or briefcase, Open a tight or new jar, Write, Carry a heavy object (over 5 kg), Turn a key, Prepare a meal, Do heavy household chores, Push open a heavy door, Place an object on a shelf above your head, Wash your back, Make the bed, Wash or blow dry your hair, Garden or do yard work, Change a lightbulb overhead, Do recreational activities which require little effort, Put on a pullover sweater, Use a knife to cut food, Do recreational activities in which you move your arm freely, Do self-hemostasis of the AVF, Manage transportation needs, Engage in sexual activities, Drive a car, Sleep in an unrestricted position	_**Write**_, _**Eat or drink**_, _**Scratch an itch**_, _**Sleep in an unrestricted position**_, Read a book, Operate a mobile phone or smart phone, Remove something from your bag, Take medicine, Operate a TV remote controller, Communicate with staff or other patients
Physical appearance	_**Wear a short-sleeved shirt**_, Enter a hot spring or public bath, Engage in sexual activities, Feel less capable, confident, or useful because of the AVF	
Worrying about AVF obstruction	_**Wear a wristwatch**_, _**Hang a bag on the arm**_, _**Bend the arm for an extended time**_, _**Wear wrist-constricting clothes**_, _**Receive an arm massage**_, _**Carry a baby or dog in the arms**_, Hold a handle strongly, _**Perform a blood pressure check**_, Carry a heavy object (over 5 kg), Do recreational activities in which you take some force or impact through your arm, _**Care not to hit the arm**_, _**Care not to rub the arm strongly**_, _**Concern the AVF is obstructed due to dehydration**_, _**Care to avoid insect bites on the arm**_, Care to protect the arm from becoming cold, Sleep in an unrestricted position	_**Sleep in an unrestricted position**_
Unusual sensation	Stiffness in the arm, shoulder, or hand apparently caused by the AVF, Pain in the arm, shoulder, or hand while performing any specific activity apparently caused by the AVF, Difficulty sleeping due to pain in the arm, shoulder, or hand apparently caused by the AVF, Puncture site itchiness, Listlessness in the shoulder after dialysis, Weakness in the arm, shoulder, or hand apparently caused by the AVF, Pain in the arm, shoulder, or hand at rest apparently caused by the AVF	

Fig. 5 Questionnaire items classified into 4 categories: 1) those that do not compress the arm but become restricted when motor function of the arm declines (Motor function), 2) those related to physical appearance (Physical appearance), 3) those that can compress and/or damage the arm, causing restriction out of worry for AVF obstruction (Worrying about AVF obstruction), and 4) those related to unusual sensation (Unusual sensation). Bold, underlined, and italicized items had an overall average score of 2 or more. AVF: Arteriovenous Fistula

during dialysis [1]. However, patients who regularly wear a wristwatch or hang things on the arm in their occupation or hobbies may instead be recommended to have the AVF in the dominant arm.

This study has several limitations. First, all participants were Japanese. Consideration of differences in race, religion, lifestyle, and physique will be needed when extrapolating these findings abroad. Second, patients who did not fulfill all eligibility criteria (especially poor PS or undergoing non-AVF dialysis) were excluded. Patients with poor PS have different lifestyles, and so our results may not have applied. Patients undergoing dialysis from a non-AVF site (especially those using catheters) may also not have been applicable to our results [22]. Moreover, the questionnaire was long and took considerable time to complete, causing some patients to decline participation. There was a possibility that only cooperative patients were selected for this study, which might have generated selection bias. Third, there were no patients with steal syndrome or sore finger syndrome resulting from their AVF in the study, which might limit the applicability of our results on patients with such after-effects of AVF creation.

Fourth, the response rate was low for several question items (especially "engage in sexual activities") that might have created information bias. Fifth, no controls were tested for comparisons with normal individuals. Lastly, particularly in the comparisons between the DA-group and nDA-group, statistical power may have been insufficient for some items due to small sample size. We are currently planning a larger, controlled study based on the items identified in this study.

Conclusions

The presence of an AVF impairs some motor functions by connection to the dialysis machine during dialysis but generally does not affect motor behaviors during non-dialysis, at which time some activities are limited by worry about damage to the AVF. Patients having an AVF in the dominant arm tend to experience activity difficulties during dialysis, while those with an AVF in the non-dominant arm are more prone to restrictions during non-dialysis. The results of this study will help with patient explanation prior to AVF creation and more optimal selection of the AVF arm.

Abbreviations
AVF: Arteriovenous Fistula; DA-group: Dominant Arm group; DASH: Disability of the Arm, Shoulder, and Hand; nDA-group: non Dominant Arm group; PS: Performance Status; RR: Response Rates

Acknowledgements
The authors sincerely thank the physicians, engineers, and nurses at Kanno Dialysis and Vascular Access Clinic and Jishukai Ueda Kidney Clinic.

Funding
No funding received.

Authors' contributions
YH*, KS*, KH*, KF, and YY planned the study, collected and analyzed the data, and wrote the article. *These 3 authors are co-first authors and contributed equally to this work. YK planned the study and wrote the article. All authors have read and approved the final manuscript.

Competing interests
The authors declare that they have no competing interests.

References
1. Vascular Access 2006 Work Group. Clinical practice guidelines for vascular access. Am J Kidney Dis. 2006;48(Suppl 1):S176–247.
2. Vascular Access Work Group Committee. Guidelines of vascular access construction and repair for chronic hemodialysis. J Jpn Soc Dial Ther. 2011; 44:855–937 (in Japanese).
3. Rehfuss JP, Berceli SA, Barbey SM, He Y, Kubilis PS, Beck AW, et al. The spectrum of hand dysfunction after hemodialysis fistula placement. Kidney Int Rep. 2017;2:332–41.
4. Domenick Sridharan N, Fish L, Yu L, Weisbord S, Jhamb M, Makaroun MS, et al. The associations of hemodialysis access type and access satisfaction with health-related quality of life. J Vasc Surg. 2018;67:229–35.
5. Al-Thani H, El-Menyar A, Al-Thani N, Asim M, Hussein A, Sadek A, et al. Characteristics, management, and outcomes of surgically treated arteriovenous fistula aneurysm in patients on regular hemodialysis. Ann Vasc Surg. 2017;41:46–55.
6. Kamyar MM, Saeed Modaghegh MH, Kazemzadeh G. Limb complaints after autogenous arteriovenous fistula creation in chronic hemodialysis patients. Semin Vasc Surg. 2016;29:172–7.
7. Abram HS. Psychiatric reflections on adaptation to repetitive dialysis. Kidney Int. 1974;6:67–72.
8. Hong Yan QIN, Ping JIA, Hui LIU. Nursing strategies for patients with chronic renal failure undergoing maintenance hemodialysis treatment by arteriovenous fistula. Iran J Public Health. 2016;45:1270–5.
9. Oken MM, Creech RH, Tormey DC, Horton J, Davis TE, McFadden ET, et al. Toxicity and response criteria of the eastern cooperative oncology group. Am J Clin Oncol. 1982;5:649.
10. Imaeda T, Uchiyama S, Wada T, Okinaga S, Sawaizumi T, Omokawa S, et al. Reliability, validity, and responsiveness of the Japanese version of the patient-rated wrist evaluation. J Orthop Sci. 2010;15:509–17.
11. Fissell RB, Fuller DS, Morgenstern H, Gillespie BW, Mendelssohn DC, Rayner HC, et al. Hemodialysis patient preference for type of vascular access: variation and predictors across countries in the DOPPS. J Vasc Access. 2013; 14:264–72.
12. Pisoni RL, Zepel L, Port FK, Robinson BM. Trends in US vascular access use, patient preferences, and related practices: an update from the US DOPPS practice monitor with international comparisons. Am J Kidney Dis. 2015;65: 905–15.
13. Jose MD, Marshall MR, Read G, Lioufas N, Ling J, Snelling P, et al. Fatal Dialysis vascular access hemorrhage. Am J Kidney Dis. 2017;70:570–5.
14. Mahmud SN, Baloch BK, Safdar M, Saeed M. Spontaneous Rupture and Dissection of aspergillus infected arteriovenous fistula. J Coll Physicians Surg Pak. 2016;26:116–7.
15. Imaizumi T, Hasegawa T, Nomura A, Sasaki S, Nishiwaki H, Ozeki T, et al. Association between Staphylococcus aureus bacteremia and hospital mortality in hemodialysis patients with bloodstream infection: a multicenter cohort from Japanese tertiary care centers. Ther Apher Dial. 2017;21:354–60.
16. Lopes AA, Bragg J, Young E, Goodkin D, Mapes D, Combe C, et al. Depression as a predictor of mortality and hospitalization among hemodialysis patients in the United States and Europe. Kidney Int. 2002;62: 199–207.
17. Fukuhara S, Green J, Albert J, Mihara H, Pisoni R, Yamazaki S, et al. Symptoms of depression, prescription of benzodiazepines, and the risk of death in hemodialysis patients in Japan. Kidney Int. 2006;70:1866–72.
18. Mapes DL, Lopes AA, Satayathum S, McCullough KP, Goodkin DA, Locatelli F, et al. Health-related quality of life as a predictor of mortality and hospitalization: the Dialysis outcomes and practice patterns study (DOPPS). Kidney Int. 2003;64:339–49.
19. Yamamoto Y, Hayashino Y, Yamazaki S, Akiba T, Akizawa T, Asano Y, et al. Depressive symptoms predict the future risk of severe pruritus in haemodialysis patients: Japan Dialysis outcomes and practice patterns study. Br J Dermatol. 2009;161:384–9.
20. Shioura M, Handedness in Normal Subjects RH. Sogo. Rehabilitation. 1988; 16:391–3 (in Japanese).
21. Hirota M, Nakamura M, Nakamura M, Gotoh M, Sawada Y. The role of upper extremities during kitchen knife cutting: comparing one-hand and two-hand motions. J Japanese Occup Ther Assoc. 2010;29:733–42 (in Japanese).
22. Quinn RR, Lamping DL, Lok CE, Meyer RA, Hiller JA, Lee J, et al. The vascular access questionnaire: assessing patient-reported views of vascular access. J Vasc Access. 2008;9:122–8.

13

High rates of central obesity and sarcopenia in CKD irrespective of renal replacement therapy – an observational cross-sectional study

Jutta Dierkes[1]* , Helene Dahl[1], Natasha Lervaag Welland[1], Kristina Sandnes[1], Kristin Sæle[2], Ingegjerd Sekse[2] and Hans-Peter Marti[1,2]

Abstract

Background: Poor nutritional status of patients with renal disease has been associated with worsening of renal function and poor health outcomes. Simply measuring weight and height for calculation of the body mass index does however not capture the true picture of nutritional status in these patients. Therefore, we measured nutritional status by BMI, body composition, waist circumference, dietary intake and nutritional screening in three groups of renal patients.

Methods: Patients with chronic kidney disease not on renal replacement therapy (CKD stages 3–5, $n = 112$), after renal transplantation ($n = 72$) and patients treated with hemodialysis ($n = 24$) were recruited in a tertiary hospital in Bergen, Norway in a cross-sectional observational study. Dietary intake was assessed by a single 24 h recall. All patients underwent nutritional screening, anthropometric measurements, body composition measurement andfunctional measurements (hand grip strength). The prevalence of overweight and obesity, central obesity, sarcopenia, sarcopenic obesity and nutritional risk was calculated.

Results: Central obesity and sarcopenia were present in 49% and 35% of patients, respectively. 49% of patients with central obesity were normal weight or overweight according to their BMI. Factors associated with central obesity were a diagnosis of diabetes and increased fat mass, while factors associated with sarcopenia were age, female gender, number of medications. An increase in the BMI was associated with lower risk for sarcopenia.

Conclusion: Central obesity and sarcopenia were present in renal patients at all disease stages. More attention to these unfavorable nutritional states is warranted in these patients.

Keywords: ESRD, Renal disease, Nutritional status, Sarcopenia

Background

Worldwide, the prevalence of patients treated for chronic kidney disease is increasing. Improvements in therapy have improved the outcomes of chronic kidney disease and renal replacement therapy, such as hemodialysis and transplantation, leading to higher numbers of patients who represent with increased number of comorbidities [1]. Diet and nutritional status play a major role in chronic renal disease, as loss of renal function has a major impact on nutritional metabolism and its regulation, as the progression of disease can be modified by diet and nutritional status, and dietary measures can reduce the burden of comorbidities such as hypertension, diabetes mellitus, and risk of cardiovascular disease [2].

Nutritional status can be affected by both over- and undernutrition. Obesity and especially diabetes mellitus are strong risk factors to develop renal disease [3]. Overweight and obesity are common features of diabetes mellitus, and especially central obesity, with increased visceral fat accumulation and waist circumference, is associated with

* Correspondence: jutta.dierkes@uib.no
[1]Department of Clinical Medicine, Center for Nutrition, University of Bergen, Jonas Lies vei 68, 5021 Bergen, Norway
Full list of author information is available at the end of the article

unfavorable metabolic changes and increased risk of diabetes mellitus and cardiovascular disease [4, 5].

On the other hand, during dialysis, the risk to develop malnutrition or protein-energy wasting (PEW), due to insufficient energy and protein intake or increased losses, is increased and poses an important risk factor for increased morbidity and mortality. Patients on hemodialysis often suffer from lack of appetite and increased catabolism, which can lead to undernutrition if not adequately diagnosed and treated [6].

As chronic kidney disease and end-stage renal disease are especially common among older subjects, common age related changes in metabolism and body composition are also observed in patients with kidney disease. Changes in body composition associated with aging affect an increase of fat mass and a decrease of lean body mass. Skeletal muscles are especially affected and aging is associated with a decrease of muscle mass and strength, also called sarcopenia. Sarcopenia has been identified as a major risk factor for frailty, which itself is a risk factor for mortality in dialysis patients [7], falls and other unfavorable health outcomes. As it affects skeletal muscles, it can also occur in obese patients ('sarcopenic obesity'). Estimates of body composition and sarcopenia can be made either with DEXA or with bioelectrical impedance assessment (BIA) methods [8]. BIA has the advantage of being transportable, easy to use and cheap, and studies have shown that BIA estimates are comparable to DEXA estimates of lean body mass [9, 10]. Muscle strength can be measured by functional measurements and the measurement of hand grip strength with handheld dynamometers has been widely used [11, 12].

Patients in hospitals are a vulnerable group for developing undernutrition. It has been estimated that about every third patient admitted to hospitals in Western countries is undernourished or at risk of undernutrition as assessed by screening tools [13]. Nutritional screening usually focuses on body mass, recent weight losses, loss of appetite and disease-related conditions [14]. In many Norwegian hospitals, the screening tool NRS2002 is used. This tool can also be used in patients attending outpatient clinics such as CKD and patients with a kidney transplant.

Thus, nutritional status can be measured in different dimensions: over- and undernutrition, the distribution of fat mass, changes in body composition associated with aging and disease (loss of muscle mass, sarcopenia) or nutritional risk. However, in clinical praxis, nutritional status is often defined by body mass index only which is based on weight and height measurements but does not take into account body composition (skeletal muscle mass) and fat distribution. We propose that a single measurement will not be able to capture these different dimensions of nutritional status. In addition, renal patients require dietary advice and treatment that is adapted to the patients' stage of renal disease and that changes during the course of the disease. Therefore, the aim of the current study was to investigate the feasibility and meaning of different dimensions of nutritional status assessment by anthropometry, body composition measurement, dietary assessment, functional measurements of muscle strength and nutritional screening in patients with renal disease ranging from CKD stage 3 to pre-dialysis, hemodialysis and renal transplant patients.

Methods

Patients, consent and ethics

This is a cross-sectional, single center observational study conducted at the Haukeland University Hospital, Bergen Norway. Adult patients with renal disease were eligible for inclusion into the study, which was conducted at the dialysis unit and the outpatient clinic of the Section of Nephrology at the Department of Medicine. During 2014–2017, outpatients from the Section of Nephrology were recruited to the study after signing informed consent (November 2014 to February 2015: $n = 24$ patients with hemodialysis (selected by consent from $n = 74$ patients), August to December 2015: $n = 112$ patients with chronic kidney disease stage 3 to 5 (selected by consent from $n = 183$ CKD patients without renal replacement therapy), and September 2016 to January 2017: $n = 72$ patients with a renal transplant (selected by consent from $n = 249$ patients)) Included patients were compared regarding age and sex to the total patient group, and in dialysis patients, regarding time on dialysis and dialysis treatments and no significant deviations were found (data not shown).

The study was conducted in accordance with principles of the Declaration of Helsinki and was approved by the Regional Committee for Medical and Health Research Ethics at the University of Bergen (REK Vest, No. 2014/ 1790).

Study procedures

For renal transplant patients and CKD patients, all patients were informed about the study by mail prior to their regular outpatient visit. During the visit, they were asked whether they were interested to participate in a study on dietary habits, nutritional status and health. Eligible patients were patients providing informed consent, 18 years or older, and able to communicate either in Norwegian or English. Reasons for exclusion were refusal of informed consent, language problems or cognitive decline. After informed consent, these patients filled in a questionnaire about lifestyle habits and disease history, underwent a single 24 h dietary recall, measurement of hand grip strength, anthropometric measurements (weight, height, skinfolds, waist and upper arm circumference), body composition measurement by bioelectrical impedance, and donated an extra blood and urine sample for later analyses.

Patients treated with hemodialysis were asked during dialysis whether they wanted to participate in the study. After providing informed consent, a new appointment for the data collection was scheduled with the routine blood sampling. Identical questionnaires and procedures were used as for renal transplant patients and CKD patients. All functional, body composition and anthropometric measurements were made after dialysis.

All measurements were conducted by clinical dieticians trained in anthropometric measurements and dietary recall. Information about disease history including comorbidities, medication and blood pressure were obtained from the patients' records.

Bioelectrical impedance analysis (BIA)

Body composition was measured by a single frequency (50 KHz) tetrapolar BIA 101 Aniversary Sport Edition (AKERN). The measurements were usually performed on the non-dominant side of the body, unless the patients had a fistula on this side of the body. All jewelry, clocks and belts were removed. Patients were usually non-fasting. The current–injector electrode was placed on the dorsum of the hand, just above the phalangeal-metacarpal joint and on the ventral side of the foot just below the transverse arch. Detector electrodes were placed on the dorsal side of the wrist, midline and in line with the pisiform bone, and across the ankle in line with the medial malleolus. Patients with a pacemaker or an implantable cardioverter-defibrillator were not investigated by BIA. In this way, resistance and reactance values were obtained in Ohms, and in addition the phase angle. The total fat free mass (FFM) in kg and fat mass (FM, in kg and in % of body weight) were calculated using a formula of Deurenberg 1989 [15].

$$FFM = 6.520 \times 100 \times height^2/resistance + 3.8 \times gender + 10.9$$

(height in m, resistance at 50 kHz in Ω, gender with male = 1 and female = 0).

For the calculation of appendicular lean mass (ALM), the following formula (Macdonald 2006) was used (ALM):

$$ALM_{BIA} = -11.626 + (0.292 \times height^2/resistance) \\ +(0.06983 \times reactance) + (0.08553 \times height) \\ +(-2.092 \times gender) + (-0.05 \times age)$$

(height in cm; resistance and reactance at 50 kHz (Ω); gender, 0 = male, 1 = female; age in years).

The obtained ALM was used for the calculation of the skeletal muscle index (ALM/Ht²). Cut-off values in men of ≤8.87 kg/m² and in women of ≤6.42 kg/m² were

applied (in addition to low hand grip strength) for the definition of sarcopenia [8].

Hand grip strength was measured using a hand held dynamometer (JAMAR, Sammons Preston, Bolingbrook, IL, USA) in triplicate. Both average and maximum hand grip strength was recorded. For the definition of sarcopenia, a cut off of 30 kg in men and 20 kg in women was applied [16].

Diagnosis of sarcopenia was made when the patient fulfilled the definition for both ALM/ht² and HGS.

Weight (while wearing light clothing and no shoes) and height (without shoes) was measured using the same type of scales and stadiometer (Seca model 877, and model 217, Seca, Hamburg, Germany). The body mass index (BMI) was then calculated, and the patients were classified as either underweight (BMI < 18.5 kg/m²), normal weight (BMI 18.5–24.99 kg/m²), overweight (BMI 25.0–29.99 kg/m²), or obese (BMI ≥ 30 kg/m²). In addition, a patient was identified as having central obesity when the waist circumference was > 102 cm in males and > 88 cm in females, regardless of the patient's BMI.

Nutritional screening was performed using NRS2002 which is an established tool for patients in hospitals and used routinely in Haukeland University Hospital [13]. The screening is based on 4 initial questions (BMI < 20.5 kg/m², weight loss during the last three months, reduced food intake during the last week, presence of severe illness?). If any question was answered with yes, the interviewer continued to the main screening with questions regarding both nutritional status and disease status. Both sections are graded with a score from 0 to 3, with increasing scores in relation to severity of disease and deterioration of nutritional status. Patients aged 70 years or older received an extra score. A score ≥ 3 identifies patients at nutritional risk for malnutrition [17].

Dietary intake was assessed by a single 24 h dietary recall. The patients were asked about food and drink intake the day before the appointment and the interviewer went through all meals and possible consumption between meals, using a standardized interview guideline [18]. Portion size was estimated using a booklet with four different portion sizes demonstrated or in household measurements or no. of items consumed. Data were entered in the online dietary tool 'Kostholdsplanleggeren.no' which is based on the official Norwegian food composition table and edited by the Norwegian Food Safety authority and the Norwegian directorate of health.

Patients were also asked whether they followed dietary restrictions and if so, they were asked to specify them. In addition, the number of prescribed medications was noted.

Laboratory data were taken from the patients' routine blood samples which were usually taken the same day as the appointment. Laboratory variables were analyzed in the central laboratory of the Haukeland University hospital which is ISO 15189 certified. Variables of interest were hemoglobin, albumin, C-reactive protein, creatinine in serum, and urinary albumin excretion rate (in spot urine, per mmol creatinine). The estimated glomerular filtration rate (eGFR) was calculated using the CKD-Epi equation [19].

Statistical analysis

Each group of patients was analyzed separately. Differences between continuous variables were tested with either the t-test or the Mann Whitney U test, and between categorical variables were tested by the Chi squared or the Fisher's exact test. Differences between the patients' groups were tested with analysis of variance or Kruskal-Wallis test. Associations between continuous variables were investigated by Spearman's rho correlation analysis.

Logistic regression was used to explore factors associated with central obesity and sarcopenia. SPSS (version 25) was used for the statistical calculations. A p-value of 0.05 was regarded as significant.

Results

Age and sex distribution of the selected patients were similar to the patient cohort of kidney patients treated at the Hospital.

Patient characteristics are depicted in Table 1. In brief, patients with CKD were older than ESRD-HD and renal transplant patients, and the distribution of men and women was similar in the three patient groups. Renal function was best in the renal transplant group, with higher eGFR and lower albumin excretion than in the CKD patients. Patients in the ESRD-HD group were at median 2 years on dialysis (reflecting the short waiting time for a kidney transplant in Norway of less than one year), and in renal transplant patients, at median almost 9 years were gone after transplantation. The prevalence of hypertension and diabetes was highest in the ESRD-HD group and lowest in the renal transplant group, with highly significant differences. Albumin concentrations were lowest in the ESRD-HD group, but only five of 24 patients in this group showed low albumin levels (< 38 g/L).

The average BMI was highest in the CKD group, followed by the renal transplant and the ESRD-HD group.

Table 1 Characteristics of the patients with different stages of renal disease (CKD chronic kidney disease; ESRD-HD end-stage renal disease treated with hemodialysis; renal transplant: recipients of a renal transplant)

	CKD $N = 112$	ESRD-HD $N = 24$	Renal transplant $N = 72$	P (ANOVA) Kruskal Wallis test
Age	66 (51, 76)	63 (50, 76)	60 (49, 67)	0.04
Sex (m/f)	79/33 (71%/29%)	17/7 (71%/29%)	51/21 (71%/29%)	0.999
Body mass index (kg/m²)	27.4 (23.9, 31.0)	24.7 (21.8, 27.5)	26.0 (24.0, 29.3)	0.02
Hypertension n (%)	82 (92%)	23 (96%)	28 (39%)	< 0.001
Diabetes mellitus n (%)	33 (30%)	11 (46%)	11 (15%)	< 0.001
Current smoking n (%)	17 (15%)	3 (12%)	8 (11%)	0.104
No. of prescribed medication[a]	7 (4, 9)	14 (12, 17)	9 (7, 11)	< 0.001
eGFR[b] (ml/min/1.73m²)	28 (18, 38)	6 (5, 8)	53 (38, 73)	< 0.001
CKD stages n (1–3/4/5)	44/52/16	0/0/24	59/11/1	
Systolic blood pressure (mmHg)	134 (125, 145)	159 (142, 175)[c]	130 (120, 140)	< 0.001
Diastolic blood pressure (mmHg)	80 (70, 82)	67 (61, 77)[c]	80 (71, 82)	< 0.001
Years on dialysis	–	2 (1–4)	–	
Years since renal transplant	–	–	8.9 (5.9, 15.5)	
Serum creatinine (μmol/L)	209 (159, 278)	656 (560, 844)	114 (96, 164)	< 0.001
Serum urea (mmol/L)	16 (11.2, 20.0)	23 (19, 28)	9.3 (6.7, 13.8)	< 0.001
Hemoglobin (g/L)	12.9 ± 1.6	11.9 ± 1.6	13.6 ± 1.9	< 0.001
Serum albumin (g/L)	44 (41, 45)	40.5 (38, 43)	43 (41, 45)	0.001
Serum C-reactive protein (mg/L)	3 (1, 6)	3 (1, 16)	2 (1, 4)	0.08
HbA1c (%)	5.8 (5.5, 6.3)	5.8 ± 1.2	5.7 (5.5, 6.1)	0.12
Urinary albumin (mg/mmol Crea)	30 (5, 104)	–	2.7 (0.9, 17.0)	< 0.001

[a]Medication and supplements described in The Norwegian Pharmaceutical Product Compendium (Felleskatalogen AS)
[b]eGFR was calculated using CKD-Epi equation [18]
[c]pre dialysis, median (IQR)

CKD patients also showed the highest prevalence of obesity (BMI > 30 kg/m^2, 33%) and central obesity (increased waist circumference, 53%), followed by the renal transplant group (22% and 50%, respectively) and the ESRD-HD group (4% and 39%, respectively). In the renal transplant group, there were 3 patients (all female) who were underweight with a BMI < 18.5 kg/m^2 (Fig. 1a). Applying higher BMI cut-offs for underweight as suggested in patients with renal disease [20], resulted in higher numbers: BMI < 23 kg/m^2 was observed in 21 (19%) of the CKD patients, 13 (18%) of the transplant group and 9 (37.5%) of the ESRD-HD group.

Nutritional and functional data are shown in Table 2. Nutritional risk and sarcopenia were most prevalent in the ESRD-HD group with 33% being at nutritional risk by NRS2002 screening and 42% diagnosed as having sarcopenia (low skeletal muscle index plus low hand grip strength). Nutritional risk was rare in the CKD and renal transplant group (3% and 7%, respectively). Patients at nutritional risk were either underweight ($n = 2$), normal weight ($n = 9$) or overweight ($n = 5$). In CKD and renal transplant patients, sarcopenia was almost as prevalent as in the ESRD-HD group. Overall, only 29% of patients in the CKD group, 39% in the ESRD-HD group and 31% of patients in the renal transplant group had neither sarcopenia nor central obesity (Fig. 1b).

Dietary intake was assessed by a single 24 h dietary recall (Table 2). Neither dietary energy nor protein intakes were significantly different across patient groups. On average, protein intake exceeded 0.8 g/kg BW, the recommended amount of protein in the CKD and renal transplant patients [21], respectively, and was lower than recommended (1.2 g/kg body weight) in the ESRD-HD group [22]. In addition, the energy intake was on average lower than the expected dietary energy requirement, and even if underreporting of dietary intake was considered, the dietary intake was well below the recommended dietary intake (30–35 kcal/kg/d) [22, 23].

About half of the patients mentioned that they were following dietary restrictions ($n = 107$, 74 men and 33 women). While most patients from the ESRD-HD group had restrictions ($n = 19$, 79%), CKD and renal transplant patients had less often dietary restrictions ($n = 55$, 49%, and $n = 27$, 38%, respectively). Most restrictions were on salt and fluid ($n = 35$), or phosphate/potassium intake ($n = 20$), or patients followed multiple (protein, salt, potassium, phosphate, fluid) restrictions ($n = 40$). Restrictions on energy intake were only mentioned by two patients specifically. Overall, dietary restrictions had little effect on dietary intake (data not shown).

Sarcopenia was significantly associated with higher age, lower mean upper arm circumference, lower phase angle by BIA, lower serum levels of creatinine and hemoglobin, higher CRP, but not with differences in serum albumin, BMI or waist circumference. While absolute protein intake was lower in sarcopenic patients, there were no differences in g protein intake per kg body weight or in energy intake (data not shown). There was no difference in patient group, or presence of central obesity (Table 2 and Fig. 1b).

In a multivariate logistic regression model, age, female gender, and number of prescribed medications were significantly associated with a higher risk for sarcopenia and higher fat mass or body mass index were associated with lower risk, while type of renal disease, comorbidities like diabetes mellitus or hypertension were not significantly associated with risk for sarcopenia (Table 3).

Central obesity, as defined by increased waist circumference, was observed in 102 patients. Remarkably, 50 patients (49%) with increased waist circumference had a BMI either in the normal range or in the overweight category and would therefore not be classified as obese by BMI only. In the multivariate logistic regression model, higher fat mass and diabetes mellitus were associated with central obesity. (Table 4). In CKD patients and renal transplant patients, urinary albumin excretion rate was also significantly associated with central obesity (data not shown).

Sarcopenia and obesity defined by a BMI exceeding 30 kg/m^2 was only observed in 12 CKD patients and one renal transplant patient, but sarcopenia with concurrent increased waist circumference was frequent and affected

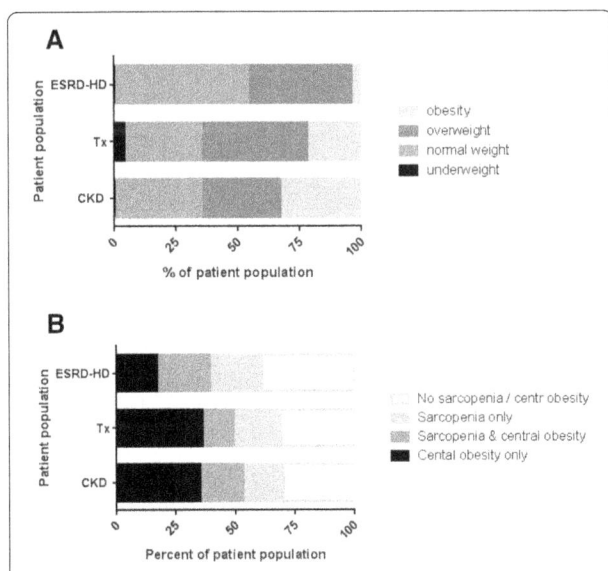

Fig. 1 Nutritional status of patients according to stage of kidney disease (CKD chronic kidney disease; ESRD-HD end-stage renal disease treated with hemodialysis; Tx: recipients of a renal transplant) and established BMI cut-offs (**a**) and according to sarcopenia, central obesity and sarcopenic obesity (**b**). Sarcopenia was defined by low skeletal muscle index and low hand grip strength, central obesity according to waist circumference and sarcopenic obesity as presence of sarcopenia and central obesity

Table 2 Nutritional data and functional data of patients with renal disease according to stage of renal disease (CKD chronic kidney disease; ESRD-HD end-stage renal disease treated with hemodialysis; renal transplant: recipients of a renal transplant)

	CKD $N = 112$	ESRD-HD $N = 24$	Renal transplant $N = 72$	P (ANOVA) Kruskal Wallis test
Weight (kg)	82.1 ± 18.6	72.5 ± 12.4	79.0 ± 15.0	0.04
BMI (kg/m^2)	27.8 ± 5.1	24.7 ± 3.7	26.7 ± 4.5	0.02
Resistance (Ω)	475 ± 80	509 ± 67	487 ± 86	0.104
Reactance (Ω)	48 ± 11	45 ± 14	50 ± 13	0.215
Phase angle (°)	5.76 ± 1.19	5.0 ± 1.4	5.86 ± 1.03	0.027
Appendicular lean mass (kg)[a]	21.3 ± 5.2	19.6 ± 5.3	21.4 ± 4.8	0.274
Skeletal muscle index (ALM/Ht^2, kg/m^2)[b]	7.1 (6.3, 7.6)	6.6 (5.7, 7.6)	7.6 (6.2, 8.0)	0.077
Fat mass (kg)	27.4 (19.8, 35.1)	22.4 (13.9, 27.1)	25.2 (15.9, 34.8)	0.102
Fat mass (% of weight)	33.6 (27.4, 39.1)	29.0 (21.4, 34.5)	32.9 (23.4, 41.1)	0.256
Fat free mass (kg)	53.3 (45.8, 61.6)	49.5 (44.9, 54.8)	55.2 (43.3, 59.9)	0.385
Waist circumference (cm)	99.2 ± 14.4	95.9 ± 13.6[c]	98.0 ± 14.3	0.47
Mid upper arm circumference (cm)	32.6 ± 4.8	29.0 ± 3.6	30.5 ± 3.4	< 0.001
Biceps skinfold (mm)	15 (10, 21)	8 (4, 11)	7 (5, 12)	< 0.001
Triceps skinfold (mm)	23 (17, 30)	14 (10, 19)	18 (12, 26)	< 0.001
Dietary intake (Kcal/d)	1730 (1380, 2120)	1700 (1230, 1927)	1794 (1303, 2087)	0.635
Dietary intake (Kcal/kg bw/d)	22 (16, 29)	23 (17, 30)	21 (18, 28)	0.875
Dietary protein (g/d)	76 (56, 96)	71 (60, 80)	78 (59, 103)	0.238
Dietary protein (g/kg bw/d)	0.95 (0.73, 1.23)	1.00 (0.77, 1.23)	0.96 (0.79, 1.38)	0.493
Handgrip strength average (kg)	30 ± 12	28 ± 12	30 ± 11	0.66
Handgrip strength maximum (kg)	32 ± 13	31 ± 13	32 ± 11	0.75
Knee extension average (N)	173 ± 52	–	183 ± 37	0.234
Knee extension maximum (N)	184 ± 54	–	195 ± 39	0.235
Nutritonal risk (NRS2002)	3 (3%)	8 (33%)	5 (7%)	< 0.001
Sarcopenia[d]	41 (37%)	10 (42%)	23 (32%)	0.642
Central obesity	58 (53%)	9 (39%)[c]	35 (50%)	0.490

Data are shown as median with interquartile range or as mean with standard deviation
[a]appendicular lean mass was calculated according to MacDonald et al. [10]
[b]Skeletal mass index calculated from appendicular lean mass divided by height squared
[c]$n = 23$
[d]BIA measurements were performed in 101 CKD patients, 23 ESRD-HD patients and 69 renal transplant patients due to contraindications present. In patients with missing BIA measurements, sarcopenia was defined by low hand grip strength only

20 CKD patients (18%), 5 ESRD-HD patients (22%) and 9 renal transplant patients (13%) (Fig. 1B).

Discussion

This study aimed to investigate nutritional status of patients with renal disease at different stages. There was a particular interest in the concurrent occurrence of low muscle mass and accumulation of fat mass, as has been described to be typical for patients with kidney disease but which is less obvious from routine weight measurements.

The main findings were that 1) Obesity was frequent in CKD and renal transplant patients. Increased waist circumference, indicating central obesity affected almost half of all patients in all patient groups, 2) A substantial proportion of patients on hemodialysis was found to be at nutritional risk, while the proportion of patients at

nutritional risk was low in CKD and renal transplant patients, 3) Sarcopenia was present in about one third of the patients. Low skeletal mass index and low appendicular lean muscle mass were present in almost all patients with ESRD and in ¾ of CKD patients, while low hand grip strength was present in more than a third of all patients across renal disease stages, 4) Sarcopenic obesity, defined as the concurrence of central obesity with increased waist circumference and sarcopenia was frequent. Sarcopenic obesity with BMI > 30 kg/m^2 was less frequently observed, and not at all in the ESRD-HD patients.

Thus, the study revealed a number of nutritional problems in patients with kidney disease, spanning over- and undernutrition and nutritional quality. These problems need to be carefully addressed during treatment as they

Table 3 New

Odds ratio (95% confidence interval)	
Multivariate logistic regression with Sarcopenia as dependent variable	
CKD patients (reference)	
ESRD-HD	0.31 (0.08, 1.25)
Renal transplant	0.80 (0.35, 1.83)
Gender (female =1)	2.87 (1.27, 6.48)
Age (per year increase)	1.10 (1.06, 1.14)
Prescribed medications (per no. increase)	1.19 (1.07. 1.32)
BMI (per unit increase)	0.92 (0.85, 0.99)

may affect disease progression, metabolic control, and quality of life.

The high rate of high BMI but also of central obesity in the CKD and renal transplant patients reflects both the overall high prevalence of overweight and obesity in the general population and disease-specific reasons [24]. Diabetes mellitus type 2, which is usually associated with overweight and obesity, was frequent especially in the CKD patients (30%). It has been shown that obesity itself is a risk factor for the development of CKD and the progression of the disease [3, 25]. Overweight and obesity in renal transplant patients is a known problem due to weight gain after transplantation [26, 27].

Other studies have also reported high prevalence of overweight and obesity in patients with CKD [28, 29]. Similar to data of the present study, the British patients with central obesity had higher prevalence of cardiovascular risk factors.

The concurrent finding of low ALM and overweight/obesity puts a challenge on all approaches of weight reduction in these patients. Body weight reduction is the sum of reductions in fat mass and in fat-free mass, which usually outweigh about 20% of lost weight [30]. Although reduction of fat mass is warranted in overweight and obese CKD and renal transplant patients for improvement of metabolic control, especially in patients with diabetes mellitus, any diet would also compromise the maintenance of muscle mass. Protein-rich diets have been recommended in weight loss studies due to their effects on satiety and maintenance of muscle mass [31, 32], however, CKD patients are advised not to increase their protein intake [22, 33]. Thus,

Table 4 New

Odds ratio (95% confidence interval)	
Multivariate logistic regression with 'central obesity' as dependent variable	
CKD patients (reference)	
ESRD-HD	2.12 (0.55, 8.18)
Renal transplant	2.00 (0.71, 5.62)
Diagnosis of diabetes mellitus	3.10 (1.20, 8.03)
Fat mass (increase in 1 kg)	1.29 (1.20, 1.39)

approaches involving increase of physical activity and targeted muscle training are warranted in combination with weight reduction diets.

In the present study, we did not observe differences in dietary intake between the patient groups. A careful evaluation of the 24 h recalls revealed underreporting especially in the obese patients, who had lower energy intakes than lean or overweight patients. This is a known phenomenon [34, 35] that should be acknowledged in the evaluation of dietary intake [36]. As obesity (and thus underreporting) was much more prevalent in CKD and renal transplant patients than in the ESRD-HD patients, it can be argued that probably the true energy intake was lower in ESRD-HD than in CKD and renal transplant. A sensitivity analysis, where all patients with BMI > 30 kg/m^2 were removed showed that average energy intake increased in CKD and renal transplant, but there were still no significant differences between the patient groups (data not shown).

The high prevalence of sarcopenia can both be attributed to the age of the patients which was on average over 60, and the kidney disease in conjunction with the common comorbidities in these patients. We did not assess physical activity in the patients, but it can be assumed that many of them had a sedentary lifestyle as reported by others [37] and which is also associated with low muscle muss and muscle strength. As sarcopenia is associated with lower quality of life [38, 39], more attention should be awarded to the condition and lifestyle changes to slow down the process should be encouraged [40].

Protein intake is a major concern in renal disease. While CKD patients are advised to limit their protein intake, ESRD-HD patients should have a high protein intake of 1.2 g/kg body weight. Protein intake was similar in the three patient groups, indicating on average high protein intake in CKD patients and low protein intake in ESRD-HD. A protein intake of less than 0.8 g/kg BW was reported in 26% of the patients with ESRD, and was associated with nutritional risk in this group of patients. Protein intake of less than 0.6 g/kg BW was reported in 20% of CKD patients. More focus on nutritional education including dietary protein at all stages of renal disease would probable enable more patients to follow a diet adequate in protein.

The study had several advantages and limitations. Advantages of the present study were that the study patients represent typical and well-documented patients with renal disease of a tertiary hospital, the comprehensive assessment of nutritional status, including nutritional screening, anthropometric measurements, body composition measurement and clinical variables combined with dietary assessment. Three different groups of patients suffering from kidney diseases with or without renal replacement therapy were included which allows to mirror the development of nutritional status during the course of the disease. All analyses have been made in a highly standardized way.

Among the limitations, it has to be mentioned that the study lacked an assessment of physical activity, that underreporting limited the use of the dietary data, and that future studies should also include a follow up to investigate the importance of nutritional status on the course of the disease. The number of patients on hemodialysis is rather low and this makes it difficult to draw more general conclusions. Also, we did not include patients on peritoneal dialysis. Other limitations that apply include that we did not have a non-CKD, age-matched control group, and no 24-h urine samples due to logistic reasons e.g. to assess normalised protein catabolic rate (nPCR) as a more objective marker for protein intake. Another limitation is the single 24-h recall, which is less accurate than two or more 24-h recalls. The cut-off values for sarcopenia were derived from a population without kidney disease, and the applicability to renal patients may be questioned.

In conclusion, the study showed that nutritional problems are highly prevalent at all stages of renal disease, with sarcopenia and obesity being the most prevalent conditions in CKD and renal transplant patients, while ESRD-HD patients also show a high prevalence of nutritional risk. The high prevalence of central obesity and sarcopenic obesity warrants attention.

Future studies should focus on treatment of obesity in renal disease with concurrent focus on maintenance of muscle mass. Most urgently, all CKD patients with stages ≥3 should strongly be advised to increase their physical activity in formalized programs especially for reduction of central obesity and sarcopenia.

Conclusion

The present study shows that nutritional disturbances are common in patients with chronic kidney disease, with a predominance of sarcopenia and central obesity. These cannot easily measured by weight and height, but need determination of body composition and waist circumference. As both are associated with unfavorable health outcomes, these additional measurements are strongly recommended in patients with chronic kidney disease regardless of renal replacement therapy.

Acknowledgements
We thank all patients who have contributed to the study and the physicians at the Department of Nephrology for referring the patients to the study.

Authors' contributions
JD and HPM designed the study, HD, NLW, KS1, KS2, IS contributed to data collection and analysis, JD, HD, NLW and KS1 performed the statistical analysis, and the primary manuscript preparation. All authors contributed to the writing process and reviewed the manuscript. JD has the primary responsibility for the final content. All authors read and approved the final manuscript.

Competing interests
The authors declare that they have no competing interests. The results presented in this paper have not been published elsewhere in whole or in part, except in abstract form.

Author details
[1]Department of Clinical Medicine, Center for Nutrition, University of Bergen, Jonas Lies vei 68, 5021 Bergen, Norway. [2]Department of Nephrology, Haukeland University Hospital, Jonas Lies vei 65, 5021 Bergen, Norway.

References
1. Jha V, Garcia-Garcia G, Iseki K, Li Z, Naicker S, Plattner B, et al. Chronic kidney disease: global dimension and perspectives. Lancet. 2013;382(9888): 260–72.
2. Nazar CM. Significance of diet in chronic kidney disease. J Nephropharmacol. 2013;2:37–43.
3. Cao X, Zhou J, Yuan H, Wu L, Chen Z. Chronic kidney disease among overweight and obesity with and without metabolic syndrome in an urban Chinese cohort. BMC Nephrol. 2015;16:85.
4. Feller S, Boeing H, Pischon T. Body mass index, waist circumference, and the risk of type 2 diabetes mellitus : implications for routine clinical practice. Dtsch Arztebl Int. 2010;107:470–6.
5. Pischon T, Boeing H, Hoffmann K, Bergmann M, Schulze MB, Overvad K, et al. General and abdominal adiposity and risk of death in Europe. N Engl J Med. 2008;359:2105–20.
6. Ikizler TA, Cano NJ, Franch H, Fouque D, Himmelfarb J, Kalantar-Zadeh K, et al. Prevention and treatment of protein energy wasting in chronic kidney disease patients: a consensus statement by the International Society of Renal Nutrition and Metabolism. Kidney Int. 2013;84:1096–107.
7. Kallenberg MH, Kleinveld HA, Dekker FW, van Munster BC, Rabelink TJ, van Buren M, et al. Functional and cognitive impairment, frailty, and adverse health outcomes in older patients reaching ESRD-A systematic review. Clin J Am Soc Nephrol. 2016;11:1624–39.
8. Cruz-Jentoft AJ, Baeyens JP, Bauer JM, Boirie Y, Cederholm T, Landi F, et al. Sarcopenia: European consensus on definition and diagnosis: report of the European working group on sarcopenia in older people. Age Ageing. 2010; 39:412–23.
9. Steihaug OM, Gjesdal CG, Bogen B, Ranhoff AH. Identifying low muscle mass in patients with hip fracture: validation of Biolectrical impedance analysis and anthropometry compared to dual energy X-ray absorptiometry. J Nutr Health Aging. 2016;20:685–90.
10. Macdonald JH, Marcora SM, Jibani M, Roberts G, Kumwenda MJ, Glover R, et al. Bioelectrical impedance can be used to predict muscle mass and hence improve estimation of glomerular filtration rate in nondiabetic patients with chronic kidney disease. Nephrol Dial Transplant. 2006;21:3481–7.
11. Leal VO, Mafra D, Fouque D, Anjos LA. Use of handgrip strength in the assessment of the muscle function of chronic kidney disease patients on dialysis: a systematic review. Nephrol Dial Transplant. 2011;26:1354–60.
12. Norman K, Stobaus N, Gonzalez MC, Schulzke JD, Pirlich M. Hand grip strength: outcome predictor and marker of nutritional status. Clin Nutr. 2011;30:135–42.
13. Tangvik RJ, Tell GS, Guttormsen AB, Eisman JA, Henriksen A, Nilsen RM, et al. Nutritional risk profile in a university hospital population. Clin Nutr. 2015;34:705–11.
14. van der Schueren MA v B-d, Guaitoli PR, Jansma EP, de Vet HC. Nutrition screening tools: does one size fit all? A systematic review of screening tools for the hospital setting. Clin Nutr. 2014;33:39–58.
15. Deurenberg P, Weststrate JA, van der Koy K. Body composition canges assesed by bioelectrical impedance measurements. Am J Clin Nutr. 1989;49:401–3.
16. Lauretani F, Russo CR, Bandinelli S, Bartali B, Cavazzini C, Di Iorio A, et al. Age-associated changes in skeletal muscles and their effect on mobility: an operational diagnosis of sarcopenia. J Appl Physiol (1985). 2003;95:1851–60.

17. Kondrup J, Allison SP, Elia M, Vellas B, Plauth M. ESPEN guidelines for nutrition screening 2002. Clin Nutr. 2003;22:415–21.

18. Blanton CA, Moshfegh AJ, Baer DJ, Kretsch MJ. The USDA automated multiple-pass method accurately estimates group total energy and nutrient intake. J Nutr. 2006;136:2594–9.

19. Levey AS, Stevens LA, Schmid CH, Zhang YL, Castro AF, 3rd, Feldman HI, et al. A new equation to estimate glomerular filtration rate. Ann Intern Med 2009;150:604–612.

20. Fouque D, Kalantar-Zadeh K, Kopple J, Cano N, Chauveau P, Cuppari L, Franch H, Guarnieri G, Ikizler TA, Kaysen G, Lindholm B, Massy Z, Mitch W, Pineda E, Stenvinkel P, Treviño-Becerra A, Wanner C. A proposed nomenclature and diagnostic criteria for protein-energy wasting in acute and chronic kidney disease. Kidney Int. 2008 Feb;73(4):391–8.

21. Kidney Disease. Improving global outcomes (KDIGO) CKD work group. KDIGO clinical practice guideline for the evaluation and management of chronic kidney disease. Kidney Int Suppl. 2013;3:1–150.

22. Wright M, Jones C. Renal association clinical practice guideline on nutrition in CKD. Nephron Clin Pract. 2011;118(Suppl 1):c153–64.

23. Shah A, Bross R, Shapiro BB, Morrison G, Kopple JD. Dietary energy requirements in relatively healthy maintenance hemodialysis patients estimated from long-term metabolic studies. Am J Clin Nutr. 2016;103:757–65.

24. Midthjell K, Lee CM, Langhammer A, Krokstad S, Holmen TL, Hveem K, et al. Trends in overweight and obesity over 22 years in a large adult population: the HUNT study, Norway. Clin Obes. 2013;3:12–20.

25. Burton JO, Gray LJ, Webb DR, Davies MJ, Khunti K, Crasto W, et al. Association of anthropometric obesity measures with chronic kidney disease risk in a non-diabetic patient population. Nephrol Dial Transplant. 2012;27:1860–6.

26. de Oliveira CM, Moura AE, Goncalves L, Pinheiro LS, Pinheiro FM, Jr., Esmeraldo RM. Post-transplantation weight gain: prevalence and the impact of steroid-free therapy. Transplant Proc 2014;46:1735–1740.

27. Wissing KM, Pipeleers L. Obesity, metabolic syndrome and diabetes mellitus after renal transplantation: prevention and treatment. Transplant Rev (Orlando). 2014;28:37–46.

28. Evans PD, McIntyre NJ, Fluck RJ, McIntyre CW, Taal MW. Anthropomorphic measurements that include central fat distribution are more closely related with key risk factors than BMI in CKD stage 3. PLoS One. 2012;7:e34699.

29. Silva MI, Vale BS, Lemos CC, Torres MR, Bregman R. Body adiposity index assess body fat with high accuracy in nondialyzed chronic kidney disease patients. Obesity (Silver Spring). 2013;21:546–52.

30. Krieger JW, Sitren HS, Daniels MJ, Langkamp-Henken B. Effects of variation in protein and carbohydrate intake on body mass and composition during energy restriction: a meta-regression 1. Am J Clin Nutr. 2006;83:260–74.

31. Cava E, Yeat NC, Mittendorfer B. Preserving healthy muscle during weight loss. Adv Nutr. 2017;8:511–9.

32. Wycherley TP, Moran LJ, Clifton PM, Noakes M, Brinkworth GD. Effects of energy-restricted high-protein, low-fat compared with standard-protein, low-fat diets: a meta-analysis of randomized controlled trials. Am J Clin Nutr. 2012;96:1281–98.

33. Bellizzi V, Conte G, Borrelli S, Cupisti A, De Nicola L, Di Iorio BR, et al. Controversial issues in CKD clinical practice: position statement of the CKD-treatment working group of the Italian Society of Nephrology. J nephrol. 2017;30:159–70.

34. Avesani CM, Kamimura MA, Draibe SA, Cuppari L. Is energy intake underestimated in nondialyzed chronic kidney disease patients? J Ren Nutr. 2005;15:159–65.

35. Johansson G, Wikman A, Ahren AM, Hallmans G, Johansson I. Underreporting of energy intake in repeated 24-hour recalls related to gender, age, weight status, day of interview, educational level, reported food intake, smoking habits and area of living. Public Health Nutr. 2001;4:919–27.

36. Subar AF, Freedman LS, Tooze JA, Kirkpatrick SI, Boushey C, Neuhouser ML, et al. Addressing current criticism regarding the value of self-report dietary data. J Nutr. 2015;145:2639–45.

37. Cupisti A, D'Alessandro C, Finato V, Del Corso C, Catania B, Caselli GM, et al. Assessment of physical activity, capacity and nutritional status in elderly peritoneal dialysis patients. BMC Nephrol. 2017;18:180.

38. Manrique-Espinoza B, Salinas-Rodriguez A, Rosas-Carrasco O, Gutierrez-Robledo LM, Avila-Funes JA. Sarcopenia is associated with physical and mental components of health-related quality of life in older adults. J Am Med Dir Assoc 2017;18(7):636.e1-.e5.

39. Alston H, Burns A, Davenport A. Loss of appendicular muscle mass in haemodialysis patients is associated with increased self-reported depression, anxiety and lower general health scores. Nephrology (Carlton). 2017.

40. Painter P, Marcus RL. Assessing physical function and physical activity in patients with CKD. Clin J Am Soc Nephrol. 2013;8:861–72.

14

Deleterious effects of dialysis emergency start, insights from the French REIN registry

Alain Michel[1][*] ⓘ, Adelaide Pladys[2,3], Sahar Bayat[2,4], Cécile Couchoud[5], Thierry Hannedouche[6] and Cécile Vigneau[1,7,8]

Abstract

Background: Emergency start (ES) of dialysis has been associated with worse outcome, but remains poorly documented. This study aims to compare the profile and outcome of a large cohort of patients starting dialysis as an emergency or as a planned step in France.

Methods: Data on all patients aged 18 years or older who started dialysis in mainland France in 2012 or in 2006 were collected from the Renal Epidemiology and Information Network and compared, depending on the dialysis initiation condition: ES or Planned Start (PS). ES was defined as a first dialysis within 24 h after a nephrology visit due to a life-threatening event. Three-year survival were compared, and a multivariate model was performed after multiple imputation of missing data, to determine the parameters independently associated with three-year survival.

Results: In 2012, 30.3% of all included patients (n = 8839) had ES. Comorbidities were more frequent in the ES than PS group (≥ 2 cardiovascular diseases: 39.2% vs 28.8%, p < 0.001). ES was independently associated with worse three-year survival (57% vs. 68.2%, p = 0.029, HR 1.10, 95% CI 1.01–1.19) in multivariate analysis. Among ES group, a large part had a consistent previous follow-up: 36.4% of them had ≥3 nephrology consultations in the previous year. This subgroup of patients had a particularly high comorbidity burden. ES rate was stable between 2006 and 2012, but some proactive regions succeeded in reducing markedly the ES rate.

Conclusion: ES remains frequent and is independently associated with worse three-year survival, demonstrating that ES deleterious impact is never overcome. This study shows that a large part of patients with ES had a previous follow-up, but high comorbidity burden that could favor acute decompensation with life-threatening conditions before uremic symptoms appearance. This suggests the need of closer end-stage renal disease follow-up or early dialysis initiation in these high-risk patients.

Keywords: Emergency start, Survival, Outcome, ESRD, Dialysis, France

Background

Differently from recent trends in the USA [1] and in overall European Union [2], the number of incident patients with End-Stage Renal Disease (ESRD) in France continues to progress, with a steadily rise of 2.2% per year between 2006 and 2012, mainly due to diabetes 2-related ESRD [3].

Preparing patients for renal replacement therapy (RRT) is a challenge for nephrologists whose role is to convince them about the asymptomatic end stage of a vital organ, help them choosing the most appropriate RRT modality, prepare a dialysis access, manage anemia

* Correspondence: alain.michel@chu-rennes.fr
[1]CHU Pontchaillou, Service de néphrologie, 2 rue H Le Guilloux, 35033 Rennes cedex, France
Full list of author information is available at the end of the article

and nutritional support, and assess their suitability for renal transplantation waitlisting. Late referral to nephrologists (defined as a referral < 3–4 months before RRT initiation) has been associated with poorer outcome, prolonged initial hospitalization, higher risk of all-cause death [4–7], and increased costs for the health care system [8]. In France, strong efforts have been made to promote the early referral of patients with chronic kidney disease (CKD), including information to general practitioners about CKD, definition of national guidelines for renal care and referral, and implementation of health networks between hospitals and general practitioners [9].

Once referred, current guidelines recommend delaying dialysis initiation until the occurrence of uremic symptoms, degradation of nutritional status, uncontrolled hypertension, volume overload, threatening acid-base or electrolytes disorders [10]. For some patients, acute pulmonary oedema or threatening electrolytes disorders appear before uremic symptoms, that lead to start dialysis in emergency conditions. The impact of starting dialysis in emergency conditions ("Emergency Start" (ES)) has not been widely studied. A previous French epidemiologic study [11] based on the 2006 Renal Epidemiology and Information Network (REIN) data, pointed out that ES was associated with a worse one-year survival rate than "Planned Start" (PS) of dialysis (74.2% for ES vs. 87.4% for PS, $p < 0.001$). Some other studies also have reported worse outcomes associated with unplanned dialysis start [12, 13], but no strong data is available about the profile of patients starting dialysis in emergency conditions, and the factors leading to ES. Moreover, the group of patients exhibiting an ES is probably heterogeneous and deserve to be better described, in order to enhance their management.

The aim of this study was to compare the clinical status and outcomes of dialysis incident patients in 2012 mainland France according to the dialysis initiation condition (ES or PS), and to analyze the ES group. In addition, patients who started dialysis in 2006 or 2012 were compared to determine whether the ES rates, profile and outcomes changed during this interval.

Methods
Study population
This study was based on data from the REIN registry. This registry started in 2002, and progressively extended to the 22 metropolitan French regions and 5 overseas territories. All French patients with ESRD are registered, including those who undergo preemptive kidney transplantation. Patients with acute kidney injury requiring dialysis are not included in the registry. If unclear, chronic kidney failure is defined by a persistent requirement of dialysis after 45 days of RRT (REIN guidelines).

All incident patients aged 18 years or older who started long-term RRT in one of the 22 metropolitan regions in 2012 (or in the 16 regions included in 2006) were included, if the dialysis initiation status (PS or ES) was described. Patients who underwent preemptive kidney transplantation and patients on dialysis after loss of a functional transplant were not included because they were not considered as incident patients (REIN guidelines). Patients from overseas territories were excluded because of the significant differences in demographic characteristics (higher rate of diabetes and hypertension) and clinical practices compared with mainland France.

Collected data
The proportion of ES among the included patients was calculated, globally and for each region. ES was defined

as a first dialysis session within 24 h after a nephrology visit, for life threatening conditions, including acute pulmonary edema, severe hyperkalemia or acidosis, uremic confusion or pericarditis. This applied also to patients with a previous follow-up and presenting with an acute complication. However, the exact cause of dialysis start was not recorded in the registry.

For both groups (ES or PS), the following baseline (i.e., at dialysis initiation) data were collected: age, sex, primary renal disease, nutritional status, comorbidities, walking disability, and ESRD management (place of care, modalities). The number of previous nephrology visits within 1 year before dialysis start was also registered. Primary renal diseases were grouped in three categories, depending on the form of renal function impairment: acute nephropathy (including CKD exacerbation or flare), slowly progressive nephropathy, or unknown (see Additional file 1).

Then, the same data were compared between ES patients who started dialysis in 2006 and in 2012 (in the same 16 regions included in the REIN registry in 2006). Only, the number of nephrology visits in the last year before dialysis was not compared because this item was not recorded in the registry in 2006.

Statistical analysis
Patients' baseline characteristics were expressed as frequencies and percentages for categorical variables, and as median and interquartile values (IQR) for continuous variables. Demographic and clinical features were described by subgroups and compared using the Chi-square test, according to the initiation timing and the year of dialysis start: ES vs PS in 2012; ES in 2012 vs ES in 2006. Moreover, subgroups of 2012 ES patients were also distinguished and compared depending on the number of nephrology visits within 1 year before dialysis start (if available): no previous visit vs ≥3 visits. Missing data were presented in tables for the descriptive results when > 10%. Before the analyze of each event of interest, missing data were handled by multiple imputation method.

Three-year survival and cox regression
All patients who started dialysis in 2012 were included in the analyses (three-year follow-up was completed for all included patients). Patient survival was assessed from dialysis initiation up to 3 years after dialysis initiation. Kaplan Meier survival curves were plotted for each group and log-rank tests were used to compare three-year survival of the groups. The Cox regression method was used to evaluate the association between patients' characteristics and three-year survival. All variables associated with the outcome in the unadjusted model ($p < 0.2$) (were included in the adjusted model. All variables

with a p-value < 0.05 in the final adjusted model were considered as statistically significant. To deal with the problem of missing data, the Multiple Imputation by Chained Equations (MICE) procedure [14] was used for each variable before Cox regression. The process was repeated for all variables with missing values and to stabilize the results, the procedure was repeated for ten cycles to produce a single imputed dataset. Finally, the whole procedure was iterated five times to obtain five imputed datasets.

Statistical analyses were performed with the Stata 13.1 software (College Station, Texas, USA).

Results

Comparison of the 2012 incident patients depending on the dialysis start condition (ES or PS)

A total of 8839 patients were included and represented 91% of all incident patients in mainland France in 2012 (9% were excluded because the dialysis initiation status was missing). Among them, 30.3% experienced an ES. The baseline characteristics of the ES and PS groups are presented in Table 1. There was no significant difference in sex and age between the ES and PS groups. Patients experimenting an ES had significantly more comorbidities: 39.2% had ≥ 2 cardiovascular diseases compared with 28.8% in the PS group ($p < 0.001$), and there was a higher proportion of smokers and respiratory disease, cirrhosis, or cancer in ES group. BMI repartition showed a higher proportion of extreme rates, and a larger part of ES patients had a serum albumin concentration < 30 g/l. The first RRT technique for patients with ES was almost always hemodialysis (98.2% for ES vs 86.6% for PS, $p < 0.001$) and required most often a central venous catheter placement at initiation (85.4% vs 43.3%, $p < 0.001$).

The three-year survival rate (Kaplan-Meier curves) was significantly lower in the ES than in the PS group (57% vs 68.2%, $p < 0.001$) (Fig. 1). After adjustment for age, sex, comorbidities, nutritional status, pre-dialysis anemia management, baseline eGFR, vascular access and dialysis start condition (ES or PS), ES remained an independent risk factor of death within 3 years from dialysis start (Hazard Ratio 1.10, 95% CI 1.01–1.19) in the multivariate analysis (Table 2). Causes of death were similar in ES and PS groups (Additional file 1: Table S2). About first dialysis management, the use of central venous catheter was independently and strongly associated with worse three-year survival (HR 1.41, 95% CI 1.30–1.54).

Some data provided insights into the patients' management before dialysis start. In the ES group, 26.5% of patients were using an erythropoiesis-stimulating agent (ESA) and 20.5% had an arteriovenous fistula at dialysis initiation, thereby demonstrating a previous follow-up

(Table 1). Moreover, among patients for whom the data was available (1240/2678), 36.4% of patients in the ES group visited the nephrologist three time or more in the year before dialysis initiation. The analysis of the characteristics of patients in the ES group with ≥ 3 previous visits (Table 3) revealed a particularly high proportion of patients with diabetes (53.4%), cardiovascular (54.3% had ≥ 2 cardiovascular diseases) and respiratory diseases (22.8%). Interestingly, 78.5% of them had a slowly progressive kidney disease, and they exhibited an ES with a median eGFR of 8.9 ml/min/1.73m^2, close from patients of the PS group. The three-year survival rate was significantly lower in the ES group with ≥ 3 previous visits than in PS group (56.1% vs 68.2%, $p < 0.001$) (Fig. 2). Conversely, patients in the ES group without previous nephrology consultation were younger and with less comorbidities, starting dialysis with low eGFR (median 6.2 ml/min/1.73m^2); their three-year survival rate was 58.4%.

Comparison between the 2012 and 2006 data

Next, data on 6119 patients who started dialysis in 2006 (92.6% of all incident patients in the 16 regions included in the REIN registry at that time) were compared with the data on the 7084 patients from the same regions who started dialysis in 2012.

ES proportion was similar in both years: 29.2% in 2012 and 28.4% in 2006 ($p = 0.282$). Nevertheless, the detailed comparison by region showed large local differences (Additional file 1: Table S3). Some regions did manage to reduce the ES percentage from 2006 to 2012 (e.g., in Lorraine, the ES rate dropped from 49.8% in 2006 to 19.5% in 2012).

The clinical profile of patients with ES remained similar, with high comorbidity level (Table 4). The proportion of some comorbidities were even higher in 2012 than in 2006: 17.6% of patients had a respiratory disease in 2012 vs. 14.1% in 2006 ($p = 0.001$), and 25.5% had serum albumin concentration < 30 g/l in 2012 vs. 19.6% in 2006, $p = 0.004$.

Discussion

This large epidemiologic study, based on prospectively collected data from the REIN registry shows that in France, the ES rate is very high (about 30% of all incident dialysis patients in 2012) and remained stable between 2006 and 2012. This result is consistent with studies on other European and North-American cohorts [15, 16] that highlighted the difficulty in reducing ES rate, despite the development of multidisciplinary management for ESRD [17].

Our study shows unequivocally that ES is associated with worse prognosis than PS (three-year survival: 57% for ES vs 68.2% for PS, $p < 0.001$), indicating that ES

Table 1 Characteristics of dialysis incident patients in mainland France in 2012, according to the dialysis initiation condition: planned start or emergency start

| | Planned start ($n = 6161$; 69.7%) | Emergency start ($n = 2678$; 30.3%) | |
	n (%)	n (%)	p
Men	3918 (63.6)	1736 (64.8)	0.268
Age, y (mean ± SD)	67.9 ± 18.8	67.8 ± 16.4	0.65
Primary renal disease			< 0.001
Acute nephropathy	478 (7.8)	407 (15.2)	
Slowly progressive nephropathy	4454 (72.3)	1668 (62.3)	
Unknown	1229 (19.9)	603 (22.5)	
Serum albumin < 30 g/dl	981 (15.9)	669 (25)	< 0.001
Missing	1090 (17.7)	563 (21)	
BMI (kg/m^2)			< 0.001
< 18.5	254 (4.1)	158 (5.9)	
18.5–25	1908 (31)	865 (32.3)	
> 25	2658 (43.1)	987 (36.9)	
Missing	1341 (21.8)	668 (24.9)	
Smoking status			0.006
Current smoker	594 (9.6)	277 (10.3)	
Former smoker	1464 (23.8)	658 (24.6)	
Never smoker	3209 (52.1)	1237 (46.2)	
Missing	894 (14.5)	506 (18.9)	
Respiratory disease	725 (11.8)	457 (17.1)	< 0.001
Hepatic disease	127 (2.1)	80 (3)	0.005
Active malignancy[a]	636 (10.3)	394 (14.7)	< 0.001
Diabetes	2459 (39.9)	1105 (41.3)	0.229
Type 1	162 (6.6)	47 (4.3)	0.006
Type 2	2280 (92.7)	1051 (95.1)	
Cardiovascular diseases[b]			< 0.001
0	2995 (48.6)	1055 (39.4)	
1	1390 (22.6)	573 (21.4)	
2	895 (14.5)	479 (17.9)	
≥ 3	881 (14.3)	571 (21.3)	
Mobility			< 0.001
Totally dependent for transfers	216 (3.5)	209 (7.8)	
Need assistance for transfers	638 (10.4)	407 (15.2)	
Walk without help	4718 (76.6)	1760 (65.7)	
First dialysis modality			< 0.001
HD/HDF	5333 (86.6)	2628 (98.2)	
APD/CAPD	828 (13.4)	49 (1.8)	
Vascular access at initiation			
Central venous catheter	2115 (34.3)	2286 (85.4)	< 0.001
Arteriovenous fistula (used or not)	3291 (53.4)	566 (21.1)	< 0.001
Pre-dialysis anemia management			
Hemoglobin < 10 g/dl	2660 (43.2)	1628 (60.8)	< 0.001
ESA therapy	2860 (46.4)	709 (26.5)	< 0.001

Table 1 Characteristics of dialysis incident patients in mainland France in 2012, according to the dialysis initiation condition: planned start or emergency start *(Continued)*

	Planned start (*n* = 6161; 69.7%)	Emergency start (*n* = 2678; 30.3%)	
	n (%)	*n* (%)	p
Residual eGFR ml/min/1.73m^2 (median, IQR)	9.2 (7.2–12.1)	8.05 (5.5–11.4)	< 0.001
Missing	725 (11.8)	355 (13.3)	
Waitlisted at dialysis initiation (< 80 years)	580 (12.1)	37 (1.8)	< 0.001

[a] Active malignancy: solid tumors or hematological malignancies
[b] Cardiovascular diseases: myocardial infarction, arrhythmias, coronary insufficiency, heart failure, arteritis of the lower limbs, cerebrovascular accident
BMI Body Mass Index, *HD* hemodialysis, *HDF* hemodiafiltration, *APD* automated peritoneal dialysis, *CAPD* continuous ambulatory peritoneal dialysis, *ESA* erythropoietin stimulating agent, *eGFR* estimated glomerular filtration rate

deleterious effect is never overcome. Indeed, after full adjustment, ES was still an independent risk factor for death at 3 year (HR 1.10, 95% CI 1.01–1.19). Our results confirm previous studies in smaller cohorts of French dialyzed patients showing that ES is associated with early mortality on dialysis [16, 18]. Similarly, Descamp et al. demonstrated in a monocentric study that ES was the major confounding factor explaining the over-mortality of hemodialysis compared with peritoneal dialysis as first RRT modality, and ES was the only factor strongly associated with early mortality in dialysis [16]. Moreover, the STARRT study showed that the benefits of early referral to a nephrologist are lost in the case of "suboptimal" dialysis start (i.e., not starting with the planned modality or as an inpatient or with a central venous catheter) [12, 13]. Furthermore, ES is associated with poor quality of life and a substantial heavier healthcare burden [15].

Due to ES deleterious impact, it is important to precise the profile of ES patients, in order to improve their management. Our data bring some insights on the clinical profile of patients exhibiting an ES. Compared with patients in the PS group, these patients had higher comorbidity burden, especially cardiovascular diseases. Moreover, within the ES group, we could distinguish two discrete subgroups based on previous nephrology care: on one hand, patients without pre-dialysis care (no previous nephrology consultation), who experimented ES with low residual renal function because of an acute kidney injury or an undiagnosed ESRD. On the other hand, patients with consistent pre-dialysis care (≥3 consultations in the previous year), who probably initiated the RRT preparation (confirmed by arteriovenous fistula and the use of ESA), but presented a life-threatening event before the appearance of uremic symptoms. They mainly have slowly progressive nephropathy, but a particularly high comorbidity burden that could lead to an acute decompensation of their cardiovascular or respiratory condition at quite high eGFR. Patients in the ES group with ≥3 visits have worse three-year survival than patients in the PS group in our study (56.1% vs 68.2%, *p* < 0.001).

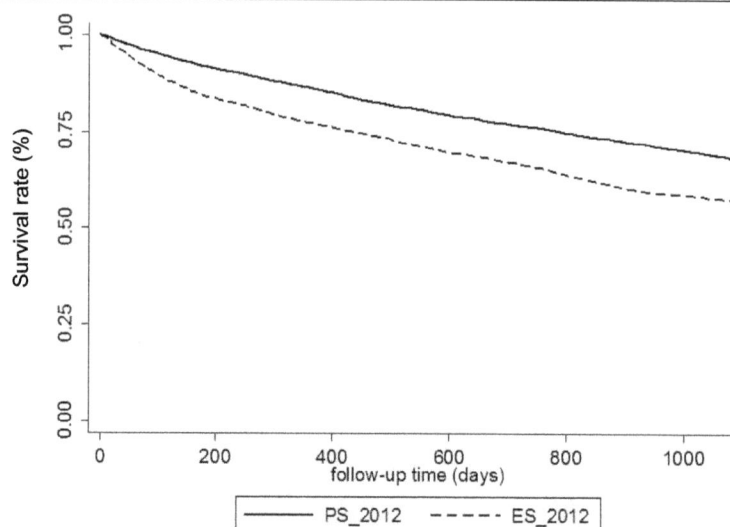

Fig. 1 Kaplan Meier survival curves of dialysis incident patients in 2012 according to the dialysis initiation condition: planned start (PS_2012, full line) or emergency start (ES_2012, dashed line)

Table 2 Factors associated with three-year mortality on multivariate analysis in 2012 incident patients ($n = 8839$)

Multivariate Cox model	HR	95% CI	p
Women (vs Men)	0.96	0.88–1.04	0.311
Age (vs 18–45 years)			
45–60	2.70	1.96–3.71	< 0.001
60–75	4.99	3.70–6.73	< 0.001
≥ 75	8.51	6.32–11.46	< 0.001
Albumin < 30 (vs ≥30 g/dl)	1.32	1.19–1.46	< 0.001
Hemoglobin (vs [10–12] g/dl)			
< 10	1.16	1.07–1.26	< 0.001
> 12	0.99	0.88–1.12	0.908
BMI (vs 23–25 kg/m^2)			
< 18.5	1.41	1.14–1.74	0.002
18.5–23	1.22	1.08–1.37	0.001
≥ 25	0.92	0.82–1.03	0.138
Diabetes (vs No)	1.09	1.01–1.18	0.025
Respiratory disease (vs No)	1.22	1.12–1.34	< 0.001
Active malignancy (vs No)	1.76	1.60–1.93	< 0.001
Hepatic disease (vs No)	2.01	1.66–2.43	< 0.001
Cardiovascular diseases (vs 0)			
1	1.31	1.19–1.45	< 0.001
2	1.54	1.39–1.72	< 0.001
≥ 3	1.78	1.60–1.97	< 0.001
Walking disability (vs Walk without help)			
Totally dependent for transfers	2.24	1.95–2.57	< 0.001
Need assistance for mobility	1.70	1.55–1.86	< 0.001
eGFR (vs [5–10]ml/min/1.73m^2)			
< 5	0.99	0.85–1.15	0.860
[10–15]	1.17	0.99–1.37	0.058
≥ 15	1.39	1.17–1.65	< 0.001
1st RRT on PD (vs HD)	1.37	1.21–1.54	< 0.001
1st RRT on catheter (vs No)	1.41	1.30–1.54	< 0.001
Emergency start (vs planned start)	1.10	1.01–1.19	0.029

BMI Body Mass Index; Active malignancy: solid tumors or hematological malignancies; Cardiovascular diseases: myocardial infarction, arrhythmias, coronary insufficiency, heart failure, arteritis of the lower limbs, cerebrovascular accident; *RRT* Renal Replacement Therapy, *PD* Peritoneal Dialysis; *HD* Hemodialysis; *HR* Hazard Ratio; *95%CI* 95%Confidence Interval

These findings corroborate the results of the only other study on this topic, performed in 184 Canadian patients. In this study, the group of patients with previous follow-up but unplanned start had a significantly worse one-year survival rate than patients with planned first dialysis. Congestive heart failure and higher BMI were independently associated with the risk of unplanned dialysis start (i.e., initiated as inpatient) [17]. These and our findings suggest that the ESRD

Table 3 Characteristics of patients in the ES group in 2012, according to the number of nephrology consultations in the year before starting dialysis

	No previous consultation 550/1240 (44.4%)	≥3 previous consultations 451/1240 (36.4%)	
	n (%)	n (%)	p
Men	360 (65.5)	316 (70.1)	0.121
Age, y (mean ± SD)	65 ± 18.06	69.2 ± 15.3	< 0.001
Primary renal disease			< 0.001
Acute nephropathy	145 (26.3)	31 (6.8)	
Slowly progressive nephropathy	236 (42.9)	354 (78.5)	
Unknown	169 (30.7)	66 (14.6)	
Serum Albumin < 30 g/l	172 (31.3)	109 (24.2)	0.017
Missing	59 (10.7)	67 (14.9)	
BMI (kg/m^2)			< 0.001
< 18.5	54 (9.8)	23 (5.1)	
18.5–25	219 (39.8)	154 (34.1)	
> 25	186 (33.8)	213 (47.2)	
Missing	91 (16.5)	61 (13.5)	
Smoking status			0.003
Current smoker	91 (16.5)	45 (10)	
Former smoker	143 (26)	152 (33.7)	
Never smoker	216 (39.3)	165 (36.6)	
Missing	100 (18.2)	89 (19.7)	
Respiratory disease	72 (13.1)	103 (22.8)	< 0.001
Hepatic disease	24 (4.4)	12 (2.7)	0.353
Active malignancy[a]	109 (19.8)	51 (11.3)	0.001
Diabetes	173 (31.5)	241 (53.4)	< 0.001
Cardiovascular diseases[b]			< 0.001
0	254 (46.2)	120 (26.6)	
1	125 (22.7)	86 (19.1)	
2	78 (14.2)	101 (22.4)	
≥ 3	93 (16.9)	144 (31.9)	
Mobility			0.262
Totally dependent for transfers	48 (8.7)	32 (7.1)	
Need assistance for transfers	84 (15.3)	57 (12.6)	
Walk without help	377 (68.5)	317 (70.3)	
First dialysis modality			0.027
HD/HDF	543 (98.7)	436 (96.7)	
APD/CAPD	7 (1.3)	15 (3.3)	
Vascular access at initiation			
Central venous catheter	537 (97.6)	301 (66.7)	< 0.001
Arteriovenous fistula (used or not)	30 (5.5)	207 (45.9)	< 0.001
Pre-dialysis anemia management			
Hemoglobin < 10 g/dl	406 (73.8)	251 (55.7)	< 0.001
ESA therapy	30 (5.5)	251 (55.7)	< 0.001
Residual eGFR ml/min/1.73m^2 (median, IQR)	6.2 (4.2–9.3)	8.9 (6.7–11.7)	< 0.001
Missing	73 (13.3)	30 (6.7)	

[a] Active malignancy: solid tumors or hematological malignancies
[b] Cardiovascular diseases: myocardial infarction, arrhythmias, coronary insufficiency, heart failure, arteritis of the lower limbs, cerebrovascular accident
BMI Body Mass Index, *HD* hemodialysis, *HDF* hemodiafiltration, *APD* automated peritoneal dialysis, *CAPD* continuous ambulatory peritoneal dialysis, *ESA* erythropoietin stimulating agent, *eGFR* estimated glomerular filtration rate

management of patients with high comorbidity burden needs to be improved and question the suitability of the current recommended strategy of dialysis initiation at the uremic symptomatic stage for these high-risk patients.

This is apparently in contradiction with the recent evidence-based guidelines on "late initiation". However, these recommendations are based on the IDEAL cohort, a highly selected subgroup of younger, relatively "healthy" patients with a careful follow-up and, consequently, they may not fully apply to patients with high comorbidity burden. Controlled trials are needed to determine whether early dialysis initiation could avoid ES and improve survival in this specific group of patients. Another way of improvement is to optimize the attendance of pre-dialysis clinics, and to increase the ESRD follow-up frequency [19]. Indeed, Singhal et al. underlined that "cumulative care" (number of nephrology consultations) and "consistent critical period care" (defined as ≥3 consultations during the 6 months before dialysis initiation) are more relevant than the classic "early referral", and are independently associated with better survival [20].

Even if a part of ES remains unavoidable (acute kidney injuries), reducing the proportion of ES is not a desperate cause: some regions in France managed to decrease ES rate from 2006 to 2012. For example, the Lorraine region set up a city-hospital nephrology network (Nephrolor) and increased the volume of information given to the general practitioners. ES proportion dropped from 49.8% in 2006 to 19.5% in 2012. This example indicates that ES high rate is not inevitable, but a proactive ESRD care policy is needed.

The main limitations of our study are linked to the nature of a registry-based epidemiologic work. First, the definition of "ES" remains open to criticism. The REIN registry classifies as ES any first dialysis occurring within 24 h after a nephrology consultation because of a life-threatening complication. The problem of not standardized terminology about unplanned dialysis start is still unsolved. Mendelssohn proposed the term of "suboptimal initiation", defined as starting dialysis as an inpatient or with a central venous catheter, or not with the planned dialysis modality [15]. However, we consider this definition inappropriate because many patients, mostly elderly, are not eligible to arteriovenous fistula or refuse it, but may start dialysis on a catheter in a planned setting.

Another limitation concerns the "previous visit" item, which was added in the registry only in 2009. However, this information was available only for 45% (n = 2797) of all 2012 incident patients included in our study. Therefore, the conclusions based on this information must be interpreted cautiously. Finally, the REIN registry does not record the specific cause of dialysis start, which could be useful to better identify the patients' profile and ES context.

Conclusions

Our study shows that in mainland France, the absolute rate of ES is still high (about 30% of all incident patients) and didn't decrease between 2006 and 2012. After full

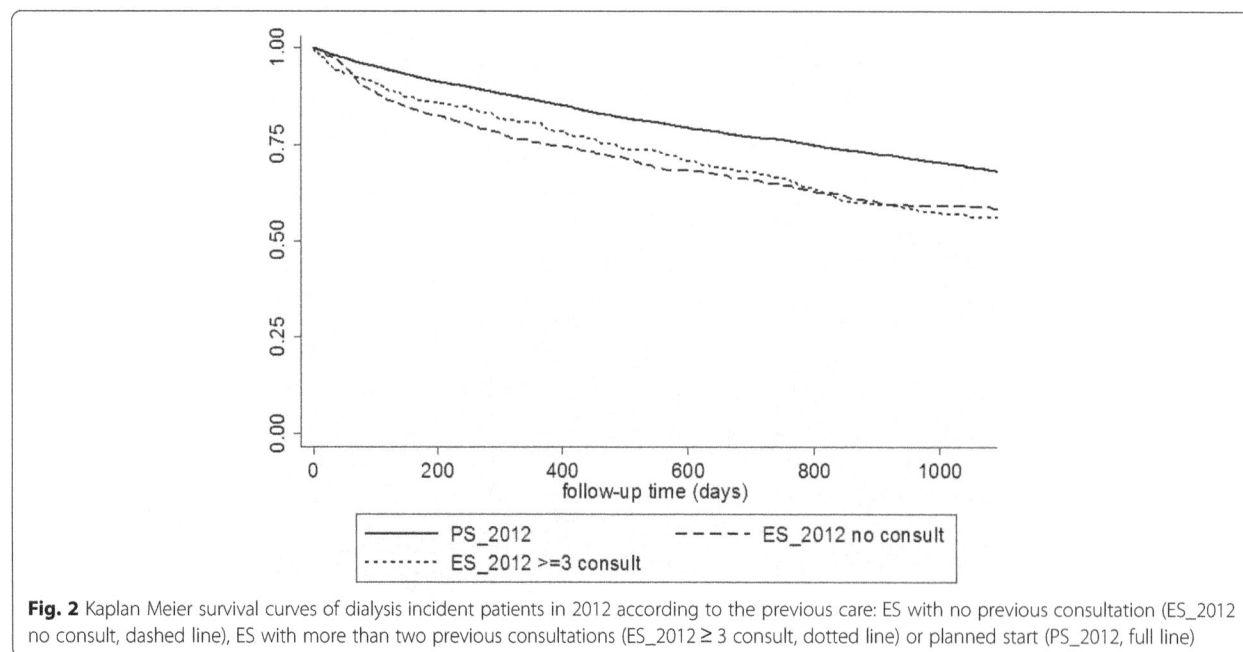

Fig. 2 Kaplan Meier survival curves of dialysis incident patients in 2012 according to the previous care: ES with no previous consultation (ES_2012 no consult, dashed line), ES with more than two previous consultations (ES_2012 ≥ 3 consult, dotted line) or planned start (PS_2012, full line)

Table 4 Characteristics of patients in ES group in 2006 and 2012 (16 French regions)

	ES 2006	ES 2012	
	n (%)	n (%)	p
Emergency start rate n (%)	1736/6119 (28.4)	2070/7084 (29.2)	0.282
Men	1060 (61.1)	1339 (64.7)	0.021
Age, y (mean ± SD)	67.2 ± 16.4	67.4 ± 16.6	0.62
Primary renal disease			0.55
Acute nephropathy	278 (16)	321 (15.5)	
Slowly progressive nephropathy	1032 (59.5)	1266 (61.2)	
Unknown	426 (24.5)	483 (23.3)	
Serum Albumin < 30 g/l	340 (19.6)	528 (25.5)	0.004
Missing	535 (30.8)	487 (23.5)	
BMI (kg/m^2)			0.026
< 18.5	83 (4.8)	116 (5.6)	
18.5–25	584 (33.6)	603 (29.2)	
> 25	581 (33.5)	749 (36.2)	
Missing	488 (28.1)	602 (29.1)	
Smoking status			0.002
Current smoker	168 (9.7)	205 (9.9)	
Former smoker	357 (20.6)	481 (23.2)	
Never smoker	966 (55.6)	981 (47.4)	
Missing	245 (14.1)	403 (19.5)	
Respiratory disease	244 (14.1)	364 (17.6)	0.001
Hepatic disease	41 (2.4)	65 (3.1)	0.146
Active malignancy[a]	217 (12.5)	303 (14.6)	0.056
Diabetes	666 (38.4)	853 (41.2)	0.145
Cardiovascular diseases[b]			0.763
0	705 (40.6)	840 (40.6)	
1	397 (22.9)	449 (21.7)	
2	290 (16.7)	348 (16.8)	
≥ 3	344 (19.8)	433 (20.9)	
Mobility			0.86
Totally dependent for transfers	166 (9.6)	190 (9.2)	
Need assistance for transfers	333 (19.2)	389 (18.8)	
Walk without help	1237 (71.3)	1491 (72)	
First dialysis modality			< 0.001
HD/HDF	1683 (96.9)	2033 (98.2)	
APD/CAPD	53 (3.1)	37 (1.8)	
Vascular access at initiation			
Central venous catheter	1455 (83.8)	1782 (86.1)	0.001
Arteriovenous fistula (used or not)	419 (24.1)	432 (20.9)	0.016
Pre-dialysis anemia management			
Hemoglobin < 10 g/dl	920 (53)	1218 (58.8)	0.001
ESA therapy	496 (28.6)	507 (24.5)	0.289
Residual eGFR ml/min/1.73m^2 (median, IQR)	7.23 (5.1–10)	7.75 (5.4–10.7)	0.001
Missing	368 (21.2)	398 (19.2)	
Waitlisted at dialysis initiation (< 80 years)	10 (0.7)	31 (2)	0.004

[a] Active malignancy: solid tumors or hematological malignancies
[b]Cardiovascular diseases: myocardial infarction, arrhythmias, coronary insufficiency, heart failure, arteritis of the lower limbs, cerebrovascular accident
BMI Body Mass Index, HD hemodialysis, HDF hemodiafiltration, APD automated peritoneal dialysis, CAPD continuous ambulatory peritoneal dialysis, ESA erythropoietin stimulating agent, eGFR estimated glomerular filtration rate

adjustment, ES remains independently associated with higher three-year mortality risk. A substantial proportion of ES was observed in patients with regular previous follow-up but high comorbidity burden, suggesting acute decompensation as the cause of ES. More data are needed to identify patients at risk of ES and improve their pre-dialysis management, in order to avoid ES and its deleterious consequences.

Abbreviations
BMI: Body Mass Index; CKD: Chronic Kidney Disease; eGFR: Estimated glomerular filtration rate; ES: Emergency start; ESA: Erythropoietin stimulating agent; ESRD: End Stage Renal Disease; PS: Planned start; REIN: Renal Epidemiology and Information Network; RRT: Renal replacement therapy

Acknowledgments
The authors thank all REIN registry participants, especially nephrologists and data managers in charge of data collection and quality control. The dialysis centers participating in the registry are fully listed in the REIN annual report https://www.agence-biomedecine.fr/Le-programme-REIN).
The authors thank Elisabetta Andermarcher for reviewing english language.

Funding
This study was not financially supported.

Authors' contributions
AM and CV designed the study; CC provided access to the REIN registry data; AP collected data and performed statistical analyses; AM and AP performed data analysis and manuscript writing. All authors reviewed the manuscript and approved the final draft.

Competing interests
The authors declare that they have no competing interests.

Author details
[1]CHU Pontchaillou, Service de néphrologie, 2 rue H Le Guilloux, 35033 Rennes cedex, France. [2]EHESP, Département d'Epidémiologie et de Biostatistiques, Rennes, France. [3]Université Rennes 1, UMR CNRS 6290, Rennes, France. [4]EA MOS EHESP, Rennes, France. [5]Registre REIN, Agence de la biomédecine, La Plaine Saint Denis, France. [6]Faculté de médecine de Strasbourg, Hôpitaux universitaires de Strasbourg, 1 place de l'Hôpital, 67091 Strasbourg cedex, France. [7]Université de Rennes 1, 2 av prof L Bernard, 35000 Rennes, France. [8]Inserm (Institut national de la santé et de la recherche médicale), IRSET, U1085, SFR Biosit, 9 Avenue du Professeur Léon Bernard, 35000 Rennes, France.

References
1. USRDS 2015 Incidence, prevalence, patient characteristics, and treatment modalities [internet]. Available from: http://www.usrds.org/2015/view/v2_01.aspx [cited 2016 Feb 25].
2. Pippias M, Jager KJ, Kramer A, Leivestad T, Sánchez MB, Caskey FJ, et al. The changing trends and outcomes in renal replacement therapy: data from the ERA-EDTA Registry. Nephrol Dial Transplant. 2016;31(5):831-41.
3. Vigneau C, Kolko A, Stengel B, Jacquelinet C, Landais P, Rieu P, et al. Ten-years trends in renal replacement therapy for end-stage renal disease in mainland France: Lessons from the French Renal Epidemiology and Information Network (REIN) registry. Nephrol Ther. 2017;13(4):228-35.
4. Chan MR, Dall AT, Fletcher KE, Lu N, Trivedi H. Outcomes in patients with chronic kidney disease referred late to nephrologists: a meta-analysis. Am J Med. 2007;120:1063–1070.e2.
5. Maynard C, Cordonnier D. The late referral of diabetic patients with kidney insufficiency to nephrologists has a high human and financial cost: interdisciplinary communication is urgently needed. Diabetes Metab. 2001;27:517–21.

6.   Stack AG. Impact of timing of nephrology referral and pre-ESRD care on mortality risk among new ESRD patients in the United States. Am J Kidney Dis Off J Natl Kidney Found. 2003;41:310–8.

7.   Winkelmayer WC, Owen WF, Levin R, Avorn J. A propensity analysis of late versus early nephrologist referral and mortality on Dialysis. J Am Soc Nephrol. 2003;14:486–92.

8.   Lee J, Lee JP, Park JI, Hwang JH, Jang HM, Choi J-Y, Kim Y-L, Yang CW, Kang S-W, Kim N-H, Kim YS, Lim CS. CRC for ESRD investigators: early nephrology referral reduces the economic costs among patients who start renal replacement therapy: a prospective cohort study in Korea. PLoS One. 2014;9:e99460.

9.   Frimat L, Siewe G, Loos-Ayav C, Briançon S, Kessler M, Aubrège A. Insuffisance rénale chronique : connaissances et perception par les médecins généralistes. Néphrologie Thérapeutique. 2006;2:127–35.

10. Kidney Disease. Improving global outcomes (KDIGO) CKD work group. KDIGO 2012 clinical practice guideline for the evaluation and Management of Chronic Kidney Disease. Kidney Int Suppl. 2013;3:4.

11. Chantrel F, Lassalle M, Choucoud C, Frimat L. Démarrage d'un traitement par dialyse chronique en urgence. Quels patients? Quelles conséquences? Bull Épidémiologique Hebd BEH. 2010;(9-10). http://opac.invs.sante.fr/index.php?lvl=notice_display&id=790.

12. Mendelssohn DC, Curtis B, Yeates K, Langlois S, MacRae JM, Semeniuk LM, Camacho F, McFarlane P. Investigators for the SS: suboptimal initiation of dialysis with and without early referral to a nephrologist. Nephrol Dial Transplant. 2011;26:2959–65.

13. Hughes SA, Mendelssohn JG, Tobe SW, McFarlane PA, Mendelssohn DC. Factors associated with suboptimal initiation of dialysis despite early nephrologist referral. Nephrol Dial Transplant Off Publ Eur Dial Transpl Assoc Eur Ren Assoc. 2013;28:392–7.

14. Sterne JAC, White IR, Carlin JB, Spratt M, Royston P, Kenward MG, Wood AM, Carpenter JR. Multiple imputation for missing data in epidemiological and clinical research: potential and pitfalls. BMJ. 2009;338:b2393.

15. Mendelssohn DC, Malmberg C, Hamandi B. An integrated review of "unplanned" dialysis initiation: reframing the terminology to "suboptimal" initiation. BMC Nephrol. 2009;10:22.

16. Descamps C, Labeeuw M, Trolliet P, Cahen R, Ecochard R, Pouteil-Noble C, Villar E. Confounding factors for early death in incident end-stage renal disease patients: role of emergency dialysis start. Hemodial Int. 2011;15:23–9.

17. Brown PA, Akbari A, Molnar AO, Taran S, Bissonnette J, Sood M, Hiremath S. Factors associated with unplanned Dialysis starts in patients followed by nephrologists: a Retropective cohort study. PLoS One. 2015;10:e0130080.

18. Couchoud C, Moranne O, Frimat L, Labeeuw M, Allot V, Stengel B. Associations between comorbidities, treatment choice and outcome in the elderly with end-stage renal disease. Nephrol Dial Transplant. 2007;22:3246–54.

19. Buck J, Baker R, Cannaby A-M, Nicholson S, Peters J, Warwick G. Why do patients known to renal services still undergo urgent dialysis initiation? A cross-sectional survey. Nephrol Dial Transplant Off Publ Eur Dial Transpl Assoc - Eur Ren Assoc. 2007;22:3240–5.

20. Singhal R, Hux JE, Alibhai SMH, Oliver MJ. Inadequate predialysis care and mortality after initiation of renal replacement therapy. Kidney Int. 2014;86:399–406.

15

Meeting patients where they are: improving outcomes in early chronic kidney disease with tailored self-management support (the CKD-SMS study)

Kathryn Havas[1,2]* , Clint Douglas[1] and Ann Bonner[1,2,3]

Abstract

Background: To achieve optimal health outcomes, people with chronic kidney disease must make changes in their everyday lives to self-manage their condition. This can be challenging, and there is a need for self-management support interventions which assist people to become successful self-managers. While interventions have been developed, the literature in this area is sparse and limited by lack of both individualisation and sound theoretical basis. The aim of this study was to implement and evaluate the Chronic Kidney Disease-Self-Management Support intervention: a theory-based, person-centred self-management intervention for people with chronic kidney disease stages 1–4.

Methods: A single-sample, pre-post study of an individualised, 12-week intervention based upon principles of social-cognitive theory and person-centred care was conducted with patients attending outpatient renal clinics in Queensland, Australia ($N = 66$). Data were collected at T0 (pre-intervention) and T1 (post-intervention). Primary outcomes were self-efficacy and self-management behaviour.

Results: There were significant, small-to-medium improvements in primary outcomes (self-efficacy: mean difference + 0.8, 95% CI 0.3–1.2, $d = 0.4$; self-management behaviour: mean difference + 6.2, 95% CI 4.5–7.9, $d = 0.8$). There were further significant improvements in secondary outcomes (blood pressure, disease-specific knowledge, physical activity, fruit and vegetable consumption, alcohol consumption, health-related quality of life, psychological distress, and communication with healthcare providers), with effect sizes ranging from negligible to large (all $ps < .05$).

Conclusions: Social-cognitive theory shows promise as a framework for providing effective person-centred self-management support to patients within this population, and longer-term evaluation is needed.

Keywords: Chronic kidney disease, Self-management, Self-care, Person-centred care, Patient-centred care, Intervention, Patient education

* Correspondence: kathryn.havas@qut.edu.au
[1]School of Nursing, Queensland University of Technology, Victoria Park Rd, Kelvin Grove, Brisbane, QLD 4059, Australia
[2]NHMRC Chronic Kidney Disease Centre for Research Excellence, University of Queensland, St Lucia, Australia
Full list of author information is available at the end of the article

Background

Chronic kidney disease (CKD) is a significant burden to those with the disease [1] and healthcare systems [2]. Prevalence is rising, due to increasing rates of diabetes, obesity, and hyptertension [3], and this is predicted to continue [4], with variation across different socioeconomic groups [5]. Burden is particularly high in end-stage kidney disease (ESKD), which requires expensive, time-consuming kidney replacement therapies (KRT; dialysis or transplantation). In earlier stages of CKD, there is an opportunity for interventions to slow progression and improve outcomes. Effective self-management (in areas including diet, physical activity, medication, and smoking and alcohol reduction) impacts health outcomes [6, 7]; therefore, interventions which improve adherence in these areas have potential to improve outcomes for people with CKD. However, self-management support (SMS) intervention studies for people with CKD, especially earlier stages, are rare and limited by methodological and reporting issues [8–10]. Furthermore, difficulties have been identified in recruiting [10, 11] and sustaining [12, 13] participation. The current study builds upon the extant literature to address some of these problems, drawing on patient preferences for SMS and a theoretical framework for behavioural change. The personalised intervention reported here (the Chronic Kidney Disease Self-Management Support program – CKD-SMS) aimed to meet patients where they are, developing goals and tailoring support to improve knowledge, skills, and confidence in self-managing CKD in ways that are congruent with their current knowledge, skills, and engagement with regard to managing their health.

Despite the importance of theory-driven intervention [14], efforts to improve CKD self-management have been largely atheoretical [8]. Additionally, not all behaviour change theories are suited to guide SMS. Some fail to account for the role of emotional states, assuming instead that all behaviour has purely a rational basis [15, 16]. One effective way of improving CKD self-management is by improving self-efficacy (confidence in ability [17]) to manage the disease [18, 19]. Social-cognitive theory (SCT [17]) provides a framework for mechanisms of change in a self-efficacy-based model of behaviour. Within a SCT framework (see Fig. 1), self-efficacy is at the heart of behaviour change, and amount of change in behavioural, psychological, and clinical outcomes depends on factors including baseline knowledge and skills, past experiences self-managing, and available coping resources.

Attempts have been made to deliver SCT-based self-management interventions within the CKD literature. However, these have been underdeveloped in attempts to manipulate self-efficacy, tending to focus on only one mechanism of self-efficacy change (including studies focused solely on verbal persuasion, the weakest mechanism [17]), or have not described theoretical reasons for change at all [10]. Furthermore, these studies (like the broader CKD literature) are limited by design and reporting problems [8–10]. A major gap is lack of individualisation, as the CKD population are heterogeneous in terms of support needs and capacity to participate in interventions [20, 21]. Additionally, patient activation (engagement with self-management and treatment [22]) in chronic illness is developmental, passing through several stages

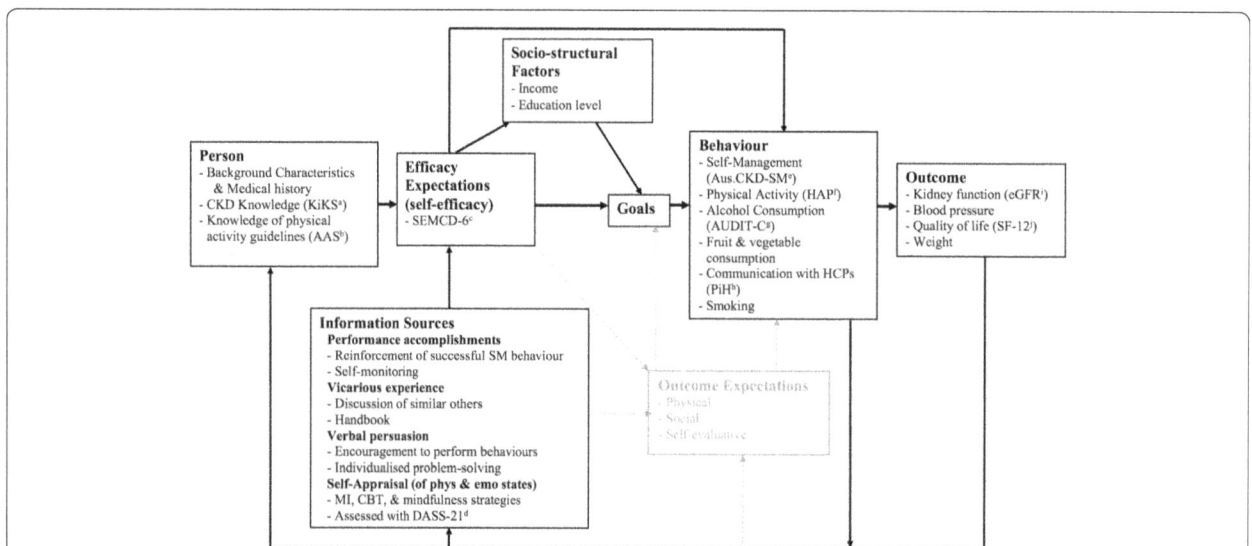

Fig. 1 SCT model (adapted from [19]. [a]Kidney Knowledge survey [31]; [b]Four items from the Active Australia Survey [33]; [c]Self-Efficacy for Managing Chronic Disease 6-Item Scale [29]; [d]Depression, Anxiety, and Stress Scales 21-Item Version [32]; [e]CKD Self-Management Instrument Australian version [30]; [f]Human Activity Profile [35]; [g]Alcohol Use Disorders Identification Test Consumption Questions Scale [37]; [h]Two items from Partners in Health Scale [36]; [i]SF-12v2, Australian version [34]

(from understanding that participation is important, to ability to maintain effective self-management under stress).

In contrast to a "one-size-fits-all" approach, a person-centred approach [23] to SMS requires an understanding of support desires of the target population and a willingness to take into account individual circumstances, capacity, activation, and motivation while working collaboratively with patients to generate and work towards personally meaningful and attainable goals. People at different stages of activation are likely to benefit from different types of SMS to improve self-efficacy, ranging from basic education to complex problem-solving and skill-development [22]. This exploratory study aimed to evaluate a person-centred, theory-based intervention to improve self-management in people with stage 1–4 CKD (the CKD-SMS). It was hypothesised that the CKD-SMS would lead to increased self-efficacy, CKD knowledge, and engagement in desirable behaviours (CKD self-management, physical activity, fruit and vegetable consumption, and effective communication with healthcare providers (HCPs)), as well as reduction in emotional distress and undesirable behaviours (smoking and alcohol consumption). According to SCT, this should lead to improvements in CKD outcomes (blood pressure (BP), health-related quality of life (HRQoL), weight, and estimated glomerular filtration rate (eGFR)).

Methods
Design and participants
This study was a prospective, single-sample, pre-post design. This design was selected over a randomised-controlled trial (RCT) due to aforementioned known challenges with recruitment and participant retention amongst this population, which are such that recruiting and retaining a sample to adequately power a 2×2 research design was not feasible. Furthermore, the flexibility that is inherent in a person-centred intervention required flexible appointment and rescheduling options, which are incompatible with a highly controlled RCT design. One-sample, repeated-measures designs are common in this field due to the above reasons (e.g., [24–27]), while those studies which have chosen an RCT design cite their small sample sizes as a weakness [28, 29]. Pre-post designs make valuable contributions to the literature when experimental designs are not feasible due to practical constraints such as these [30]. The Transparent Reporting of Evaluations with Nonrandomized Designs (TREND) statement was used to guide reporting [31], and the Template for Intervention Description and Replication (TIDieR) [32] was used to ensure adequate intervention description. Fifty-six participants were required to have 95% power to detect a medium effect ($d = 0.50$ [33]) in a paired t-test, assuming a 5% significance level (two-tailed; calculated using G*Power [34]). These estimates were based upon results of Su and colleagues [19] who used the same primary outcome (the Self-Efficacy for Managing Chronic Disease 6-Item Scale; SEMCD-6) with a similar population to evaluate a SCT-based intervention. Allowing for approximately 30% attrition, we recruited 78 participants.

Patients who attended five nephrologists' clinics across two public sector outpatient renal clinics in Queensland, Australia were screened by clinic staff for eligibility. These sites are general nephrology outpatient clinics, where patients are typically referred by their General Practitioner or family physician when their eGFR decreases below 60 mL/min/1.73m^2 or sometimes earlier in the case of sudden kidney function deterioration. Inclusion criteria were: diagnosis of CKD; eGFR ≥25 mL/min/1.73m^2 (so participants would not have commenced pre-dialysis education); ≥18 years of age; and ability to understand English. Exclusion criteria were: cognitive impairment which would inhibit participation (as determined by clinic staff); inability to be followed up (> 60 km from researcher's location); and already receiving extensive CKD SMS through select Queensland clinics known to provide enhanced SMS as part of their renal care. Participant recruitment and participation can be seen in Fig. 2. Data were collected at T0 (baseline) and T1 (13 weeks; 1 week after intervention completion). Due to financial constraints, blinded data collection was not possible.

Procedure
Recruitment took place between April and December 2016, with follow-up completion in March 2017. Flyers were sent with appointment letters, and verbal consent was obtained for the researcher to approach when patients attended appointments. A systematic recruitment protocol was implemented whereby all eligible patients were approached consecutively by a male or female researcher and provided study information prior to consenting. Participants commenced study instruments, which took approximately 20–30 min to complete, and finalised these at first intervention appointment. The principal investigator, a researcher in CKD self-management with a background in psychology, delivered intervention sessions over a 12-week period. One week after final intervention session, participants completed study questionnaires again face-to-face with the researcher.

Intervention: The CKD-SMS
The intervention was highly individualised, based upon principles of person-centred care (PCC) and SCT. Expert input was sought (from nephrologists, renal nurses, academic specialists in CKD, and people with CKD) regarding intervention and resource design. The design of the CKD-SMS was also informed by our previous work investigating SMS desires of people with CKD [20, 21], conducted

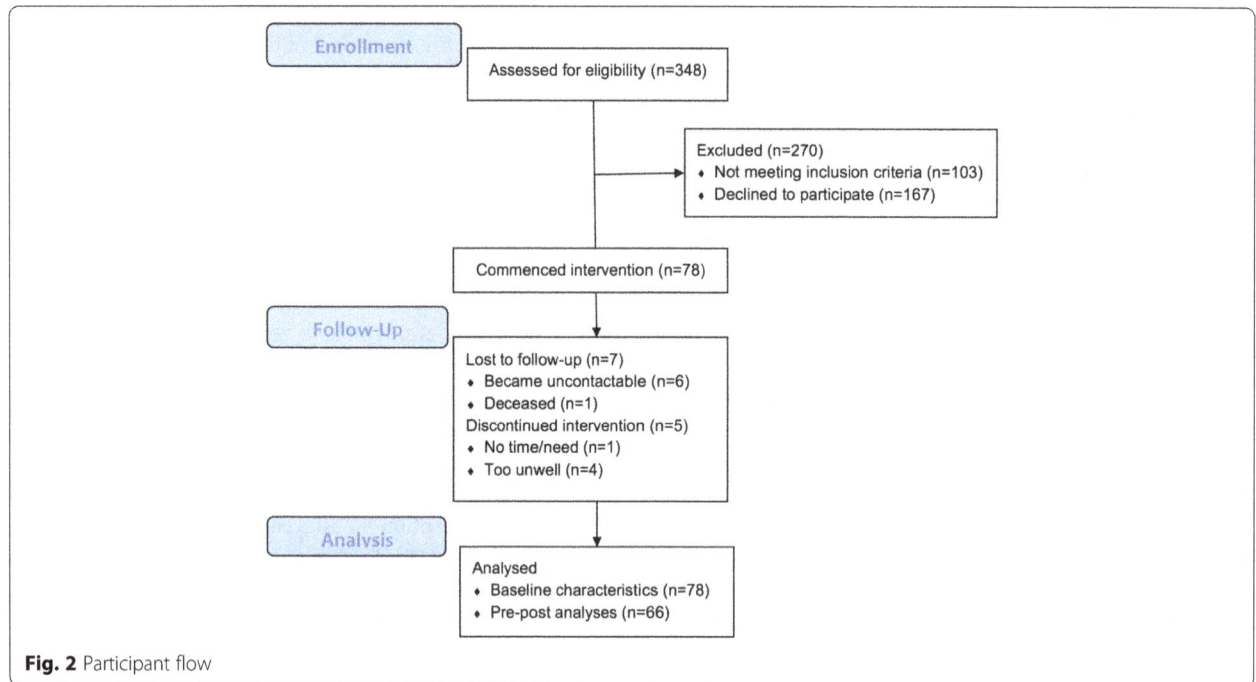

Fig. 2 Participant flow

with the explicit goal of informing intervention development. An outline of the purposes and procedures of CKD-SMS sessions can be seen in Additional file 1.

Participants engaged in two face-to-face intervention sessions with the principal researcher, at week 1 and week 12, which took place in a mutually convenient location (most often the participant's home or workplace, 80.8%). Length of these sessions ranged from 20 to 90 min ($M = 44$ min), dependent upon individual need. Between face-to-face sessions, participants nominated preferred frequency of phone sessions (weekly, fortnightly, or monthly), with most (71.2%) opting for monthly sessions. Phone sessions ranged from five to 60 min, but were mostly brief ($M = 12$ min). At the first session, participants and researcher collaborated to generate individualised goals in areas including: diet; physical activity; communication with HCPs and engagement with treatment; emotional distress; maintaining roles; and understanding CKD and laboratory results. During the course of the intervention, techniques from SCT (performance accomplishment reinforcement, vicarious experience, and verbal persuasion) were used to assist participants achieve their goals, as were motivational interviewing, cognitive-behavioural, and mindfulness techniques as appropriate (see Additional file 2 for examples of how these strategies were used).

Participants were given a handbook (adapted with permission from Kidney Health Australia's "Living with Reduced Kidney Function" handbook [35]) to accompany the intervention, which was used to prompt discussion. Participants also received self-monitoring and note-taking handouts,[1] and were encouraged to request further resources. Participants were encouraged to invite family members or friends to attend sessions if desired. One week after the final face-to-face intervention session, participants completed study questionnaires again face-to-face with the researcher.

Intervention Fidelity

All included participants engaged in at least two telephone sessions and two face-to-face sessions during the intervention period. However, during the program, there were 23 instances of participant failure to attend a scheduled face-to-face appointment and 15 instances in which participants were unable to be contacted for scheduled telephone sessions (despite multiple attempts). The person-centred nature of the program meant that flexibility was possible and most participants were able to be followed up and to continue participation in the program.

Outcomes and measurement

We hypothesised that the CKD-SMS would improve behavioural and patient outcomes, with associated increased knowledge and self-efficacy and reduced emotional distress. Study measures are detailed in Table 1. Primary outcomes were self-efficacy and self-management, assessed using the SEMCD-6 [36] and the Australian version of the Chronic Kidney Disease Self-Management Instrument (Aus.CKD-SM) [37], respectively. Secondary outcomes were: HRQoL; CKD knowledge; emotional distress; understanding of physical activity guidelines and engagement in physical activity; fruit and vegetable consumption; communication

Table 1 Study instruments

Outcome	Instrument	Reliability/Validity	Items and Scoring
Background and Clinical Details	Background and clinical details	N/A	10 items assessing background characteristics; 13 items assessing clinical characteristics.
Comorbidity	Charlson Comorbidity Index (CCI) [45]	Valid in predicting risk of death from comorbid disease [45].	Combines age and number of pre-determined, serious comorbidities into a single index. All participants in this study started with a minimum score of 2 for CKD.
CKD Knowledge	Kidney Knowledge Survey (KiKS) [38]	Adequate internal consistency (Kuder-Richardson-20 = .7) [38]; investigates knowledge of important CKD topics such as function, treatment, and BP targets. α = .7 and .8 in current study.	28 multiple-choice items; Maximum score = 28.
Understanding of Physical Activity Guidelines	Four items from Active Australia Survey (AAS) [40]	Assesses understanding of/agreement with physical activity guidelines. Overall instrument has good-excellent reliability (Spearman's Rho 0.5–0.8) [44], and items used showed high reliability in this study (α = .9).	4 Likert Scale items (1 = *Strongly Disagree* – 5 = *Strongly Agree*); Maximum score = 20.
Self-Efficacy to Manage Chronic Disease	Self-Efficacy for Managing Chronic Disease (SEMCD-6) [36]	High internal consistency (α = .9), scales upon which instrument is based sensitive to change in disease-related self-efficacy in response to intervention [36]. α = .9 and .9 in current study.	6 items scored 1–10. Overall scale score = mean of items 1–10.
Depression, Anxiety, and Stress	Depression Anxiety Stress Scales (DASS-21) [39]	Distinguishes well between psychological disorders and has good-excellent internal consistency (α = .9) [73]. α = .8 – > .9 in current study.	21 Likert Scale items (0 = *Never* – 3 = *Almost Always*). Three subscales and overall scale. Scores reported are for 21-item version and must be doubled to be compared to 42-item version scores or cut-offs.
CKD Self-Management Behaviour	Chronic Kidney Disease Self-Management Instrument – Australian Version (Aus.CKD-SM) [37]	Adequate internal consistency (α = .7–.85) [37]. α = .6–.9 in current study.	17 Likert Scale items (1 = *Never* – 4 = *Always*). Four subscales and overall scale.
Physical Activity	Human Activity Profile (HAP) [42]	Used extensively in chronic disease research [74]; adequate test-retest reliability (α = .8), content validity [42]. α = .8 - . > 9 in current study.	94 items rated *"still doing"*, *"stopped doing"* and *"never did"*. Maximum activity score, adjusted activity score, and four research subscales.
Alcohol Use	Alcohol Use Disorders Identification Test-Consumption Questions (AUDIT-C) [44]	Effective in detection of heavy drinking and alcohol abuse or dependence [44]. α = .7 in current study.	Three multiple-choice questions with five response options scored 0–4; Maximum score 12; clinical cut-off of 3 for women and 4 for men.
Fruit and Vegetable Consumption	Two questions about fruit and vegetable consumption yesterday	Directly assesses consumption of fruit and vegetable on previous day.	Two questions assessing serves of fruit and vegetables eaten on previous day, added together for total.
Communication with Healthcare Providers	Two items from the Partners in Health Scale (PiH) [43]	Overall scale has demonstrated construct and face validity and internal consistency (α = .9) and inter-rater reliability [43]. α = .6 and .8 in current study.	Two Likert Scale items (0 = *Never* – 8 = *Always*). Maximum score = 16.
Health-Related Quality of Life	Short Form Health Survey-12-Item Australian v2; (SF-12) [75]	Conceptually and empirically validated [76]; adequate test-retest reliability (α = .8–.9).	12 Likert Scale items (scales vary from 3- to 5-point). Eight subscales contribute to two overall composite scores.

with HCPs; alcohol use; and physiological measures (BP, weight, and eGFR). Additional instruments were: demographic and clinical record form (T0 only); the Kidney Knowledge Survey (KiKS) [38]; the Depression, Anxiety, and Stress Scales 21-Item Version (DASS-21) [39]; four items from the Active Australia Survey (AAS) [40] assessing understanding of physical activity guidelines; the SF-12v2 (Australian version) [41]; the Human Activity Profile (HAP) [42]; two items from the Partners in Health Scale (PiH) [43]; two questions assessing fruit and vegetable consumption; and the Alcohol Use Disorders Test Consumption Questions Scale (AUDIT-C) [44]. Available clinical information at T0 and T1 was gathered from electronic medical records. The Charlson Comorbidity Index (CCI) [45] was used to calculate comorbidity score.

Data analysis

Data were analysed using IBM SPSS Statistics version 23 [46]. Descriptive statistics were generated for background and clinical data, and T0 and T1 results on patient-reported instruments and clinical measures were compared. Descriptive statistics are presented as frequencies and/or range, mean (M) or median (Mdn), and standard deviation (SD) or interquartile range (IQR), as appropriate. Where data met assumptions, paired-samples t-tests were conducted to assess change. Where data did not meet assumptions, non-parametric equivalent tests (Wilcoxon Signed-Rank tests) were conducted. Between-groups t-tests and Fisher's exact tests were performed to assess for baseline differences between those who completed the intervention and those who did not. Mean differences (Diff) and 95% confidence intervals (CI), along with effect sizes (d or r) and statistical significance (at $p < .05$) are reported for all pre-post-intervention analyses.

Results
Sample characteristics and participant flow
Background and clinical characteristics of the original sample ($N = 78$) can be seen in Tables 2 and 3. Slightly over half the sample were female, and age ranged from 25 to 84, with a mean of 57.6. Most participants were born in Australia and predominantly spoke English at home, and two participants identified as Aboriginal or Torres Strait Islander (ATSI). Approximately half (47.4%) of participants had a high-school or lower level of education and the same number were currently employed. Most had CKD stage 2 or 3, and a third had been living with CKD for 10 years or longer, while some had been diagnosed as recently as 4 months ago.

At baseline, the only difference across background and clinical characteristics and scores on questionnaires between those who completed the intervention and those who did not was that non-completers reported more effective communication with HCPs ($p = .04$).

Intervention outcomes
All participants displayed improvement in one or more outcomes between T0 and T1. Details of overall group pre-post intervention changes can be seen in Table 4. Participants identified one or more goals, the most common being overall self-management support (identified 30 times) and knowledge (identified 22 times). The highest percentage of improvement in identified areas was attained for those who set goals of improving knowledge (86.4%) or overall self-management (80.0%).

Self-efficacy and self-management behaviour
Comparison of T0 and T1 SEMCD-6 mean scores revealed that participants' self-efficacy to manage CKD improved significantly (Diff = 0.8, CI = 0.3–1.2, $p = .001$), though the effect size was small ($d = 0.4$). Scores on the Aus.CKD-SM indicated that engagement in CKD self-management behaviours also increased during the study period, with significant improvement in scores on the overall instrument (Diff = 6.2, CI = 4.5–7.9, $p < .001$) and all individual subscales (self-integration; seeking support; adherence to lifestyle modifications; and problem-solving; all ps < .001), with effects ranging from small (for seeking support; $d = 0.4$) to medium (for all other subscales and overall instrument, ds ranging from 0.5 to 0.8). Almost all participants (63; 95.5%) displayed improvement in one or both primary outcomes.

CKD knowledge
Change in mean scores on the KiKS revealed significant improvement in CKD knowledge over the course of the intervention ($p < .001$), with a large effect size ($d = 0.8$).

Knowledge of physical activity guidelines and engagement in physical activity
Understanding of physical activity guidelines increased significantly over the study period ($p = .02$), with a small effect size ($d = 0.4$). Similarly, mean scores on the HAP indicated engagement in physical activity also increased. At T1, participants were engaging in more strenuous activities than they were at T0 ($p = .01$), and more physical activity overall ($p = .02$), though effect sizes were negligible (ds = 0.2), with improvements concentrated in entertainment/social and independent exercise domains.

Health-related quality of life
Participants demonstrated significant improvement in physical aspects of HRQoL over the study period. Overall physical wellbeing (PCS) improved significantly ($p = .01$), with a small effect size ($d = 0.30$), while there was

Table 2 Background characteristics

Variable	Frequency (%)
Gender	
Male	31 (39.7)
Female	47 (60.3)
Age Range: 25–84 *M* = 57.6 SD = 16.7	
25–39	14 (17.9)
40–59	25 (32.1)
60–79	33 (42.3)
≥ 80	6 (7.7)
Place of Birth	
Australia	54 (69.2)
New Zealand	4 (5.1)
South-east Asia	4 (5.1)
Europe	6 (7.7)
Other	10 (12.8)
Main Language	
English	73 (93.6)
Other	5 (6.4)
ATSI[a] Status	
Identifies as Aboriginal	2 (2.6)
Identifies as neither ATSI	76 (97.4)
Marital Status	
Single	15 (19.2)
Married/Defacto	50 (64.1)
Divorced	11 (14.1)
Widowed	2 (2.6)
Years of Education Range: 0[b] – 24 *M* = 12.9 SD = 3.9	
Highest Educational Qualification Attained	
Less than Grade 10 Equivalent	8 (10.4)
Grade 10 or Equivalent	22 (28.6)
Grade 12 or Equivalent	7 (9.1)
TAFE Qualification/Certificate/Diploma	21 (27.3)
Undergraduate Degree (Bachelors)	14 (18.2)
Masters Degree	3 (3.9)
Doctoral Degree (Including PhD)	2 (2.6)
Annual Household Income	
< $20,000	10 (12.8)
$20,000 - $39,999	23 (29.5)
$40,000 - $59,999	8 (10.3)
$60,000 - $79,999	7 (9.0)
$80,000 - $99,999	8 (10.3)
$100,000 - $119,999	9 (11.5)
$120,000+	6 (7.7)
Don't Know/Would Rather not say	7 (9.0)
Employment Status	

Table 2 Background characteristics *(Continued)*

Variable	Frequency (%)
Unemployed	9 (11.5)
Casual	2 (2.6)
Part Time	8 (10.3)
Full Time	25 (32.1)
Retired	32 (41.0)
Other (Employed)	2 (2.6)

[a]*ATSI* Aboriginal or Torres Strait Islander
[b]One participant reported receiving no formal education during her youth in Southeast Asia

no significant change in mental aspects of HRQoL (MCS; $p = .43$, $d = 0.11$).

Communication with healthcare providers

Participants' self-reported communication with HCPs improved significantly between T0 and T1 ($p = .01$), with a small effect size ($d = 0.3$).

Fruit and vegetable consumption, alcohol use, and smoking

Fruit and vegetable intake improved significantly over the study period, evidenced by self-reported serves consumed on the day prior to assessment ($p < .001$), with a large effect size ($d = 1.7$). Alcohol consumption decreased significantly ($p = .01$), though effect size was negligible ($d = 0.1$). There was no change in cigarettes per day amongst the four smokers.

Emotional distress

There were significant reductions in overall emotional distress as assessed by the DASS-21 between T0 and T1 ($p < .001$), with a large effect size ($r = .7$). These improvements were concentrated in the areas of depression ($p = .03$) and stress ($p = .01$), with medium effect sizes for both subscales ($rs = .3$).

Blood pressure

T0 and T1 BP data was available for 39 participants. Significant improvement was seen in systolic ($p < .01$) and diastolic ($p = .02$) measurements, with medium effect sizes ($ds = 0.7$ and 0.6, respectively). Percentage of participants at target ($\leq120/80$) remained stable (88.5%).

Discussion

Through a person-centred, theory-based approach to SMS, this exploratory study demonstrates improved behavioural and patient outcomes among people with stages 1–4 CKD. As postulated by SCT, this was associated with improvements in knowledge, emotional distress, and self-efficacy. The person-centred, flexible approach meant not only that a wide range of people (including those with physical

Table 3 Clinical characteristics

Variable	Frequency (%)
CKD Stage	
1	12 (15.6)
2	22 (28.6)
3A	15 (19.5)
3B	20 (26.0)
4	8 (10.4)
eGFR[a] Range: 25- > 90 *M* = 57.5 SD = 22.3	
Creatinine μmol/L Range: 48–259 *M* = 116.3 SD = 45.4	
Time Since Diagnosis (Self-Reported) Range: 4 months – 33 years *Mdn* = 5 years QR = 26.3–120.0 (months)	
≤ 12 months	11 (14.5)
12 years 1 month - 3 years	13 (17.1)
3 years, 1 month - 5 years	15 (19.7)
5 years, 1 month < 10 years	12 (15.8)
≥ 10 years	25 (32.9)
Unknown	2 (2.6)
Cause of CKD	
Renovascular	13 (16.9)
Glomerulonephritis	13 (16.9)
Diabetes Mellitus (I or II)	12 (15.6)
Systemic Lupus Erythematosus	8 (10.4)
Other	25 (32.5)
Unknown	6 (7.8)
Charlson Comorbidity Index Score Range: 2–11 *Mdn* = 5.5 IQR = 3.3–8.0	
2–5	36 (50.0)
6–9	31 (43.1)
10+	5 (6.9)
Smoking Status	
Non-smoker	43 (55.1)
Ex-smoker	28 (35.9)
Current Smoker	7 (9.0)
Current Medications Range: 1–14 *Mdn:* 6	

[a]CKD-EPI Creatinine Equation [77]

disabilities such as quadriplegia, blindness, and limb amputation and those with English as their second language, as well as full-time workers with busy schedules) were able to participate, but also that personally meaningful goals were able to be worked towards in order to achieve overall improvements in self-efficacy and self-management. PCC as standard in SMS would mean support was directed where it was needed, a more efficient use of time and resources. The heart failure (HF) literature provides support for this idea, with studies demonstrating that, when delivered as intended, PCC improves patient outcomes and decreases disease burden [47, 48].

Individuals are experts on their lives, yet people with chronic disease often do not feel that HCPs value their knowledge and insight regarding their condition [49]. In this study, those with lower self-efficacy at baseline chose more intensive intervention schedules, demonstrating awareness of need for support. SMS in CKD has historically been delivered and evaluated from the perspective of HCPs, focusing on what they know to be important and assuming that provision of disease-specific information will lead to improved self-management [8, 50–52], while failing to account for the complexity of chronic disease self-management from the perspective of their patients. Multiple reviews of CKD self-management intervention studies have been published in recent years [8–10, 53], however, they consistently reach similar conclusions: that studies are limited and difficult to review due to large variation in samples, methodologies, and outcomes. In chronic disease, the burden of disease-management is overwhelmingly with the individual, and it is crucial that support processes are in place to set up and maintain effective self-management. In the field of SMS for these diseases, meaningful change for individuals is what is important, and flexibility in intervention and evaluation protocols is going to be necessary in order for this support to reach those who need it most. In contrast to repeated attempts to synthesise overall results of studies in this field, meta-analyses of individual patient data provide techniques which can help to ascertain what works for whom, and under what conditions, rather than continually trying to synthesise disparate studies [54].

After receiving the individualised CKD-SMS, participants displayed overall improvements on several outcomes. Both primary outcomes improved significantly, with small to medium effect sizes. We also found significant improvement in several secondary outcomes. The pattern of findings is consistent with a SCT model of CKD self-management [17, 55, 56], indicating that the intervention led to changes in knowledge and self-efficacy via multiple sources (education, performance accomplishments, vicarious experience, verbal persuasion, and self-appraisal) which led to changes in behaviour and outcomes. Testing of our SCT model was beyond the scope of this study, but it has provided a framework for future research by proposing a model for self-management in CKD which is empirically testable using standardised measures. In addition to elements assessed in this study, several participants desired assistance with sleep (i.e., training in sleep hygiene), and this was provided during intervention sessions and by way of additional resources. This may be an area that is important to include as an outcome in future studies.

Inclusion of goal-setting and awareness of general SMS needs in planning and implementing person-centred

Table 4 Pre-post changes in primary and secondary outcomes

	Time – Mean (SD)				
	Baseline	12 weeks	Diff (95% CI)	d	p
Person Variables					
KiKS	17.0 (5.0)	20.7 (3.8)	3.7 (2.7–4.8)	0.8	<.001
Understanding of Physical Activity Guidelines	16.4 (2.5)	17.2 (2.3)	0.9 (0.1–1.6)	0.4	.02
Self-Efficacy					
SEMCD-6	6.7 (2.1)	7.44 (1.9)	0.8 (0.3–1.2)	0.4	<.01
Emotional Distress/Self-Appraisal					
DASS-21					
Depression[ab]	4.2[c] (4.1[d])	3.0[c] (3.3[d])	1.2 (0.1–2.1)	0.3[e]	.03
Anxiety[ab]	4.6[c] (4.1[d])	4.4[c] (4.1[d])	0.2 (−0.91–1.3)	0.1[e]	.70
Stress[ab]	5.7[c] (4.2[d])	4.5[c] (3.6[d])	1.2 (0.3–2.1)	0.3[e]	.01
Behaviour					
Aus.CKD-SM	47.0 (8.7)	53.2 (7.5)	6.2 (4.5–7.9)	0.8	<.001
Self-Integration	13.7 (3.3)	15.8 (2.9)	2.2 (1.5–2.9)	0.7	<.001
Seeking Support	8.3 (2.7)	9.2 (2.7)	1.0 (0.4–1.5)	0.4	<.001
Adherence to Lifestyle Modifications	12.4 (2.8)	13.7 (2.7)	1.4 (0.8–2.0)	0.5	<.001
Problem-Solving	12.7 (2.7)	14.4 (2.1)	1.7 (1.1–2.3)	0.7	<.001
HAP					
Maximum Activity Score	69.2 (15.6)	72.0 (14.8)	2.8 (0.6–5.0)	0.2	.01
Adjusted Activity Score	59.4 (21.5)	62.4 (19.3)	3.0 (0.6–5.3)	0.2	.02
Self-care	7.5 (1.6)	7.5 (1.5)	< 0.1 (−0.2–0.2)	< 0.1	.89
Personal/Household Work	18.7 (6.6)	19.4 (5.9)	0.7 (− < 0.1–1.5)	0.1	.06
Entertainment/Social	9.5 (2.8)	10.0 (2.6)	0.5 (< 0.1–0.9)	0.2	.04
Independent Exercise	8.0 (6.5)	9.2 (6.8)	1.2 (0.1–2.2)	0.2	.04
AUDIT-C	2.4 (2.7)	2.0 (2.3)	0.3 (0.1–0.6)	0.1	.01
Fruit and Vegetables Consumed Yesterday[a]	2.3 (1.5)	6.3 (3.0)	4.0 (3.3–4.8)	1.7	<.001
Communication with HCPs[f]	13.4 (2.9)	14.3 (2.3)	0.7 (0.2–1.6)	0.3	.01
Cigarettes per day (n = 4)	16.3 (4.8)	16.3 (4.8)	0.0 (−6.5–6.5)	< 0.001	.99
Outcomes					
eGFR (n = 46)	55.2 (24.1)	51.3 (24.2)	3.9 (1.0–6.9)	0.7	.01
BP (n = 39) 88.5% at target (T0 and T1)					
Systolic	129.6 (23.3)	120.7 (15.8)	8.9 (2.9–14.9)	0.7	<.01
Diastolic	74.8 (11.1)	70.5 (9.6)	4.3 (0.9–7.8)	0.6	.01
SF12					
PCS	41.3 (11.1)	44.5 (8.7)	3.2 (0.9–5.4)	0.3	.01
MCS	51.9 (9.8)	50.9 (9.6)	−1.1 (−3.8–1.6)	0.1	.43
Weight (n = 37)	87.4 (30.6)	87.8 (30.6)	−0.4 (−1.1–0.4)	0.3	.32

SD standard deviation, Diff mean difference, CI confidence interval

d = Effect size (small ≥0.2; medium ≥0.5; large ≥0.8 [40])

[a] n = 56

[b] Wilcoxon Signed-Rank test results reported to deal with effects of violations of t-test assumptions

[c] Median

[d] IQR

[e] r = Effect size (small ≥0.1; medium ≥0.3; large ≥0.5 [40])

[f] n = 65

intervention is crucial, as it has been identified that outcome measures often do not even match goals of people with chronic diseases [57]. On an individual, goal-focused level, the areas of greatest improvement were for knowledge and overall self-management. That said, all participants demonstrated improvement in one or more outcomes, indicating that person-centred intervention has the potential to improve patient outcomes overall. This is consistent with previous research across various chronic diseases, which has determined that interventions that are tailored to patient activation [58], preferences [47], values and goals [59], and/or individual circumstances [60] and aligned with principles of PCC [61] can lead to improved patient outcomes. Additionally, HF research has indicated that compatibility of prescribed self-management tasks with life goals is unsurprisingly associated with adherence [62].

The findings of this study are consistent with those of previous research which have indicated that self-management interventions can lead to improved outcomes (see [8–10, 53] for reviews and limitations). Improvements in BP provide physiological evidence of participant-reported behaviour change, although, as renal function deteriorates, more pharmacological intervention to control BP is required. Smoking behaviour did not improve, however only four smokers participated, and each indicated an unwillingness quit. Smoking cessation is challenging, requiring both readiness and often intensive, targeted intervention [63]. Despite positive outcomes, kidney function declined during the study, although there are multiple possible explanations for this. First, it must be noted that T1 eGFR was only available for participants who were required to see their nephrologist at least every 3 months ($n = 46$), indicating faster kidney function decline. Second, effect from lifestyle modifications takes significant time – longer than the three-month follow-up in this study [64]. Third, understanding about those who are likely to experience CKD progression is emerging, and interventions to slow decline warrant further research.

This research indicates that delivery of individualised, person-centred, theory-based self-management support has potential to help patients with CKD to achieve clinical targets and better health and quality of life outcomes. While our focus was the development of a person-centred intervention, future implementation research is needed to examine its scalability in clinical practice. Elsewhere we report on participants' perspectives of the CKD-SMS intervention, which support this approach as highly useful and helpful in managing their CKD [65]. Yet we acknowledge the systems barriers to change that reduce uptake of person-centred innovation in healthcare [66]. There are opportunities for this intervention to be delivered at existing nurse-led CKD clinics (e.g., [67]), or by nurses alongside routine clinical appointments at outpatient clinics. There is also potential

for practices such as this to attract additional funding, with the current international focus on PCC in healthcare practice [68, 69]. Self-management support desires of people with CKD identified by our previous work [20, 21] could also be used in healthcare contexts to guide goal-setting and development over time. Those with poorer relationships with their HCPs and greater complexity in terms of treatment regimens and comorbidities are likely to need more support than those who feel supported by their HCPs and/or have less complex health problems. People with CKD have to live and manage their condition in an environment fraught with illness and treatment complexity and inconsistency. Person-centred care provides an opportunity to support patients within their complex healthcare environment, and findings from the HF literature demonstrating that PCC helps alleviate feelings of illness-related complexity and ambiguity indicate that it can be effective in doing so [70]. Recognition that people with chronic disease frequently suffer from multiple comorbidities (increasing complexity and rendering advice focused on one discrete illness unhelpful [71]) is also crucial. Government bodies are starting to recognise the importance of integrated care, and to provide subsidies for a HCP in a patient advocate role who has a holistic understanding of individual patients [72].

This study was limited by the fact that data were collected by the researcher who delivered the intervention, which may have encouraged response bias. Selection bias is also possible due to the study design, and may have favoured patients who were motivated to engage in self-management. We were unable to report data on non-consenting patients, however we would expect the intervention effects to be even greater in a more diverse sample. A further limitation of the study was its pre-post design, which does not allow for comparison to an active control group (e.g., one in which participants receive pure information with no SCT or PCC elements). There is an opportunity for future research to build on this study, using longer term evaluations of programs such as the CKD-SMS to assess maintenance of behaviour change and effects on clinical outcomes and disease progression, and also to investigate effects of an intervention such as this in comparison to an active control group. Other constructs not captured in this study such as social support may also be built into the SCT model proposed here.

Conclusions

CKD research has generally proceeded in ways that ignore the complexity of self-managing chronic illness – both in the design of interventions and the reporting of study outcomes. In doing so, it has fallen short of developing models that are meaningful to people with CKD, and failed to provide practitioners with the kind of knowledge needed to best support patients. There are several systematic reviews that are inconclusive or do not provide information about how to optimise SMS to meet patient needs. This study is an important step in moving the field forward: demonstrating improved outcomes in early stage CKD by adopting a person-centred approach to SMS. It also supports SCT as a useful framework to guide future interventions. People with CKD have diverse needs and associated complex comorbidity. It is important to consider individual circumstances, needs and goals, as well as current level of activation, when providing SMS to this population.

Endnotes
[1]Handbook and handouts available from lead author upon request.

Abbreviations
BP: Blood pressure; CKD: Chronic kidney disease; CKD-SMS: The chronic kidney disease self-management support intervention; ESKD: End-stage kidney disease; HF: Heart failure; KRT: Kidney replacement therapy; PCC: Person-centred care; SCT: Social-cognitive theory

Acknowledgements
The authors acknowledge the support of the staff at Queensland Kidney Health Services sites and at Kidney Health Australia in developing and conducting this research and the assistance of Vincent Tam as a recruitment and data collection research assistant.

Funding
This work was supported by the Australian Government and the Queensland University of Technology in the form of an Australian Postgraduate Award, and by the National Health and Medical Research Council Chronic Kidney Disease Centre for Research Excellence by way of a supervisor scholarship. These funding bodies had no involvement in study design; collection, analysis, or interpretation of data; the writing of the report; or in the decision to submit the article for publication.

Authors' contributions
Conception and design: KH, AB, CD; data collection and intervention delivery: KH; data analysis and interpretation: KH, AB, CD; manuscript drafting and revisions: KH, AB, CD. All authors have read and approved the final manuscript. KH will act as overall guarantor for the manuscript.

Competing interests
The authors declare that they have no competing interests.

Author details
[1]School of Nursing, Queensland University of Technology, Victoria Park Rd, Kelvin Grove, Brisbane, QLD 4059, Australia. [2]NHMRC Chronic Kidney Disease Centre for Research Excellence, University of Queensland, St Lucia, Australia. [3]Visiting Research Fellow, Kidney Health Service, Metro North Hospital and Health Service, Brisbane, Australia.

References
1. Almutary H, Bonner A, Douglas C. Symptom burden in chronic kidney disease: a review of recent literature. J Ren Care. 2013;39(3):140–50.
2. World Health Organization. Disease burden by cause, age, sex, by Country and by Region, 2000–2015. Geneva: WHO; 2016.
3. Levin A, Tonelli M, Bonventre J, Coresh J, Donner J-A, Fogo AB, Fox CS, Gansevoort RT, Heerspink HJL, Jardine M, et al. Global kidney health 2017 and beyond: a roadmap for closing gaps in care, research, and policy. Lancet. 2017;390:1888–917.
4. World Health Organization. Projections of mortality and causes of death, 2015 and 2030. Geneva: WHO; 2013.
5. Webster AC, Nagler EV, Morton RL, Masson P. Chronic kidney disease. Lancet. 2017;389(10075):1238–52.
6. Devins GM, Mendelssohn DC, Barre PE, Binik YM. Predialysis psychoeducational intervention and coping styles influence time to dialysis in chronic kidney disease. Am J Kidney Dis. 2003;42(4):693–703.
7. Stenberg U, Haaland-Overby M, Fredriksen K, Westermann KF, Kvisvik T. A scoping review of the literature on benefits and challenges of participating in patient education programs aimed at promoting self-management for people living with chronic illness. Patient Educ Couns. 2016;99(11):1759–71.
8. Bonner A, Havas K, Douglas C, Thepha T, Bennett P, Clark R. Self-management programmes in stages 1-4 chronic kidney disease: a literature review. J Ren Care. 2014;40(3):194–204.
9. Lee M, Wu S, Hsieh N, Tsai J. Self-management programs on eGFR, depression, and quality of life among patients with chronic kidney disease: a meta-analysis. Asian Nurs Res (Korean Soc Nurs Sci). 2016;10(4):255–62.
10. Welch J, Johnson M, Zimmerman L, Russell CL, Perkins SM, Decker B. Self-management interventions in stages 1 to 4 chronic kidney disease: an integrative review. West J Nurs Res. 2015;37(5):652–78.
11. Jacobson Vann JC, Hawley J, Wegner S, Falk RJ, Harward DH, Kshirsagar AV. Nursing intervention aimed at improving self-management for persons with chronic kidney disease in North Carolina Medicaid: a pilot project. Nephrol Nurs J. 2015;42(3):239.
12. Byrne J, Khunti K, Stone M, Farooqi A, Carr S. Feasibility of a structured group education session to improve self-management of blood pressure in people with chronic kidney disease: an open randomised pilot trial. British Med J Open. 2011;1(2):e000381.
13. Williams A, Manias E, Liew D, Gock H, Gorelik A. Working with CALD groups: testing the feasibility of an intervention to improve medication self-management in people with kidney disease, diabetes, and cardiovascular disease. Renal Soc Australas J. 2012;8(2):62–9.
14. Glanz K, Bishop DB. The role of behavioral science theory in development and implementation of public health interventions. Annu Rev Public Health. 2010;31(1):399–418.
15. Fishbein M, Ajzen I. Predicting and changing behavior: the reasoned action approach. New York: Psychology Press; 2010.
16. Janz NK, Becker MH. The health belief model: a decade later. Health Educ Behav. 1984;11(1):1–47.
17. Bandura A. Self-efficacy: toward a unifying theory of behavioral change. Psychol Rev. 1977;84(2):191–215.
18. Aliasgharpour M, Shomali M, Moghaddam MZ, Faghihzadeh S. Effect of a self-efficacy promotion training programme on the body weight changes in patients undergoing haemodialysis. J Ren Care. 2012;38(3):155–61.
19. Su C, Lu X, Chen W, Wang T. Promoting self-management improves the health status of patients having peritoneal dialysis. J Adv Nurs. 2009;65(7):1381–9.
20. Havas K, Bonner A, Douglas C. Self-management support for people with chronic kidney disease: patient perspectives. J Ren Care. 2016;42(1):7–14.
21. Havas K, Douglas C, Bonner A. Person-centred care in chronic kidney disease: a cross-sectional study of patients' desires for self-management support. BMC Nephrol. 2017a;18(1):17.
22. Hibbard JH, Stockard J, Mahoney ER, Tusler M. Development of the patient activation measure (PAM): conceptualizing and measuring activation in patients and consumers. Health Serv Res. 2004;39(4p1):1005–26.
23. Gerteis M, Edman-Levitan S, Daley J, Delbanco T. Through the patient's eyes: understanding and promoting patient-centered care. San Francisco: Jossey-Bass; 1993.
24. Kazawa K, Moriyama M. Effects of a self-management skills-acquisition program on pre-dialysis patients with diabetic nephropathy. Nephrol Nurs J. 2013;40(2):141.
25. Walker R, Marshall M, Polaschek N. A prospective clinical trial of specialist renal nursing in the primary care setting to prevent progression of chronic kidney: a quality improvement report. BMC Fam Pract. 2014;15:155.
26. Campbell KL, Ash S, Bauer JD. The impact of nutrition intervention on quality of life in pre-dialysis chronic kidney disease patients. Clin Nutr. 2008; 27(4):537–44.
27. Yen M, Huang JJ, Teng HL. Education for patients with chronic kidney disease in Taiwan: a prospective repeated measures study. J Clin Nurs. 2008; 17(21):2927–34.

28. Chen S-H, Tsai Y-F, Sun C-Y, Wu IW, Lee C-C, Wu M-S. The impact of self-management support on the progression of chronic kidney disease--a prospective randomized controlled trial. Nephrol Dial Transplant. 2011; 26(11):3560–6.

29. Flesher M, Woo P, Chiu A, Charlebois A, Warburton DE, Leslie B. Self-management and biomedical outcomes of a cooking, and exercise program for patients with chronic kidney disease. J Ren Nutr. 2011;21(2):188–95.

30. Watson R, McKenna H, Cowman S, Keady J. Nursing research: designs and methods. London: Elsevier Health Sciences UK; 2008.

31. Des Jarlais DC, Lyles C, Crepaz N, The TREND group. Improving the reporting quality of nonrandomized evaluations of behavioral and public health interventions: the TREND statement. Am J Public Health. 2004;94(3):361–6.

32. Hoffmann TC, Glasziou PP, Boutron I, Milne R, Perera R, Moher D, Altman DG, Barbour V, Macdonald H, Johnston M, et al. Better reporting of interventions: template for intervention description and replication (TIDieR) checklist and guide. BMJ. 2014;348:g1687.

33. Cohen J. Statistical power analysis for the behavioral sciences. 2nd ed. Hillsdale: Lawrence Erlbaum Associates; 1988.

34. Faul F, Erdfelder E, Lang A, Buchner A. G*power 3: a flexible statistical power analysis program for the social, behavioral, and biomedical sciences. Behav Res Methods. 2007;39(2):175–91.

35. Kidney Health Australia. Living with reduced kidney function: a handbook for self management of chronic kidney disease. Australia: Kidney Health Australia; 2008.

36. Lorig KR, Sobel DS, Ritter PL, Laurent D, Hobbs M. Effect of a self-management program on patients with chronic disease. Eff Clin Pract : ECP. 2001;4(6):256.

37. Wembenyui C, Bonner A, Douglas C. Examining patients' knowledge about chronic kidney disease in a primary health care setting. Queensland: Renal Society of Australasia 44th annual conference; 2016.

38. Wright JA, Wallston KA, Elasy TA, Ikizler TA, Cavanaugh KL. Development and results of a kidney disease knowledge survey given to patients with CKD. Am J Kidney Dis. 2011;57(3):387–95.

39. Lovibond SH, Lovibond PF. Manual for the depression anxiety stress scales. 2nd ed. Sydney: Psychology Foundation; 1995.

40. Australian Institute of Health and Welfare. The active Australia survey: a guide and manual for implementation, analysis and reporting. Canberra: Australian institute of health and welfare; 2003.

41. Ware JE, Kosinski M, Bjorner JB, Turner-Bowker DM, Gandek B, Maruish ME. SF-36v2 health survey: Administration guide for clinical trial investigators. Lincoln: QualityMetric Incorporated; 2008.

42. Fix A, Daughton D. Human activity profile professional manual. Odessa: Psychological Assessment Resources, Inc; 1988.

43. Battersby MW, Ask A, Reece MM, Markwick MJ, Collins JP. The Partners in Health scale: the development and psychometric properties of a generic assessment scale for chronic condition self-management. Aus J Prim Health. 2003;9(3):41–52.

44. Bush K, Kivlahan DR, McDonell MB, Fihn SD, Bradley KA. The AUDIT alcohol consumption questions (AUDIT-C): an effective brief screening test for problem drinking. Ambulatory care quality improvement project (ACQUIP). Alcohol use disorders identification test. Arch Intern Med. 1998;158(16):1789–95.

45. Charlson M, Szatrowski TP, Peterson J, Gold J. Validation of a combined comorbidity index. J Clin Epidemiol. 1994;47(11):1245–51.

46. Corp IBM. SPSS for mac. 23.0 ed. Armonk: IBM Corp; 2015.

47. Brännström M, Boman K. Effects of person-centred and integrated chronic heart failure and palliative home care. PREFER: a randomized controlled study. Eur J Heart Fail. 2014;16(10):1142–51.

48. Hansson E, Ekman I, Swedberg K, Wolf A, Dudas K, Ehlers L, Olsson L-E. Person-centred care for patients with chronic heart failure – a cost–utility analysis. Eur J Cardiovasc Nurs. 2016;15(4):276–84.

49. Zoffmann V, Harder I, Kirkevold M. A person-centered communication and reflection model: sharing decision-making in chronic care. Qual Health Res. 2008;18(5):670–85.

50. Granger BB, Sandelowski M, Tahshjain H, Swedberg K, Ekman I. A qualitative descriptive study of the work of adherence to a chronic heart failure regimen: patient and physician perspectives. J Cardiovasc Nurs. 2009;24(4):308–15.

51. Lake AJ, Staiger PK. Seeking the views of health professionals on translating chronic disease self-management models into practice. Patient Educ Couns. 2010;79(1):62–8.

52. Sadler E, Wolfe CD, McKevitt C. Lay and health care professional understandings of self-management: a systematic review and narrative synthesis. SAGE Open Med. 2014;2(0). https://doi.org/10.1177/2050312114544493.

53. Lin M-Y, Liu MF, Hsua L-F, Tsai P-S. Effects of self-management on chronic kidney disease: a meta-analysis. Int J Nurs Stud. 2017;74:128–37.

54. Jonkman NH, Groenwold RHH, Trappenburg JCA, Hoes AW, Schuurmans MJ. Complex self-management interventions in chronic disease unravelled: a review of lessons learned from an individual patient data meta-analysis. J Clin Epidemiol. 2017;83:48–56.

55. Bandura A. Health promotion by social cognitive means. Health Educ Behav. 2004;31(2):143–64.

56. Curtin RB, Walters BAJ, Schatell D, Pennell P, Wise M, Klicko K. Self-efficacy and self-management behaviors in patients with chronic kidney disease. Adv Chronic Kidney Dis. 2008;15(2):191–205.

57. Gardner T, Refshauge K, McAuley J, Goodall S, Hubscher M, Smith L. Patient led goal setting in chronic low back pain-what goals are important to the patient and are they aligned to what we measure? Patient Educ Couns. 2015;98(8):1035–8.

58. Hibbard JH, Greene J, Tusler M. Improving the outcomes of disease management by tailoring care to the patient's level of activation. Am J Manag Care. 2009;15(6):353–60.

59. Lundgren J, Andersson G, Dahlstrom O, Jaarsma T, Kohler AK, Johansson P, Institutionen för medicin och h, Medicinska f, Hjärt- och M, Institutionen för beteendevetenskap och l, et al. Internet-based cognitive behavior therapy for patients with heart failure and depressive symptoms: a proof of concept study. Patient Educ Couns. 2015;98(8):935–42.

60. Lion KC, Mangione-Smith R, Britto MT. Individualized plans of care to improve outcomes among children and adults with chronic illness: a systematic review. Care Manag J. 2014;15(1):11–25.

61. Ekman I, Wolf A, Olsson L-E, Taft C, Dudas K, Schaufelberger M, Swedberg K. Effects of person-centred care in patients with chronic heart failure: the PCC-HF study. Eur Heart J. 2012;33(9):1112–9.

62. Zhang KM, Dindoff K, Arnold JMO, Lane J, Swartzman LC. What matters to patients with heart failure? The influence of non-health-related goals on patient adherence to self-care management. Patient Educ Couns. 2015;98(8):927–34.

63. Australian Government Department of Health and Ageing. Smoking cessation guidelines for Australian general practice. Australia: The Royal Australian College of General Practitioners; 2012.

64. Enworom CD, Tabi M. Evaluation of kidney disease education on clinical outcomes and knowledge of self-management behaviors of patients with chronic kidney disease. Nephrol Nurs J. 2015;42(4):363–73.

65. Havas K, Douglas C, Bonner A. Closing the loop in person-centered care: patient experiences of a chronic kidney disease self-management intervention. Patient Prefer Adherence. 2017;11:1963–73.

66. Brummel-Smith K, Butler D, Frieder M, Gibbs N, Henry M, Koons E, Loggers E, Porock D, Reuben DB, Saliba D, et al. Person-centered care: a definition and essential elements. J Am Geriatr Soc. 2016;64(1):15–8.

67. Coleman S, Havas K, Ersham S, Stone C, Taylor B, Graham A, Bublitz L, Purtell L, Bonner A. Patient satisfaction with nurse-led chronic kidney disease clinics: a multicentre evaluation. J Ren Care. 2017;43(1):11–20.

68. Australian Commission on Safety and Quality in Healthcare. Patient-centred care: Improving quality and safety through partnerships with patients and consumers. Sydney: Australian Commission on Safety and Quality in Healthcare; 2011.

69. NHS England. Putting patients first - The NHS England business plan for 2013/14–2015/16. London: The Stationery Office; 2013.

70. Dudas K, Olsson L-E, Wolf A, Swedberg K, Taft C, Schaufelberger M, Ekman I. Uncertainty in illness among patients with chronic heart failure is less in person-centred care than usual care. Eur J Cardiovasc Nurs. 2013;12(6):521–8.

71. Bowling CB, Vandenberg AE, Phillips LS, McClellan WM, Johnson TMI, Echt KV. Older patients' perspectives on managing complexity in CKD self-management. Clin J Am Soc Nephrol. 2017;12:635–43.

72. Bayliss EA, Balasubramianian BA, Gill JM, Stange KC. Perspectives in primary care: implementing patient-centered care coordination for individuals with multiple chronic medical conditions. Ann Fam Med. 2014;12(6):500–3.

73. Antony MM, Bieling PJ, Cox BJ, Enns MW, Swinson RP. Psychometric properties of the 42-item and 21-item versions of the depression anxiety stress scales in clinical groups and a community sample. Psychol Assess. 1998;10(2):176–81.

16

Activation of RAAS in a rat model of liver cirrhosis: no effect of losartan on renal sodium excretion

A. D. Fialla[1]* (ID), O. B. Schaffalitzky de Muckadell[1], P. Bie[3] and H. C. Thiesson[2]

Abstract

Background: Liver cirrhosis is characterized by avid sodium retention where the activation of the renin angiotensin aldosterone system (RAAS) is considered to be the hallmark of the sodium retaining mechanisms. The direct effect of angiotensin II (ANGII) on the AT-1 receptor in the proximal tubules is partly responsible for the sodium retention. The aim was to estimate the natriuretic and neurohumoral effects of an ANGII receptor antagonist (losartan) in the late phase of the disease in a rat model of liver cirrhosis.

Methods: Bile duct ligated (BDL) and sham operated rats received 2 weeks of treatment with losartan 4 mg/kg/day or placebo, given by gastric gavage 5 weeks after surgery. Daily sodium and potassium intakes and renal excretions were measured.

Results: The renal sodium excretion decreased in the BDL animals and this was not affected by losartan treatment. At baseline the plasma renin concentration (PRC) was similar in sham and BDL animals, but increased urinary excretion of ANGII and an increase P-Aldosterone was observed in the placebo treated BDL animals. The PRC was more than 150 times higher in the losartan treated BDL animals ($p < 0.001$) which indicated hemodynamic impairment.

Conclusions: Losartan 4 mg/kg/day did not increase renal sodium excretion in this model of liver cirrhosis, although the urinary ANGII excretion was increased. The BDL animals tolerated Losartan poorly, and the treatment induced a 150 times higher PRC.

Keywords: Sodium retention, Bile duct ligation, ANGII antagonists, Liver cirrhosis, Aldosterone

Background

Liver cirrhosis is characterized by avid sodium retention, where several mechanisms are considered to be responsible. Impaired renal sodium handling is partly due to increased angiotensin II (ANGII) as well as aldosterone levels and its action at the proximal, distal and collecting tubules in the kidneys. Both ANGII and aldosterone are expected to be increased in cirrhosis secondary to the central vasodilation, reduced effective blood volume, where the neurohumoral response maintain blood pressure [1]. ANGII exerts its action mainly through the AT-1 receptor and leads to constriction of the renal artery and increases sodium reabsorption in the proximal tubule [2]. Secondly, ANGII promotes aldosterone release from the adrenal gland which in concert with ANGII regulates the hydro-electrolytic balance [3]. The action of an AT1 receptor antagonist (losartan) is anticipated to be an increased renal sodium excretion and reduced aldosterone release. The bile duct ligated (BDL) rat model of cirrhosis is characterized by portal hypertension and sodium retention [4]. The activity of RAAS has in this model been found contradictory; normal renin coexisting with either low or high levels of aldosterone [4, 5] or coexisting increased levels of renin, ANGII and aldosterone [6]. One study found increased levels of intrarenal components of RAAS irrespective of the systemic RAAS [7]. Although systemic RAAS activation does not fully explain the sodium retention in the BDL model, the sodium excreting effects of losartan, an ANGII receptor antagonist, has previously been

* Correspondence: adam@health.sdu.dk
[1]Department of Gastroenterology and Hepatology, Odense University Hospital, Sdr Boulevard, 5000 Odense C 29 Odense, Denmark
Full list of author information is available at the end of the article

demonstrated where long term treatment in the early course of disease did not increase sodium excretion [8] whereas low doses in the late phase given short term increased sodium excretion [9].

Yet has to be explored, whether long-term treatment with ANGII receptor antagonists may improve sodium excretion in the late phase of the diseases where formation of ascites is frequent. It is hypothesized, that long-term treatment with losartan increases sodium excretion in the BDL model of cirrhosis in the late course of disease by direct blockage of the AT1 receptor and reduction of aldosterone secretion.

Methods

Animals and surgical protocol

The experimental model used is the common bile duct ligated rat (BDL) [10, 11]. Male Wistar rats (17 weeks) were obtained from M&B /Ejby, Denmark. The animals where randomized to BDL or sham surgery., and the group allocation was blinded to the investigator. They were given a 0.2% sodium and 1.0% potassium diet (Altromin 1324;Altromin International, Lage, Germany) and had free access to tap water. Food was administered as granules in metabolic cages to avoid spillage into the urine collection vials. For surgery the animals were anesthetized by subcutaneous injection of fentanyl citrate (0.25 mg/kg), fluanosone (8 mg/kg), and diazepam (4 mg/kg). In BDL rats the common bile duct was isolated, ligated and 0.5 cm was excised. In sham rats the common bile duct was isolated, manipulated and left intact. Postoperative pain was treated with buprenorphin subcutaneously (0.1 mg/kg). At the end of the treatment protocols the rats were anaesthetized by CO_2 inhalation shortly before decapitation and trunk blood was collected for analysis. Organs were removed and weighed. Ascites volume was estimated by aspiration of free fluid from the abdominal cavity. In two BDL rats invasive blood pressure measurement was performed. The Danish Animal Experiments Inspectorate approved all experimental procedures and all animals were treated according to the "Guide for the Care and Use of Laboratory Animals".

The experimental design

Four groups consisting of two BDL groups ($n = 20$) and two sham groups ($n = 16$) were followed for 34 days after surgery after which they were placed in individual metabolic cages. Day 35, baseline measures were obtained and treatment initialized on day 36. The animals were treated with a daily dose of losartan (Cozaar©, MSD, Denmark; 4 mg/kg) or placebo (tap water) for 14 days (Fig. 1).The treatment was blinded to the investigator of the results. The treatment was administered by gastric gavage twice a day. Na^+, K^+, water intake and excretion and ANGII excretion were measured daily. Animals that did not complete the 2 week 24 h collections were excluded from the data analysis.

Plasma and urine analyses

Hormones: Plasma renin concentration (PRC) was measured by radioimmunoassay as previously described [12]. ANGII in urine was determined using a specific antibody (Ab-5-030682) as previously described [13]. Plasma aldosterone was measured with a commercial kit (Coat-A-Count Aldosterone, DPC, Los Angeles). *Biochemistry*: S-Bilirubin, S-Albumin, S-creatinine were analyzed using Cobas Mira Plus analyzer (Roche Diagnostics, Basel). Platelet count, leucocytes, hematocrit and hemoglobin were analyzed on a Celltaca MEK-6108 K (Nihon Kohden, Tokyo, Japan). *Electrolytes in urine and plasma* were determined by flame photometry (IL 943 flame photometer; Instrumentation Labatory, Milan, Italy) Osmolality was measured by freezing point depression (Osmomat 030D; Gonotec, Berlin, Germany). *Calculations:* Sodium and potassium excretion were calculated as the urinary excretion normalized to the body weight on a daily basis. The renal sodium and potassium retention was calculated as the intake minus urinary excretion. *Blood pressure measurement:* Blood pressure was measured with the TA11PA-C40 transmitter (Data Sciences International, St. Paul, Mn, USA), which was implanted in the abdominal aorta under general anesthesia one week before the

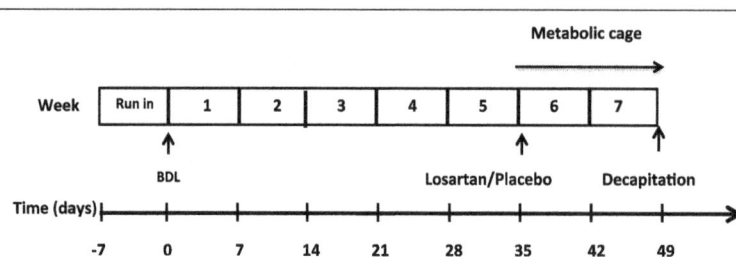

Fig. 1 Study design

start of data collection. In conscious animals measurements were recorded every minute for 24 h a day for 4 days a week in all 7 weeks. The systolic and diastolic blood pressures were recorded, whereas mean arterial pressure and heart rate were calculated. The multiple blood pressure recordings where reported as mean and SD at the end of week 1 and the end of week 7. Dataquest A.R.T software, version 2.10 was applied (Data Sciences International, St. Paul, Mn, USA).

Statistical analysis

Water intake, food intake, urine volume, sodium and potassium intake, sodium and potassium excretion were all reported as summary measures for the first and second week after treatment initiation (week 6 + 7). The sodium and potassium excretion is given as the excretion/intake. Results are given as mean ± standard error of the mean (SEM). For group comparison the Kruskal-Wallis test with post test was applied. Calculations were performed Graph Pad/Prism 5.2, When comparing groups, the difference within the sham -operated animals as well as the BDL animal was analyzed as well as the difference between the BDL animals and their respective sham operated controls. Sample size calculation was not performed, since the experiment was initially explorative.

Results

Animal characteristics

The number of rats completing the protocol was 8 out of 10 in BDL + placebo group and 6 out 10 in the BDL + losartan group. In the BDL + placebo group 2 animal died on day 7 after treatment due to intraperitoneal bleeding. Both animals had ascites. In the BDL losartan group 1 animal was found dead on day 6 due to intraperitoneal bleeding. 3 animals where terminated on day 5, 10 and 14 according to the rules of animal welfare. One animal had ascites. All the sham operated rats completed the protocol. Preoperative weight was similar in all four groups. The final ascites free weight (dry) was significantly reduced in the BDL animals compared to their respective controls. Ascites developed in 7/8 rats in the BDL+ placebo group and in 3/6 animals in the BDL + losartan group. In the sham operated animals the spleen, the liver, the kidneys and the heart were all smaller than in the BDL animals. The spleen was significantly smaller in the losartan treated BDL animals compared to the placebo treated BDL animals. S-bilirubin and B-leucocytes were significantly higher in the BDL animals and S-albumin as well as the platelet count was lower compared to the sham controls. P-potassium was higher in the losartan treated BDL animals compared to the placebo treated BDL animals (Table 1).

Food and water intake

The sham-operated animals ate significantly more than the BDL animals. This was consistent with higher intake of sodium and potassium in the sham animals compared to the BDL animals. Water intake was similar in all four groups (Table 2).

Sodium and potassium excretion

During week 6 after surgery the renal sodium excretion was decreased in the BDL animals (sham+ placebo: 0.80 ± 0.02 vs. BDL+ placebo: 0.72 ± 0.03, $p < 0.05$, Fig. 2a). Losartan treatment did not affect the sodium excretion in the BDL animals compared to placebo (BDL + losartan: 0.77 ± 0.02, $p > 0.05$, Fig. 2a). At week 7 after BDL the renal sodium excretion was even lower in the BDL (sham + placebo: 0.85 ± 0.03 vs. BDL + placebo: 0.68 ± 0.04, $p < 0.001$, Fig. 2b). This was not affected by losartan treatment (BDL + losartan: 0.72 ± 0.03 $p > 0.05$, Fig. 2b). During week 6 after BDL the renal potassium excretion increased in the BDL animals (sham + placebo: 0.91 ± 0.02 vs. BDL + placebo: 0.99 ± 0.02, $p < 0.001$, Fig. 2c). Losartan treatment tended to decrease the potassium excretion and it was similar to the sham animals (sham + losartan 0.91 ± 0.01 vs. BDL losartan 0.95 ± 0.02, $p > 0.05$, Fig. 2c). During week 7 the urinary potassium excretion was similar in all four groups (Fig. 2d).

Neurohumoral activity and hemodynamics

The PRC was similar in the two placebo groups (sham: 4.7 ± 0.2 vs. BDL: 4.3 ± 1.1 10^{-5}GU/ml, $p > 0.05$, Fig. 3a). Treatment with losartan increased PRC markedly (BDL + losartan: 769.3 ± 143.7 10^{-5}GU/ml, $p < 0.001$, Fig. 3a). The urinary excretion of ANG II was increased in placebo treated BDL group compared to the sham control (sham+ placebo: 9.8 ± 0.4 vs. BDL+ placebo: 24.9 ± 1.0 pg/µl, $p < 0.001$). Losartan treatment increased ANGII excretion further in the BDL animals compared to the placebo treated BDL group (BDL + losartan: 35.4 ± 1.5 pg/µl, $p < 0.01$, Fig. 3b). BDL induced an increase in P-Aldosterone as expected (sham+ placebo: 16.4 ± 3.0 vs. BDL + placebo vs. BDL+ placebo: 123 ± 25.7 pg/ml, $p < 0.001$, Fig. 3c). Although ANGII excretion was increased in the losartan treated animals there was a trend of a lower P-Aldosterone in these animals compared to the placebo treated BDL animals (Fig. 3c). Considering the aldosterone/PRC ratio the aldosterone response to renin stimulus losartan treatment of the BDL animals markedly reduced the ratio (BDL + losartan: 0.01 ± 0.03 vs. BDL+ placebo: 43.5 ± 31.7, $p < 0.001$, Fig. 3d).

Invasive blood pressure was measured in two BDL operated animals, one placebo treated and one losartan treated. After onset of treatment with losartan there was a decrease in blood pressure of approximately 25% compared to baseline in the losartan

Table 1 Demografic and biochemical data

	Unit	Sham + placebo	Sham + losartan	BDL + placebo	BDL + losartan
Initial number rats	N	8	8	10	10
Mortality	N	0	0	3	6
Rats with/ without ascites	N	0\8	0\8	7\1	3\3
Preoperative weight	g	237 ± 5	243 ± 9	240 ± 4	237 ± 7
Final weight	g	346 ± 14	366 ± 15	325 ± 5	317 ± 9
Final weight (dry)	g	346 ± 14	366 ± 15	317 ± 6	314 ± 8
Weight gain (dry)	g	109 ± 13†	123 ± 12†	77 ± 5	77 ± 8
Liver	(g/100gBW)	3.37 ± 0.17†††	3.31 ± 0.05†††	7.41 ± 0.37	7.09 ± 0.22
Spleen	(g/100gBW)	0.19 ± 0.01†††	0.19 ± 0.004†††	0.62 ± 0.02	0.50 ± 0.05*
Kidney	(g/100gBW)	0.56 ± 0.08††	0.60 ± 0.01†	0.76 ± 0.01	0.80 ± 0.03
Heart	(g/100GBW)	0.27 ± 0.01†	0.25 ± 0.01††	0.33 ± 0.02	0.28 ± 0.02
Adrenal gland	(g/100gBW)	0.016 ± 0.001	0.015 ± 0.001	0.018 ± 0.001	0.018 ± 0.001
B-Haemoglobin	mmol/L	9.7 ± 0.1	9.7 ± 0.1	9.6 ± 0.4	9.9 ± 0.6
B-Haematocrit	%	47 ± 1	46 ± 1	49 ± 1	49 ± 3
B-Leucocytes	10*9/L	5.8 ± 0.4†††	6.3 ± 0.3†††	26.0 ± 2.3	23.9 ± 4.7
B-Platelets	10*9/L	791 ± 33	769 ± 41	567 ± 113	597 ± 56
S-Bilirubin	µmol/l	1.3 ± 0.16†††	0.8 ± 0.17†††	188.6 ± 10.8	227.3 ± 18.6
S-Albumin	µmol/l	667.3 ± 35.7†††	607.6 ± 23.1†	475.0 ± 25.2	514.8 ± 18.4
S-Creatinine	µmol/l	17.6 ± 0.6	16.3 ± 2.1	18.3 ± 1.3	21.5 ± 2.6
P-Osmolality	mOsm/kg	305 ± 2	306 ± 2	300 ± 1	304 ± 2
P-Sodium	mmol/l	139 ± 1.0	139 ± 0.8	141 ± 0.4	140 ± 0.9
P-Potassium	mmol/l	6.3 ± 0.2	6.5 ± 0.4	5.8 ± 0.2	7.1 ± 0.5*

Values are given as mean ± SEM. *$p < 0.05$: BDL placebo vs. BDL losartan. $^\dagger p < 0.05$: Sham vs. BDL, $^{\dagger\dagger}p < 0.01$ Sham vs. BDL, $^{\dagger\dagger\dagger}p < 0.001$: Sham vs. BDL

treated rat whereas the blood pressure remained practically unchanged in the placebo treated BDL rat. BDL + losartan: 95.7 ± 23.2 to 74.1 ± 7.0 mmHg vs. BDL+ placebo: 114.8 ± 18.6 to 111.7 ± 4.7 mmHg (week 1 vs. week 7).

Discussion

The treatment with losartan 4 mg/kg did not improve sodium excretion in the BDL rat model of cirrhosis in the late course of disease. As the smaller spleen size reflects reduced portal hypertension, and fewer animals had ascites in

Table 2 Water, food,electrolyte intake and electrolyte excretion in sham and BDL animals

	Unit		Sham + placebo	Sham + losartan	BDL + placebo	BDL + losartan
Water intake	ml/100 g BW*24 h	Week 6	9.8 ± 0.2	9.9 ± 0.1†	9.7 ± 0.3	9.9 ± 0.5
		Week 7	9.7 ± 0.2	9.9 ± 0.2†	9.2 ± 0.3	10.6 ± 0.6
Food intake	µg/100 g BW*24 h	Week 6	21.4 ± 0.3†††	21.6 ± 0.4†††	16.8 ± 0.6	17.4 ± 0.5
		Week 7	20.8 ± 0.3†††	21.1 ± 0.3†††	15.3 ± 0.4	15.7 ± 0.5
Sodium intake	µmolNa/100 g BW*24 h	Week 6	586 ± 9†††	580 ± 9†††	483 ± 17	504 ± 12
		Week 7	554 ± 9†††	553 ± 7†††	430 ± 11	459 ± 10
Potassium intake	µmolK/100 g BW*24 h	Week 6	1697 ± 25†††	1679 ± 27†††	1398 ± 49	1460 ± 35
		Week 7	1604 ± 27†††	1599 ± 21†††	1243 ± 32	1327 ± 46
Diureses	ml/100 g BW*24 h	Week 6	5.0 ± 0.1	5.1 ± 0.1	5.8 ± 0.2	5.8 ± 0.4
		Week 7	5.2 ± 0.2	5.3 ± 0.2	5.7 ± 0.3	6.8 ± 0.5
Osmolality	mOsm/kg	Week 6	1.50 ± 0.03	1.52 ± 0.04	1.36 ± 0.06	1.42 ± 0.06
		Week 7	1.39 ± 0.04†††	1.41 ± 0.04†††	1.21 ± 0.06	1.08 ± 0.05

Values given as mean ± sem, $^{\dagger\dagger}p < 0.01$ Sham vs. BDL, $^{\dagger\dagger\dagger}p < 0.001$: Sham vs. BDL

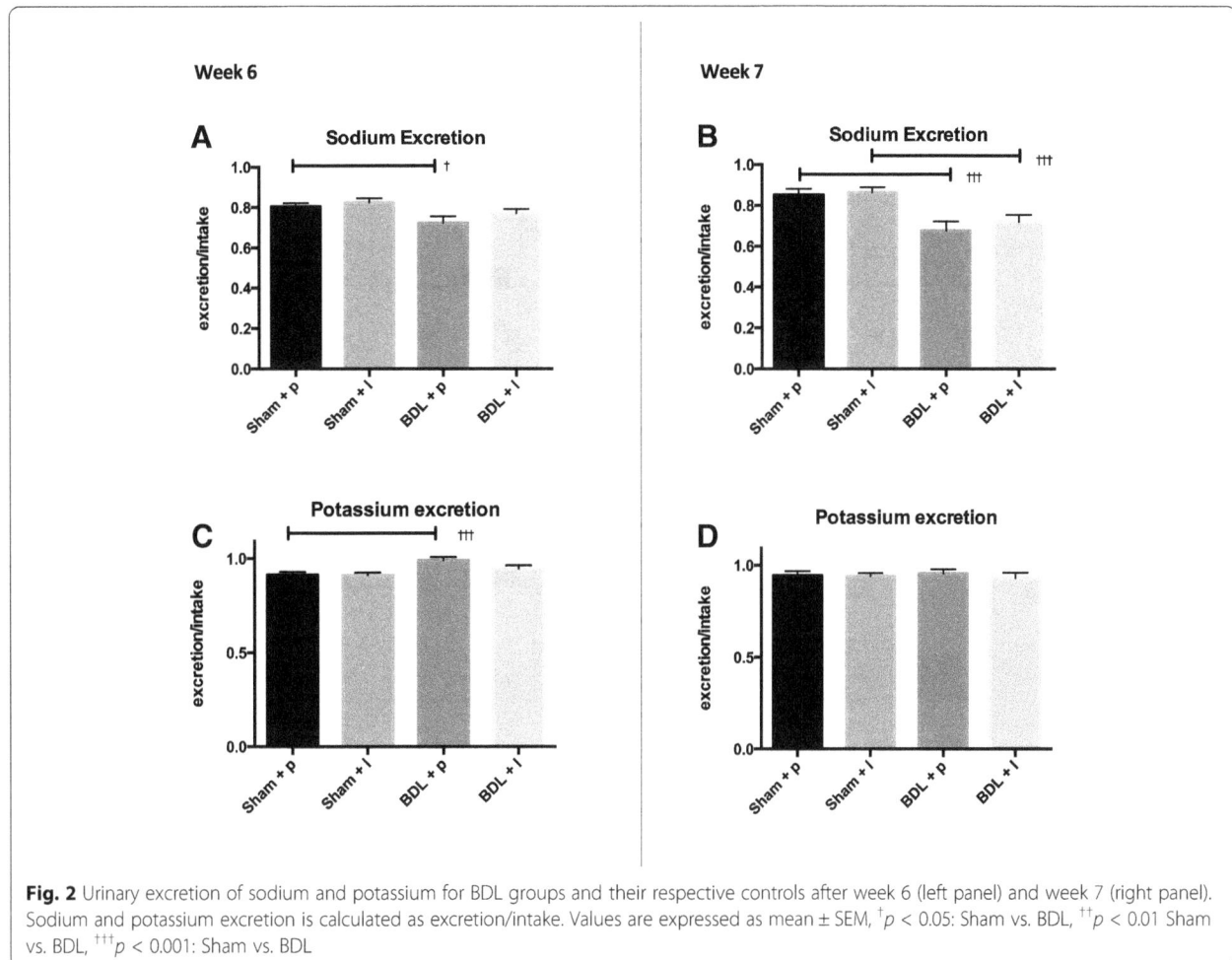

Fig. 2 Urinary excretion of sodium and potassium for BDL groups and their respective controls after week 6 (left panel) and week 7 (right panel). Sodium and potassium excretion is calculated as excretion/intake. Values are expressed as mean ± SEM, [†]$p < 0.05$: Sham vs. BDL, [††]$p < 0.01$ Sham vs. BDL, [†††]$p < 0.001$: Sham vs. BDL

the losartan treated animals, some effect of losartan may have been present. The otherwise normal PRC in BDL rats increased 150 fold after losartan, which may be due to losartan-induced hypotension. This is supported by the 25% decrease in blood pressure in a single rat after losartan. We demonstrated elevated urinary ANGII levels reflecting an importance of intrarenal RAS in the BDL rat, which was further increased after losartan. The chosen dose of losartan blocked the AT-1 receptor efficiently as demonstrated by the trend towards reduced p-Aldosterone levels and reduced PRC/Aldosterone ratio. The renal sodium retention in the BDL animals was evident at week 6 and 7 after surgery. This is coherent with the fact that the animals develop ascites in the late phase of the disease [10]. Apart from the possible hemodynamic effect of losartan, the increase of PRC in the sham+losartan group might reflect the loss of angiotensin type 1 receptor mediated negative feedback on renin secretion by losartan. It is supported by the fact that renal angiotensin levels in BDL + losartan were higher than in BDL + placebo.

The increased potassium excretion in the BDL animals during the 6th week after surgery is explained by increased P-Aldosterone in the diseased animals. This was not found in the terminal phase of the disease (week 7). However as we did not measure fecal electrolyte excretions we are not able to calculate the precise balances of sodium and potassium. We have previously shown that BDL rats have significantly higher intestinal potassium and sodium excretions as compared to their controls at the end of week 7 and similar renal potassium excretions [11]. The fecal sodium and potassium excretions at the end of week 6 have not previously been studied.

In a previous study enhanced sodium excretion was found when losartan was given at dose of 0.5 mg/kg/day for one week starting at week 5 after surgery, whereas 10 mg/kg/day lead to deterioration of renal function and more pronounced sodium retention than seen in the control animals [9]. In a second study, long term treatment of losartan 5 and 10 mg/kg/day was given during early course of disease for 4 weeks in BDL model, and for 9 weeks the CCl_4 model. Both doses were well tolerated in the CCl_4 model but induced significantly reduced blood pressure in the BDL model. None of the doses improved sodium excretion [8]. In a preliminary study in

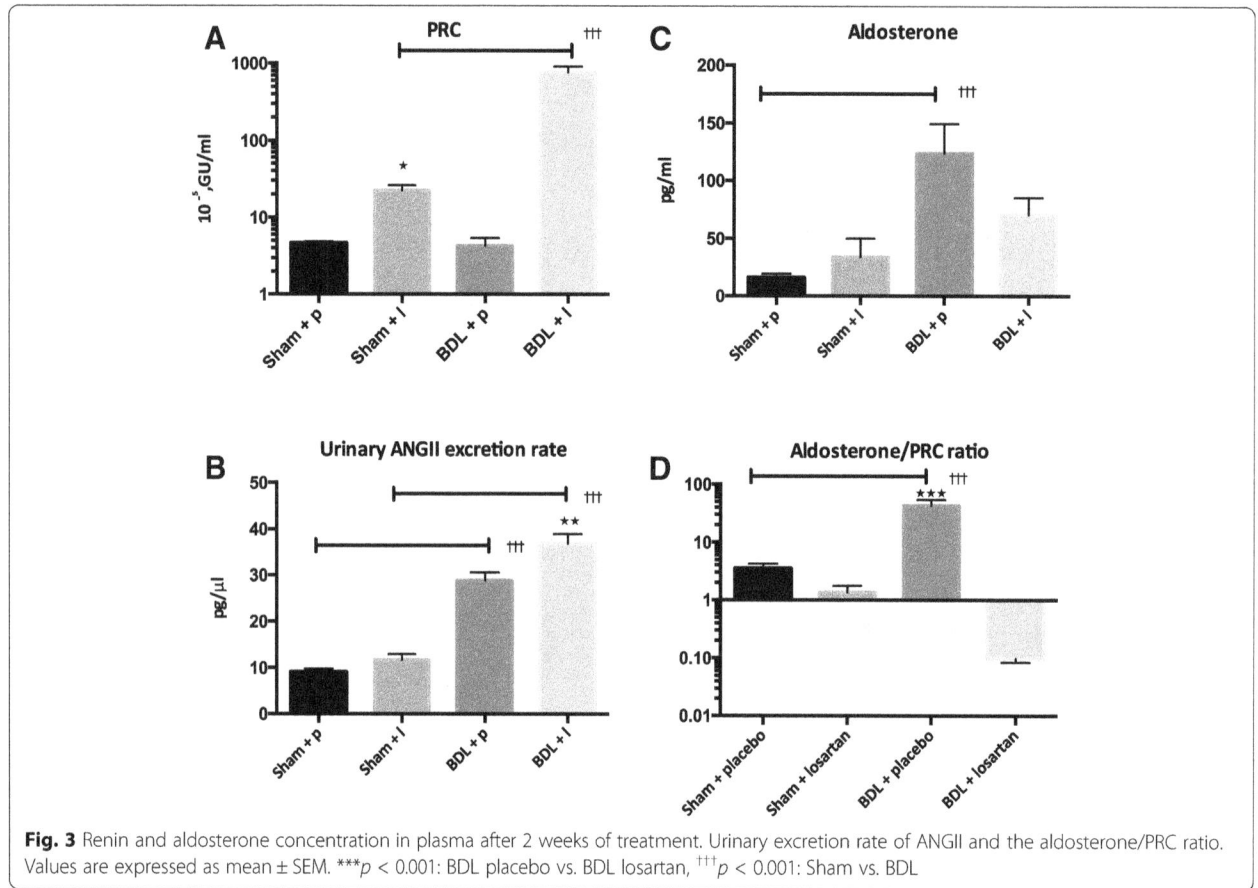

Fig. 3 Renin and aldosterone concentration in plasma after 2 weeks of treatment. Urinary excretion rate of ANGII and the aldosterone/PRC ratio. Values are expressed as mean ± SEM. ***p < 0.001: BDL placebo vs. BDL losartan, †††p < 0.001: Sham vs. BDL

the BDL model, 10 mg/kg/day induced a marked decrease in blood pressure, whereas a dose of 6 mg/kg day for 1 week at week 3 after surgery was well tolerated and reduced portal pressure [14]. The acute response to losartan infusion decreased MAP significantly at the doses 10 mg/kg and 30 mg/kg but not 3 mg/kg at week 5 [14]. In this study a dose of 4 mg/kg divided in two was anticipated to be sufficient to block the ANGII effect in the kidneys and at the same time be tolerated. Yet it seemed that the dosage of 4 mg/kg of losartan in the present study was poorly tolerated in the BDL rats. Judging from the PRC response in the BDL-losartan group this hypotensive effect was pronounced. The suggested hypotensive effect of the dosage used was also evident in the blood pressure measurement in a single rat in which it was reduced by 25%. However blood pressure measurement in only one animal is not sufficient to support this conclusion. Other indicators of profound side effects of the losartan treatment were found in the BDL rats. The mortality was higher and the P-Potassium was higher. Summing up these effects, there is an indication of a pronounced hemodynamic impairment in this animal model of cirrhosis [15]. Although this proposed mechanism and role of hemodynamic deterioration is based on incomplete data we find it plausible.

Intolerability to losartan in the BDL model could be explained by the biliary elimination of losartan of 50–60% [16], where the metabolite is pharmacologically more active. Severe cholestasis develops in the BDL model, and accumulation of losartan metabolites may be partly responsible for deleterious hemodynamic and succeeding renal deterioration [17].

In a series of human experiment the role of ANGII antagonist in treatment of sodium retention has been explored. In a dose-response study renal sodium retention was recovered by 7.5 mg losartan in patients with preascitic cirrhosis. A decrease in mean arterial pressure was observed when treated with 10 mg losartan [18]; and the sodium retention induced by erect posture was blunted by 7.5 mg of losartan [19]. Patients treated with transjugular intrahepatic portosystemic shunt (TIPS), reducing or normalizing portal pressure [20], still show impaired sodium handling similar to that of patients with pre-ascitic cirrhosis [21]. Treatment with losartan 7.5 mg given to patients treated with TIPS improved sodium excretion during upright position [22]. The effects of the low dose of losartan were attributed to the intrarenal component of ANGII. A short term dose of 25 mg of losartan given to compensated and decompensated cirrhotic patients has been shown to improve natriuresis without renal impairment [23]. We measured urinary ANG II as an indicator of intrarenal RAAS activation. We demonstrated that despite normal PRC, the placebo treated rat BDL rat has elevated urinary ANG II level indicating increased intrarenal RAAS activation, which support a role of intrarenal RAAS activation in cirrhosis. The role of ANGII receptor antagonists in the treatment of sodium retention is not yet established. Emerging evidence suggests ANGII receptor antagonists as effective treatment of both portal hypertension as well as liver fibrosis, thus the deleterious renal effect is of concern [24, 25].

Conclusions

Losartan 4 mg/kg/day did not increase sodium excretion in this model of liver cirrhosis although the intrarenal ANGII was increased. However losartan reduced spleen size, and the presence of ascites. Losartan induced increased urinary excretion of ANGII and trend towards reduced aldosterone response indicating sufficient blockage of the receptor. However, losartan was not well tolerated in the BDL animals, and the expected effect on sodium excretion was not seen, on the contrary, a 150-fold increase in PRC was induced. The effect of an ANGII antagonist has not previously been studied in the late phase of the disease and there fore this study provided important information about the potential deleterious effects of the treatment. Lower doses of losartan in the same model would have explored the possibility of natriuretic effects in this stage of disease.

Abbreviations
ANGII: Angiotensin II; BDL: Bile duct ligation.; PRC: Plasma renin concentration.; RAAS: Renin angiotensin aldosterone systeme.

Acknowledgements
To Claus Bistrup for assistance with blood pressure monitoring.

Funding
The first author is funded by the Region of Southern Denmark. The funding body had no role in the design of the study and collection, analysis, or interpretation of data or in writing the manuscript.

Authors contributions
Protocol: ADF, HT, PB, SDM, Performed experiment: ADF, HT, data analysis: ADF, HT, PB, SDM, draft of manuscript: ADF. All the authors read and approved the final version of the manuscript.

Competing interests
The authors declare that they have no competing interests.

Author details
[1]Department of Gastroenterology and Hepatology, Odense University Hospital, Sdr Boulevard, 5000 Odense C 29 Odense, Denmark. [2]Department of Nephrology, Odense University Hospital, Odense, Denmark.

[3]Cardiovascular and Renal Research, University of Southern Denmark, Odense, Denmark.

References
1. Sola E, Gines P. Renal and circulatory dysfunction in cirrhosis: current management and future perspectives. J Hepatol. 2010;53:1135–45.
2. Lumbers ER. Angiotensin and aldosterone. Regul Pept. 1999;80:91–100.
3. Lavoie JL, Sigmund CD. Minireview: overview of the renin-angiotensin system--an endocrine and paracrine system. Endocrinology. 2003;144:2179–83.
4. Martinez-Prieto C, Ortiz MC, Fortepiani LA, Ruiz-Macia J, Atucha NM, Garcia-Estan J. Haemodynamic and renal evolution of the bile duct-ligated rat. Clin Sci (Lond). 2000;98:611–7.
5. Thiesson HC, Jensen BL, Bistrup C, Ottosen PD, McNeilly AD, Andrew R, Seckl J, Skott O. Renal sodium retention in cirrhotic rats depends on glucocorticoid-mediated activation of mineralocorticoid receptor due to decreased renal 11beta-HSD-2 activity. Am J Physiol Regul Integr Comp Physiol. 2007;292:R625–36.
6. Yang YY, Lin HC, Huang YT, Lee TY, Hou MC, Lee FY, Liu RS, Chang FY, Lee SD. Effect of 1-week losartan administration on bile duct-ligated cirrhotic rats with portal hypertension. J Hepatol. 2002;36:600–6.
7. Ubeda M, Matzilevich MM, Atucha NM, Garcia-Estan J, Quesada T, Tang SS, Ingelfinger JR. Renin and angiotensinogen mRNA expression in the kidneys of rats subjected to long-term bile duct ligation. Hepatology. 1994;19:1431–6.
8. Croquet V, Moal F, Veal N, Wang J, Oberti F, Roux J, Vuillemin E, Gallois Y, Douay O, Chappard D, et al. Hemodynamic and antifibrotic effects of losartan in rats with liver fibrosis and/or portal hypertension. J Hepatol. 2002;37:773–80.
9. Heller J, Trebicka J, Shiozawa T, Schepke M, Neef M, Hennenberg M, Sauerbruch T. Vascular, hemodynamic and renal effects of low-dose losartan in rats with secondary biliary cirrhosis. Liver Int. 2005;25:657–66.
10. Kountouras J, Billing BH, Scheuer PJ. Prolonged bile duct obstruction: a new experimental model for cirrhosis in the rat. Br J Exp Pathol. 1984;65:305–11.
11. Accatino L, Contreras A, Berdichevsky E, Quintana C. The effect of complete biliary obstruction on bile secretion. Studies on the mechanisms of postcholestatic choleresis in the rat. J Lab Clin Med. 1981;97:525–34.
12. Poulsen K, Jorgensen J. An easy radioimmunological microassay of renin activity, concentration and substrate in human and animal plasma and tissues based on angiotensin I trapping by antibody. J Clin Endocrinol Metab. 1974;39:816–25.
13. Bie P, Sandgaard NC. Determinants of the natriuresis after acute, slow sodium loading in conscious dogs. Am J Physiol Regul Integr Comp Physiol. 2000;278:R1–r10.
14. Heller J, Shiozawa T, Trebicka J, Hennenberg M, Schepke M, Neef M, Sauerbruch T. Acute haemodynamic effects of losartan in anaesthetized cirrhotic rats. Eur J Clin Investig. 2003;33:1006–12.
15. Cervenka L, Wang CT, Navar LG. Effects of acute AT1 receptor blockade by candesartan on arterial pressure and renal function in rats. Am J Phys. 1998;274:F940–5.
16. Christ DD, Wong PC, Wong YN, Hart SD, Quon CY, Lam GN. The pharmacokinetics and pharmacodynamics of the angiotensin II receptor antagonist losartan potassium (DuP 753/MK 954) in the dog. J Pharmacol Exp Ther. 1994;268:1199–205.
17. Bomzon A, Rosenberg M, Gali D, Binah O, Mordechovitz D, Better OS, Greig PD, Blendis LM. Systemic hypotension and decreased pressor response in dogs with chronic bile duct ligation. Hepatology. 1986;6:595–600.
18. Girgrah N, Liu P, Collier J, Blendis L, Wong F. Haemodynamic, renal sodium handling, and neurohormonal effects of acute administration of low dose losartan, an angiotensin II receptor antagonist, in preascitic cirrhosis. Gut. 2000;46:114–20.
19. Wong F, Liu P, Blendis L. The mechanism of improved sodium homeostasis of low-dose losartan in preascitic cirrhosis. Hepatology. 2002;35:1449–58.
20. Skeens J, Semba C, Dake M. Transjugular intrahepatic portosystemic shunts. Annu Rev Med. 1995;46:95–102.
21. Wong W, Liu P, Blendis L, Wong F. Long-term renal sodium handling in patients with cirrhosis treated with transjugular intrahepatic portosystemic shunts for refractory ascites. Am J Med. 1999;106:315–22.
22. Therapondos G, Hol L, Benjaminov F, Wong F. The effect of single oral low-dose losartan on posture-related sodium handling in post-TIPS ascites-free cirrhosis. Hepatology. 2006;44:640–9.

23. Yang YY, Lin HC, Lee WC, Hou MC, Lee FY, Chang FY, Lee SD. One-week losartan administration increases sodium excretion in cirrhotic patients with and without ascites. J Gastroenterol. 2002;37:194–9.
24. Grace JA, Herath CB, Mak KY, Burrell LM, Angus PW. Update on new aspects of the renin-angiotensin system in liver disease: clinical implications and new therapeutic options. Clin Sci (Lond). 2012;123:225–39.
25. Tandon P, Abraldes JG, Berzigotti A, Garcia-Pagan JC, Bosch J. Renin-angiotensin-aldosterone inhibitors in the reduction of portal pressure: a systematic review and meta-analysis. J Hepatol. 2010;53:273–82.

17

Value of reduced glomerular filtration rate assessment with cardiometabolic index: insights from a population-based Chinese cohort

Hao-Yu Wang[1†], Wen-Rui Shi[1†], Xin Yi[2], Shu-Ze Wang[3], Si-Yuan Luan[4] and Ying-Xian Sun[1*]

Abstract

Background: Recent studies have suggested that cardiometabolic index (CMI), a novel estimate of visceral adipose tissue, could be of use in the evaluation of cardiovascular risk factors. However, the potential utility and clinical significance of CMI in the detection of reduced estimated glomerular filtration rate (eGFR) remains uncertain. The purpose of this study was to investigate the usefulness of CMI in assessing reduced eGFR in the general Chinese population.

Methods: This cross-sectional analysis included 11,578 participants (mean age: 53.8 years, 53.7% females) from Northeast China Rural Cardiovascular Health Study (NCRCHS) of general Chinese population (data collected from January 2013 to August 2013). CMI was calculated by triglyceride to high density lipoprotein cholesterol ratio multiply waist-to-height ratio. Reduced eGFR was defined as eGFR< 60 ml/min per 1.73m^2. Multivariate regressions were performed to determine CMI's association with eGFR value and eGFR reduction, ROC analyses were employed to investigate CMI's discriminating ability for decreased eGFR.

Results: The prevalence of reduced eGFR was 1.7% in males and 2.5% in females. CMI was notably more adverse in reduced eGFR groups, regardless of genders. In fully adjusted multivariate linear models, each 1 SD increment of CMI caused 3.150 ml/min per 1.73m^2 and 2.411 ml/min per 1.73m^2 loss of eGFR before CMI reached 1.210 and 1.520 in males and females, respectively. In logistic regression analyses, per 1 SD increase of CMI brought 51.6% additional risk of reduced eGFR in males while caused 1.347 times of risk in females. After divided into quartiles, people in the top quartile of CMI had higher adjusted ORs of having reduced eGFR, with ORs of 4.227 (1.681, 10. 627) and 3.442 (1.685–7.031) for males and females respectively. AUC of CMI was revealed to be 0.633 (0.620–0.646) in males and 0.684 (0.672–0.695) in females.

Conclusions: Higher CMI was independently associated with greater burden of reduced eGFR, highlighting VAT distribution and dysfunction as a potential mechanism underlying the association of obesity with kidney damage and adverse cardiovascular outcomes. The findings from this study provided important insights regarding the potential usefulness and clinical relevance of CMI in the detection of reduced eGFR among general Chinese population.

Keywords: Cardiometabolic index, Dyslipidemia, Obesity, Reduced eGFR, Sex-specific, Visceral adipose tissue

* Correspondence: yxsun_cmu1h@163.com
†Hao-Yu Wang and Wen-Rui Shi contributed equally to this work.
[1]Department of Cardiology, The First Hospital of China Medical University, 155 Nanjing North Street, Heping District, Shenyang 110001, China
Full list of author information is available at the end of the article

Background

Chronic kidney disease (CKD) was a disease with heterogeneous etiology that caused 15.8 deaths per 100,000 people worldwide in 2013 and was estimated to attack 119.5 million Chinese people in the year of 2012 [1, 2]. Besides, CKD has been identified to be related with multiple cardiovascular risk factors like hypertension and diabetes mellitus (DM), revealing its close association with cardiovascular health [3, 4]. Therefore, CKD has brought great burden to the health-care work and economy [5, 6]. Knowing the poor outcomes and high cost that caused by CKD as a worldwide public health problem, it is a good choice to focus on the early detection of reduced estimated glomerular filtration rate (eGFR) for avoiding the progression of CKD. Accordingly, early detection of reduced eGFR is critically needed for timely CKD prevention and overall improvement in prognosis.

There is an wealthy evidence that dyslipidemia and obesity are strongly related to the deterioration of renal function, even in the early stage [7, 8]. Dyslipidemia in CKD often exhibits a pattern of increased triglyceride (TG) levels and decreased high density lipoprotein cholesterol (HDL-C) levels [7]. Findings revealed that increased TG level was significantly correlated with CKD [9–11]. Furthermore, as a combination of 2 characteristics of dyslipidemia in CKD, TG to HDL-C ratio (TG / HDL-C) has also been identified to strongly associated with decline of eGFR in participants without CKD and rapid decrement of eGFR in participants with CKD [12–14]. Obesity is another condition that strongly correlated with decreased eGFR or CKD [8, 15]. As the most widely used index of obesity, body mass index (BMI) was revealed to correlated with reduced eGFR, CKD and end stage renal disease (ESRD) [16, 17]. However, BMI did not take abdominal obesity into consideration when reflecting obesity status. Therefore, some indexes such as waist circumference (WC) and waist-to-height ratio (WHtR) were designed to be measurements of central obesity [18]. And they have already showed strong associations with CKD [19–22]. Nevertheless, comparisons between BMI, WC and WHtR did not provide sufficient evidence for anyone of them to be a premier marker of CKD with great sensitivity or specificity [19–22]. Moreover, indexes of abdominal obesity were insufficient to detecting visceral adipose tissue (VAT), which was elucidated to possess a more adverse effect on CKD development than subcutaneous adipose tissue (SAT) [23, 24]. However, when cooperating with aforementioned indexes of dyslipidemia, their strength to discriminating VAT got reinforcement [24]. Taken together, combination of dyslipidemia and abdominal obesity could improve the identification of VAT and therefore refine the detecting of reduced eGFR.

Recently, a novel marker named "cardiometabolic index (CMI)" has been put forward by Ichiro Wakabayashi [25]. CMI can be considered as an ideal marker to recognize VAT because of its integration of dyslipidemia and abdominal obesity. This emerging marker has been shown in several studies to be a useful screening tool for various populations, identifying those with a deteriorated metabolic profile and higher risk for cardiovascular disease, such as left ventricular geometry abnormalities, hyperuricemia, diabetes, hypertension, and ischemic stroke [25–29]. It is unclear, however, if CMI can be an identifier of reduced eGFR, independent of cardiovascular risk factors and hypertension. Accordingly, the present study was designed to test whether or not higher CMI increase the risk of reduced eGFR in the general Chinese population.

Methods

Study population

This study was part of a large cross-sectional population-based epidemiological investigation that described the prevalence, incidence, and natural history of cardiovascular risk factors among 11,956 permanent residents (≥35 years of age) in rural areas of China from January 2012 to August 2013. The full details regarding the design and rationale of the study were extensively described elsewhere [26, 30, 31]. Briefly, the study adopted a multistage, stratified random cluster-sampling scheme. In the first stage, 3 counties (Dawa, Zhangwu, and Liaoyang County) were selected from the eastern, southern, and northern region of Liaoning province. In the second stage, 1 town was randomly selected from each county (a total of 3 towns). In the third stage, 8 to 10 rural villages from each town were randomly selected (a total of 26 rural villages). Participants with pregnancy, malignant tumor, or mental disorder were excluded from the present study. The study protocol complied with the Second Helsinki Declaration (and recent amendments) and was approved by the Ethics Committee of China Medical University (Shenyang, China), and all study participants provided written informed consent. Patients with missing data for any of CMI components or other variables analyzed in the study (n = 378) were excluded. Accordingly, the final study cohort was composed of 11,578 subjects.

Data collection and measurements

Detailed process about data collection and measurements was described by previous publications from our research team that involved in the same survey as this study [26, 30, 31]. Cardiologists and nurses completed a training and passed a test before they were allowed to conduct the questionnaire which collected information about demographic data, health-related behavior, anthropometric parameters, dietary condition, current medicine usage condition, history of cardiovascular disease (CVD).

A carefully designed questionnaire was used to collect data from subjects. A central steering committee with a subcommittee conducted the quality control of the information collection process. Subjects were divided into two groups: Han and others. Education level was regarded as three ordinal groups: primary school or below, middle school, high school or above. Three ordinal groups (≤5000 CNY, 5000–20,000 CNY, > 20,000 CNY) were utilized to represent the family annual income level. Diet score was calculated according to the collected information about vegetable and meat consumption, a lower score meant lower meat consumption and higher vegetable consumption. Detailed information about diet score has been reported in a prior study from our team [32]. Physical activity level was acquired in both work and off hours, and divided into three levels (low, middle, high). Messages of current smoking and alcohol intake status were collected through a series of questions about smoking and drinking history of participants. Medicine usage such as anti-hypertensive, anti-diabetic and lipid-lowering drugs was recorded in the questionnaire as well. History of CVD included coronary heart disease, arrhythmia, heart failure, and stroke. Meanwhile, history of kidney disease was defined as nephritis, kidney dysfunction, renal stones, renal tumor, and autoimmune kidney disease.

After subjects completed a 5 min rest in sitting position with relaxation, two randomly selected trained medical staffs performed the blood pressure measurements for them. Three consecutive readings were recorded and their mean value was taken into statistical analyses.

With regard to the measurements of anthropometric indices, subjects were requested to wear in light clothing without shoes. Standard weight was measured to the nearest 0.1 kg by using a calibrated digital scale. Subjects held in a standing position when a calibrated stadiometer was used to quantify their standard height to the nearest 0.1 cm. As for the measurement of WC, elastic measuring tapes was used to get the readings in a horizontal position at 1 cm above the umbilicus. All of the above measurements were performed twice and their mean values were used for analyses.

Detailed delineation of the process of storage and methods of laboratory measurements was reported in our previous studies [26, 30, 31]. Briefly, fasting (12 h overnight) blood samples were collected through venipuncture. And these samples were separated and frozen at − 20 °C within 1 h after the collection, and then transported to a laboratory with certification for examination. An Olympus AU 640 auto analyzer (Olympus, Kobe, Japan) was used for biochemical analyses. All laboratory equipment was calibrated and blinded duplicate samples were used.

Definitions

BMI was calculated as mean weight divided by mean height squared (kg/m^2). WHtR was acquired as WC divided by mean height. CMI was obtained by the following equation [25]: CMI = TG/HDL-C × WHtR. lipid accumulation product (LAP) was calculated according to the sex-specific formula [33]: LAP = TG (mmol/L) × [WC (cm)-58] for females and LAP = TG (mmol/L) × [WC (cm)-65] for males. And visceral adiposity index (VAI) was determined by using the following formula [34]: Males: VAI = [WC / 39.68 + (1.88 × BMI)] × (TG / 1.03) × (1.31 / HDL); Females: VAI = [WC / 36.58 + (1.89 × BMI)] × (TG / 0.81) × (1.52/HDL).

eGFR was calculated according to CKD-EPI equation [35]. Reduced eGFR was defined as eGFR < 60 ml/min per 1.73m^2 [36]. Diagnostic criteria of hypertension were mean systolic blood pressure (SBP) equal to or greater than 140 mmHg and/or diastolic blood pressure (DBP) at least 90 mmHg and/or participants who were on anti-hypertensive medications or self-reported previous diagnosed hypertension [37]. Diagnosis of diabetes based on the American Diabetes Association criteria: fasting plasma glucose (FPG) ≥ 7.0 mmol/L and/or self-reported previous diagnosis history or receiving plasma glucose lowering therapy [38].

Statistical analyses

Analyses were performed in a sex-specific manner. Continuous variables were expressed as mean values ± standard deviation (SD) or as median (interquartile range) if appropriate. Categorical variables were depicted as frequencies (percentages). Continuous variables were compared between groups with Student's t test or Mann-Whitney test according to their distribution, in the meantime, categorical variables were also compared between groups by using χ^2 test [39]. As for the comparison of ordinal categorical variables (education level, family annual income, physical activity), rank-sum test was performed in order to get full utilization of the ordinal information. Before inferential analyses, CMI values were log transformed due to highly skewed distributions. The chi-square linear-by-linear association test was used to reveal linear trends across the quartiles of CMI for percentages of prevalence of reduced eGFR. Multivariate linear regression analysis was conducted to evaluate the independent effect of CMI on eGFR value. And logarithmic likelihood ratio test was employed to compare the one-line linear regression model with a two-piecewise linear model. Furthermore, multivariate logistic regression analysis was performed to explore the isolated association of CMI as a continuous variable and as quartiles with the prevalence of reduced eGFR. Sex-specific odds ratios (ORs) for every SD change of CMI to identify the risk of reduced eGFR were acquired, the results were displayed as ORs and 95% confidence intervals (95% CI). Lastly, receiver-operating characteristic (ROC) curve was employed to investigate the optimal cut-off value of CMI to detect the presence of reduced eGFR. Area under the curve (AUC) was used to compare the discriminating ability of CMI and other indexes. All of the statistical analyses involved were performed by SPSS 25.0 software (IBM corp), statistical software packages R (http://www.R-project.org, The R Foundation) and EmpowerStats (http://www.empowerstats.com, X&Y Solutions, Inc., Boston, MA), Prism 7.0 software (Graphpad software, Inc) and MedCalc version 18.5 (MedCalc software, Belgium), a two-tailed P value less than 0.05 indicated statistical significant.

Results

After excluding ineligible participants, we finally took 11,578 subjects into analyses, the results were shown in Table 1. Of these subjects, 46.3% were males. The mean age of total population was 53.8 years while people with eGFR decrement were elder than their counterparts in both genders. The prevalence of reduced eGFR was 1.7% in males while females exhibited a higher rate of 2.5%. As for the demographic information, education level, family annual income, diet score and physical activity exhibited significant lower levels in patients with reduced eGFR. Contradictorily, female patients were more likely to smoke at present but male patients tended not to be a current smoker. Only males showed significant difference on alcoholic status between groups, but the results revealed that normal eGFR subjects had greater possibility to be a current drinker. With regard to laboratory test results, FPG, serum uric acid, TG and TG/HDL-C confirmed a remarkable augmentation among eGFR decrement patients, together with a dramatically decline of HDL-C in patients. SBP, height, WC, WHtR showed great increment when comparing CKD patients with their counterparts regardless of sex. But DBP only exhibited higher level in male patients while less weight was specific to female patients. Prevalence of hypertension and diabetes were noticeable higher among subjects with reduced eGFR for both genders, and the usages of anti-hypertensive, anti-diabetic and lipid-lowering drug were more popular in reduced eGFR group. Concordantly, the prevalence of cardiovascular and kidney diseases history showed dramatic augmentation in eGFR reduction patients of both genders. Within our expectation, patients with reduced eGFR of both genders experienced pronounced increment of CMI, VAI as well as LAP.

Quartile analyses revealed gradient correlation between CMI and prevalence of reduced eGFR, as displayed in Fig. 1. When comparing the top quartile with the bottom one, males exhibited a 6.0-fold change for the probability of eGFR reduction while females showed a higher fold change of 8.2. Both genders confirmed linear trends of prevalent eGFR reduction across quartiles of CMI (all P for trend< 0.001).

Results of linear regression analyses identified robust negative association between CMI with eGFR. As presented in Table 2, logarithmic likelihood ratio test identified the association between CMI and eGFR was non-linear in both genders after adjustment of age, race, education level, family annual income, diet score, physical activity, current smoking, alcohol intake, hypertension, diabetes, antihypertensive drug, antidiabetic drug, lipid-lowering drug, history of cardiovascular and kidney diseases. In the full model of males, the two-piecewise linear model revealed a rapid decrease of eGFR value along with the early increase of normalized CMI, with a β value of − 3.150 (− 3.589, − 2.712). However, when normalized CMI reached 1.113 (equaled to 1.210 of CMI), the change of eGFR shifted to a mild increase, with a β value of 1.906 (0.675, 3.138). Similarly, in the complete model of females, the eGFR also suffered a loss of 2.411 ml/min per 1.73m² for each SD increase of CMI before normalized CMI arrived to 1.472 (equaled to 1.520 of CMI). But after that, the eGFR began to have a increment of 2.268 ml/min per 1.73m² along with every single unit increase of normalized CMI.

Logistic regression analyses confirmed the intensive relationship between CMI with reduced eGFR, the results were arranged in Table 3. In males, per 1 SD increase of CMI still caused 52% of additional risk for eGFR reduction after adjusting all included cofounders. When divided into quartiles, highest quartile of CMI displayed 4.2 times risk for developing eGFR decrement compared with lowest category in the full model, and there was a significant linear trend for the risk of eGFR reduction across the quartiles of CMI (P for trend< 0.001). Similar results were observed in female participants, risk of eGFR reduction got an elevation of 34.7% for every single SD increment of CMI. Furthermore, the ORs for top quartile compared with bottom group was 3.442 (1.685–7.031), and the linear trend across quartiles also existed (P for trend< 0.001). We further conducted a test for the interaction between genders and CMI, and the results displayed to be insignificant, identifying the robust association between CMI and reduced eGFR across genders.

ROC analyses showed a significant AUC value of CMI for discriminating eGFR reduction, the results were summarized in Table 4. In males, our findings displayed that CMI possessed the greatest AUC (AUC: 0.633, 95% CI: 0.620–0.646) among various indexes, statistically significantly higher than that of LAP (AUC 0.633 vs. 0.606, P = 0.036) and BMI (AUC 0.633 vs. 0.544, P = 0.004), and there was also a trend for CMI to be superior than VAI (0.627, 0.614–0.640). Meanwhile, CMI showed a

Table 1 Characteristics of participants with reduced eGFR stratified by sex

Variables	Males (n = 5360)			Females (n = 6218)		
	Reduced eGFR (n = 90)	Normal eGFR (n = 5270)	P value*	Reduced eGFR (n = 155)	Normal eGFR (n = 6063)	P value*
Age (years)	68.78 ± 10.41	54.11 ± 10.64	< .001	68.69 ± 8.87	52.99 ± 10.08	< .001
Race (Han) (%)	87 (96.7)	4987 (94.6)	0.394	152 (98.1)	5747 (94.8)	0.068
Education level (%)			< .001			< .001
Primary school or below	57 (63.3)	2177 (41.3)		135 (87.1)	3398 (56.0)	
Middle school	26 (28.9)	2487 (47.2)		18 (11.6)	2187 (36.1)	
High school or above	7 (7.8)	606 (11.5)		2 (1.3)	478 (7.9)	
Income level (CNY) (%)			< .001			< .001
≤ 5000	28 (31.1)	693 (13.1)		41 (26.5)	680 (11.2)	
5000 – 20,000	45 (50.0)	2827 (53.6)		77 (49.7)	3361 (55.4)	
> 20,000	17 (18.9)	1750 (33.2)		37 (23.9)	2022 (33.3)	
Diet score	2.24 ± 0.96	2.55 ± 1.10	0.008	1.68 ± 1.03	2.15 ± 1.11	< .001
Physical activity (%)			< .001			< .001
Low	52 (57.8)	1158 (22.0)		100 (64.5)	2133 (35.2)	
Middle	36 (40.0)	3817 (72.4)		42 (27.1)	3587 (59.2)	
High	2 (2.2)	295 (5.6)		13 (8.4)	343 (5.7)	
Current smoking (%)	28 (31.1)	3030 (57.5)	< .001	43 (27.7)	987 (16.3)	< .001
Current alcohol intake (%)	14 (15.6)	2421 (45.9)	< .001	3 (1.9)	180 (3)	0.452
FPG (mmol/L)	5.74 (5.35 – 6.67)	5.60 (5.22 – 6.09)	0.010	5.78(5.30 – 7.05)	5.49 (5.12 – 5.99)	< .001
Serum uric acid (μmol/L)	447.52 ± 122.56	331.80 ± 81.34	< .001	363.21 ± 94.01	253.06 ± 64.66	< .001
TG (mmol/L)	1.41 (1.10 – 2.07)	1.22 (0.86 – 1.88)	0.006	1.86 (1.30 – 2.55)	1.24 (0.89 – 1.88)	< .001
HDL-C (mmol/L)	1.21 ± 0.27	1.41 ± 0.42	< .001	1.35 ± 0.41	1.41 ± 0.34	0.018
TG/HDL-C	1.19 (0.80 – 2.11)	0.91 (0.57 – 1.57)	< .001	1.42 (0.92 – 2.24)	0.92 (0.59 – 1.51)	< .001
SBP (mmHg)	161.58 ± 26.32	143.36 ± 22.43	< .001	154.16 ± 26.14	139.79 ± 23.87	< .001
DBP (mmHg)	89.01 ± 16.20	83.69 ± 11.71	0.003	82.57 ± 14.77	80.52 ± 11.41	0.088
Height (cm)	164.08 ± 5.56	166.46 ± 6.35	< .001	152.91 ± 5.91	155.69 ± 6.06	< .001
Weight (kg)	68.52 ± 12.06	68.61 ± 11.10	0.940	58.08 ± 10.64	60.33 ± 10.11	0.006
BMI (kg/m²)	25.36 ± 3.65	24.72 ± 3.54	0.091	24.77 ± 3.95	24.86 ± 3.76	0.778
WC (cm)	87.05 ± 10.36	83.74 ± 9.75	0.003	84.07 ± 10.37	81.20 ± 9.71	< .001
WHtR	0.53 ± 0.06	0.50 ± 0.06	< .001	0.55 ± 0.07	0.52 ± 0.06	< .001
hypertension (%)	74 (82.2)	2818 (53.5)	< .001	120 (77.4)	2907 (47.9)	< .001
diabetes (%)	22 (24.4)	508 (9.6)	< .001	41 (26.5)	629 (10.4)	< .001
Anti-hypertensive drug (%)	50 (55.6)	641 (12.2)	< .001	73 (47.1)	989 (16.3)	< .001
Anti-diabetic drug (%)	13 (14.4)	148 (2.5)	< .001	20 (12.9)	278 (4.6)	< .001
Lipid-lowering drug (%)	7 (7.8)	159 (3.0)	0.021	12 (7.7)	202 (3.3)	0.003
history of CVD (%)	46 (51.1)	781 (14.8)	< .001	62 (40.0)	1092 (18.0)	< .001
history of kidney disease	5 (5.6)	60 (1.1)	< .001	11 (7.1)	77 (1.3)	< .001
eGFR (ml/min per 1.73m²)	54.81 (46.46 – 57.67)	95.44 (87.00 – 103.44)	< .001	52.90 (46.89 – 57.47)	93.23 (82.89 – 103.29)	< .001
LAP (cm·mmol/L)	31.88 (18.63 – 51.35)	21.79 (10.62 – 43.35)	0.001	44.94 (26.00 – 77.56)	27.84 (16.00 – 50.25)	< .001
VAI	1.51 (1.00 – 2.60)	1.12 (0.68 – 1.98)	< .001	2.68 (1.78 – 4.17)	1.67 (1.06 – 2.78)	< .001
CMI	0.62 (0.41 – 1.10)	0.45 (0.27 – 0.82)	< .001	0.81 (0.49 – 1.26)	0.47 (0.29 – 0.81)	< .001

Data are expressed as mean ± standard deviation(SD) or median (interquartile range) and numbers (percentage) as appropriate. Income level: family annual income; *CNY* Chinese currency (1CNY = 0.15 USD), *SBP* systolic blood pressure, *DBP* diastolic blood pressure, *FPG* fasting plasma glucose, *CVD* cardiovascular disease, includes coronary heart disease, arrhythmia, heart failure, and stroke; Kidney disease: includes nephritis, kidney dysfunction, renal stones, renal tumor, and autoimmune kidney disease. Body mass index; *WC* waist circumference, *WHtR* waist-to-height ratio, *TG* triglyceride, *HDL-C* high density lipoprotein cholesterol, *TG/HDL-C* triglyceride to high density lipoprotein cholesterol ratio, *eGFR* estimated glomerular infiltration rate, *LAP* lipid accumulation product, *VAI* visceral adiposity index, *CMI* cardiometabolic index
*Comparisons of category variables between groups were tested by chi-square test or rank-sum test (ordinal category variables) and comparisons for continuous variables between groups were tested by Student's t or Mann-Whitney test

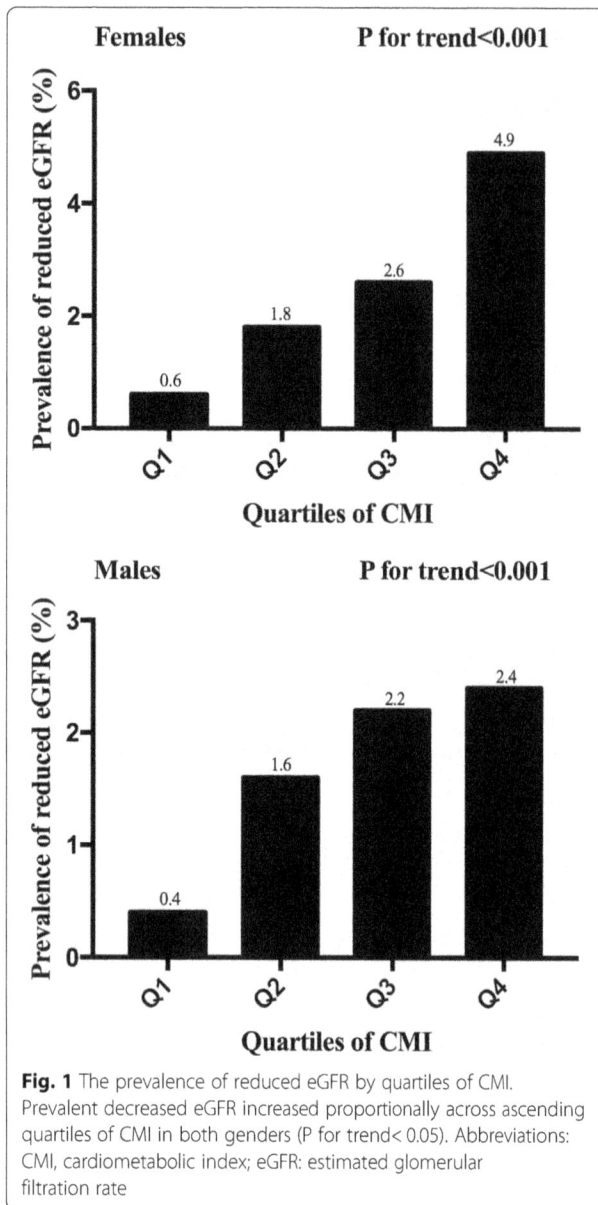

Fig. 1 The prevalence of reduced eGFR by quartiles of CMI.
Prevalent decreased eGFR increased proportionally across ascending
quartiles of CMI in both genders (P for trend< 0.05). Abbreviations:
CMI, cardiometabolic index; eGFR: estimated glomerular
filtration rate

sensitivity of 88.9% and a specificity of 37.1%. In females, CMI had an AUC (AUC: 0.684, 95% CI: 0.672–
0.695) which was comparable to that of VAI (AUC: 0.688,
95% CI: 0.676–0.699, P value for difference = 0.148) and
statistically significantly greater than that of LAP (AUC
0.684 vs 0.660, $P = 0.047$), WC (AUC 0.684 vs 0.588,
$P < 0.001$) and BMI (AUC 0.684 vs 0.500, $P < 0.001$). Furthermore, CMI exhibited the greatest sensitivity (89.0%) in
this gender. However, the specificity was still low and was
given to 39.8%.

Discussion

Our study showed that in this large, community-based
cohort of middle-aged Chinese individuals, CMI, a
novel measure of VAT, was independently and robustly

associated with the presence of reduced eGFR in both
genders. CMI could reflect not only VAT but also pathologic process that resulted in impaired kidney function,
thus provided a clinical clue for related basic researches.
As our results revealed the potential of CMI as a screening marker of reduced eGFR, further understanding of the
underlying pathophysiology should improve strategies to
prevent and potentially reverse detrimental kidney failure
and cardiovascular outcomes, especially in people with
poor socioeconomic conditions.

Dyslipidemia is a condition that always appears in the
development of CKD, even in the early stage of eGFR
reduction, and the major components of dyslipidemia in
CKD has been revealed to be increased TG level and
decreased HDL-C level [7]. Indexes that represent this
specific pattern has been identified to have a strong correlation with CKD. For instance, Hou et al. revealed that TG
level was closely associated with mildly decreased eGFR
even among middle aged or elderly Chinese population. It
was worthy to note that this relationship existed when TG
level was still in the normal range. This finding gave us an
implication that increased TG level could appear in the
early process of decreased eGFR [9]. Lee et al. identified
hypertriglyceridemia as an independent risk factor of progressed CKD, confirmed the association persistent in middle and late stage of CKD [11]. Furthermore, Tozawa et al.
and Shimizu et al. provided compelling evidences that TG
had an independent effect to increase the risk of eGFR
decrement from longitudinal studies, Tozawa et al. also
identified HDL-C positively related to eGFR value and revealed TG had an impact on the development of proteinuria [10, 40]. Apart from above investigations, researches
also identified the utility of TG/HDL-C in identifying
eGFR reduction as it incorporated both TG and HDL-C
level. Ho et al. demonstrated the correlation between TG/
HDL-C with CKD, and Wen et al. even showed the advantage of TG/HDL-C when compared with TG alone with
respect to the development of CKD, confirmed our aforementioned hypothesis [13, 14]. However, there was one
point that worth to be mentioned, although TG/HDL-C
had a robust association with CKD, it was not an ideal
marker of eGFR reduction due to its low sensitivity and
specificity [13].

As another condition that always accompany with
CKD, obesity is related to multiple risk factors of CKD,
such as hypertension and diabetes [41, 42]. Its direct
association with CKD has been evaluated through indexes. As the most widely used index of obesity, BMI
has already been elucidated to have a connection with
new-onset CKD, CKD progression and end stage renal
failure [16, 17, 43]. However, since BMI do not consider
adipose tissue distribution, there is no doubt that BMI is
unsuitable for reflecting the relationship between obesity
phenotype with CKD. Therefore, indexes of abdominal

Table 2 Evaluation of the impact of CMI on eGFR value with the use of piecewise linear regression[a]

		Unadjusted	MV adjusted
Males			
Linear model	β Value (95% CI) P value	−1.850 (−2.259, −1.440) < 0.001	−2.214 (−2.561, −1.866) < 0.001
Non-linear model	Breakpoint (K)	1.024	1.113
	β 1 (<K) (95% CI) P value	−3.324 (−3.863, − 2.786) < 0.001	−3.150 (−3.589, − 2.712) < 0.001
	β 2 (>K) (95% CI) P value	3.777 (2.371, 5.182) < 0.001	1.906 (0.675, 3.138) 0.002
	Logarithmic likelihood ratio test P value	< 0.001	< 0.001
Females			
Linear model	β Value (95% CI) P value	−4.046 (−4.438, −3.654) < 0.001	−1.914 (−2.262, − 1.566) < 0.001
Non-linear model	Breakpoint (K)	1.34	1.472
	β 1 (<K) (95% CI) P value	−5.001 (−5.472, −4.530) < 0.001	−2.411 (− 2.813, − 2.010) < 0.001
	β 2 (>K) (95% CI) P value	2.478 (0.636, 4.320) 0.008	2.268 (0.547, 3.988) 0.010
	Logarithmic likelihood ratio test P value	< 0.001	< 0.001

Abbreviations: *CMI* cardiometabolic index, *OR* odds ratio, *95% CI* 95% confidence interval. Linear model: model that presumes the association between CMI and eGFR is linear. Non-linear model: model that presumes the association between CMI and eGFR is non-linear and has breakpoint. Unadjusted: no adjustment; MV adjusted: multivariable adjusted model, includes age, race, education level, family annual income, physical activity, current smoking, current alcohol intake, hypertension, diabetes, antihypertensive drug, antidiabetic drug, lipid-lowering drug, history of cardiovascular disease and kidney disease. [a]Two-step linear regression model was applied to explore the non-linear association between CMI and eGFR

obesity such as WC and WHtR have been investigated for their associations with CKD. Among them, WHtR was found to have greatest application potential for detecting CKD by several studies [19, 20]. Theoretically, by using height to standardize WC value, WHtR was design to be a superior reflection of abdominal obesity since people with different height were supposed to have different standard WC value. Nevertheless, studies did not support any of these indexes to be an eligible marker with great sensitivity or specificity for detection of reduced eGFR [19–22]. Meanwhile, studies found that VAT contributed more to CKD than SAT [23]. Indexes like WC hadd no power to distinguish VAT from SAT alone but could recognize VAT correctly when working

together with TG [24, 44]. Taking all above messages together, we can speculate that indexes contain information about dyslipidemia and abdominal obesity should do better in the identification of VAI and be able to refine the recognition of eGFR reduction.

Indexes that integrate both abdominal obesity and dyslipidemia has been proposed. Determined by WC and TG levels, LAP was put forward for recognizing cardiovascular risk [33], and it has also been identified to possess a stronger association with CKD than BMI, WC and WHtR [45]. Later, a concept named VAI was posited as an indicator of cardiometabolic risk with an additional consideration of HDL-C and BMI when compared with LAP [34]. In recent studies, VAI showed strong association with

Table 3 Sex-specific logistic regression models for reduced eGFR with CMI

	Males				Females				P for interaction
	Unadjusted OR (95% CI)	P value	MV adjusted OR (95% CI)	P value	Unadjusted OR (95% CI)	P value	MV adjusted OR (95% CI)	P value	
CMI (Per 1 SD increase)	1.467 (1.211, 1.777)	< 0.001	1.516 (1.182, 1.943)	0.001	1.760 (1.519, 2.040)	< 0.001	1.347 (1.122, 1.618)	0.001	0.172
Quartiles of CMI									
Quartile 1	1.000		1.000		1.000		1.000		
Quartile 2	3.711 (1.500, 9.182)	0.005	2.717 (1.061, 6.957)	0.037	2.835 (1.372, 5.856)	0.005	2.285 (1.069, 4.888)	0.033	
Quartile 3	5.092 (2.112, 12.273)	< 0.001	3.867 (1.551, 9.640)	0.004	4.187 (2.090, 8.387)	< 0.001	2.509 (1.204, 5.225)	0.014	
Quartile 4	5.439 (2.267, 13.052)	< 0.001	4.227 (1.681, 10.627)	0.002	7.939 (4.091, 15.408)	< 0.001	3.442 (1.685, 7.031)	< 0.001	
P value for trend		< 0.001		0.001		< 0.001		< 0.001	

MV indicates multivariable, *OR* odds ratio, *CI* confidence interval, *CMI* cardiometabolic index. Cut points for CMI: Men: ≤ 0.27, > 0.27 and ≤ 0.46, > 0.46 and ≤ 0.83, > 0.83; Women: ≤ 0.30, > 0.30 and ≤ 0.48, > 0.48 and ≤ 0.82, > 0.82. MV model adjusted for age, race, education level, family annual income, diet score, physical activity, current smoking, current alcohol intake, hypertension, diabetes, antihypertensive drug, antidiabetic drug, lipid-lowering drug, history of cardiovascular disease (coronary heart disease, arrhythmia, heart failure, and stroke) and kidney disease (nephritis, kidney dysfunction, renal stones, renal tumor, and autoimmune kidney disease)

Table 4 AUC for indexes to discriminate eGFR reduction in females and males

Variables	AUC (95%CI)	P value	Cut-off according to Youden's index	Sensitivity (%)	Specificity (%)
Males					
CMI	0.633 (0.620–0.646)[a,c]	< 0.001	> 0.35	88.9%	37.1%
VAI	0.627 (0.614–0.640)[c]	< 0.001	> 0.83	90.0%	34.7%
LAP	0.606 (0.593–0.619)[c]	< 0.001	> 18.33	77.8%	43.6%
WC	0.589 (0.576–0.602)[c]	0.001	> 79.1	83.3%	35.0%
BMI	0.544 (0.531–0.558)	0.135	> 22.02	88.9%	22.8%
Females					
CMI	0.684 (0.672–0.695)[a,b,c]	< 0.001	> 0.39	89.0%	39.8%
VAI	0.688 (0.676–0.699)[a,b,c]	< 0.001	> 1.69	80.0%	50.4%
LAP	0.660 (0.648–0.672)[b,c]	< 0.001	> 36.12	65.2%	61.8%
WC	0.588 (0.576–0.600)[c]	< 0.001	> 84.20	52.9%	64.0%
BMI	0.500 (0.488–0.513)	0.995	≤ 27.81	76.1%	20.1%

Abbreviations: *AUC* area under the ROC curve, *95% CI* 95% confidence interval, *CMI* cardiometabolic index, *VAI* visceral adiposity index, *LAP* lipid accumulation product, *WC* waist circumference, *BMI* body mass index
[a]indicates a significant larger as compared to LAP;
[b]indicates a significant larger as compared to WC;
[c]indicates a significant larger as compared to BMI

CKD and greater potential as a marker of eGFR reduction than LAP as well as traditional anthropometric indexes [45, 46]. However, these two novel indexes still have limitations. Both LAP and VAI have sex-specific equations, and VAI has a sophisticated algorithm, these will increase the complexity of calculation. As for LAP, information about HDL-C is not utilized, which is an important aspect of dyslipidemia in CKD. Moreover, height info is also wasted by LAP, but people with different height should have different WC standard. Last but not least, although VAI possessed a greater discriminative power than LAP and other indexes, it still failed to reach satisfying sensitivity and specificity values, thus its value for becoming a marker of eGFR reduction is limited [46].

CMI is a young index which was posited by Ichiro Wakabayashi in 2015 [25]. Different from LAP and VAI, it reflects both characteristics of dyslipidemia in CKD and accurate central obesity status through a simple, generalized eq. CMI has also been identified to correlate with multiple cardiovascular risk factors, implicated to have a great potential in screening related diseases [25–29]. Since many of these diseases has been identified to be risk factors of CKD [16, 47–50], we hypothesize that CMI correlates with reduced eGFR and is capable of being a premier indicator of eGFR decrement. In our present study, regression analyses revealed the intensive and direct associations of CMI with eGFR value and eGFR reduction in both genders, confirming above hypothesis. Moreover, we observed a breakpoint in the association between CMI and eGFR value, which meant the change of eGFR shifted from decrease to increase after CMI reached certain value. And this phenomenon was robust and persistent across genders. Although the exact mechanism underlying this

paradoxical phenomenon is still unclear, some previous findings can also give us a clue for possible explanations. While obesity was commonly considered to associate with the decline of eGFR [8, 15], studies also found a protective effect of obesity on CKD patients [51, 52], and this protective effect could be explained by the evidence that excessive adipose tissue might temper the deleterious effects of inflammatory factors by sequestering them [53, 54]. Consistent with this theory, the breakpoint was located at high levels of CMI (> 75 percentile) in each gender, which meant that the protective effect became more predominant than the destructive effect only when fatty tissue accumulated to a sufficient volume. Another possible explanation was the residual confounders. Although we had adjusted several factors that related to CMI and eGFR, there were still some confounders that we did not take into our regression equations. Therefore, some uncovered confounding factors could influence our results and caused this paradox. In order to validate the paradox founded in the present study, studies with prospective design and consideration of more modifiers are needed in the future.

Further, we confirmed the association between CMI and reduced eGFR was positive and strong. We found that the risk of reduced eGFR was proportionally increased across the quartiles of CMI, which was different from the breakpoint phenomenon in the association between CMI and eGFR value. Given that the breakpoint of CMI located behind the 75 percentile in both genders, we could easily figure out that the limited increase of eGFR in CMI levels above the breakpoint has minimal effect on the whole inverse trend of CMI with reduced kidney function (eGFR< 60 ml/min per 1.73m^2). We also noticed that males had a slightly higher risk of developing reduced eGFR when compared with their female counterparts. But the interaction test revealed that this disadvantage was statistically insignificant. However, although we could not conclude that males were under greater risk of reduced eGFR, we still elucidated that CMI had a robust association with eGFR reduction in both genders, identifying the utility and stability of CMI for the risk stratification of reduced eGFR.

Findings from ROC analyses provided compelling evidence for CMI to be a screening marker of CKD. In males, CMI possessed greatest AUC value, although it did not have a significant larger discriminating ability than VAI, the simple and generalized equation for both sexes would be a vantage. With a sensitivity of 88.9%, CMI demonstrated its capability to function well in the screening test, since more suspicious patients should be positive in this kind of examination. It was worthy to note that neither of CMI, VAI and LAP had a significant greater AUC than WC, which was beyond our expectation, this could be explained by the lacking of sample size since the absolute number and prevalence of reduced eGFR were much lower in males than in females. Further studies are needed to validate this intriguing finding. In females, CMI did an even better job as it performed better than other indexes significantly except VAI. Although exhibited a negligible disadvantage in discriminating eGFR reduction, CMI showed a much higher sensitivity than VAI, thus the applicative value for CMI was still superior than VAI among females. In conclusion, with great discriminative ability and high sensitivity value, CMI showed its potential for becoming an economic screening marker to filter out people with reduced eGFR.

Mounting evidence has emerged to reveal the mechanism under the association between CMI with CKD. First, mechanism of dyslipidemia in CKD has already been elucidated. Hypertriglyceridemia is a multifactorial phenomenon, and is partially due to diminished catabolism. This reduction is an outcome of depressed lipoprotein lipase (LPL) activity, which is responsible for the hydrolysis of TG [55]. And the decreased LPL activity has been identified to be caused by secondary hyperparathyroidism induced insulin resistance (IR) and excess of lipase inhibitors like apolipoprotein (Apo) C-III in the progression of CKD [56, 57]. For another aspect, hepatic Apo A-I gene expression and hepatic lecithin cholesterol acyl transferase (LCAT) mRNA expression are downregulated during the course of CKD, and then this change attributes to a lower plasma Apo A-I level and decreased LCAT activity [58, 59]. Since Apo A-I is an essential functional component of HDL-C [60], the concentration of HDL-C in blood is consequently decreased. Similarly, the normal function

of HDL-C is also impaired because of inadequate LCAT activity, which is important in the process of transporting cholesterol to HDL in peripheral tissues [60]. Second, basic research has also revealed the intrinsic mechanism between obesity with CKD. Adipocytes produce a series of factors, such as angiotensinogen, precursor of angiotensin II and leptin, which may trigger glomerular hypertension through local renin-angiotensin-aldosterone system (RAAS) or sympathetic system, then leading to the decrease of eGFR [8]. Furthermore, inflammation involves in the association between obesity with CKD as well, macrophages are found to accumulate in the kidney of obese animals in the effect of angiotensin [61]. Some inflammatory cytokines such as interleukin-6 (IL-6) and Tumor necrosis factor-α (TNF-α) have also been implicated in obesity-related CKD [62]. Therefore, obesity could promote the progression of renal disease through several, partially overlapping mechanisms. Sum up above two points, as composites of CMI, dyslipidemia and obesity have experiment confirmed relationship with CKD. Thus, the association between CMI with reduced eGFR observed in our study has a concrete foundation from basic researches.

There are still some limitations in our study that needed to be mentioned. First, due to the cross-sectional design, our work can only provide evidence about the strong association between CMI and reduced eGFR, but information about the causality of this relationship need further prospective studies to confirm. Second, it has an inherent limitation of not being a randomized study. Although multivariable adjustments were performed for potential confounding factors, a possible effect of unmeasured variables such as C-reactive protein cannot be excluded. Third, our study participants were recruited from rural area of northeast of China, whether the results can be applied to populations of different areas or races require more studies to investigate. Finally, our diagnosis based on a single biochemistry test, the creatinine value could be influenced by uncertain factors, thus the accuracy of eGFR could be mildly disturbed.

Conclusions

In summary, our work was the first study to reveal the relationship between CMI and reduced eGFR which was independent of prevalent CVD, medication used, and conventional cardiovascular risk factors. Thus, these data provide strong evidence of a unique, independent and economic role of CMI in a high burden of kidney disease. These findings have important implications for guiding primordial prevention and understanding the mechanisms underlying VAT-mediated renal injury.

Abbreviations
AUC: Area under the curve; BMI: Body mass index; CI: Confidence internal; CKD: Chronic kidney disease; CMI: Cardiometabolic index;

CVD: Cardiovascular disease; DBP: Diastolic blood pressure; DM: Diabetes mellitus; eGFR: Estimated glomerular filtration index; ESRD: End stage renal disease; FPG: Fasting plasma glucose; HDL-C: High density lipoprotein cholesterol; IL: Interleukin; IR: Insulin resistance; LAP: Lipid accumulation product; LCAT: Lecithin cholesterol acyl transferase; LPL: Lipoprotein lipase; NCRCHS: Northeast China Rural Cardiovascular Health Study; NO: Nitric oxide; ORs: Odds ratios; RAAS: Renin-angiotensin-aldosterone system; ROC: Receiver operating characteristic curve; SAT: Subcutaneous adipose tissue; SBP: Systolic blood pressure; SD: Standard deviation; TG: Triglyceride; TG/HDL-C: Triglyceride to high density lipoprotein cholesterol ratio; TNF-α: Tumor necrosis factor alpha; VAI: Visceral adiposity index; VAT: Visceral adipose tissue; WC: Waist circumference; WHtR: Waist to height ratio

Acknowledgements

We would like to express our gratitude to all those who exert their effects in achieving this study.

Funding

This study was supported by grants from the "Thirteenth Five-Year" program funds (The National Key Research and Development Program of China, Grant #2017YFC1307600). The founder provided financial support for our survey, but do not interfere the design, operation and analysis of the study.

Authors' contributions

In this study, HYW and WRS did the study design, statistical analyses and results interpretation. XY, SZW and SYL participated as analyzing and resolving difficulties of analytic strategies and results discussion. Finally, YXS functioned as final reviewer who gave constructional suggestions for the interpretation of data. The corresponding author was YXS. All authors have read and approved the manuscript.

Competing interests

The authors declare that they have no competing interests.

Author details

[1]Department of Cardiology, The First Hospital of China Medical University, 155 Nanjing North Street, Heping District, Shenyang 110001, China. [2]Department of Cardiovascular Medicine, Beijing Moslem Hospital, Beijing 100054, China. [3]Department of Computational Medicine and Bioinformatics, University of Michigan, 100 Washtenaw Avenue, Ann Arbor, MI 48109, USA. [4]West China School of Medicine, Sichuan University, #37 Guoxue Alley, Chengdu 610041, China.

References

1. Global, regional, and national age-sex specific all-cause and cause-specific mortality for 240 causes of death, 1990–2013: a systematic analysis for the Global Burden of Disease Study 2013. Lancet 2015;385:117–71.
2. Zhang L, Wang F, Wang L, Wang W, Liu B, Liu J, et al. Prevalence of chronic kidney disease in China: a cross-sectional survey. Lancet. 2012;379:815–22.
3. Horowitz B, Miskulin D, Zager P. Epidemiology of hypertension in CKD. Adv Chronic Kidney Dis. 2015;22:88–95.
4. Levey A, Astor B, Stevens L, Coresh J. Chronic kidney disease, diabetes, and hypertension: what's in a name? Kidney Int. 2010;78:19–22.
5. Nugent R, Fathima S, Feigl A, Chyung D. The burden of chronic kidney disease on developing nations: a 21st century challenge in global health. Nephron Clin Pract. 2011;118:c269–77.
6. Luyckx V, Tonelli M, Stanifer J. The global burden of kidney disease and the sustainable development goals. Bull World Health Organ. 2018;96:414–22D.
7. Hager M, Narla A, Tannock L. Dyslipidemia in patients with chronic kidney disease. Rev Endocr Metab Disord. 2017;18:29–40.
8. Mallamaci F, Tripepi G. Obesity and CKD progression: hard facts on fat CKD patients. Nephrol Dial Transplant. 2013;28:iv105–iv8.
9. Hou X, Wang C, Zhang X, Zhao X, Wang Y, Li C, et al. Triglyceride levels are closely associated with mild declines in estimated glomerular filtration rates in middle-aged and elderly Chinese with normal serum lipid levels. PLoS One. 2014;9:e106778.
10. Shimizu M, Furusyo N, Mitsumoto F, Takayama K, Ura K, Hiramine S, et al. Subclinical carotid atherosclerosis and triglycerides predict the incidence of chronic kidney disease in the Japanese general population: results from the Kyushu and Okinawa population study (KOPS). Atherosclerosis. 2015;238:207–12.
11. Lee P, Chang H, Tung C, Hsu Y, Lei C, Chang H, et al. Hypertriglyceridemia: an independent risk factor of chronic kidney disease in Taiwanese adults. Am J Med Sci. 2009;338:185–9.
12. Tsuruya K, Yoshida H, Nagata M, Kitazono T, Iseki K, Iseki C, et al. Impact of the triglycerides to high-density lipoprotein cholesterol ratio on the incidence and progression of CKD: a longitudinal study in a large Japanese population. Am J Kidney Dis. 2015;66:972–83.
13. Ho C, Chen J, Chen S, Tsai Y, Weng Y, Tsao Y, et al. Relationship between TG/HDL-C ratio and metabolic syndrome risk factors with chronic kidney disease in healthy adult population. Clin Nutr. 2015;34:874–80.
14. Wen J, Chen Y, Huang Y, Lu Y, Liu X, Zhou H, et al. Association of the TG/HDL-C and non-HDL-C/HDL-C ratios with chronic kidney disease in an adult Chinese population. Kidney Blood Press Res. 2017;42:1141–54.
15. Kramer H, Luke A, Bidani A, Cao G, Cooper R, McGee D. Obesity and prevalent and incident CKD: the hypertension detection and follow-up program. Am J Kidney Dis. 2005;46:587–94.
16. Fox C, Larson M, Leip E, Culleton B, Wilson P, Levy D. Predictors of new-onset kidney disease in a community-based population. JAMA. 2004;291:844–50.
17. Ejerblad E, Fored C, Lindblad P, Fryzek J, McLaughlin J, Nyrén O. Obesity and risk for chronic renal failure. J Am Soc Nephrol. 2006;17:1695–702.
18. Bacopoulou F, Efthymiou V, Landis G, Rentoumis A, Chrousos G. Waist circumference, waist-to-hip ratio and waist-to-height ratio reference percentiles for abdominal obesity among Greek adolescents. BMC Pediatr. 2015;15:50.
19. He Y, Li F, Wang F, Ma X, Zhao X, Zeng Q. The association of chronic kidney disease and waist circumference and waist-to-height ratio in Chinese urban adults. Medicine (Baltimore). 2016;95:e3769.
20. Lin C-H, Chou C-Y, Lin C-C, Huang C-C, Liu C-S, Lai S-W. Waist-to-height ratio is the best index of obesity in association with chronic kidney disease. Nutrition. 2007;23:788–93.
21. Odagiri K, Mizuta I, Yamamoto M, Miyazaki Y, Watanabe H, Uehara A. Waist to height ratio is an independent predictor for the incidence of chronic kidney disease. PLoS One. 2014;9:e88873.
22. Dong Y, Wang Z, Chen Z, Wang X, Zhang L, Nie J, et al. Comparison of visceral, body fat indices and anthropometric measures in relation to chronic kidney disease among Chinese adults from a large scale cross-sectional study. BMC Nephrol. 2018;19:40.
23. Madero M, Katz R, Murphy R, Newman A, Patel K, Ix J, et al. Comparison between different measures of body fat with kidney function decline and incident CKD. Clin J Am Soc Nephrol. 2017;12:893–903.
24. Després J, Lemieux I, Bergeron J, Pibarot P, Mathieu P, Larose E, et al. Abdominal obesity and the metabolic syndrome: contribution to global cardiometabolic risk. Arterioscler Thromb Vasc Biol. 2008;28:1039–49.
25. Wakabayashi I, Daimon T. The "cardiometabolic index" as a new marker determined by adiposity and blood lipids for discrimination of diabetes mellitus. Clin Chim Acta. 2015;438:274–8.
26. Wang H, Chen Y, Sun G, Jia P, Qian H, Sun Y. Validity of cardiometabolic index, lipid accumulation product, and body adiposity index in predicting the risk of hypertension in Chinese population. Postgrad Med. 2018;130:325–33.
27. Wang H, Sun Y, Li Z, Guo X, Chen S, Ye N, et al. Gender-specific contribution of cardiometabolic index and lipid accumulation product to left ventricular geometry change in general population of rural China. BMC Cardiovasc Disord. 2018;18:62.
28. Wang H, Chen Y, Guo X, Chang Y, Sun Y. Usefulness of cardiometabolic index for the estimation of ischemic stroke risk among general population in rural China. Postgrad Med. 2017;129:834–41.
29. Dursun M, Besiroglu H, Otunctemur A, Ozbek E. Association between cardiometabolic index and erectile dysfunction: a new index for predicting cardiovascular disease. Kaohsiung J Med Sci. 2016;32:620 3.

30. Li Z, Guo X, Zheng L, Yang H, Sun Y. Grim status of hypertension in rural China: results from Northeast China rural cardiovascular health study 2013. J Am Soc Hypertens. 2015;9:358–64.

31. Wang H, Li Z, Guo X, Chen Y, Chen S, Tian Y, et al. Contribution of non-traditional lipid profiles to reduced glomerular filtration rate in H-type hypertension population of rural China. Ann Med. 2018;50:249–59.

32. Chen S, Guo X, Dong S, Li Z, Sun Y. Relationship between lifestyle factors and hyperhomocysteinemia in general Chinese population: a cross-sectional study. Postgrad Med. 2017;129:216–23.

33. Kahn H. The "lipid accumulation product" performs better than the body mass index for recognizing cardiovascular risk: a population-based comparison. BMC Cardiovasc Disord. 2005;5:26.

34. Amato M, Giordano C, Galia M, Criscimanna A, Vitabile S, Midiri M, et al. Visceral adiposity index: a reliable indicator of visceral fat function associated with cardiometabolic risk. Diabetes Care. 2010;33:920–2.

35. Levey A, Stevens L, Schmid C, Zhang Y, Castro A, Feldman H, et al. A new equation to estimate glomerular filtration rate. Ann Intern Med. 2009;150: 604–12.

36. Stevens P, Levin A. Evaluation and management of chronic kidney disease: synopsis of the kidney disease: improving global outcomes 2012 clinical practice guideline. Ann Intern Med. 2013;158:825–30.

37. Chobanian A, Bakris G, Black H, Cushman W, Green L, Izzo J, et al. The seventh report of the joint National Committee on prevention, detection, evaluation, and treatment of high blood pressure: the JNC 7 report. JAMA. 2003;289:2560–72.

38. 2. Classification and Diagnosis of Diabetes. Diabetes Care. 2018;41:S13–27.

39. Zhang Z. Univariate description and bivariate statistical inference: the first step delving into data. Ann Transl Med. 2016;4:91.

40. Tozawa M, Iseki K, Iseki C, Oshiro S, Ikemiya Y, Takishita S. Triglyceride, but not total cholesterol or low-density lipoprotein cholesterol levels, predict development of proteinuria. Kidney Int. 2002;62:1743–9.

41. Seravalle G, Grassi G. Obesity and hypertension. Pharmacol Res. 2017;122:1–7.

42. DeFronzo R, Ferrannini E, Groop L, Henry R, Herman W, Holst J, et al. Type 2 diabetes mellitus. Nat Rev Dis Primers. 2015;1:15019.

43. Yun HR, Kim H, Park JT, Chang TI, Yoo TH, Kang SW, et al. Am J Kidney Dis. 2018;72(3):400-10.

44. Britton K, Fox C. Ectopic fat depots and cardiovascular disease. Circulation. 2011;124:e837–41.

45. Dai D, Chang Y, Chen Y, Chen S, Yu S, Guo X, et al. Int J Environ Res Public Health. 2016;13(12).

46. Chen Y, Lai S, Tsai Y, Chang S. Visceral adiposity index as a predictor of chronic kidney disease in a relatively healthy population in Taiwan. J Ren Nutr. 2018;28:91–100.

47. Garofalo C, Borrelli S, Pacilio M, Minutolo R, Chiodini P, De Nicola L, et al. Hypertension and prehypertension and prediction of development of decreased estimated GFR in the general population: a meta-analysis of cohort studies. Am J Kidney Dis. 2016;67:89–97.

48. Tsioufis C, Kokkinos P, Macmanus C, Thomopoulos C, Faselis C, Doumas M, et al. Left ventricular hypertrophy as a determinant of renal outcome in patients with high cardiovascular risk. J Hypertens. 2010;28:2299–308.

49. Masson P, Webster A, Hong M, Turner R, Lindley R, Craig J. Chronic kidney disease and the risk of stroke: a systematic review and meta-analysis. Nephrol Dial Transplant. 2015;30:1162–9.

50. Bellinghieri G, Santoro D, Mallamace A, Savica V. Sexual dysfunction in chronic renal failure. J Nephrol. 2008;21(Suppl 13):S113–7.

51. Naderi N, Kleine C, Park C, Hsiung J, Soohoo M, Tantisattamo E, et al. Obesity paradox in advanced kidney disease: from bedside to the bench. Prog Cardiovasc Dis. 2018;61:168–81.

52. Park J, Ahmadi SF, Streja E, Molnar MZ, Flegal KM, Gillen D, et al. Obesity paradox in end-stage kidney disease patients. Prog Cardiovasc Dis. 2014;56:415–25.

53. Mohamed-Ali V, Goodrick S, Bulmer K, Holly J, Yudkin J, Coppack S. Production of soluble tumor necrosis factor receptors by human subcutaneous adipose tissue in vivo. Am J Phys. 1999;277:E971–5.

54. Drechsler C, Wanner C. The obesity paradox and the role of inflammation. J Am Soc Nephrol. 2016;27:1270–2.

55. KORN E. Clearing factor, a heparin-activated lipoprotein lipase. II. Substrate specificity and activation of coconut oil. J Biol Chem. 1955;215:15–26.

56. Vaziri N, Wang X, Liang K. Secondary hyperparathyroidism downregulates lipoprotein lipase expression in chronic renal failure. Am J Phys. 1997;273: F925–30.

57. Vaziri N, Liang K. Down-regulation of tissue lipoprotein lipase expression in experimental chronic renal failure. Kidney Int. 1996;50:1928–35.

58. Vaziri N, Deng G, Liang K. Hepatic HDL receptor, SR-B1 and Apo A-I expression in chronic renal failure. Nephrol Dial Transplant. 1999;14:1462–6.

59. Vaziri N, Liang K, Parks J. Down-regulation of hepatic lecithin:cholesterol acyltransferase gene expression in chronic renal failure. Kidney Int. 2001; 59:2192–6.

60. Zannis V, Chroni A, Krieger M. Role of apoA-I, ABCA1, LCAT, and SR-BI in the biogenesis of HDL. J Mol Med. 2006;84:276–94.

61. Ma L, Corsa B, Zhou J, Yang H, Li H, Tang Y, et al. Angiotensin type 1 receptor modulates macrophage polarization and renal injury in obesity. Am J Physiol Renal Physiol. 2011;300:F1203–113.

62. Spoto B, Zoccali C. Spleen IL-10, a key player in obesity-driven renal risk. Nephrol Dial Transplant. 2013;28:1061–4.

18

Influence of exogenous growth hormone administration on circulating concentrations of α-klotho in healthy and chronic kidney disease subjects: a prospective, single-center open case-control pilot study

Aaltje Y. Adema[1], Camiel L. M. de Roij van Zuijdewijn[1], Joost G. Hoenderop[2], Martin H. de Borst[3], Piet M. Ter Wee[1], Annemieke C. Heijboer[4], Marc G. Vervloet[1,5*] and for the NIGRAM consortium,

Abstract

Background: The CKD-associated decline in soluble α-Klotho (α-Klotho) levels is considered detrimental. Some studies suggest a direct induction of α-Klotho concentrations by growth hormone (GH). In the present study, the effect of exogenous GH administration on α-Klotho concentrations in a clinical cohort with mild chronic kidney disease (CKD) and healthy subjects was studied.

Methods: A prospective, single-center open case-control pilot study was performed involving 8 patients with mild CKD and 8 healthy controls matched for age and sex. All participants received subcutaneous GH injections (Genotropin®, 20 mcg/kg/day) for 7 consecutive days. α-Klotho concentrations were measured at baseline, after 7 days of therapy and 1 week after the intervention was stopped.

Results: α-Klotho concentrations were not different between CKD-patients and healthy controls at baseline (554 (388–659) vs. 547 (421–711) pg/mL, $P = 0.38$). Overall, GH therapy increased α-Klotho concentrations from 554 (405–659) to 645 (516–754) pg/mL, $P < 0.05$. This was accompanied by an increase of IGF-1 concentrations from 26.8 ± 5.0 nmol/L to 61.7 ± 17.7 nmol/L ($P < 0.05$). GH therapy induced a trend toward increased α-Klotho concentrations both in the CKD group (554 (388–659) to 591 (358–742) pg/mL ($P = 0.19$)) and the healthy controls (547 (421–711) pg/mL to 654 (538–754) pg/mL ($P = 0.13$)). The change in α-Klotho concentration was not different for both groups (P for interaction $= 0.71$). α-Klotho concentrations returned to baseline levels within one week after the treatment ($P < 0.05$).

Conclusions: GH therapy increases α-Klotho concentrations in subjects with normal renal function or stage 3 CKD. A larger follow-up study is needed to determine whether the effect size is different between both groups or in patients with more severe CKD.

Keywords: α-Klotho, Growth hormone, Chronic kidney disease

* Correspondence: m.vervloet@vumc.nl
[1]Department of Nephrology, VU University Medical Center, De Boelelaan 1117, 1081, HV, Amsterdam, The Netherlands
[5]Amsterdam Cardiovascular Sciences (ACS), Amsterdam, The Netherlands
Full list of author information is available at the end of the article

Background

The excessively high cardiovascular (CV) risk in patients with chronic kidney disease (CKD) is only partially explained by the higher prevalence of traditional risk factors [1]. Therefore, other CKD-related factors are believed to play a causal role, such as deregulation of the fibroblast growth factor 23 (FGF23)-Klotho-vitamin D axis [2]. The anti-aging α-Klotho protein was discovered in 1997 following manipulation of its gene [3]. α-Klotho is predominantly synthesized in the distal tubular epithelial cells of the kidneys and in lower levels in the proximal tubule [4]. The extracellular domain is cleaved and released into extracellular fluid, including blood, cerebrospinal fluid and urine [3]. As CKD progresses, α-Klotho concentrations decrease [5]. Lower α-Klotho concentrations are associated with progressive CKD [5], higher prevalence of cardiovascular disease [6], arterial stiffness [7] and vascular calcification [8]. Animal studies showed that restoration of α-Klotho reduces oxidative stress, attenuates hypertension, ameliorates cardiac hypertrophy and prevents endothelial dysfunction [9–12]. Therefore, increasing α-Klotho concentrations may be a legitimate goal in CKD patients in order to slow down or even reverse these processes. However, clinical long-term exogenous supplementation of the relatively large α-Klotho-protein (130 kDa) might be an option for the far future in human and therefore upregulation of the endogenous production of α-Klotho might be more feasible, at least in the predialysis phase, as the kidney is the primary production site of α-Klotho. Several recent studies assessed different experimental options to up-regulate endogenous α-Klotho [13–21]. In humans, the use of angiotensin-receptor blockers (ARBs) and vitamin D were shown to increase α -Klotho concentrations to some extend [21, 22]. However, despite the widespread use of vitamin D en ARBs in patients with CKD, the frequency of CV events and mortality in patients with CKD remains high. Recent data showed a complex relationship between growth hormone (GH) and α-Klotho concentrations [23]. Whether IGF-1 or GH directly affects α-Klotho concentrations is still unknown, although small pilot studies showed that GH replacement therapy in both children and adults with GH deficiency increased α-Klotho concentrations [24, 25]. However, the effect of administration of exogenous GH on the α-Klotho concentration in subjects with CKD and healthy controls is unknown.

In the present study, the effect of subcutaneous GH therapy on α-Klotho concentrations in subjects with or without mild CKD is investigated in a prospective, single-center open-label case-control pilot study.

Methods

Participants and intervention

In total, 18 subjects (12 men and 6 women) with or without CKD stage 3 (creatinine clearance of 30–60 mL/min/1.73m^2 according to the Chronic Kidney Disease Epidemiology Collaboration (CKD-EPI)) were included in the period of January 2015 until March 2016 from the outpatient clinic of nephrology in the VU medical center. Subjects were matched for age and sex, to allow an adequate comparison between those with and without CKD. Exclusion criteria were the use of immunosuppressive agents, GH suppletion, oestrogens, corticosteroids, androgens, or anabolic steroids. Furthermore, subjects with any pituitary disease, history of malignancy, respiratory disorder or obstructive sleep apnoea syndrome, known thyroidal disease, active vasculitis, heart failure, severe hepatic disease, chronic systemic infections, uncontrolled hypertension, diabetes mellitus, malnutrition, autosomal dominant polycystic kidney disease, single kidney or a BMI > 30 kg/m^2 were also excluded. All included subjects received subcutaneous GH injections (Genotropin®, 20 mcg/kg/day) for 7 consecutive days. The primary end point was the change in α-Klotho concentrations after 7 days of GH-administration. Secondary endpoint was the potential difference in change of α-Klotho concentration between patients with CKD and healthy subjects.

Assays

Non-fasting blood samples and first morning spot urine were drawn at baseline, after 7 days of treatment and 1 week after the treatment stopped. Collected material was stored at − 80 °C until use. No additional freeze-thaw cycles were needed. IGF-1 was measured in serum samples using an immunochemiluminescent assay (Liaison, DiaSorin®). Concentrations of creatinine, phosphate, C-reactive protein, glucose, albumin and calcium were measured in heparin samples (Cobas, Roche Diagnostics). Urine creatinine, calcium, phosphate and albumin were measured in first morning spot urine samples (Cobas, Roche Diagnostics). Fractional excretion of phosphate was calculated using spot urine samples. α-Klotho was measured in − 80 °C stored heparin samples using a α-Klotho immunoassay (IBL international GmbH, Hamburg, Germany) with an intra-assay variation of < 5% and an inter assay variation < 7.5% [26]. C-terminal FGF23 was measured in EDTA-plasma using ELISA (Immutopics) [27] with an intra-assay variation of < 5% and an inter assay variation < 10%. Tubular maximal reabsorption of phosphate normalized to GFR (TmP/GFR) was used as an index of the renal threshold for phosphate excretion, calculated from values in serum and spot urine according to the nomogram by Walton and Bijvoet [28].

Statistical analysis

Baseline characteristics are shown as mean (standard deviation), median (interquartile range (IQR)) or number (percentage), when appropriate. Normally distributed numerical variables were compared using an unpaired T-test, nonparametric data with a Mann-Whitney U test and categorical variables by a Chi-square test. Longitudinal data were analysed with linear mixed models (LMM) with a random intercept, a random slope or both, based on the lowest Aikaike's

Information Criterion. For all analyses, an autoregressive covariance matrix was used. All model assumptions were checked and not violated. To test whether the effect of growth hormone administration on α-Klotho was different for CKD patients or healthy controls, a LMM was fitted with an interaction term between time and group. A p-value < 0.05 was considered statistically significant. All analyses were performed using IBM SPSS Statistics software version 20 (IBM Inc., IL, USA) (Additional file 1).

Results

Characteristics study population

All subjects, except one tolerated the administration of GH well. One male subject in the CKD subgroup discontinued the study due to complaints of headache. Furthermore, 1 male subject in the healthy control subgroup was withdrawn due to a serious adverse event (SAE) during the study. This SAE, a hospital admission for pain and acute kidney injury due to an obstructive kidney stone, was not related to study procedures. Thus, data on 16 subjects were analysed, 8 patients in the CKD-group and 8 in the healthy control group. This study adheres to the CONSORT guidelines (Fig. 1). Mean age of the participants was 46 years old (ranging from 25 to 59 years old). Mean eGFR in the CKD-subgroup was 57 ± 17 mL/min/1.73 m^2). As can be seen in Table 1, baseline characteristics are comparable

between the two groups, except for eGFR by definition of the groups.

IGF-1 concentrations

After 7 days of GH suppletion therapy (GHST), IGF-1 concentrations, as indicator of GH therapy bioactivity, increased from 26.8 ± 5.0 nmol/L to 61.7 ± 17.7 nmol/L ($P < 0.05$). Mean IGF-1 concentrations increased from 26.3 ± 2.8 nmol/L to 59.8 ± 20.5 nmol/L ($P < 0.05$) and from 27.3 ± 6.8 nmol/L to 63.6 ± 15.6 nmol/L ($P < 0.05$) in the CKD-group and healthy controls respectively. The increase in IGF-1 concentrations was not different over time between the CKD subgroup and the healthy controls, (P for interaction = 0.71, Table 2).

Effect of subcutaneous growth hormone therapy on circulating α-klotho concentrations

At baseline, α-Klotho concentrations were not statistically significant different between CKD-patients and healthy controls (Table 1, $p = 0.38$). Median α-Klotho concentrations increased from 554 (IQR 405–659) to 645 (IQR 516–754) pg/mL ($P = 0.05$). As can be seen by Fig. 2a, the variability in response is rather high. α-Klotho concentrations increased from 554 (IQR 388–659) to 591 (IQR 358–742) pg/mL ($P = 0.19$) and from 547 (IQR 421–711) pg/mL to 654 (IQR 538–754) pg/mL

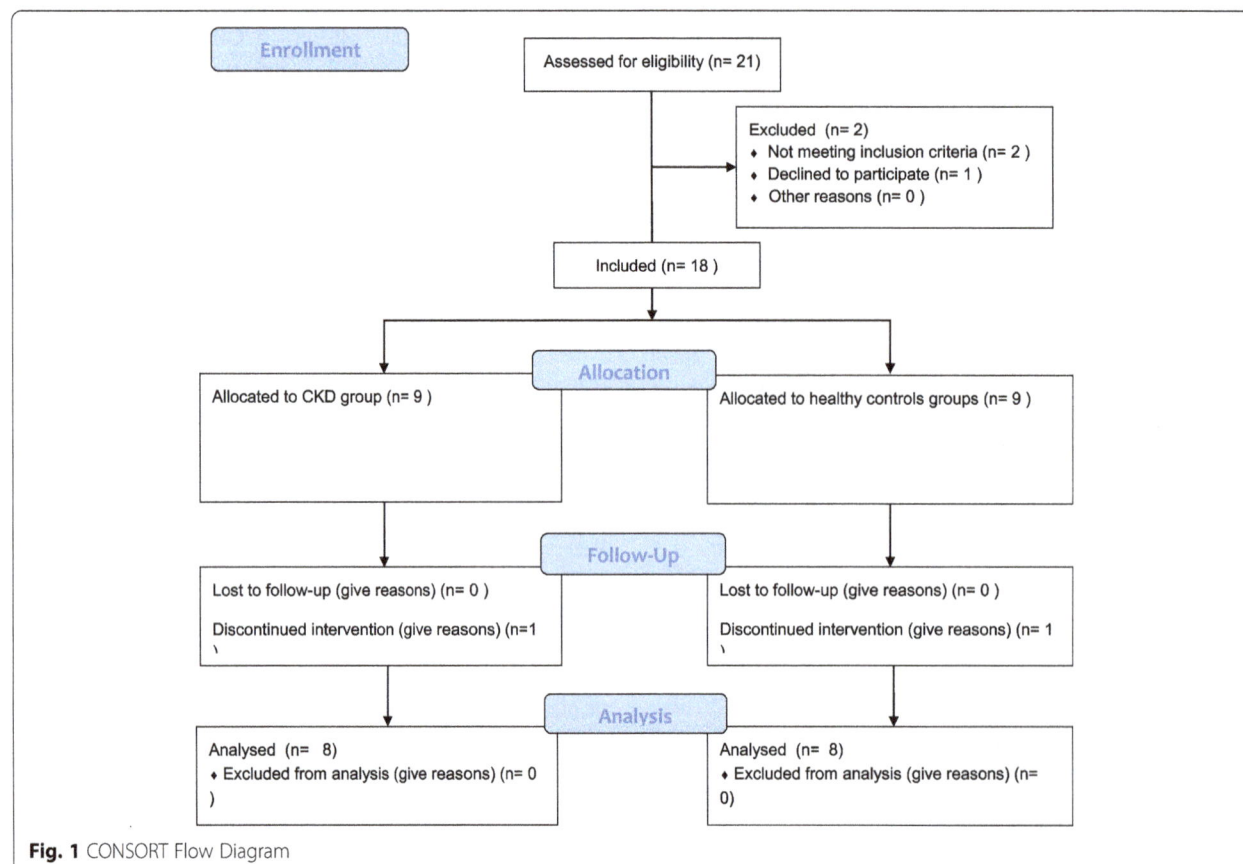

Fig. 1 CONSORT Flow Diagram

Table 1 Baseline characteristics of the participants[a]

	CKD stage III (n = 8)	Healthy controls (n = 8)	p for difference
Age (years)	46.9 ± 12.9	44.5 ± 11.4	0.70
Male, no. (%)	5 (62.5)	5 (62.5)	1.00
BMI (kg/m^2)	23.5 ± 2.8	25.3 ± 2.9	0.23
Smokers, no. (%)	1 (12.5)	0 (0)	0.30
SBP (mmHg)	134 ± 13	133 ± 10	0.87
DBP (mmHg)	82 ± 11	78 ± 6	0.33
eGFR# (ml/min/1.73 m2)	57 ± 17	100 ± 8	< 0.01
IGF-1 (nmol/L)	26.3 ± 2.8	27.3 ± 6.8	0.71
Serum phosphate (mmol/L)	0.89 ± 0.16	1.01 ± 0.16	0.16
PTH (pmol/L)	7.3 ± 3.1	4.7 ± 1.2	0.05
25(OH)D3 (nmol/L)	70 ± 20	76 ± 30	0.69
cFGF23 (RU/mL) (median + IQR)	100 (77–127)	92 (80–105)	0.57
CRP < 10 (mg/L)	8 (100%)	8 (100%)	n/a
Albumin (g/L)	38.3 ± 2.1	38.0 ± 2.3	0.82
α-Klotho (pg/mL) (median + IQR)	554 (388–659)	547 (421–711)	0.57

[a]Values are expressed as mean ± SD, unless specified otherwise. *IQR* interquartile range
[b]Estimated GFR expressed using the Chronic Kidney Disease Epidemiology Collaboration (CKD-EPI) equation

($P = 0.13$) in the CKD and the healthy subgroup respectively. The difference in change of α-Klotho concentration was not statistically significant between the two subgroups (p for interaction = 0.71). All α-Klotho concentrations returned to baseline levels within one week after the treatment being stopped (Fig. 2a).

Figure 2: The effect of endogenous growth hormone therapy on serum α-klotho and cFGF23 concentrations
Serum cFGF23, serum phosphate, urinary phosphate excretion, TmP/GFR and PTH

Median of cFGF23 changed from 96.5 RU/mL (IQR: 80.3–120.5) to 126.0 RU/mL (IQR: 105.5–138.8; $p < 0.05$, Fig. 2b). In the CKD subgroup, median cFGF23 changed from 99.5 RU/mL (IQR: 77.3–127.3) to 132.5 (IQR: 112.0–138.8) ($P < 0.05$) and in healthy controls from 92.0 RU/mL (IQR: 80.3–105.3) to 114.0 RU/mL (IQR: 101.8–137.8) (P < 0.05). The rate of change in cFGF23 concentrations was not different between the two subgroups (P for interaction = 0.74, Table 2).

Serum phosphate concentrations, urinary phosphate excretion, the TmP/GFR and PTH did not change significantly in the entire cohort or both individual groups (Table 2).

Discussion
The main finding of our study is that GH therapy increases serum α-Klotho concentrations in subjects with normal kidney function or stage 3 CKD. α-Klotho concentrations increased in both subgroups, although within subgroups the increase did not reach statistical significance, most likely due to small subgroup size.

These results are in line with previous studies showing that GH therapy increases α-Klotho concentrations in GH deficient, paediatric and adult patients [24, 25]. Although the increment of α-Klotho concentrations was more prominent in the small study group of Locher et al.. However, they included GH-deficient subjects whereas in the present study GH-sufficient subjects were included. It is conceivable that an additional increment of α-Klotho concentrations is more difficult to achieve if IGF-1 concentrations are already sufficient.

Previous studies have convincingly shown that α-Klotho concentrations decrease as kidney function declines [29]. However, both α-Klotho and FGF23 concentrations in our patients of the CKD subgroup, which are classified as mild-moderate CKD according to the CKD-EPI were not significantly different from the healthy controls at baseline. This underlines the literature that shows that eGFR loss and decrease of serum α-Klotho concentrations do not parallel [30], and may depend on the ELISA used [26]. Moreover, there is oversampling in the CKD-subgroup close to stage 2 CKD, where soluble α-Klotho concentrations may be maintained in the normal range. Importantly, our study was underpowered to make firm statements about differences between the two subgroups.

Our findings show that α-Klotho concentrations are modifiable using administration of exogenous GH in a clinical cohort of subjects with mild CKD and healthy subjects. This increase may be of clinical relevance for patients with CKD in terms of CKD progression and cardiovascular risk as animal studies show that even small increases in α-Klotho concentrations are protective

Table 2 Time-related results within and between groups

	Entire cohort		Patients with CKD		Healthy controls		P interaction (time*group)
	Absolute change after 1 week of growth hormone administration (95% CI)	P	Absolute change after 1 week of growth hormone administration (95% CI)	P	Absolute change after 1 week of growth hormone administration (95% CI)	P	
IGF-1 (nmol/L)	34.9 (27.5–42.3)	< 0.01	33.5 (21.8–45.2)	< 0.01	36.4 (25.4–47.3)	< 0.01	0.71
Phosphate (mmol/L)	0.04 (−0.04–0.12)	0.34	−0.02 (−0.16–0.12)	0.78	0.10 (0.00–0.19)	0.05	0.15
Urinary phosphate excretion (mmol/L)	4.94 (−3.73–13.62)	0.25	−2.99 (−9.56–3.58)	0.34	12.88 (−3.10–28.9)	0.11	0.06
TMP/GFR (mmol/L)	0.06 (−0.04–0.17)	0.22	0.01 (−0.09–0.12)	0.78	0.11 (−0.08–0.30)	0.23	0.35
PTH (pmol/L)	−0.19 (−1.09–0.70)	0.66	−0.94 (−2.64–0.77)	0.26	0.55 (−0.18–1.28)	0.13	0.10
cFGF23 (RU/mL)	26.1 (15.7–36.6)	< 0.01	27.9 (12.3–43.5)	0.01	24.4 (8.0–40.8)	0.01	0.74
α-Klotho (pg/mL)	81.1 (1.7–160.4)	0.05	96.4 (−52.2–245.0)	0.19	65.8 (−20.8–152.3)	0.13	0.71

95%CI = 95% confidence interval. P interaction (time*group) is the interaction term between the CKD group and healthy controls

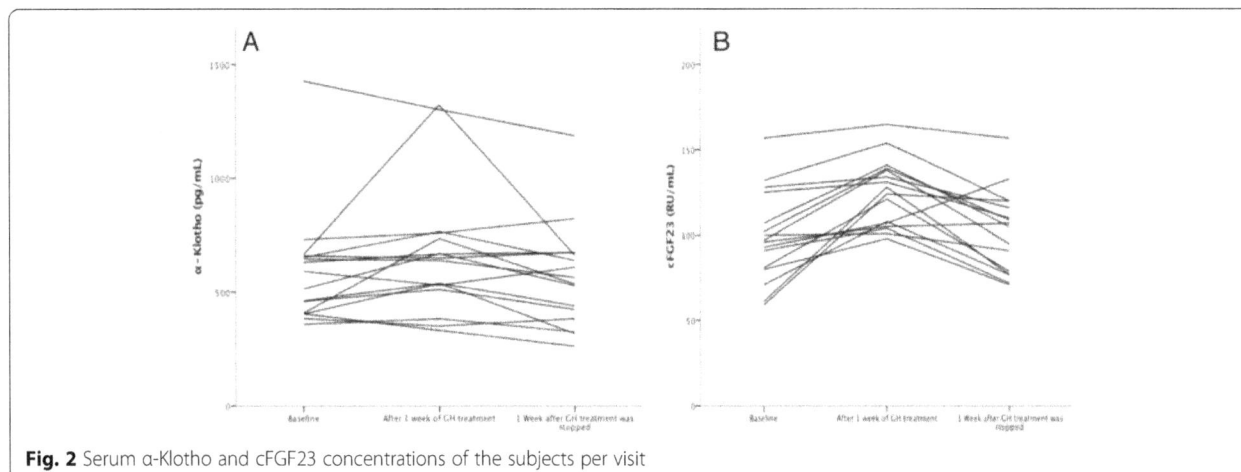

Fig. 2 Serum α-Klotho and cFGF23 concentrations of the subjects per visit

for remnant kidney function and attenuates cardiovascular intermediate endpoints [13, 31–33]. Obviously, this concept requires clinical studies to be confirmed.

Despite the reduced bioactivity of GH and IGF-1 observed in CKD, there is a valid rationale for the use of GH in this setting. Indeed, treatment with GH results in a decrease of serum IGFBP-1 concentrations and a marked increase in serum insulin, IGF-1, IGFBP-3 and IGFBP-5 concentrations, which subsequently leads to a marked increase in IGF-1 bioactivity [34, 35]. In a previous study exogenous GH therapy had no effect on all-cause mortality and cardiovascular morbidity and mortality in haemodialysis patients [36]. Although at that time its possible effect on α-Klotho was unknown. It is unlikely that major increments of α-Klotho did occur in these patients with end-stage kidney disease as the kidneys are the principal source of α-Klotho [37]. Moreover, the study was terminated early, none of the subjects completed the study and follow-up was short. On the contrary, some small short-term studies tested the effect of GH therapy in earlier stages of CKD and noted that GH therapy significantly improved LDL-cholesterol, phosphate and capillary blood flow, however no significant effect was demonstrated on intermediate endpoints, namely total peripheral vascular resistance and cardiac output [38, 39]. It would be very interesting to apply GH suppletion in well-powered studies including patients with CKD stage 4 and 5, not on dialysis, as well.

The absolute increase in α-Klotho concentrations in our study population was modest. This is also exemplified by the lack of robust effect on phosphate homeostatic parameters, measured in our study, including serum phosphate concentration and urinary excretion. The study design however precludes concluding if this effect would have been stronger with a longer duration or a higher dose of administrated GH. Given the strong phenotypic similarity between α-Klotho knockout models and CKD, and the wide range of CKD-related pathologies that in experimental

studies can be attenuated by exogenous α-Klotho, additional exploration is warranted of all options that upregulate endogenous α-Klotho, including GH therapy.

In agreement with other studies, our study showed that cFGF23 increases after GH therapy [25, 40]. However, previous studies also reported an increase in serum phosphate concentrations, which was not observed in the present study. Therefore, the hypothesis from the earlier studies that GH therapy induces FGF23 production in response to increased serum phosphate concentrations is not confirmed in our study [25]. Besides a stable serum phosphate concentration, phosphate excretion did not change either, despite an increase in cFGF23 and a slight increase in α-Klotho level. The explanation for a lack of effect on renal phosphate handling is not obvious from our data, although one could speculate that GH induced cleavage of tubular α-Klotho concentrations, leaving tubular cell deprived of α-Klotho, and as such promoting FGF23 resistance. Data on the effect of GH and IGF-1 on serum phosphate concentrations are highly contradictory [41, 42]. Unfortunately, only cFGF23 was measured in this study. However, the study of Effthymiadou et al. in 23 children with a GH-deficiency showed that both cFGF23 and iFGF23 increase after GH administration [25].

Bianda et al. reported a significant increase of serum 1,25-dihydroxyvitamin D3 $(1,25-(OH)_2D_3)$ concentrations after GH- or IGF-1 therapy [41]. Serum $1,25-(OH)_2D_3$ is known to upregulate FGF23 gene expression in bone and consequent gives a rise in serum FGF23 concentrations [43–47]. Therefore, the observed increase of serum cFGF23 concentrations might be explained by an assumed GH-induced rise in serum $1,25-(OH)_2D_3$ levels. Unfortunately, vitamin D concentrations were measured only at baseline in this study. Moreover, IGF-1 and GH treatment increase markers of bone turnover like serum osteocalcin and carboxyterminal propeptide of type 1 procollagen (PICP) as indicators of osteoblast activity [41, 42]. Therefore, it is conceivable that

GH has an indirect effect through IGF-1 on bone turnover and osteoblasts, one of the cell types, besides osteocytes, that produce FGF23. It is unknown if the potential beneficial effects of an increase of α-Klotho concentrations can outweigh the assumed dismal effects of increased cFGF23 concentrations.

Besides the small sample size of this study, there are some other limitations that need to be underlined. First, the exclusion criteria for participants limit generalizability, in particular for patients with more advanced CKD. Second, the specificity of the IBL-assay used to measure α-Klotho concentration is disputed [26, 48]. We did not use the semi-quantitative precipitation-immunoblotting technique as described by Barker et al., which probably has improved specificity [29]. This method awaits external validation in a different cohort and by different laboratories. Moreover, we recently found that the ELISA used in our study performs best among currently commercially available immunoassays [26]. Unfortunately, we were not able to assess the influence of GH therapy on membrane-bound α-Klotho due to the absence of kidney biopsies in our study. Finally, a study of longer duration is needed to determine the more long-term effects of GH on α-Klotho concentrations in the CKD population, and establish a dose-response effect. Our study however was designed as a proof of concept to study the modifiability of α-Klotho by GH.

Conclusions

In conclusion, exogenous GH therapy can induce a significant increase in α-Klotho concentrations in subjects with normal kidney function or stage 3 CKD. It is unknown if this can also be accomplished in more advanced CKD. Additional studies are necessary to study whether this increase of α-Klotho concentrations improves intermediate endpoints and subsequently patient-level outcome.

Abbreviations

ARBs: Angiotensin-receptor blockers; BMI: Body mass index; CKD: Chronic kidney disease; CKD-EPI: Chronic Kidney Disease Epidemiology Collaboration; CV: Cardiovascular; eGFR: Estimated glomerular filtration rate; FGF23: Fibroblast-growth-facor-23; GH: Growth hormone; GHST: Growth hormone suppletion therapy; IGF-1: Insulin growth factor-1; IQR: Interquartile range; LMM: Linear mixed models; PTH: Parathyroid hormone; SAE: Serious adverse event; TmP/GFR: Tubular maximal reabsorption of phosphate normalized to GFR; α-Klotho: Soluble alpha-Klotho

Acknowledgements

This work is supported by a consortium grant from the Dutch Kidney Foundation (NIGRAM Consortium, Grant No. CP10.11). The NIGRAM consortium consists of the following principal investigators: R. Bindels[1], J.G. Hoenderop[1], M.H. de Borst[2], J.L. Hillebrands[2], G.J. Navis[2], P.M. ter Wee[3] and M.G. Vervloet[3#]

[1]Department of Physiology, Radboud University medical center Nijmegen, The Netherlands.
[2]Department of Internal Medicine, Division of Nephrology, University Medical Center Groningen, Groningen, The Netherlands.
[3]Department of Nephrology, VU University Medical Center, Amsterdam, The Netherlands.
Lead author of the NIGRAM consortium (m.vervloet@vumc.nl).

Funding

The NIGRAM consortium is fully supported by the Dutch Kidney Foundation. Genotropin® was supplied by Pfizer. Both, the funder and Pfizer, had no role in the study design and/or report of this trial.

Authors' contributions

AA participated in the design of the study, collection of the data, statistical analysis and made substantial contributions to the interpretation of data and drafted the article. CRZ made contributions to the statistical analysis, interpretation of the data and revising the manuscript. JH, MB and PW and AH have participated in the design of the study, interpretation of the data and revising the manuscript. MV participated in the design of the study, collection of the data and made substantial contributions to the interpretation of data and drafted the article. All authors read and approved the final manuscript.

Competing interests

A.Y. Adema: None
C.L.M. de Roij van Zuijdewijn: None
J.G. Hoenderop: None
M.H. de Borst: None
P.M. ter Wee: None
A.C. Heijboer: None
M.G. Vervloet: received financial support for research, consultancy of lecture fees from Vifor, Fresenius Medical Care Renal Pharma, Amgen, Medice, Baxter, Shire and Otsuka.

Author details

[1]Department of Nephrology, VU University Medical Center, De Boelelaan 1117, 1081, HV, Amsterdam, The Netherlands. [2]Department of Physiology, Radboud University Medical Center Nijmegen, Nijmegen, The Netherlands. [3]Department of Internal Medicine, Division of Nephrology, University Medical Center Groningen, Groningen, The Netherlands. [4]Department of Clinical Chemistry, VU University Medical Center, Amsterdam, The Netherlands. [5]Amsterdam Cardiovascular Sciences (ACS), Amsterdam, The Netherlands.

References

1. Foley RN, Parfrey PS, Sarnak MJ. Epidemiology of cardiovascular disease in chronic renal disease. J Am Soc Nephrol. 1998;9:S16–23.
2. Olauson H, Vervloet MG, Cozzolino M, Massy ZA, Urena Torres P, Larsson TE. New insights into the FGF23-klotho axis. Semin Nephrol. 2014;34:586–97.
3. Kuro-o M, Matsumura Y, Aizawa H, Kawaguchi H, Suga T, Utsugi T, Ohyama Y, Kurabayashi M, Kaname T, Kume E, et al. Mutation of the mouse klotho gene leads to a syndrome resembling ageing. Nature. 1997;390:45–51.
4. Hu MC, Shi M, Zhang J, Pastor J, Nakatani T, Lanske B, Razzaque MS, Rosenblatt KP, Baum MG, Kuro-o M, Moe OW. Klotho: a novel phosphaturic substance acting as an autocrine enzyme in the renal proximal tubule. FASEB J. 2010;24:3438–50.
5. Kim HR, Nam BY, Kim DW, Kang MW, Han JH, Lee MJ, Shin DH, Doh FM, Koo HM, Ko KI, et al. Circulating alpha-klotho levels in CKD and relationship to progression. Am J Kidney Dis. 2013;61:899–909.
6. Semba RD, Cappola AR, Sun K, Bandinelli S, Dalal M, Crasto C, Guralnik JM, Ferrucci L. Plasma klotho and cardiovascular disease in adults. J Am Geriatr Soc. 2011;59:1596–601.
7. Kitagawa M, Sugiyama H, Morinaga H, Inoue T, Takiue K, Ogawa A, Yamanari T, Kikumoto Y, Uchida HA, Kitamura S, et al. A decreased level of serum soluble klotho is an independent biomarker associated with arterial stiffness in patients with chronic kidney disease. PLoS One. 2013;8:e56695.

8. Hu MC, Shi M, Zhang J, Quinones H, Griffith C, Kuro-o M, Moe OW. Klotho deficiency causes vascular calcification in chronic kidney disease. J Am Soc Nephrol. 2011;22:124–36.

9. Saito Y, Nakamura T, Ohyama Y, Suzuki T, Iida A, Shiraki-Iida T, Kuro-o M, Nabeshima Y, Kurabayashi M, Nagai R. In vivo klotho gene delivery protects against endothelial dysfunction in multiple risk factor syndrome. Biochem Biophys Res Commun. 2000;276:767–72.

10. Li BS, Ma HX, Wang YJ, Wu P. klotho gene attenuates the progression of hypertension and heart damage in spontaneous hypertensive rats. Zhonghua Yi Xue Yi Chuan Xue Za Zhi. 2012;29:662–8.

11. Xie J, Yoon J, An SW, Kuro OM, Huang CL. Soluble klotho protects against uremic cardiomyopathy independently of fibroblast growth factor 23 and phosphate. J Am Soc Nephrol. 2015;26:1150–60.

12. Ohta J, Rakugi H, Ishikawa K, Yang J, Ikushima M, Chihara Y, Maekawa Y, Oguro R, Hanasaki H, Kida I, et al. Klotho gene delivery suppresses oxidative stress in vivo. Geriatr Gerontol Int. 7(3):293–9.

13. Mitani H, Ishizaka N, Aizawa T, Ohno M, Usui S, Suzuki T, Amaki T, Mori I, Nakamura Y, Sato M, et al. In vivo klotho gene transfer ameliorates angiotensin II-induced renal damage. Hypertension. 2002;39:838–43.

14. Zhang H, Li Y, Fan Y, Wu J, Zhao B, Guan Y, Chien S, Wang N. Klotho is a target gene of PPAR-gamma. Kidney Int. 2008;74:732–9.

15. Yamagishi T, Saito Y, Nakamura T, Takeda S, Kanai H, Sumino H, Kuro-o M, Nabeshima Y, Kurabayashi M, Nagai R. Troglitazone improves endothelial function and augments renal klotho mRNA expression in Otsuka long-Evans Tokushima fatty (OLETF) rats with multiple atherogenic risk factors. Hypertens Res. 2001;24:705–9.

16. Yang HC, Deleuze S, Zuo Y, Potthoff SA, Ma LJ, Fogo AB. The PPARgamma agonist pioglitazone ameliorates aging-related progressive renal injury. J Am Soc Nephrol. 2009;20:2380–8.

17. Saito K, Ishizaka N, Mitani H, Ohno M, Nagai R. Iron chelation and a free radical scavenger suppress angiotensin II-induced downregulation of klotho, an anti-aging gene, in rat. FEBS Lett. 2003;551:58–62.

18. Yoon HE, Ghee JY, Piao S, Song JH, Han DH, Kim S, Ohashi N, Kobori H, Kuro-o M, Yang CW. Angiotensin II blockade upregulates the expression of klotho, the anti-ageing gene, in an experimental model of chronic cyclosporine nephropathy. Nephrol Dial Transplant. 2011;26:800–13.

19. Mitobe M, Yoshida T, Sugiura H, Shirota S, Tsuchiya K, Nihei H. Oxidative stress decreases klotho expression in a mouse kidney cell line. Nephron Exp Nephrol. 2005;101:e67–74.

20. Kuwahara N, Sasaki S, Kobara M, Nakata T, Tatsumi T, Irie H, Narumiya H, Hatta T, Takeda K, Matsubara H, Hushiki S. HMG-CoA reductase inhibition improves anti-aging klotho protein expression and arteriosclerosis in rats with chronic inhibition of nitric oxide synthesis. Int J Cardiol. 2008;123:84–90.

21. Karalliedde J, Maltese G, Hill B, Viberti G, Gnudi L. Effect of renin-angiotensin system blockade on soluble klotho in patients with type 2 diabetes, systolic hypertension, and albuminuria. Clin J Am Soc Nephrol. 2013;8:1899–905.

22. Donate-Correa J, Henriquez-Palop F, Martin-Nunez E, Perez-Delgado N, Muros-de-Fuentes M, Mora-Fernandez C, Navarro-Gonzalez JF. Effect of Paricalcitol on FGF-23 and klotho in kidney transplant recipients. Transplantation. 2016;100:2432–8.

23. Schmid C, Neidert MC, Tschopp O, Sze L, Bernays RL. Growth hormone and klotho. J Endocrinol. 2013;219:R37–57.

24. Locher R, Egger A, Zwimpfer C, Sze L, Schmid C, Christ E. Effect of growth hormone replacement therapy on soluble klotho in patients with growth hormone deficiency. Clin Endocrinol. 2015;83(4):593–5.

25. Efthymiadou A, Kritikou D, Mantagos S, Chrysis D. The effect of GH treatment on serum FGF23 and klotho in GH-deficient children. Eur J Endocrinol. 2016;174:473–9.

26. Heijboer AC, Blankenstein MA, Hoenderop J, de Borst MH, Vervloet MG. Laboratory aspects of circulating alpha-klotho. Nephrol Dial Transplant. 2013;28:2283–7.

27. Heijboer AC, Levitus M, Vervloet MG, Lips P, ter Wee PM, Dijstelbloem HM, Blankenstein MA. Determination of fibroblast growth factor 23. Ann Clin Biochem. 2009;46:338–40.

28. Walton RJ, Bijvoet OL. Nomogram for derivation of renal threshold phosphate concentration. Lancet. 1975;2:309–10.

29. Barker SL, Pastor J, Carranza D, Quinones H, Griffith C, Goetz R, Mohammadi M, Ye J, Zhang J, Hu MC, et al. The demonstration of alphaKlotho deficiency in human chronic kidney disease with a novel synthetic antibody. Nephrol Dial Transplant. 2015;30:223–33.

30. Seiler S, Wen M, Roth HJ, Fehrenz M, Flugge F, Herath E, Weihrauch A, Fliser D, Heine GH. Plasma klotho is not related to kidney function and does not predict adverse outcome in patients with chronic kidney disease. Kidney Int. 2013;83:121–8.

31. Haruna Y, Kashihara N, Satoh M, Tomita N, Namikoshi T, Sasaki T, Fujimori T, Xie P, Kanwar YS. Amelioration of progressive renal injury by genetic manipulation of klotho gene. Proc Natl Acad Sci U S A. 2007;104:2331–6.

32. Sugiura H, Yoshida T, Tsuchiya K, Mitobe M, Nishimura S, Shirota S, Akiba T, Nihei H. Klotho reduces apoptosis in experimental ischaemic acute renal failure. Nephrol Dial Transplant. 2005;20:2636–45.

33. Sugiura H, Yoshida T, Mitobe M, Yoshida S, Shiohira S, Nitta K, Tsuchiya K. Klotho reduces apoptosis in experimental ischaemic acute kidney injury via HSP-70. Nephrol Dial Transplant. 2010;25:60–8.

34. Mak RH, Cheung WW, Roberts CT Jr. The growth hormone-insulin-like growth factor-I axis in chronic kidney disease. Growth Hormon IGF Res. 2008;18:17–25.

35. Bach LA, Hale LJ. Insulin-like growth factors and kidney disease. Am J Kidney Dis. 2015;65:327–36.

36. Kopple JD, Cheung AK, Christiansen JS, Djurhuus CB, El Nahas M, Feldt-Rasmussen B, Mitch WE, Wanner C, Gothberg M, Ikizler TA. OPPORTUNITY™: a large-scale randomized clinical trial of growth hormone in hemodialysis patients. Nephrol Dial Transplant. 2011;26:4095–103.

37. Lindberg K, Amin R, Moe OW, Hu MC, Erben RG, Ostman Wernerson A, Lanske B, Olauson H, Larsson TE. The kidney is the principal organ mediating klotho effects. J Am Soc Nephrol. 2014;25:2169–75.

38. Fischer DC, Nissel R, Puhlmann A, Mitzner A, Tiess M, Schmidt R, Haffner D. Differential effects of short-term growth hormone therapy on the cardiovascular risk profile in patients with chronic kidney disease: a pilot study. Clin Nephrol. 2009;72:344–52.

39. Nissel R, Fischer DC, Puhlmann A, Holdt-Lehmann B, Mitzner A, Petzsch M, Korber T, Tiess M, Schmidt R, Haffner D. Short-term growth hormone treatment and microcirculation: effects in patients with chronic kidney disease. Microvasc Res. 2009;78:246–52.

40. Gardner J, Ashraf A, You Z, McCormick K. Changes in plasma FGF23 in growth hormone deficient children during rhGH therapy. J Pediatr Endocrinol Metab. 2011;24:645–50.

41. Bianda T, Glatz Y, Bouillon R, Froesch ER, Schmid C. Effects of short-term insulin-like growth factor-I (IGF-I) or growth hormone (GH) treatment on bone metabolism and on production of 1,25-dihydroxycholecalciferol in GH-deficient adults. J Clin Endocrinol Metab. 1998;83:81–7.

42. Bianda T, Hussain MA, Glatz Y, Bouillon R, Froesch ER, Schmid C. Effects of short-term insulin-like growth factor-I or growth hormone treatment on bone turnover, renal phosphate reabsorption and 1,25 dihydroxyvitamin D3 production in healthy man. J Intern Med. 1997;241:143–50.

43. Kolek OI, Hines ER, Jones MD, LK LS, Lipko MA, Kiela PR, Collins JF, Haussler MR, Ghishan FK. 1alpha,25-Dihydroxyvitamin D3 upregulates FGF23 Gene Expr in bone: the final link in a renal-gastrointestinal-skeletal axis that controls phosphate Transport. Am J Physiol Gastrointest Liver Physiol. 2005;289:G1036–42.

44. Shimada T, Hasegawa H, Yamazaki Y, Muto T, Hino R, Takeuchi Y, Fujita T, Nakahara K, Fukumoto S, Yamashita T. FGF-23 is a potent regulator of vitamin D metabolism and phosphate homeostasis. J Bone Miner Res. 2004;19:429–35.

45. Saito H, Maeda A, Ohtomo S, Hirata M, Kusano K, Kato S, Ogata E, Segawa H, Miyamoto K, Fukushima N. Circulating FGF-23 is regulated by 1alpha,25-dihydroxyvitamin D3 and phosphorus in vivo. J Biol Chem. 2005;280:2543–9.

46. Nishi H, Nii-Kono T, Nakanishi S, Yamazaki Y, Yamashita T, Fukumoto S, Ikeda K, Fujimori A, Fukagawa M. Intravenous calcitriol therapy increases serum concentrations of fibroblast growth factor-23 in dialysis patients with secondary hyperparathyroidism. Nephron Clin Pract. 2005;101:c94–9.

47. Hansen D, Rasmussen K, Pedersen SM, Rasmussen LM, Brandi L. Changes in fibroblast growth factor 23 during treatment of secondary hyperparathyroidism with alfacalcidol or paricalcitol. Nephrol Dial Transplant. 2012;27:2263–9.

48. Pedersen L, Pedersen SM, Brasen CL, Rasmussen LM. Soluble serum klotho levels in healthy subjects. Comparison of two different immunoassays. Clin Biochem. 2013;46:1079–83.

19

Transport of neutral IgG2 versus anionic IgG4 in PD: implications on the electrokinetic model

Anneleen Pletinck, Wim Van Biesen*ⓘ, Clement Dequidt and Sunny Eloot

Abstract

Background: It is debated whether transperitoneal membrane transport of larger (charged) molecules in peritoneal dialysis can be partially governed by the electrokinetic model. In this model, it is postulated that streaming potentials are generated across the capillary wall by forced filtration of an ionic solution, for example transcapillary ultrafiltration induced by osmotic forces as in peritoneal dialysis. We investigated the presence of streaming potentials in the process of transperitoneal transport in Peritoneal Dialysis (PD) patients by measuring ratios of dialysate concentrations of IgG2 (neutral) and IgG4 (negative), both 150kD, under different conditions of transcapillary ultrafiltration.

Methods: Adult PD patients randomly got two consecutive dwells of 120 min each, with either 2 L Physioneal 1.36% or 3.86% glucose dialysis fluid (Baxter, USA) as their first dwell. A blood sample was taken at the test start, and dialysate samples were taken at 5, 15, 30, 60 and 120 min. IgG2 and IgG4 concentrations were measured (ELISA) and ratios calculated.

Results: In 10 patients (65 ± 17 years, 20 ± 17 months on dialysis), drained volume after 120 min was different between the 1.36% (1950 [1910; 2020] mL) and 3.86% (2540 [2380; 2800] mL) glucose dwells ($P = 0.007$). At none of the time points and irrespective of glucose concentration, a significant difference was found between the IgG2/IgG4 ratios at any time point.

Conclusion: Our data failed to demonstrate a difference in the transport ratios of two macromolecules with same molecular weight but different charge, as would be expected by the electrokinetic model, and this despite sufficient differences in transcapillary ultrafiltration.

Clinical trial registry: Belgian Registration Number B670201523397 (20/1/2015); prospective randomized trial.

Keywords: Peritoneal Dialysis, Transperitoneal membrane transport, Immunoglobulin, Three pore theory, Elektrokinetic model

Background

Within the electrokinetic model, streaming potentials are generated across a filter by forced filtration of an ionic solution [1]. The force and direction of the induced electrical field are in theory determined by the amount of flux through the filter pores, and add another transport force through electrophoresis, influencing the passage of charged macromolecules across the pores [2]. This hypothetical electrokinetic force

was previously not considered to be present across capillary walls. It is usually observed that capillary walls are negatively charged, and the electrical field should thus be positive on the outside and negative on the inside of the capillary wall. As most plasma proteins (e.g. albumin) are negatively charged, the polarity of such electrical field would result in increased transcapillary transport. In reality, these negatively charged molecules appear to be repelled from the pores towards the capillary lumen, which would presume the presence of a reversed streaming potential [3]. Whereas this seems plausible from the theoretical

* Correspondence: Wim.vanbiesen@ugent.be
Nephrology Division, Ghent University Hospital, C. Heymanslaan 10, 9000 Ghent, Belgium

perspective, and fits with observational data, its occurrence in real life is still a matter of debate. Recently, the presence of reversed streaming potentials was reported in the glomerular membrane of Necturus [4] and the bovine lens basement membrane [5].

In peritoneal dialysis (PD) it is accepted that solute transport across the peritoneal membrane can be modelled by the three pore model [6], where the transport barrier consists of a serial coupling of two distinct systems: the interendothelial slits of the capillary wall itself, and the matrix of the interstitial tissue in which the capillary is imbedded. This results in a much longer diffusion distance than for example in a human glomerulus [7]. As a consequence, transport over the peritoneal membrane behaves more like that in a gel column, whereas transport in the human glomerulus behaves more like that of a synthetic dialyser [8]. Available evidence seems to suggest that electrostatic forces have little impact in this system. There is apparently no electrostatic charge selectivity over the peritoneal membrane [9, 10]. It has been debated whether this transport can also be governed by electrokinetic forces [11–14]. In this model, it is postulated that streaming potentials are generated across the capillary wall by forced filtration of an ionic solution, for example transcapillary ultrafiltration induced by osmotic forces as in peritoneal dialysis. Accordingly, transport of solutes with the same molecular weight but different charge (e.g. IgG2 & IgG4) would be different at different time points during the dwell, an effect that would be further enhanced when transcapillary ultrafiltration is enhanced by using hypertonic glucose.

If this electrokinetic model exists in the peritoneal membrane, it will alter our understanding of transperitoneal transport, potentially opening new opportunities to use alternative osmotic agents, develop protective strategies, or detect early changes in peritoneal membrane integrity. Furthermore, a better understanding of streaming potentials would lead to a better insight in the increased transperitoneal protein loss in PD over time.

Our study therefore intends to investigate the hypothesis of the presence of (reversed) streaming potentials in the process of transperitoneal transport in PD patients by measuring dialysate IgG2/IgG4 concentration ratios, under different conditions of transcapillary ultrafiltration. These differences were induced by using non-hypertonic vs hypertonic glucose, and by measuring at different time points during the dwell, as transcapillary ultrafiltration is also decreasing with dwell time. If streaming potentials do play a role, these differences in transcapillary ultrafiltration will result in different IgG2/IgG4 ratios during the dwell, and also between the non-hypertonic and hypertonic exchanges.

Methods

Consecutive adult patients on peritoneal dialysis in the Ghent University Hospital were asked consent for participation in this prospective randomized cross-over study until 10 patients had completed the study. Exclusion criteria were active infection, pregnancy, unstable hemodynamic condition precluding use of hypertonic glucose, peritonitis in the last 4 weeks preceding the study, and age below 18. Patients with malfunctioning catheters were excluded. Malfunctioning was assessed based on medical history. In addition, when on a routine Peritoneal Equilibration Test (PET) test residual volume was more than 15%, the patient was also excluded.

The study was approved by the local Ethics Committee (Commissie voor Medische Ethiek - UZ Gent - Ref 2015/0075 - Belgian Registration Number B670201523397), and written informed consent was obtained from all participants.

Study flow is depicted in Fig. 1. Patients got two consecutive dwells of each 120 min with either 2 L Physioneal 1.36% or 2 L Physioneal 3.86% glucose dialysis fluid (Baxter, USA) as their first or second dwell. Randomisation was obtained with www.randomization.com.

A blood sample was taken from the patient before the test start, and dialysate samples were taken during each dwell at 5, 15, 30, 60 and 120 min via the peritoneal catheter. At each of these time points, the patient was first rolled from side to side to enhance optimal fluid mixing in the peritoneal cavity before 200 mL dialysate fluid was drained to diminish the impact of remaining fluid in the catheter's dead volume. Of this sample, 30 mL was sampled and put on ice for transport to the laboratory, while the remaining 170 mL were re-instilled into the peritoneal cavity. After 120 min dwell time, dialysate fluid was drained completely, and the volume checked using gravity.

Samples were immediately centrifuged at 4 °C during 10 min (3000 rpm for blood samples, and 1800 rpm for dialysate samples), after which the serum and dialysate were stored at − 80 °C until batch analysis. For all samples, IgG2 and IgG4 concentrations were estimated using commercially available ELISAs (platinum ELISA,

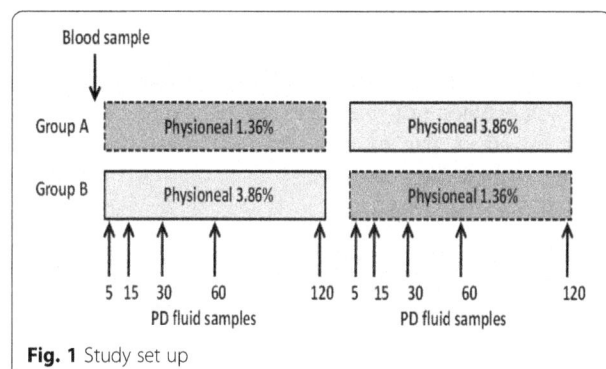

Fig. 1 Study set up

eBioscience, USA). Preliminary tests were performed to check the most optimal dilution of the samples for the respective ELISAs; for serum, dilutions were needed of 1/500,000 (IgG2) and 1/5000 (IgG4), and for dialysate fluid dilutions were 1/500 (IgG2) and 1/10 (IgG4 at time point 5, 15, and 30 min) and 1/50 (IgG4 at time point 60 and 120 min).

For each time point and in each patient, the ratio of IgG2 over IgG4 concentrations was calculated.

Specificity

The IgG2 and IgG4 assays detect both natural and recombinant human IgG2 and IgG4 respectively. No cross reactivity or interference of circulating factors of the immune system was detected. The curves obtained by serial dilutions of the dialysate was parallel to the standard curve.

Sensitivity

The limit of detection of resp. human IgG2 and IgG4 defined as the analyte concentration resulting in an absorbance significantly higher than that of the dilution medium (mean plus 2 standard deviations) was determined to be resp. 0.25 ng/ml and 0.1 ng/ml (mean of 4 independent assays).

Precision

The intra-assay coefficient of variation for serum samples was 3.6% for IgG2 and IgG4. The intra-assay coefficient of variation for dialysate samples was 4.3% for IgG2 and 5.9% for IgG4.

Statistical methods

Statistical analyses were performed with SPSS 23 (IBM©). To compare results from the 1.36% to 3.86% dwell, patients were considered their own control, so a paired non-parametric analysis was applied (Wilcoxon Signed Rank test for non-normally distributed data). For the evolution of IgG2/IgG4 over the dwell time, a repeated measures Friedman analysis was applied. We also constructed a general linear model for ratio of IgG2/IgG4, including patient identification, osmotic tonicity and time points as covariates, and interaction terms for tonicity and time points.

No formal sample size calculation was performed, as this was deemed not reliable as no data were available to estimate effect size or standard deviation and patients served as their own controls.

Results

Ten patients (2 women; 4 with diabetes mellitus), 65 ± 17 years of age, 20 ± 17 months on dialysis, and with a residual renal function of 9.7 ± 5.6 mL/min/1.73m² at the time of the study were included. Drained volume

after 120 min was different between the 1.36% and the 3.86% glucose dwells: i.e. 1950 [1910; 2020] mL versus 2540 [2380;2800] mL, respectively ($P = 0.007$).

Serum concentrations were 1.7 [0.8; 2.9] mg/mL for IgG2 and 1.3 [0.2;2.4] mg/mL for IgG4.

IgG2/IgG4 concentration ratios in dialysate are shown in Table 1 and Fig. 2 for the different time points during the PD test sessions, and for the different used PD fluids, i.e. Physioneal 1.36% versus 3.86%. At none of the time points, a significant difference was found between the 1.36% and the 3.86% ratios (Table 1). In none of the patients a difference in IgG2/IgG4 ratio was found at different time points of the dwell, neither when using the 1.36 nor the 3.86% solution.

In the general linear model ($p < 0.001$, $R^2 = 0.022$,), only patient identification but not use of hypertonic vs non-hypertonic bags or timepoint of dwell had an impact on IgG2/IgG4 ratio (Table 2).

Raw data for individual patients of concentrations of IgG2 and IgG4 in serum and in dialysate at different time points for the hypertonic and non-hypertonic exchanges are presented in Tables 3 and 4. Figure 3 represents the evolution during the dwell of IgG2, IgG4 and the IgG2/IgG4 ratio for individual patients.

Discussion

This paper evaluates the plausibility that transperitoneal transport of macromolecules is governed by an electrokinetic force induced by reversed streaming potentials. In our experiments we failed to demonstrate a difference in the transport ratios of two macromolecules with the same molecular weight but with a different charge (neutral IgG2 and negatively charged IgG4), as would be expected if such electrokinetic forces would be present, and this despite the fact that sufficient differences were obtained in transcapillary ultrafiltration by using two different osmotic strengths of glucose. Also, no difference could be observed between the transport ratios at different time points, in contrast to what would be expected if the electrokinetic model would apply, as transcapillary ultrafiltration decreases during the dwell.

The electrokinetic model of transcapillary transport has been a subject of debate for a long time [11–14].

Table 1 IgG2/IgG4 ratios at different time points during the PD test session with Physioneal 1.36% and Physioneal 3.86%

Time (min)	Physioneal 1.36%	Physioneal 3.86%	P-value
5	2.4 [1.5; 10.6]	3.2 [1.3; 10.6]	1.00
15	2.3 [1.3; 9.1]	2.5 [1.2; 8.9]	1.00
30	2.3 [1.4; 9.2]	2.2 [1.3; 8.2]	0.13
60	2.1 [1.2; 7.9]	2.3 [1.3; 8.7]	1.00
120	1.9 [1.1; 8.5]	2.1 [1.1; 8.9]	0.73

Median [interquartile range]

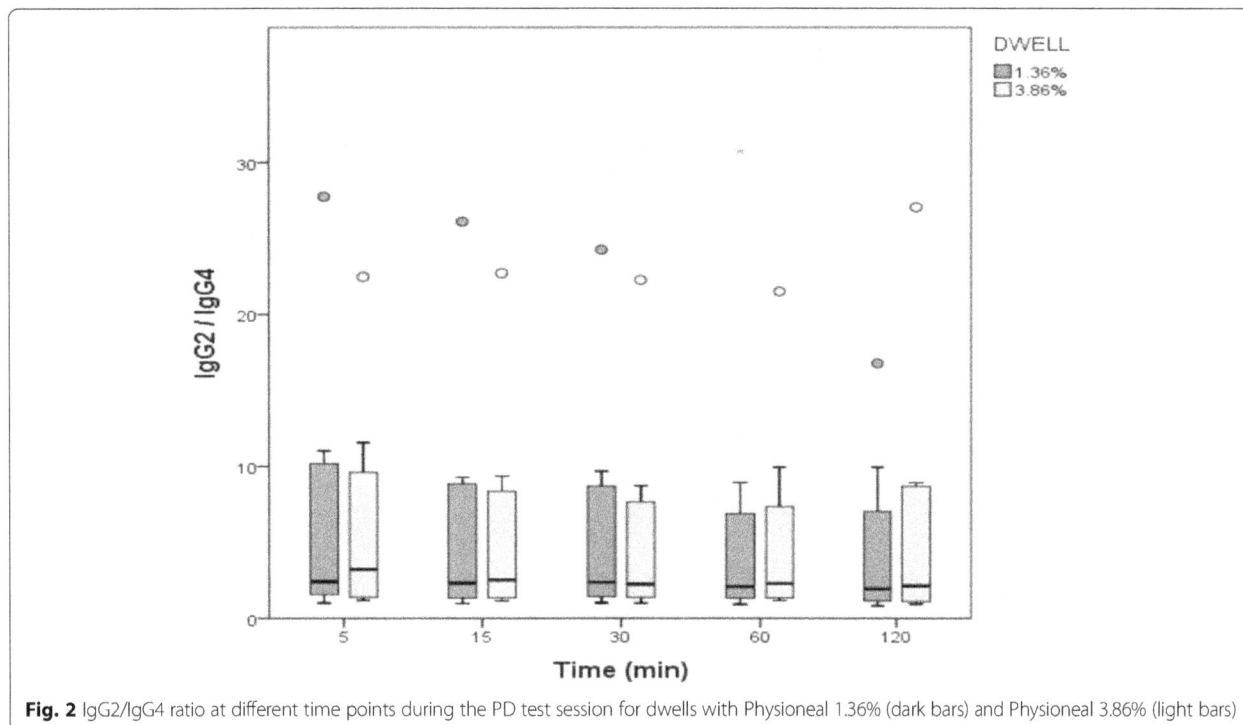

Fig. 2 IgG2/IgG4 ratio at different time points during the PD test session for dwells with Physioneal 1.36% (dark bars) and Physioneal 3.86% (light bars)

Proponents of the model claim that the model is able to explain several observations that cannot be explained otherwise by other models [3]. The pathophysiology of proteinuria for example is so far not completely explained by one of the existing models. Most strikingly, it is difficult to explain why proteins are not clogging up the pores of the glomerulus; existence of reverse streaming potentials would provide a sufficient explanation for this [1, 2]. So far, the presence of reverse streaming potentials over the glomerular basement membrane has only been demonstrated in mudpuppy (Necturus) [4]. However, it has been argued that the anatomical structure of the glomerulus of Necturus is much

different from that in humans, and that as such it is difficult to make extrapolations to the human situation. The glomerular filtration barrier in Necturus is 10 fold thicker than in humans (3.5 μm vs 0.3 μm), and has a more "tissue like" appearance [12]. Also in the bovine lens basement membrane, the other setting where streaming potentials have been observed, the filtration barrier is much thicker, and has a tissue like structure.

In peritoneal dialysis, there is an observation of higher transperitoneal protein transport in conditions of inflammation [15, 16]. Whereas it is tempting to explain this by an increased recruitment of capillaries, and thus higher availability of large pores, adjusting for surface

Table 2 General linear model for IgG2/IgG4 ratio

Source	Type III Sum of Squares	df	Mean Square	F	Sig.
Corrected Model	1040,462[a]	5	208,092	4620	,001
Intercept	6375	1	6375	,142	,708
Tonicity	7999	1	7999	,178	,675
Timepoint	7579	1	7579	,168	,683
Tonicity * timepoint	8309	1	8309	,184	,669
Patient identification	499,674	1	499,674	11,094	,001
timepoint * patient identification	2015	1	2015	,045	,833
Error	3603,201	80	45,040		
Total	8061,235	86			
Corrected Total	4643,663	85			

Table 3 dialysate concentrations for IgG2 and IgG4 at different timepoints for the different glucose strengths

PatientN°	dwell	Time point	IgG2 (ng/ml)	IgG4 (ng/ml)	Ratio (IgG2/IgG4)
1	1,36%	5	5824,5	3772,9	1, 54
		15	6746,5	5239,7	1, 29
		30	8210,5	5573,6	1, 47
		60	11,730,5	10,122	1, 16
		120	14,743,5	13,771	1, 07
	3,86%	5	2455,9	1733,8	1, 42
		15	3344,1	2185,2	1, 53
		30	4464,6	3043,9	1, 47
		60	5014,5	3670,8	1, 37
		120	6808,0	6290	1, 08
2	1,36%	5	9411,0	4465	2, 11
		15	12,267,5	5136,1	2, 39
		30	16,719,5	6263,2	2, 67
		60	20,711,0	10,830,5	1, 91
		120	33,158,0	17,144,5	1, 93
	3,86%	5	4321,2	1745,9	2, 48
		15	7379,0	3371,3	2, 19
		30	8311,0	4307	1, 93
		60	10,110,5	6497	1, 56
		120	14,258,0	8826,5	1, 62
3	1,36%	5	1028,6	93,335	11, 02
		15	1551,4	167	9, 29
		30	2284,8	236,06	9, 68
		60	3461,4	387,02	8, 94
		120	6653,0	668,75	9, 95
	3,86%	5	1994,5	172,41	11, 57
		15	3157,1	336,96	9, 37
		30	3868,1	442,99	8, 73
		60	5520,0	554,5	9, 95
		120	7742,5	916,15	8, 45
4	1,36%	5	870,5	/	/
		15	1294,4	/	/
		30	1732,4	/	/
		60	2317,0	/	/
		120	3979,2	/	/
	3,86%	5	1933,7	/	/
		15	2425,8	/	/
		30	2663,9	/	/
		60	2977,1	/	/
		120	4251,7	/	/
5	1,36%	5	1243,1	133,23	9, 33
		15	1454,8	172,31	8, 44
		30	1701,4	220,51	7, 72
		60	1995,6	414,62	4, 81

Table 3 dialysate concentrations for IgG2 and IgG4 at different timepoints for the different glucose strengths *(Continued)*

PatientN°	dwell	Time point	IgG2 (ng/ml)	IgG4 (ng/ml)	Ratio (IgG2/IgG4)
		120	2706,5	658,97	4, 11
	3,86%	5	2793,9	365,08	7, 65
		15	3064,0	417,25	7,34
		30	2745,9	417,16	6, 58
		60	2813,2	591,48	4, 76
		120	3832,0	429,14	8, 93
6	1,36%	5	2322,8	2347,4	0, 99
		15	2703,9	2817,2	0, 96
		30	3528,3	3515,1	1, 00
		60	4134,3	4605	0, 90
		120	5747,5	7067	0, 81
	3,86%	5	2455,5	2125,6	1, 16
		15	2721,1	2423,5	1, 12
		30	2563,9	2614	0, 98
		60	3268,3	2860,65	1, 14
		120	4040,1	4378,95	0, 92
7	1,36%	5	672,1	435,84	1, 54
		15	878,6	668,1	1, 32
		30	1158,8	883,53	1, 31
		60	1793,4	1257,8	1, 43
		120	2564,0	2202,15	1, 16
	3,86%	5	3099,6	2373	1, 31
		15	3363,4	2987,7	1, 13
		30	3941,3	3195,9	1, 23
		60	4324,0	3469,4	1, 25
		120	4521,3	4169,65	1, 08
8	1,36%	5	374,6	/	#WAARDE!
		15	609,5	/	#WAARDE!
		30	758,1	85,828	8, 83
		60	1071,6	/	#WAARDE!
		120	1803,2	/	#WAARDE!
	3,86%	5	619,2	65,01	9, 52
		15	905,7	100,245	9, 03
		30	966,7	85,828	11, 26
		60	1071,6	165,245	6, 48
		120	1367,3	231,85	5, 90
9	1,36%	5	1027,6	387,02	2, 66
		15	1303,1	591,82	2, 20
		30	1702,0	851,32	2, 00
		60	2204,0	1002,75	2, 20
		120	3261,2	1710	1, 91
	3,86%	5	665,5	169,33	3, 93
		15	979,5	347,67	2, 82
		30	1337,8	533,77	2, 51

Table 3 dialysate concentrations for IgG2 and IgG4 at different timepoints for the different glucose strengths *(Continued)*

PatientN°	dwell	Time point	IgG2 (ng/ml)	IgG4 (ng/ml)	Ratio (IgG2/IgG4)
		60	2037,2	686,15	2, 97
		120	3241,4	1244,8	2, 60
10	1,36%	5	7565,5	272,53	27 ,76
		15	10,973,5	420,25	26, 11
		30	14,616,0	602,27	24, 27
		60	24,084,0	783	30, 76
		120	24,346,3	1451,15	16, 78
	3,86%	5	3807,8	169,33	22, 49
		15	6596,5	290,23	22, 73
		30	8999,0	403,69	22, 29
		60	12,620,5	586,42	21, 52
		120	17,677,5	653,25	27, 06

area increase does not completely abolish this effect, suggesting that inflammation alters large pore transport per se [17]. A change in electrical charge of the capillary wall, and thus in the streaming potential over the large pores, is an attractive alternative explanation. Presence of an electrokinetic model and streaming potentials could easily explain why transperitoneal leakage only occurs to a limited extent at one and, more substantially, at another moment, as the strength and direction of the electrical field would determine protein flux. It is important that this process, though also based on electrical charges, is different from pure charge selectivity, in which charged molecules cannot pass through a pore because its effective size is smaller than its actual (anatomical) size. Previous literature has demonstrated that such a charge selectivity cannot be observed in peritoneal dialysis [9]. It can be hypothesized that small and large pores are actually the same anatomical entity, but that differences in integrity of the glycocalyx or the interstitial

Table 4 Serum values for IgG2 and IgG4 for individual patients at time point 0

PatientN°	IgG2 (ng/ml)	IgG4 (ng/ml)
1	1,758,200	2,379,000
2	3,954,600	2,490,400
3	1,053,150	173,835
4	875,000	/
5	256,640	84,665
6	1,810,300	3,030,500
7	831,750	1,284,000
8	686,250	150,925
9	1,656,800	1,917,900
10	7,310,500	764,950

space will govern transport properties by differing streaming potentials. Our results however do not add credibility to the hypothesis of streaming potentials being valid in peritoneal dialysis, as no differences were observed in the kinetic behaviour of IgG2 and IgG4, and this despite sufficient differences in generated flux by using different osmolarities of dialysate, and sampling at different time points in the dwell.

Different explanations can be forwarded to explain our negative findings.

First, it might be that IgG2 and IgG4 are not suitable to test the (hypothetical) impact of the electrokinetic forces in peritoneal dialysis. Although they have a different charge, IgG2 and IgG4 both have a comparable molecular weight around 150kD, which is 3 fold higher than that of albumin. Also, albumin has a globular structure, whereas immunoglobulins have not, but can have different, more tube-like shapes. As such, the hindrance in transport purely based on sterical hindrance can be so big that eventual small charge effects as would be induced by the electrokinetic forces in the peritoneal capillary, are overruled. However, at the level of the glomerular basement membrane, IgG2/IgG4 ratio was found to be decreased in patients with glomerulonephritis as compared to healthy volunteers (nearly 3 fold) or patients with other causes of underlying kidney disease [18]. This finding was attributed to a loss of charge selectivity of the glomerular barrier due to local inflammation. IgG2/IgG4 ratios have also been used to assess glomerular charge selectivity in non-diabetic renal disease, and correlate well with albuminuria. The large pores of the glomerular basement membrane are however much smaller (80–100 Ångstrøm) than the large pores of the peritoneal membrane (200–300 Ångstrøm), so that sterical hindrance is thus less likely to be an explanation for our observations. Potentially,

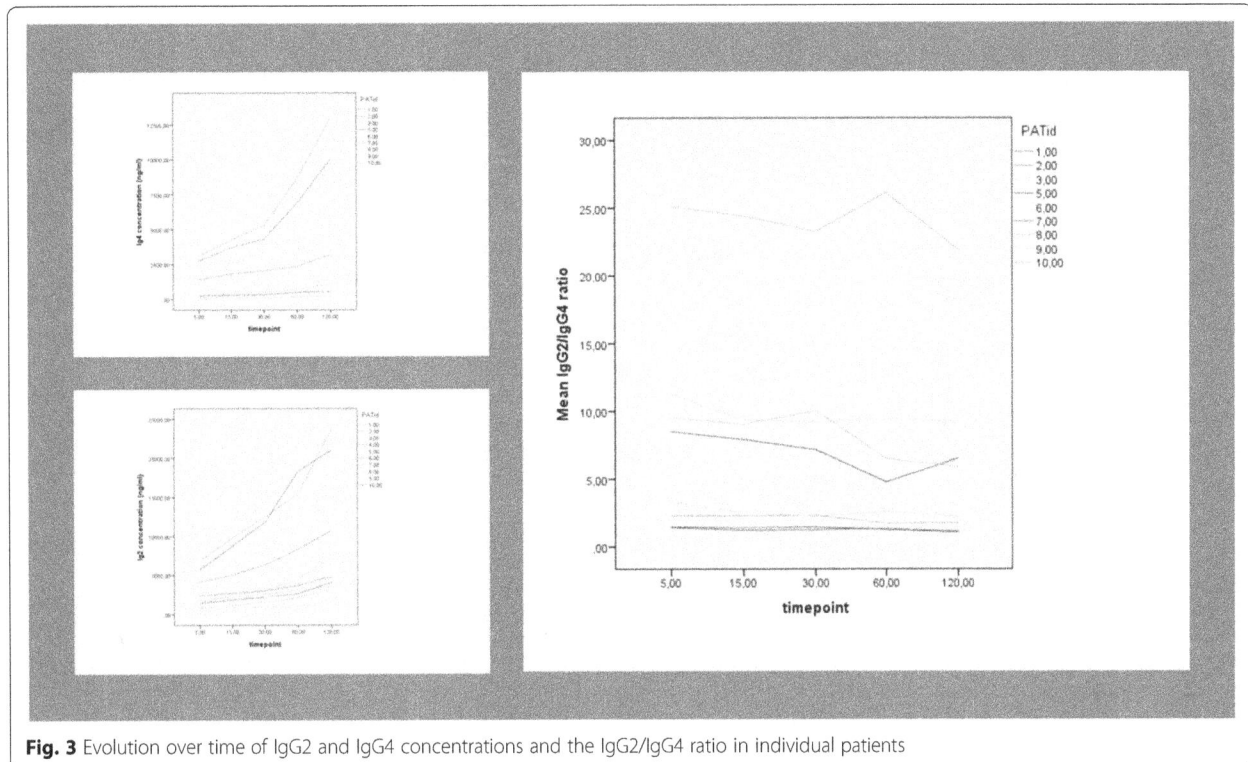

Fig. 3 Evolution over time of IgG2 and IgG4 concentrations and the IgG2/IgG4 ratio in individual patients

other pairs of endogenous or exogenous molecules should be used to test the hypothesis that the electrokinetic model is valid in peritoneal dialysis, preferentially with different ranges of molecular weight and difference in charge.

Second, it might be that the electrokinetic model cannot be applicable to peritoneal membrane transport because of huge differences between anatomical structures surrounding the capillaries of the glomerular barrier versus those of the peritoneal membrane [8]. Whereas the glomerular barrier is very thin, and allows selectivity based on size, flexibility, shape and charge, the peritoneal membrane resembles more a gel filtration model. Solute transport pathways comprise the inter-endothelial slits, coupled in series with the interstitial space, which is much larger in the peritoneal membrane than in the glomerular basement membrane. Accordingly, again, eventual small effects induced by electrokinetic forces can be masked by bigger sterical hindrance for larger molecules. Reversal of streaming potentials has however so far only been reported in thicker membranes, such as bovine lens and the glomerulus of the Necturus, which have also a distinct anatomical configuration with a more expressed interstitial space, such as present in the peritoneal membrane.

Third, it might be that we did not achieve a sufficient gradient of solute drag and transcapillary ultrafiltration. However, we actually achieved a difference in ultrafiltration of 500 mL over a 2 h dwell, which is

equivalent to a mean transcapillary ultrafiltration of around 4 mL/min. As transcapillary ultrafiltration is maximal at the beginning of the dwell, and decreases with duration of the dwell, the achieved values in the early stage of the dwell should be substantially higher than at the end. However, no difference in IgG2/IgG4 ratios at different time points was observed, neither with 1.36 or 3.86% glucose solutions.

Last, our set up might lack sufficient power to detect a meaningful difference, and sensitivity of the approach might be too low to detect a meaningful effect, especially as many other interfering forces might be at play in the clinical setting. Also Imholz et al. [19] could not find a difference in transport of larger molecules such as albumin, transferrin, IgG, IgA or alpha 2 macroglobulin after a dwell with an hypertonic vs non hypertonic glucose solution. However, in this experiment, analysis was only done after a 4 h dwell, so that any potential difference induced by streaming potentials would have been overwhelmed by cumulative diffusive transport. In addition, after 4 h, a difference in osmotically induced transcapillary ultrafiltration is unlikely to be still present, and, accordingly, no evaluation of a potential presence or absence of streaming potentials could be reasonably made in that setting. Additional experiments, using different indicator molecules, different ways to enhance convective solute drag, and larger patient groups or maybe animal models should be explored.

Conclusion

Although the electrokinetic hypothesis is appealing to help explain transcapillary transport in peritoneal dialysis, we failed to provide evidence for the existence of streaming potentials in peritoneal dialysis. More sophisticated exploration of this intriguing hypothesis is warranted.

Abbreviations

IgG2 and IgG4: Immunoglobulin 2 and Immunoglubulin 4; PD: Peritoneal Dialysis; PET: Peritoneal Equilibration Test

Acknowledgements

The authors are indebted to the dialysis nurses Nathalie Polfliet and Melanie Mouton, and to the laboratory technician Sophie Lobbestael for their technical support.

Anneleen Pletinck is a postdoctoral fellow of the Research Foundation – Flanders (FWO).

Funding

Our research unit has received an unrestricted research grant (20.000 US dollar) from the Baxter CEC (Clinical Evidence Council) grant program in 2016 for completing this research. AP is a postdoctoral fellow of the Research Foundation – Flanders (FWO). The funding body had no part in the set up of the study design, the experiments, data collection or analysis, or in the preparation and submission process of the manuscript.

Authors' contributions

All authors contributed intellectually to the concept and design of the study. AP, CD and SE performed the tests and the biochemistry. AP, SE and WVB analysed the results and wrote the first drafts of the paper. All authors contributed intellectually to the final version of the paper by adding comments, making suggestions and by proofreading. All authors read and approved the final manuscript.

Competing interests

WVB has received speaker's fees from Fresenius Medical Care, Baxter and Gambro on different occasions. The other authors declare to have no conflicts of interest relating to the content of this manuscript.

References

1. Moeller MJ. Streaming potentials as novel driving force for capillary permeability. Biophys J. 2013;104(7):1395–6.
2. Hausmann R, Grepl M, Knecht V, Moeller MJ. The glomerular filtration barrier function: new concepts. Curr Opin Nephrol Hypertens. 2012;21(4):441–9.
3. Moeller MJ, Tenten V. Renal albumin filtration: alternative models to the standard physical barriers. Nat Rev Nephrol. 2013;9(5):266–77.
4. Hausmann R, Kuppe C, Egger H, Schweda F, Knecht V, Elger M, et al. Electrical forces determine glomerular permeability. J Am Soc Nephrol. 2010;21(12):2053–8.
5. Ferrell N, Cameron KO, Groszek JJ, Hofmann CL, Li L, Smith RA, et al. Effects of pressure and electrical charge on macromolecular transport across bovine lens basement membrane. Biophys J. 2013;104(7):1476–84.
6. Rippe B. A three-pore model of peritoneal transport. Perit Dial Int. 1993; 13(Suppl 2):S35–8.
7. Rippe B, Venturoli D. Simulations of osmotic ultrafiltration failure in CAPD using a serial three-pore membrane/fiber matrix model. Am J Physiol Renal Physiol. 2007;292(3):F1035–43.
8. Rippe B, Davies S. Permeability of peritoneal and glomerular capillaries: what are the differences according to pore theory? Perit Dial Int. 2011;31(3): 249–58.
9. Buis B, Koomen GC, Imholz AL, Struijk DG, Reddingius RE, Arisz L, et al. Effect of electric charge on the transperitoneal transport of plasma proteins during CAPD. Perit Dial Int. 1996;11(6):1113–20.
10. Krediet RT, Koomen GC, Koopman MG, Hoek FJ, Struijk DG, Boeschoten EW, et al. The peritoneal transport of serum proteins and neutral dextran in CAPD patients. Kidney Int. 1989;35(4):1064–72.
11. Rippe B, Oberg CM. Point-counterpoint: pores versus an electrical field. Perit Dial Int. 2015;35(2):236.
12. Rippe B, Oberg CM. Counterpoint: defending pore theory. Perit Dial Int. 2015;35(1):9–13.
13. Moeller MJ, Point KC. Proposing the electrokinetic model. Perit Dial Int. 2015;35(1):5–8.
14. Wilkie M. Introduction to point-counterpoint: mechanisms of glomerular filtration: pores versus an electrical field. Perit Dial Int. 2015;35(1):4.
15. Zemel D, Koomen GC, Hart AA, ten Berge IJ, Struijk DG, Krediet RT. Relationship of TNF-alpha, interleukin-6, and prostaglandins to peritoneal permeability for macromolecules during longitudinal follow-up of peritonitis in continuous ambulatory peritoneal dialysis. J Lab Clin Med. 1993;122(6): 686–96.
16. Rodrigues AS, Martins M, Korevaar JC, Silva S, Oliveira JC, Cabrita A, et al. Evaluation of peritoneal transport and membrane status in peritoneal dialysis: focus on incident fast transporters. Am J Nephrol. 2007;27(1):84–91.
17. Van Biesen W, Van der Tol A, Veys N, Dequidt C, Vijt D, Lameire N, et al. The personal dialysis capacity test is superior to the peritoneal equilibration test to discriminate inflammation as the cause of fast transport status in peritoneal dialysis patients. Clin J Am Soc Nephrol. 2006;1(2):269–74.
18. Kofoed-Enevoldsen A, Foyle WJ, Fernandez M, Yudkin JS. Evidence of impaired glomerular charge selectivity in nondiabetic subjects with microalbuminuria: relevance to cardiovascular disease. Arterioscler Thromb Vasc Biol. 1996;16(3):450–4.
19. Imholz AL, Koomen GC, Struijk DG, Arisz L, Krediet RT. Effect of dialysate osmolarity on the transport of low-molecular weight solutes and proteins during CAPD. Kidney Int. 1993;43(6):1339–46.

Autosomal dominant tubulointerstitial kidney disease-UMOD is the most frequent non polycystic genetic kidney disease

Christine Gast[1,2]* ⓘ, Anthony Marinaki[3], Monica Arenas-Hernandez[3], Sara Campbell[1], Eleanor G. Seaby[2], Reuben J. Pengelly[2], Daniel P. Gale[4], Thomas M. Connor[5], David J. Bunyan[6], Kateřina Hodaňová[7], Martina Živná[7], Stanislav Kmoch[7], Sarah Ennis[2] and G. Venkat-Raman[1]

Abstract

Background: Autosomal dominant tubulointerstitial kidney disease (ADTKD) caused by mutations in the *UMOD* gene (ADTKD-UMOD) is considered rare and often remains unrecognised. We aimed to establish the prevalence of genetic kidney diseases, ADTKD and ADTKD-UMOD in adult chronic kidney disease (CKD) patients, and to investigate characteristic features.

Methods: We sent questionnaires on family history to all patients with CKD stages 3–5 in our tertiary renal centre to identify patients with inherited renal disease. Details on clinical and family history were obtained from patient interviews and clinical records. Sanger sequencing of the *UMOD* gene was performed from blood or saliva samples.

Results: 2027 of 3770 sent questionnaires were returned. 459 patients reported a family history, which was consistent with inherited kidney disease in 217 patients. 182 non-responders with inherited kidney diseases were identified through a database search. Of these 399 individuals, 252 had autosomal dominant polycystic kidney disease (ADPKD), 28 had ADTKD, 25 had Alports, and 44 were unknown, resulting in 11% of CKD 3–5 patients and 19% of end-stage renal disease patients with genetic kidney diseases. Of the unknown, 40 were genotyped, of whom 31 had findings consistent with ADTKD. 30% of unknowns and 39% of unknowns with ADTKD had *UMOD* mutations. Altogether, 35 individuals from 18 families were found to have ten distinct *UMOD* mutations (three novel), making up 1% of patients with CKD 3–5, 2% of patients with end-stage renal disease, 9% of inherited kidney diseases and 56% with ADTKD. ADTKD-UMOD was the most common genetic kidney disease after ADPKD with a population prevalence of 9 per million. Less proteinuria and haematuria, but not hyperuricaemia or gout were predictive of ADTKD-UMOD. The main limitations of the study are the single-centre design and a predominantly Caucasian population.

Conclusions: The prevalence of genetic kidney diseases and ADTKD-UMOD is significantly higher than previously described. Clinical features poorly predicted ADTKD-UMOD, highlighting the need for genetic testing guided by family history alone.

Keywords: Genetic kidney disease, Autosomal dominant tubulointerstitial kidney disease, UMOD, Prevalence

* Correspondence: Christine.gast@doctors.org.uk
[1]Wessex Kidney Centre, Queen Alexandra Hospital, Portsmouth Hospitals NHS Trust, Southwick Hill Road, Cosham, Portsmouth PO6 3LY, UK
[2]Human Genetics and Genomic Medicine, Faculty of Medicine, University of Southampton, Southampton, UK
Full list of author information is available at the end of the article

Background

Autosomal dominant tubulointerstitial kidney disease (ADTKD) is a rare genetic kidney disease. ADTKD caused by mutations in the *UMOD* gene (ADTKD-U-MOD) is the most common form of ADTKD [1, 2]. Other gene mutations causing ADTKD include mucin 1 (*MUC1*), hepatocyte nuclear factor 1 beta (*HNF1b*), renin (*REN*), and the alpha subunit of the endoplasmic reticular membrane translocon (*SEC61A1*) [3–7]. Previously known as familial juvenile hyperuricaemic nephropathy (FJHN) and uromodulin associated kidney disease (UAKD), ADTKD-UMOD is characterised by early onset hyperuricaemia and gout affecting both sexes, and the development of insidious renal failure with tubulointerstitial disease [8]. These disorders characteristically do not feature haematuria or proteinuria. Patients usually develop end stage renal disease (ESRD) between the third and sixth decade of life. However, clinical features are variable and hyperuricaemia and gout may be absent [9]. Some patients are found to have medullary renal cysts [10]. It has been shown that pathogenic *UMOD* mutations cause protein misfolding, retention in the endoplasmic reticulum (ER) and mistargeting of uromodulin in the thick ascending limb of Henle, resulting in tubulointerstitial damage through ER stress and reduced urinary uromodulin excretion [11–13]. A recent knock-in mouse model harbouring a human mutation has given insight into the pathophysiology of ADTKD-UMOD [14].

Inherited interstitial kidney diseases are underrecognised and underreported due to their lack of distinctive clinical or diagnostic histological features, lack of physician awareness and incomplete acquisition of family histories [15]. Registry data reliant on accurate diagnostic coding is known to be incomplete [16], and there is a paucity of information on the prevalence of genetic kidney diseases. Published studies suggest a prevalence of polycystic kidney disease of 5–11% and of other familial nephropathies of 4–6% amongst ESRD patients [17–21]. Registry figures for the latter are even lower between 2 and 3% [22, 23]. The UK's National Rare Disease Registry (RaDaR) lists 115 patients with ADTKD for a population of 65 million, resulting in a prevalence of 1.8 per million [24]. The published population prevalence of ADTKD-UMOD from a single Austrian study was 1.7 per million [25].

Preliminary data from our tertiary renal and transplant centre with a catchment population of 2 million had suggested that this was a gross underestimate, with a much higher in centre prevalence of ADTKD-UMOD [26]. Therefore we aimed to establish the prevalence of ADTKD-UMOD and genetic kidney diseases as a whole, and to investigate clinical and biochemical characteristics that may aid the recognition of ADTKD-UMOD.

Methods

Patient ascertainment

Questionnaires were sent to all patients in CKD stages 3–5 and all transplant recipients registered on the electronic database Proton. The one-page questionnaire asked patients to record any family members with kidney disease, their relation to the patient, their renal diagnosis (if known), the patient's own diagnosis, and their willingness to be contacted about the study (Additional File 1). Genetic kidney diseases of interest to this study were defined as monogenic diseases rather than disorders of polygenic risk alleles predisposing to kidney disease. Positive responses were reviewed.

Non-responders with CKD stages 3–5 with a family history of renal disease were identified through a search of diagnostic codes, electronic patient letters and through their nephrologists. Patient letters were reviewed for the presence of a positive family history for all non-responders with missing diagnostic codes, diagnostic codes 0 (chronic renal failure, aetiology uncertain), 30 (interstitial nephritis due to other cause, or unspecified), 40 (cystic kidney disease, type unspecified), 43 (medullary cystic kidney disease including nephronophthisis), 49 (cystic kidney disease, other specified type), 50 (hereditary/familial nephropathy type unspecified), 59 (hereditary nephropathy, other specified type) and 92 (gout).

If a genetic kidney disease was likely as suggested by a relative with a compatible diagnosis, patients were invited to participate in the study.

Patients gave written informed consent before providing a blood or saliva sample. Clinical data and pedigrees were recorded from patient interviews and clinical records.

Genetic investigations

Genomic DNA extraction from whole blood was performed by QIAamp DNA Blood Midi kit (Qiagen, Venlo, Netherlands) or the salting out method [27], and from saliva by Oragene kit (DNA Genotek, Ontario, Canada). Exons 3 to 5 of the *UMOD* gene were sequenced in an ABI 3130 XL Genetic Analyser. In three families, other *UMOD* exons had been sequenced beforehand by custom gene panel [6] or Sanger sequencing [13] at the Institute for Inherited Metabolic Disorders in Prague. Sequencing files were analysed by the software "Mutation Surveyor" (SoftGenetics, State College, PA, USA) using Genbank reference sequence NM_003361.3. Genetic variants were annotated with variant coding effects, predictive metrics of deleteriousness Polyphen-2 [28], and SIFT [29], and minor allele frequencies from the 1000 Genomes Project (1KG) [30], Exome Sequencing Project (ESP) [31] and Exome Aggregation Consortium (ExAC) [32] with ANNOVAR v2013Aug23 [33].

Exome sequencing of six samples from participants with a particularly strong family history was performed using the exome capture kits Agilent SureSelect v.5.0 (51 Mb) and Agilent Sure Select All Exon and sequenced on the HiSeq 2000 Sequencer or Illumina Genome Analyzer IIx. Reads were aligned to the reference genome (GRCh37) using Novoalign (Novocraft, 2010). Variants were called using GATK and annotated using Annovar.

Clinical confirmatory sequencing was performed using fresh blood samples.

Features associated with ADTKD-UMOD

Clinical and biochemical features were compared between patients with pathogenic *UMOD* mutations and the remaining cohort. Statistical significance was determined by the χ^2 test, Fisher's Exact test, Mann-Whitney-U test, or Kruskall-Wallis test, as appropriate, using SPSS version 24 (IBM, Armonk, NY).

Results

Patient ascertainment

3770 questionnaires on family history were sent to all patients (96% Caucasian) in CKD stages 3 to 5 and all transplant recipients registered on our electronic renal database. 2027 responses were received, corresponding to a response rate of 53.8%. 459 patients (22.6% of responders) reported a family history of kidney disease. Of these, in 217 patients (47%) an underlying genetic kidney disease was likely, in 184 patients (40%), the respective renal diagnoses for patients and relatives were apparently unrelated (e.g. diabetic nephropathy and renal cancer), and in 58 patients (13%) not enough information was available to allow an assessment (Fig. 1). The questionnaire study resulted in the identification of an additional 54 patients with genetic kidney diseases for whom either the diagnosis or coding were incomplete. Responders with an underlying genetic kidney disease were statistically younger (median age 59 versus 64 years with a reported family history and 68 years for all responders, $p < 0.001$, Kruskall-Wallis = 99.057), more likely to have ESRD (67% versus 38% for all responders, p < 0.001, $\chi^2 = 79.827$), and female (55% versus 41%, p < 0.001, $\chi^2 = 79.827$).

Amongst the non-responders, an additional 182 patients with genetic kidney diseases were identified through their nephrologists, a review of coded diagnoses and diagnoses extracted from clinic letters (Fig. 1). 38 of 61 patients (62%) with ADTKD had returned the questionnaire, and of these, 30 (79%) would have been identified by database screening.

Prevalence of genetic kidney diseases

Of the total 399 patients with genetic kidney diseases, 252 (63%) had autosomal dominant polycystic kidney disease (ADPKD), and 147 (37%) had other genetic kidney diseases. For the latter cohort, the most common diagnoses were unknown familial nephropathies, followed by ADTKD, Alport disease, familial focal segmental glomerulosclerosis (FSGS) or steroid resistant nephrotic syndrome (SRNS), and familial reflux nephropathy.

The prevalence rate of genetic kidney diseases was 11% for all CKD 3+ patients and 19% for patients with ESRD, with very similar rates obtained for responders and all patients (Table 1), confirming the effective uncovering of patients with genetic kidney diseases amongst the non-responders. Genetic kidney diseases other than ADPKD had a prevalence rate of 4% amongst CKD patients and 8% amongst ESRD patients.

UMOD mutations

Sanger sequencing of exons 3–5 of the *UMOD* gene was performed on DNA samples from 113 participants with no established conflicting genetic diagnosis. Six participants from five families with a strong family history of renal disease underwent exome sequencing before Sanger sequencing. In three families this identified pathogenic *UMOD* mutations within exons 3–5 which were confirmed to segregate with disease by Sanger sequencing.

Ten distinct heterozygous gene mutations were found in 35 participants from 18 families, all Caucasian (Table 2). Two individuals from two families carried the non-disease causing variant p.(Thr62Pro). We achieved a new diagnosis of ADTKD-UMOD in 11 individuals from seven families and confirmed ADTKD-UMOD in 24 individuals from eleven families.

28 patients had pre-existing diagnoses within the spectrum of ADTKD, 44 had unknown familial nephropathies, of whom 33 had clinical features consistent with ADTKD. Of the 44 unknown, 40 were genotyped. 30% (13/44) of the unknowns, 39% (13/33) of unknowns with ADTKD, and 57% (35/61) of all ATKD patients had *UMOD* mutations (Fig. 1). Altogether ADTKD-UMOD made up 1% (35/3770) of CKD 3+, 2% (29/1425) of ESRD, 9% (35/399) of inherited kidney diseases (24% without ADPKD), and 57% (35/61) of ADTKD. ADTKD made up 2% (61/3770) of CKD3+, 3% of ESRD (41/1425) and 15% (61/399) of inherited kidney diseases (42% without ADPKD).

Seven of the ten distinct gene mutations were published mutations and listed in the Wake Forest Inherited Kidney Disease Database for uromodulin associated kidney disease [34] (variant p.(Thr62Pro) was listed as clinically silent), and three of these were also present in the Human Gene Mutation Database (Table 3) [35].

The three novel mutations were classed as probably pathogenic in view of the patients' clinical phenotype, family history, high predictive metrics of deleteriousness

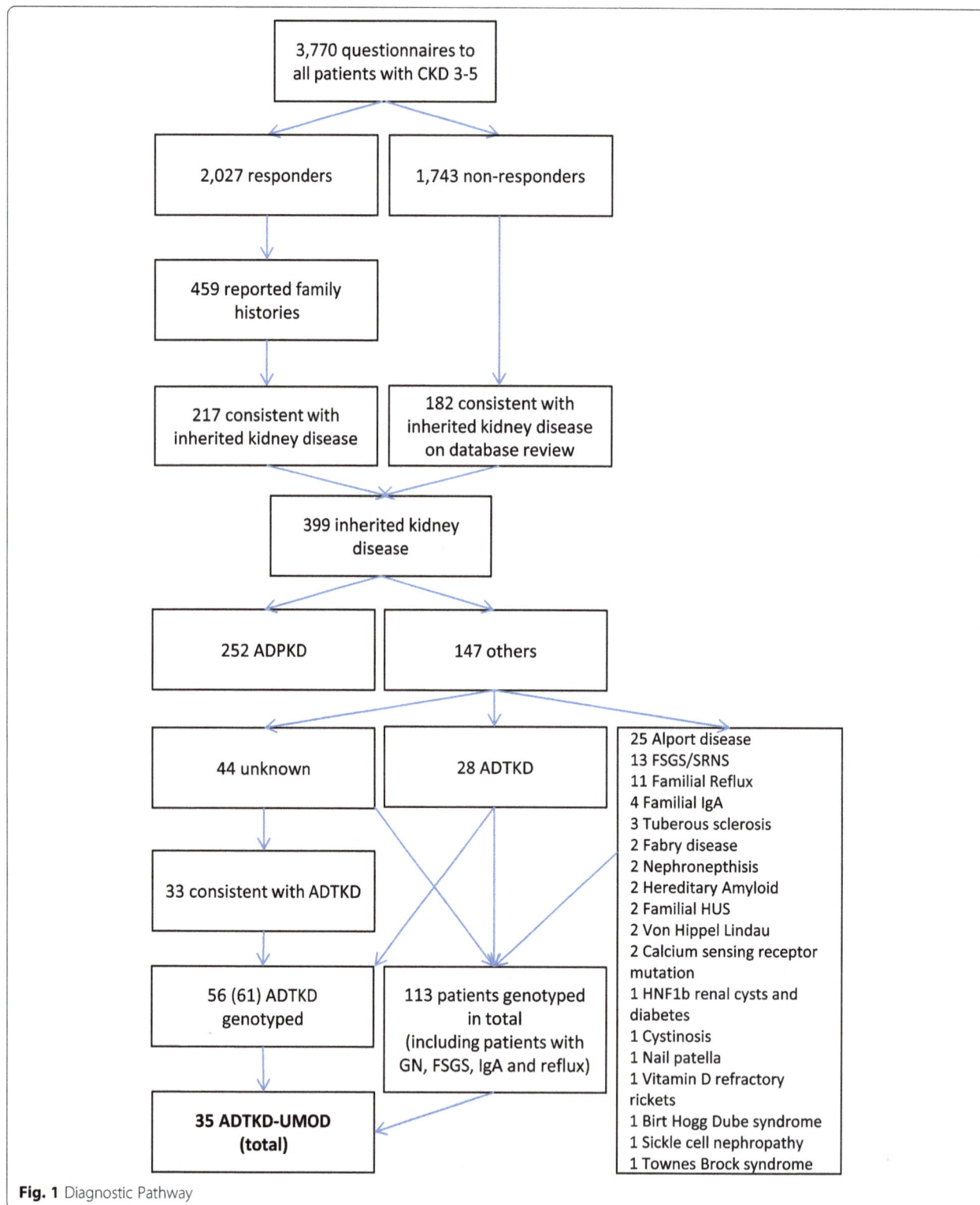

Fig. 1 Diagnostic Pathway

with Polyphen scores of 1 and SIFT scores of 0, and absence from the large population sequencing databases 1000 Genomes (1KG), Exome Sequencing Project (ESP) and Exome Aggregation Consortium (ExAC).

Mutation c.263G > T predicting *UMOD* substitution p.(Gly88Val) occurred in a patient with a diagnosis of medullary cystic kidney disease. A *UMOD* mutation had been found in a relative from another region, although the exact nature of the relative's mutation was

Table 1 Prevalence rates for genetic kidney diseases (GKD) in CKD cohort

	Responders	All Patients	Responders with ESRD	All patients with ESRD
All GKD	217/2027 = 10.7%	399/3770 = 10.6%	144/772 = 18.7%	269/1425 = 18.9%
ADPKD	140/2027 = 6.9%	252/3770 = 6.7%	88/772 = 11.4%	161/1425 = 11.3%
Other GKD (non-ADPKD)	77/2027 = 3.8%	147/3770 = 3.9%	56/772 = 7.3%	108/1425 = 7.6%
ADTKD	39/2027 = 1.9%	61/3770 = 1.6%	31/772 = 4.0%	44/1425 = 3.1%
ADTKD-UMOD	19/2027 = 0.9%	35/3770 = 0.9%	18/772 = 2.3%	27/1425 = 1.9%

unknown. Mutation c.614 T > C predicting p.(Phe205-Ser) was found in a participant with a strong family history of autosomal dominant kidney disease. As the majority of affected relatives lived abroad it was not possible to perform segregation analysis of the variant. Mutation c.860G > A predicting p.(Cys287Tyr) was found in a patient with a diagnosis of FJHN and a strong family history of kidney disease. The same mutation was confirmed in her teenage daughter, who has hyperuricaemia.

Clinical features

Clinical and biochemical parameters were compared between patients with non-polycystic genetic kidney diseases with and without *UMOD* mutations (Table 4), and between ADTKD patients with and without *UMOD* mutations (Table 5). After Bonferroni correction, patients with ADKTD-UMOD had lower protein creatinine ratios ($p < 0.001$), and a reduced presence of proteinuria ($p < 0.001$) and haematuria ($p < 0.001$) compared to all genotyped patients with genetic kidney diseases. There was no statistically significant association between ADTKD-UMOD and age at presentation, age at renal replacement therapy (RRT), gout, allopurinol use, hypertension, hyperuricaemia, uric acid levels, electrolyte abnormalities, anaemia, renal cysts, or renal size. There was a trend for a younger age at presentation for ADTKD-UMOD patients compared to ADTKD-NOS (ADTKD-not otherwise specified, i.e. *UMOD* negative), which lost its statistical significance after Bonferroni correction.

Final prevalence figures

In addition to establishing 13 new diagnoses of ADTKD-UMOD, we identified six additional patients with Alport disease through a targeted next generation sequencing panel of patients with FSGS/SRNS as described previously [36]. In total, we established 35 diagnoses of ADTKD-UMOD in our study population, and 31 diagnoses of Alport disease. 26 patients from 13 families had ADTKD of unknown genotype, and 31 patients were left with an undiagnosed genetic kidney disease.

By counting each family only once, we calculated the population prevalence of ADTKD-UMOD conservatively at 9 per million, and of ADTKD at 16 per million.

Discussion

This study identified a higher prevalence of genetic kidney diseases than previously described and found ADTKD-UMOD to be the most common genetic kidney disease after ADPKD.

Previous prevalence studies on genetic kidney diseases have largely relied on registry data and have rarely made use of genetic testing. The first study to highlight the importance of familial kidney diseases identified a prevalence of familial glomerulonephritides of 10% of all forms of glomerulonephritis in Germany [37]. An Irish cross-sectional study reported a prevalence of familial kidney diseases other than ADPKD of 4% for transplant and 5% for haemodialysis patients [17]. Similarly, 4% of ESRD patients in Newfoundland [18] and 6% of Swedish transplant patients [20] were reported to have a familial kidney disease other than ADPKD. A single-centre study from Italy established a prevalence of 4% of rare genetic disorders amongst transplant recipients with an unknown diagnosis [21]. A recent registry study of CKD patients of any stage from Australia found a prevalence of genetic kidney diseases other than ADPKD of 6% [38], but controversially included physician-ascertained congenital abnormalities of the kidneys and urinary tract (CAKUT) which constituted two thirds of genetic diagnoses.

Our prevalence of 8% for non-polycystic genetic kidney diseases amongst ESRD patients is higher than the previously published figures. We are the first to give an estimate of genetic kidney diseases amongst patients with CKD3+ of 4% (11% including ADPKD). This figure is lower than in our end-stage population consistent with our finding that patients with genetic kidney diseases were more likely to reach ESRD than patients with other diagnoses, despite being younger.

Our *UMOD* mutation analysis revealed 10 distinct pathogenic mutations in 35 participants from 18 families. Three mutations were unpublished. The presence of affected relatives with a *UMOD* mutation in two of the families makes it highly likely that these are pathogenic mutations, even in the absence of a complete segregation analysis. The third kindred had a strong family history of autosomal dominant kidney disease consistent with ADTKD-UMOD. The maximally deleterious Polyphen and SIFT scores of all three mutations and their

Table 2 *UMOD* mutation table

Study Number	Mutation (reference sequence NM_003361.3)	Protein Alteration	Family history of renal disease	Diagnosis of FJHN/ ADTKD-UMOD prior to study	Age at RRT	Hyperuricaemia	Gout
FN68 301[a]	c.202G > A	p.(Glu68Lys)	Yes	Yes	41	No	No
FN9 304[a]	c.263G > T	p.(Gly88Val)	Yes	Yes	44	Yes	No
FN2 301	c.272-274del	p.(Ser91del)	Yes	Yes	39	Yes	Yes
FN2 302	c.272-274del	p.(Ser91del)	Yes	Yes	45	Yes	No
FN2 303[a]	c.272-274del	p.(Ser91del)	Yes	Yes	58	Yes	No
FN3 301[a]	c.272-274del	p.(Ser91del)	Yes	No		Yes	No
FN3 305[a]	c.272-274del	p.(Ser91del)	Yes	No	64		No
FN3 409[a]	c.272-274del	p.(Ser91del)	Yes	No	38	No	No
FN26 301[a]	c.272-274del	p.(Ser91del)	Yes	No	56	Yes	No
FN45 304[a]	c.272-274del	p.(Ser91del)	Yes	Yes	45	Yes	No
FN45 404[a]	c.272-274del	p.(Ser91del)	Yes	Yes	51	No	Yes
FN45 405[a]	c.272-274del	p.(Ser91del)	Yes	Yes	37		No
FN65 201	c.272-274del	p.(Ser91del)	Yes	Yes	66		No
FN65 202	c.272-274del	p.(Ser91del)	Yes	Yes	59		No
FN65 203[a]	c.272-274del	p.(Ser91del)	Yes	Yes	59	Yes	No
FN65 301	c.272-274del	p.(Ser91del)	Yes	Yes		Yes	Yes
FN65 401	c.272-274del	p.(Ser91del)	Yes	Yes	47	Yes	Yes
FN65 402	c.272-274del	p.(Ser91del)	Yes	Yes		Yes	Yes
FN65 412[a]	c.272-274del	p.(Ser91del)	Yes	Yes	54	No	Yes
FN1 303[a]	c.278_289delinsCCGC CTCCT	p.(Val93_Gly97delinsAlaAlaSerCys)	Yes	No	62	Yes	No
FN24 305[a]	c.278_289delinsCCGC CTCCT	p.(Val93_Gly97delinsAlaAlaSerCys)	Yes	No	42	Yes	No
FN47 404[a]	c.278_289delinsCCGC CTCCT	p.(Val93_Gly97delinsAlaAlaSerCys)	Yes	Yes	49	Yes	No
FN77 301[a]	c.278_289delinsCCGC CTCCT	p.(Val93_Gly97delinsAlaAlaSerCys)	Yes	Yes	49	Yes	No
FN20 302	c.443G > A	p.(Cys148Tyr)	Yes	Yes	50	Yes	Yes
FN20 403	c.443G > A	p.(Cys148Tyr)	Yes	Yes		Yes	No
FN64 303[a]	c.614 T > C	p.(Phe205Ser)	Yes	No	42	Yes	Yes
FN23 302	c.629G > A	p.(Gly210Asp)	Yes	No	36	Yes	Yes
FN23 303	c.629G > A	p.(Gly210Asp)	Yes	No	46		No
FN27 304[a]	c.688 T > C	p.(Trp230Arg)	Yes	No	63	Yes	Yes
FN27 306[a]	c.688 T > C	p.(Trp230Arg)	Yes	No		Yes	Yes
FN28 302	c.688 T > C	p.(Trp230Arg)	Yes	Yes	57	Yes	Yes
FN28 401[a]	c.688 T > C	p.(Trp230Arg)	Yes	Yes		Yes	Yes
FN7 305	c.860G > A	p.(Cys287Tyr)	Yes	Yes	27	Yes	Yes
FN35 403[a]	c.917G > A	p.(Cys287Tyr)	Yes	Yes	57	Yes	No
FN35 501[a]	c.917G > A	p.(Cys287Tyr)	Yes	Yes	42	Yes	Yes

RRT renal replacement therapy, *FJHN* familial juvenile hyperuricaemic nephropathy
[a]clinically confirmed

absence from the large population databases 1KG, ESP and ExAC lend further support to this interpretation. Mutation c.184A > C predicting p.(Thr62Pro) was considered clinically silent as reported in Ensembl (SNP rs143248111) and in the Wake Forest Registry, and supported by its presence in the non-disease databases ESP and ExAC. Complete segregation analysis in the families was not possible but several affected relatives had variant p.(Thr62Pro) confirmed at another centre.

Table 3 *UMOD* mutation characteristics

Mutation	Exon	Protein alteration	Wake Forest Registry	HGMD	Polyphen	SIFT	1KG	ESP	ExAC
c.184A > C[a]	3	p.(Thr62Pro) [34]	Yes[a]	No	0.662	0.030.03 0.	–	0.0006.006	0.0004
c.202G > A	3	p.(Glu68Lys) [34]	Yes	No	0.999	0	–	–	–
c.263G > T	3	p.(Gly88Val)	No	No	1	0	–	–	–
c.272-274del	3	p.(Ser91del) [34]	Yes	No			–	–	–
c.278_289delinsCCGCCTCCT	3	p.(Val93_Gly97delins AlaAlaSerCys) [42]	Yes	Yes			–	–	–
c.443G > A	3	p.(Cys148Tyr) [10]	Yes	Yes	1	0.31	–	–	–
c.614 T > C	3	p.(Phe205Ser)	No	No	1	0	–	–	–
c.629G > A	3	p.(Gly210Asp) [34]	Yes	No	1	0	–	–	–
c.688 T > C	3	p.(Trp230Arg) [43]	Yes	Yes	1	0	–	–	–
c.860G > A	3	p.(Cys287Tyr)	No	No	1	0	–	–	–
c.917G > A	4	p.(Cys306Tyr) [34]	Yes	No	1	0	–	–	–

Mutation = *UMOD* mutation, Wake Forest Registry = inclusion in the Wake Forest School Registry of Inherited Kidney Diseases, HGMD = inclusion in the Human Gene Mutation Database. Polyphen and SIFT = predictive scores of deleteriousness, 1 KG / ESP/ ExAC = occurrence in the large sequencing projects of populations with European ancestry 1000 Genomes (1KG) and Exome Sequencing Project (ESP) and in 60,000 healthy individuals from varying ethnicities in the Exome Aggregation Consortium (ExAC). [a]clinically silent

We are likely to have underestimated the true prevalence of ADTKD-UMOD since we were only able to screen those patients with significant CKD who had been referred to tertiary renal services and their relatives. Conversely, patients with an obvious inherited kidney disease may have been referred to our service earlier than other patients in CKD stage 3. This could theoretically have led to an overestimation of ADTKD as a proportion of CKD patients, but it could not have overestimated the total prevalence figures based on the catchment population. Furthermore, when taking other possible sources of under-ascertainment into account, an overestimation of the prevalence of ADTKD appears very unlikely.

Having only sequenced exons 3–5 in the majority of patients [9, 39], we may have missed mutations in the remaining seven exons of the *UMOD* gene, where only 5% of mutations are expected to occur [40].

The incomplete response rate of 53.8% was a recognised source of incomplete ascertainment. To compensate for this, we undertook a comprehensive database search of all non-responders with missing and/or suspicious diagnostic codes. This search would have captured 79% of responders with ADTKD had they not responded. Furthermore, the prevalence rates established for responders and the cohort as a whole were very similar, indicating that any bias inherent in the different forms of patient ascertainment was likely limited, although a remaining degree of incomplete ascertainment remained.

A limitation of our study is that we have not conclusively established a prevalence for ADTKD since we have only sequenced *UMOD* as the most common underlying mutation [2] and not *MUC1* thought to be responsible for 30% of ADTKD mutations. Furthermore our prevalence rates only apply to a predominantly Caucasian population. Finally, the single centre design is a limitation, although our tertiary renal centre covers a large geographical mixed urban and rural area with a catchment population of 2 million. While a multi-centric design would be preferable, this is the first and only systematic study of the prevalence of ADTKD-UMOD amongst patients with dominant renal disease. No national or international disease registry has been based on a similar systematic approach, explaining the much lower current numbers.

To minimise any distorting local factors such as relatedness of pedigrees, our prevalence rate for ADTKD-UMOD of 9 per million was estimated conservatively by counting each family only once. If we were to count each affected patient instead, we would observe a prevalence of ADTKD-UMOD of 17.5 per million and of ADTKD of 30.5 per million.

We have shown that a simple questionnaire study on family history combined with a database search followed by genetic testing can uncover many additional cases of genetic kidney diseases in general and ADTKD-UMOD in particular.

Apart from incomplete and inadequate coding, the reason for the low published prevalence rates appears to be that genetic kidney diseases often go unrecognized [21]. This is especially true for ADTKD which has subtle phenotypic characteristics that can easily be missed [15]. While genetic tests are available for many genetic kidney diseases, they have not been commonly performed historically, because of their

Table 4 Comparison of clinical parameters between *UMOD* positive and negative patients with non-polycystic genetic kidney diseases

Clinical parameter	UMOD positive	UMOD negative	Significance level ($p < 0.0036$)
Age at presentation [years]	9–57, median 39, $n = 21$	0–80, median 35, $n = 66$	$p = 0.882$*
Age at RRT [years]	27–66, median 47, $n = 27$	9–84, median 41, $n = 61$	$p = 0.116$*
Gout	15/33 patients (45%)	30/78 (38%)	$p = 0.493$**
Allopurinol use	13/35 patients (37%)	22/78 (28%)	$p = 0.342$**
Hypertension at presentation	31/35 patients (89%)	69/78 (88%)	$p = 1.0$***
Hyperuricaemia (Uric acid > 0.35 umol/l)	24/26 patients (92%)	50/61 patients (82%)	$p = 0.328$***
Uric Acid [umol/l]	0.28–0.79, median 0.45, $n = 25$	0.12–0.85, median 0.495, $n = 60$	$p = 0.155$*
Proteinuria	8/22 patients (36%)	48/62 patients (77%)	***p = 0.0004****
Protein Creatinine Ratio [mg/g]	0–2761, median 234.5, $n = 18$	53–20,398, median = 2150, $n = 52$	***p < 0.001****
Anaemia pre RRT (Hb < 100 g/l)	4/27 patients (15%)	25/68 patients (37%)	$p = 0.036$**
Microscopic haematuria	1/27 patients (4%)	24/63 patients (38%)	***p = 0.001****
Renal cysts	4/21 patients (19%)	6/51 patients (12%)	$p = 0.463$***
Normal renal size at presentation (renal diameter > 9 cm)	11/23 patients (48%)	30/48 patients (63%)	$p = 0.241$**
Electrolyte abnormalities	6/32 patients (19%)	2/67 patients (3%)	$p = 0.013$***

A Bonferroni correction was employed to adjust the significance level for the number of performed tests (i.e. the adjusted significance level is $p < 0.05/14$)
* = Mann Whitney U, ** = χ^2, *** = Fisher's Exact test

cost and the limited availability of diagnostic centres. Rare disease registries based on genetic results are promising approaches but they still remain in their infancy.

Looking for diagnostic clues, this study has confirmed that clinical and biochemical tests need to be interpreted with caution in the diagnosis of ADTKD-UMOD. Since ADTKD-UMOD is a tubulointerstitial disease, it is not surprising that it was associated less often with haematuria and proteinuria than other genetic kidney diseases, which included familial glomerulonephritides. Despite hyperuricaemia

Table 5 Comparison of clinical parameters between *UMOD* positive and negative patients with ADTKD

Clinical parameter	UMOD positive	UMOD negative	Significance level ($p < 0.0036$)
Age at presentation [years]	9–57, median 39, $n = 21$	23–80, median 49, $n = 20$	$p = 0.024$*
Age at RRT [years]	27–66, median 47, $n = 27$	27–83, median 51.5, $n = 16$	$p = 0.606$*
Gout	15/33 patients (45%)	10/25 patients (40%)	$p = 0.678$**
Allopurinol use	13/35 patients (37%)	6/25 patients (24%)	$p = 0.281$**
Hypertension at presentation	31/35 patients (89%)	22/25 patients (88%)	$p = 1.0$***
Hyperuricaemia (Uric acid > 0.35 umol/l)	24/26 patients (92%)	15/19 patients (79%)	$p = 0.377$***
Uric Acid [mg/dl]	4.71–13.28, median 7.75, $n = 25$	4.54–12.27, median 8.07, $n = 19$	$p = 0.61$*
Proteinuria	8/22 patients (36%)	6/17 patients (35%)	$p = 0.945$**
Protein Creatinine Ratio [mg/g]	0–2761, median 234.5, $n = 18$	53–2469, median 624, $n = 14$	$p = 0.065$*
Anaemia pre RRT (Hb < 100 g/l)	4/27 patients (15%)	7/22 patients (32%)	$p = 0.185$***
Microscopic haematuria	1/27 patients (4%)	1/19 patients (5%)	$p = 1.0$***
Renal cysts	4/21 patients (19%)	4/15 patients (27%)	$p = 0.694$***
Normal renal size at presentation (renal diameter > 9 cm)	11/23 patients (48%)	12/19 patients (63%)	$p = 0.32$**
Electrolyte abnormalities	6/32 patients (19%)	1/22 patients (5%)	$p = 0.22$***

* = Mann Whitney U, ** = χ^2, *** = Fisher's Exact test

and gout being considered hallmarks of ADTKD-UMOD, there was no significant association with the disease, reflecting how common both are in a general CKD population and that they can be absent in ADTKD-UMOD [9]. Hyperuricaemia and/or gout can still be helpful when present in patients with normal renal function, especially in females and young patients [15].

As we have shown, a positive family history remains the most important diagnostic clue in the diagnosis of ADTKD-UMOD and in genetic kidney diseases in general. However, a family history may be absent in recessive diseases, in de novo mutations and where a relative's kidney disease was either not diagnosed or communicated to the rest of the family. While we recognise these limitations, we have demonstrated the usefulness of a questionnaire on family history in uncovering many undiagnosed genetic kidney diseases.

In our search for gene mutations, we performed Sanger sequencing of the UMOD gene, a targeted next generation sequencing panel of patients with FSGS/SRNS [36], and exome sequencing of selected participants. In future, next generation sequencing techniques such as (clinical) exome and whole genome sequencing are expected to largely replace conventional sequencing. They deliver more genetic information in a single assay and offer superior flexibility, as existing sequencing data can be reviewed once new pathogenic gene mutations become known. However, they bring their own significant problems of the storage and interpretation of large datasets and the interpretation of multiple novel variants. Possible solutions include the segregation analysis of variants of interest, functional studies and pooling of phenotype and genotype data in national and international efforts such as the 100,000 Genomes Project and RaDaR [24, 41]. The 31 study participants currently left with an unknown familial nephropathy will be preferentially recruited to the 100,000 Genomes Project to help uncover their underlying diagnoses which will help to further inform our disease and prevalence data.

Conclusions

This study has demonstrated that the prevalence of ADTKD, and ADTKD-UMOD in particular, is significantly higher than previously reported. Due to ADTKD's lack of distinctive clinical features, clinical suspicion should be aroused by a compatible family history alone and should lead to genetic testing. As shown, this approach is able to identify many previously unknown cases of ADTKD-UMOD, which can benefit patients in terms of prognostication, the provision of genetic counselling and the early identification of affected relatives.

Abbreviations

ADPKD: Autosomal dominant polycystic kidney disease; ADTKD: Autosomal dominant tubulointerstitial kidney disease; ADTKD-UMOD: Autosomal dominant tubulointerstitial kidney disease caused by UMOD mutations; CAKUT: Congenital abnormalities of the kidneys and urinary tract; CKD: Chronic kidney disease; ER: Endoplasmic reticulum; ESRD: End stage renal disease; FJHN: Familial juvenile hyperuricaemic nephropathy; FSGS: Focal segmental glomerulosclerosis; HNF1b: Hepatocyte nuclear factor 1 beta; MUC1: Mucin 1; RaDaR: The UK's National Rare Disease Registry; REN: Renin; RRT: Renal replacement therapy; SRNS: Steroid resistant nephrotic syndrome; UAKD: Uromodulin associated kidney disease

Acknowledgements

Abstracts based on this work were presented at the ERA-EDTA Congress 2015 and US Kidney Week 2015.

MŽ, KH and SK thank The National Center for Medical Genomics (LM2015091) for technical support with exome and gene panel sequencing. Their work was supported by grant AZV CR 17-29786A from the Ministry of Health of the Czech Republic and Charles University program UNCE 204064.

Funding

This study was funded by grants from the Wessex Kidney Centre Charitable Research Fund and the Purine Metabolic Patients' Association (PUMPA). The funding bodies had no involvement in the design of the study and collection, analysis and interpretation of data.

Authors' contributions

GVR originally conceived the design of the study, subsequently refined by CG, SC and AM; CG conducted patient recruitment, patient interviews, clinical data collection and interpretation under supervision of GVR and UMOD sequencing under AM and M A-H. KH, MZ, and SK identified UMOD mutations in three families, later confirmed by Sanger sequencing by CG. CG, RJP, and EGS conducted exome sequencing, and annotation and interpretation of genetic variants under supervision of SE. DPG and TMC performed exome sequencing of four families, DJB undertook confirmatory clinical sequencing. CG wrote the draft manuscript, which was reviewed, amended and approved by all authors.

Competing interests

The authors declare that they have no competing interests.

Author details

[1]Wessex Kidney Centre, Queen Alexandra Hospital, Portsmouth Hospitals NHS Trust, Southwick Hill Road, Cosham, Portsmouth PO6 3LY, UK. [2]Human Genetics and Genomic Medicine, Faculty of Medicine, University of Southampton, Southampton, UK. [3]Purine Research Laboratory, Guys and St Thomas' NHS Foundation Trust, London, UK. [4]UCL Centre for Nephrology, Royal Free Hospital, London, UK. [5]Oxford Kidney Unit, Churchill Hospital, Oxford, UK. [6]Wessex Regional Genetics Laboratory, Salisbury NHS Foundation Trust, Salisbury, UK. [7]Research Unit for Rare Diseases, Department of Pediatrics and Adolescent Medicine, First Faculty of Medicine, Charles University Prague, Prague, Czech Republic.

References

1. Dahan K, Devuyst O, Smaers M, Vertommen D, Loute G, Poux JM, Viron B, Jacquot C, Gagnadoux MF, Chauveau D, et al. A cluster of mutations in the UMOD gene causes familial juvenile hyperuricemic nephropathy with abnormal expression of uromodulin. J Am Soc Nephrol. 2003;14:2883–93.

2. Eckardt KU, Alper SL, Antignac C, Bleyer AJ, Chauveau D, Dahan K, Deltas C, Hosking A, Kmoch S, Rampoldi L, et al. Autosomal dominant tubulointerstitial kidney disease: diagnosis, classification, and management--a KDIGO consensus report. Kidney Int. 2015;88:676–83.

3. Kirby A, Gnirke A, Jaffe DB, Baresova V, Pochet N, Blumenstiel B, Ye C, Aird D, Stevens C, Robinson JT, et al. Mutations causing medullary cystic kidney disease type 1 lie in a large VNTR in MUC1 missed by massively parallel sequencing. Nat Genet. 2013;45:299–303.

4. Bingham C, Ellard S, van't Hoff WG, Simmonds HA, Marinaki AM, Badman MK, Winocour PH, Stride A, Lockwood CR, Nicholls AJ, et al. Atypical familial juvenile hyperuricemic nephropathy associated with a hepatocyte nuclear factor-1beta gene mutation. Kidney Int. 2003;63:1645 51.

5. Zivná M, Hůlková H, Matignon M, Hodanová K, Vylet'al P, Kalbácová M, Baresová V, Sikora J, Blazková H, Zivný J, et al. Dominant renin gene mutations associated with early-onset hyperuricemia, anemia, and chronic kidney failure. Am J Hum Genet. 2009;85:204–13.

6. Bolar NA, Golzio C, Zivna M, Hayot G, Van Hemelrijk C, Schepers D, Vandeweyer G, Hoischen A, Huyghe JR, Raes A, et al. Heterozygous loss-of-function SEC61A1 mutations cause autosomal-dominant Tubulo-interstitial and glomerulocystic kidney disease with Anemia. Am J Hum Genet. 2016;99:174–87.

7. Bleyer AJ, Kidd K, Zivna M, Kmoch S. Autosomal dominant Tubulointerstitial kidney disease. Adv Chronic Kidney Dis. 2017;24:86–93.

8. Bleyer AJ, Zivná M, Kmoch S. Uromodulin-associated kidney disease. Nephron Clin Pract. 2011;118:c31–6.

9. Bollée G, Dahan K, Flamant M, Morinière V, Pawtowski A, Heidet L, Lacombe D, Devuyst O, Pirson Y, Antignac C, Knebelmann B. Phenotype and outcome in hereditary tubulointerstitial nephritis secondary to UMOD mutations. Clin J Am Soc Nephrol. 2011;6:2429–38.

10. Hart TC, Gorry MC, Hart PS, Woodard AS, Shihabi Z, Sandhu J, Shirts B, Xu L, Zhu H, Barmada MM, Bleyer AJ. Mutations of the UMOD gene are responsible for medullary cystic kidney disease 2 and familial juvenile hyperuricaemic nephropathy. J Med Genet. 2002;39:882–92.

11. Rampoldi L, Caridi G, Santon D, Boaretto F, Bernascone I, Lamorte G, Tardanico R, Dagnino M, Colussi G, Scolari F, et al. Allelism of MCKD, FJHN and GCKD caused by impairment of uromodulin export dynamics. Hum Mol Genet. 2003;12:3369–84.

12. Williams SE, Reed AA, Galvanovskis J, Antignac C, Goodship T, Karet FE, Kotanko P, Lhotta K, Morinière V, Williams P, et al. Uromodulin mutations causing familial juvenile hyperuricaemic nephropathy lead to protein maturation defects and retention in the endoplasmic reticulum. Hum Mol Genet. 2009;18:2963–74.

13. Vylet'al P, Kublová M, Kalbácová M, Hodanová K, Baresová V, Stibůrková B, Sikora J, Hůlková H, Zivný J, Majewski J, et al. Alterations of uromodulin biology: a common denominator of the genetically heterogeneous FJHN/MCKD syndrome. Kidney Int. 2006;70:1155–69.

14. Piret SE, Olinger E, Reed AAC, Nesbit MA, Hough TA, Bentley L, Devuyst O, Cox RD, Thakker RV. A mouse model for inherited renal fibrosis associated with endoplasmic reticulum stress. Dis Model Mech. 2017;10:773–86.

15. Venkat-Raman G, Gast C, Marinaki A, Fairbanks L. From juvenile hyperuricaemia to dysfunctional uromodulin: an ongoing metamorphosis. Pediatr Nephrol. 2016;31:2035–42.

16. Venkat-Raman G, Tomson CR, Gao Y, Cornet R, Stengel B, Gronhagen-Riska C, Reid C, Jacquelinet C, Schaeffner E, Boeschoten E, et al. New primary renal diagnosis codes for the ERA-EDTA. Nephrol Dial Transplant. 2012;27:4414–9.

17. Green A, Allos M, Donohoe J, Carmody M, Walshe J. Prevalence of hereditary renal disease. Ir Med J. 1990;83:11–3.

18. Parfrey PS, Davidson WS, Green JS. Clinical and genetic epidemiology of inherited renal disease in Newfoundland. Kidney Int. 2002;61:1925–34.

19. Barbari A, Stephan A, Masri M, Karam A, Aoun S, El Nahas J, Bou Khalil J. Consanguinity-associated kidney diseases in Lebanon: an epidemiological study. Mol Immunol. 2003;39:1109–14.

20. Nyberg G, Friman S, Svalander C, Nordén G. Spectrum of hereditary renal disease in a kidney transplant population. Nephrol Dial Transplant. 1995;10:859–65.

21. Quaglia M, Musetti C, Ghiggeri GM, Fogazzi GB, Settanni F, Boldorini RL, Lazzarich E, Airoldi A, Izzo C, Giordano M, Stratta P. Unexpectedly high prevalence of rare genetic disorders in kidney transplant recipients with an unknown causal nephropathy. Clin Transpl. 2014;28:995–1003.

22. Byrne C, Steenkamp R, Castledine C, Ansell D, Feehally J. UK Renal Registry 12th Annual Report (December 2009): Chapter 4: UK ESRD prevalent rates in 2008: national and Centre-specific analyses. Nephron Clin Pract. 2010;115(Suppl 1):c41–67.

23. Hallan SI, Coresh J, Astor BC, Asberg A, Powe NR, Romundstad S, Hallan HA, Lydersen S, Holmen J. International comparison of the relationship of chronic kidney disease prevalence and ESRD risk. J Am Soc Nephrol. 2006;17:2275–84.

24. Rare Renal Information on rare kidney diseases [http://rarerenal.org/clinician-information/adtkd-clinician-information/].

25. Lhotta K, Piret SE, Kramar R, Thakker RV, Sunder-Plassmann G, Kotanko P. Epidemiology of uromodulin-associated kidney disease - results from a nation-wide survey. Nephron Extra. 2012;2:147–58.

26. Venkat Raman G, Harris K: What is the real prevalence of familial nephropathies? In *American Society of Nephrology Renal Week 2007* (ASN ed. San Francisco; 2007.

27. Miller SA, Dykes DD, Polesky HF. A simple salting out procedure for extracting DNA from human nucleated cells. Nucleic Acids Res. 1988;16:1215.

28. Adzhubei IA, Schmidt S, Peshkin L, Ramensky VE, Gerasimova A, Bork P, Kondrashov AS, Sunyaev SR. A method and server for predicting damaging missense mutations. Nat Methods. 2010;7:248–9.

29. Kumar P, Henikoff S, Ng PC. Predicting the effects of coding non-synonymous variants on protein function using the SIFT algorithm. Nat Protoc. 2009;4:1073–81.

30. Abecasis GR, Auton A, Brooks LD, DePristo MA, Durbin RM, Handsaker RE, Kang HM, Marth GT, McVean GA, Consortium GP. An integrated map of genetic variation from 1,092 human genomes. Nature. 2012;491:56–65.

31. Fu W, O'Connor TD, Jun G, Kang HM, Abecasis G, Leal SM, Gabriel S, Rieder MJ, Altshuler D, Shendure J, et al. Analysis of 6,515 exomes reveals the recent origin of most human protein-coding variants. Nature. 2013;493:216–20.

32. Karczewski KJ, Weisburd B, Thomas B, Solomonson M, Ruderfer DM, Kavanagh D, Hamamsy T, Lek M, Samocha KE, Cummings BB, et al. The ExAC browser: displaying reference data information from over 60 000 exomes. Nucleic Acids Res. 2017;45:D840–5.

33. He X, Liu GL, Xia ZK, Ren XG, Gao YF, Fan ZM, Fu YF, Fu J, Gao CL, Mao S, Chen R. Clinical and pathological study of 47 cases with Alport syndrome. Zhonghua Er Ke Za Zhi. 2008;46:914–8.

34. Bleyer A. Wake Forest Inherited Kidney Disease Registry. https://www.ncbi.nlm.nih.gov/books/NBK1356/; 1996 - present.

35. Stenson PD, Mort M, Ball EV, Shaw K, Phillips A, Cooper DN. The human gene mutation database: building a comprehensive mutation repository for clinical and molecular genetics, diagnostic testing and personalized genomic medicine. Hum Genet. 2014;133:1–9.

36. Gast C, Pengelly RJ, Lyon M, Bunyan DJ, Seaby EG, Graham N, Venkat-Raman G, Ennis S. Collagen (COL4A) mutations are the most frequent mutations underlying adult focal segmental glomerulosclerosis. Nephrol Dial Transplant. 2016;31:961–70.

37. Rambausek M, Hartz G, Waldherr R, Andrassy K, Ritz E. Familial glomerulonephritis. Pediatr Nephrol. 1987;1:416–8.

38. Mallett A, Patel C, Salisbury A, Wang Z, Healy H, Hoy W. The prevalence and epidemiology of genetic renal disease amongst adults with chronic kidney disease in Australia. Orphanet J Rare Dis. 2014;9:98.

39. Vyletal P, Bleyer AJ, Kmoch S. Uromodulin biology and pathophysiology--an update. Kidney Blood Press Res. 2010;33:456–75.

40. Moskowitz JL, Piret SE, Lhotta K, Kitzler TM, Tashman AP, Velez E, Thakker RV, Kotanko P. Association between genotype and phenotype in uromodulin-associated kidney disease. Clin J Am Soc Nephrol. 2013;8:1349–57.

41. Peplow M. The 100,000 genomes project. BMJ. 2016;353:i1757.

42. Smith GD, Robinson C, Stewart AP, Edwards EL, Karet HI, Norden AG, Sandford RN, Karet Frankl FE. Characterization of a recurrent in-frame UMOD indel mutation causing late-onset autosomal dominant end-stage renal failure. Clin J Am Soc Nephrol. 2011;6:2766–74.

43. Zaucke F, Boehnlein JM, Steffens S, Polishchuk RS, Rampoldi L, Fischer A, Pasch A, Boehm CW, Baasner A, Attanasio M, et al. Uromodulin is expressed in renal primary cilia and UMOD mutations result in decreased ciliary uromodulin expression. Hum Mol Genet. 2010;19:1985–97.

21

Effectiveness of contrast-associated acute kidney injury prevention methods; a systematic review and network meta-analysis

Khalid Ahmed[1,2]* (iD), Terri McVeigh[1], Raminta Cerneviciute[1], Sara Mohamed[1], Mohammad Tubassam[2], Mohammad Karim[3] and Stewart Walsh[1,2,4]

Abstract

Background: Different methods to prevent contrast-associated acute kidney injury (CA-AKI) have been proposed in recent years. We performed a mixed treatment comparison to evaluate and rank suggested interventions.

Methods: A comprehensive Systematic review and a Bayesian network meta-analysis of randomised controlled trials was completed. Results were tabulated and graphically represented using a network diagram; forest plots and league tables were shown to rank treatments by the surface under the cumulative ranking curve (SUCRA). A stacked bar chart rankogram was generated. We performed main analysis with 200 RCTs and three analyses according to contrast media and high or normal baseline renal profile that includes 173, 112 & 60 RCTs respectively.

Results: We have included 200 trials with 42,273 patients and 44 interventions. The primary outcome was CI-AKI, defined as ≥25% relative increase or ≥ 0.5 mg/dl increase from baseline creatinine one to 5 days post contrast exposure. The top ranked interventions through different analyses were Allopurinol, Prostaglandin E1 (PGE1) & Oxygen (0.9647, 0.7809 & 0.7527 in the main analysis). Comparatively, reference treatment intravenous hydration was ranked lower but better than Placebo (0.3124 VS 0.2694 in the main analysis).

Conclusion: Multiple CA-AKI preventive interventions have been tested in RCTs. This network evaluates data for all the explored options. The results suggest that some options (particularly allopurinol, PGE1 & Oxygen) deserve further evaluation in a larger well-designed RCTs.

Keywords: Contrast induced acute kidney injury, Contrast nephropathy, Prevention methods, Contrast associated acute kidney injury

Background

Rationale

Contrast Associated acute kidney injury (CA-AKI) also known as Contrast-induced acute kidney injury (CI-AKI) previously known as contrast induced nephropathy (CIN) is the third leading cause of hospital-acquired acute renal injury, accounting for 12% of cases [1]. It is defined as an abrupt deterioration in renal function following exposure to contrast media (CM) in the absence of other aetiological factors [2]. The absolute and relative values used to define CI-AKI vary, but are most commonly quoted as a relative increase of > 25% or an absolute increase of 0.5 mg/dL and ≥ 0.3 mg from baseline serum creatinine measurement within 1–3 (4–5 days less frequently used) of contrast exposure [3–7]. In CI-AKI, the serum creatinine level begins to rise within 24 h of contrast exposure, peaking after 72 h, and usually returning to baseline within 1–3 weeks [6].

The proposed pathophysiology of CI-AKI is acute tubular necrosis. The underlying mechanisms are thought to be vasoconstriction, leading to cellular hypoxia, or direct

* Correspondence: Khalidmd20@gmail.com
[1]Lambe Institute for Translational Research, Discipline of Surgery National University of Ireland, Galway, Republic of Ireland
[2]Department of Vascular surgery, Galway University Hospital, Galway, Republic of Ireland
Full list of author information is available at the end of the article

toxicity of contrast media to renal tubular cells [8, 9]. Multiple therapies have been postulated to prevent CI-AKI act by affecting these mechanisms or their metabolic mediators.

There is ongoing discussion about the impact of new contrast media on the size of the problem and the outcomes of prevention methods or even the existence of the problem, on the other side these conclusions were challenged as coming only from retrospective studies that does not take in account patients factors or indications for using contrast media in deferent cases with deferent baseline renal profile [10, 11].

In recent years, there have been many systematic reviews and meta-analyses for direct pair-wise comparisons of individual interventions suggested for CI-AKI prevention. With so many options explored, it is difficult to determine the treatment options most likely to show benefit in large-scale trials. Unlike conventional meta-analysis, Network facilitates simultaneous comparison of indirect relationships between multiple interventions. The network can establish an estimate of comparative efficacy between two or more treatments compared to the same control intervention [12–14]. We undertook a network-meta-analysis of preventive strategies for CA-AKI to determine the treatment most likely be beneficial based upon currently available evidence.

Methods

We conducted a systematic review and network meta-analysis in accordance with the PRISMA extension for Network Meta-Analyses [15].

Protocol and registration

No registered protocol.

Eligibility criteria

We consider all randomized controlled trials in which patients underwent a contrast-enhanced procedure with CI-AKI as a primary or secondary outcome. We evaluate studies in which a prevention method was compared to placebo, control or other intervention. Excluded from the analysis were other research designs, including non-randomised control trials; clinical trials; trials comparing different doses of the same intervention and trials using re-randomization of the same sample (Crossover design). For this review, we defined CI-AKI as an increase of more than or equal to 0.5 mg/dl and/or 25% increase in baseline serum Creatinine one to 5 days post contrast exposure [3].

Information sources

We searched for English-language trials in PubMed, Embase and Cochrane Central Register of Controlled Trials without any date restrictions. The final search was undertaken on 25th April 2017.

Search strategy and study selection

Two authors (Ahmed, Walsh) searched Electronic databases using Mesh terms "contrast nephropathy", "contrast nephropathy prophylaxis", "contrast nephropathy prevention", with the Boolean operator "OR" as appropriate. Titles and abstracts of identified studies were assessed first, with full texts reviewed thereafter. The study was included if the methodology fulfilled inclusion criterion.

Data collection

Data were recorded concerning sample size, adverse events, procedures performed, study inclusion and exclusion criteria, intervention type and dose, contrast media volume, CI-AKI definition, and contrast medium type and osmolality.

The geometry of the network

A network diagram was created using NetMetaXL tool to graphically represent the size of the trial and the number of pairwise comparisons between interventions. The size of each intervention node is proportional to a number of patients included in the trial, while the thickness of interconnecting lines is proportional to the number of pairwise comparisons between any two interventions.

Risk of bias

The Cochrane tool for risk of bias assessment (RevMan 5.3) was used to assess bias within individual studies. A bias graph was generated to portray the risk of bias overall across the included trials.

Summary measures

Odds ratios with 95% confidence intervals were calculated and presented in the form of Forest plots we generated a league table, which ranks summary estimates in order of the impact of the intervention on the primary outcome measure [10]. In the league table, interventions were ranked from those with the highest effect to the lowest. A stacked bar chart rankogram was also created to represent ranking probabilities and their uncertainty.

Analysis methods

Data with respect to events and number of patients in individual trials were prepared and entered using NetMetaXL [16], to facilitate completion of a Bayesian network meta-analysis using WinBUGS version 1.4.3 from within Microsoft excel. We used the Markov Chain Monte Carlo method of parameter estimation to obtain posterior estimates of effects. Both vague prior and informative prior results were presented in the Forest Plot.

Zero cells were adjusted using an adjusted continuity correction factor accounting for potential differences in sample size, centered around 0.5.

As NetMetaXL is a relatively new tool, we run a separate set of analyses for the same data on GeMTC R package to validate our results with no noticeable differences.

We performed analysis with both fixed effects models and random effects random-effect hierarchical models. For Bayesian computation; detailed statistical approach and diagnostics are provided in Additional file 1.

Assessment of consistency, model fit, and convergence

In NetMetaXL, 'inconsistency plot' was generated to facilitate visual assessment of conflicts between direct and indirect evidence with limitation in our analysis due to a substantial number of nodes on excel. Heterogeneity for vague and informative priors was provided within the forest plot results & Monte Carlo error < 5% of the standard deviation (SD) used to assess convergence.

For GeMTC R package Gelman-Rubin statistics used numerically and graphically to evaluate convergence while

deviance information criterion (DIC) was used for determining model fits and the model with smaller DIC value was considered better.

Additional analyses

In addition to the main analysis we performed three other analysis, the first excluding RCTs with any partial use of hyperosmolar contrast media and in the other two RCTs were divided according to baseline renal profile.

For each of the four analyses we performed sub-analysis excluding studies with zero values as corresponding effects estimates may be subject to numerical instability, generally over-estimate the effect, and that can be observed in the wide associated confidence intervals.

Results

Study selection

A total of 32,596 study titles were identified in the initial literature search, of which 200 fulfilled criteria for inclusion [4, 5, 7, 17–209] (Fig. 1). Some studies were excluded as some data were partially included or re-analyzed in a

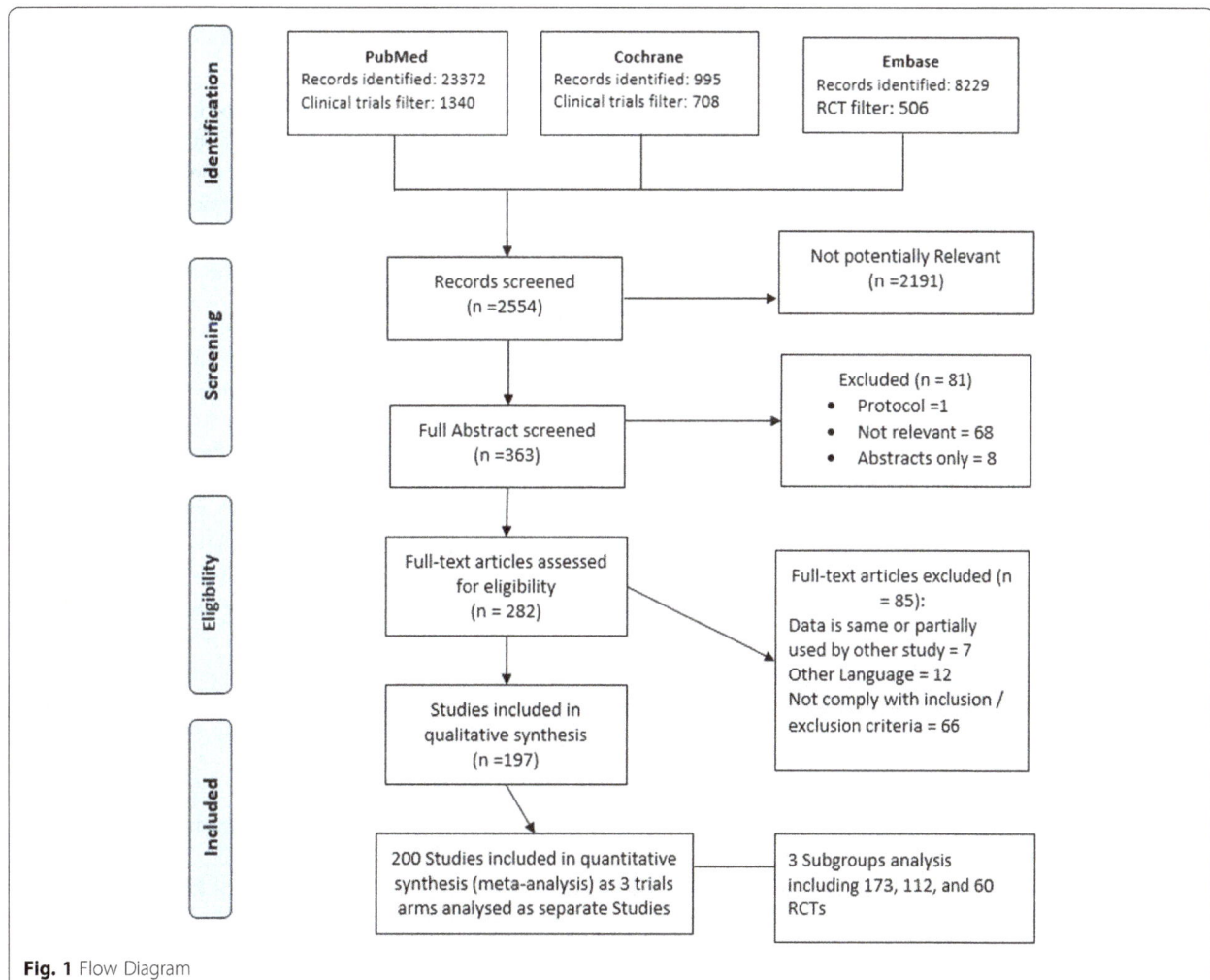

Fig. 1 Flow Diagram

follow-up study involved in our review [210–215]. A total of 32,399 studies were excluded after remove duplication the most common reasons for exclusions after full examination included observational methodology; different outcome measures, inadequate definition of CI-AKI; unclear evidence of randomization; old studies that did not comply with eligibility criteria for more than one reason [216–279]. The twelve studies published in a non-English language included those from centers in Germany [280, 281], China [282–287], Spain [288], France [289], Turkey [290] and Italy [291]. Eight further potentially suitable studies were identified in abstract form only, but were excluded as no full-text article could be identified [292–299].

Study characteristics

Additional file 2 outlines individual study characteristics (study inclusion and exclusion criteria; procedure performed; baseline renal function; definition of CI-AKI used in the study; contrast medium volume and osmolality). In total, 197studies fulfilled the inclusion criteria, including three which had multiple trial arms requiring separate analyses (Yang 2014, Kumar 2014 & Chen 2008). A total of 200 comparative analyses were therefore included in our analyses. Coronary angiography accounted for 145 (72.5%) of the contrast-dependent procedures were. Less frequently reported procedures included contrast-enhanced CT imaging (n = 16, 8%), peripheral angiography with/without angioplasty and stenting (n = 3, 1.5%) endovascular aneurysm repairs (EVAR) (n = 1, 0.5. %). Multiple procedures were included in 35 studies (17.5%). Low osmolar contrast agents were used in 111 (55.5%), iso-osmolar agents in 44 studies (22%), and hi-osmolar media in 3 studies (1.5%). Twenty-six (13%) trials permitted physician discretion in the selection of contrast media, while a further 16 (8%) did not specify the contrast medium utilized. More recent studies we observed better design with an exclusion for patients using alternative CI-AKI prevention interventions from participation or stratified those methods among arms of the trial.

Network structure

The relationship and comparisons between included studies are demonstrated in the network diagram (Fig. 2). Forty-four interventions are included in this network (Table 1).

Network geometry

Data from 42,273 patients recruited to 200 trials investigating 44 interventions were included in our analyses; a summary of network characteristics is provided in (Table 2). Nine hundred and forty-six pair-wise comparisons were possible, of which 81 used data from direct comparisons in Additional file 3. The most commonly

investigated comparisons are between N-acetylcysteine (NAC) and placebo (36 studies, 8,202patients); and intravenous normal saline and intravenous sodium bicarbonate (24 studies, 5,481patients). The interventions most commonly investigated were NAC, NaHCO3, Statins, Intravenous Hydration (I.V), and placebo or control. The characteristics of individual interventions are outlined in Additional file 3.

Risk of bias

Risk of bias assessed by two authors (Khalid, Walsh). In case of disagreement, other authors were consulted. Summary for individual studies provided in Additional file 4 while (Fig. 3) shows the risk of bias graph across all studies. Most of the studies demonstrated unclear to low risk of bias while most of the high risk of bias were observed in attrition bias domain. As the outcome measure (CA-AKI) is dependent on laboratory results it seems reasonable to assume the risk of bias attributed to blinding of outcome assessment domain was low by default.

Synthesis of results

The Renal Association, British Cardiovascular Intervention Society and the Royal College of Radiologists among many other medical bodies recommend using intravenous volume expansion as a prevention method for CA-AKI [300]. Thus, we considered intravenous hydration clinically the reference intervention in this analysis, in addition to the node size and the multiple arms within the network which make it very good comparator.

A forest plot was generated to demonstrate odds ratio generated from direct and indirect pair-wise comparisons. Effect estimates, and confidence intervals were included for both vague and informative priors using a random effects model. The overall heterogeneity for the vague prior was 0.54 (95% CI 0.41–0.69), while that for informative prior was 0.498 (95% CI 0.366–0.6403). The SUCRA (surface under the cumulative ranking curve) was utilized to generate a stacked bar chart rankogram (Fig. 4). A league table arranging summary of effect estimate, and ranking interventions according to impact on the outcome can be found in Additional file 3 in addition to the Forest Plot, characteristics of interventions and comparisons and analysis specifications. The probabilities of being ranked for the best each intervention is summarized in (Table 3) while the numerical values follow the Rankogram results the list of interventions in the first column follow the league table hierarchy and a good example is Allopurinol which included in 4 studies ranked best in both Rankogram (0.9647) and League Table while Silymarin was 3rd (0.7934) and last respectively and was included in one study.

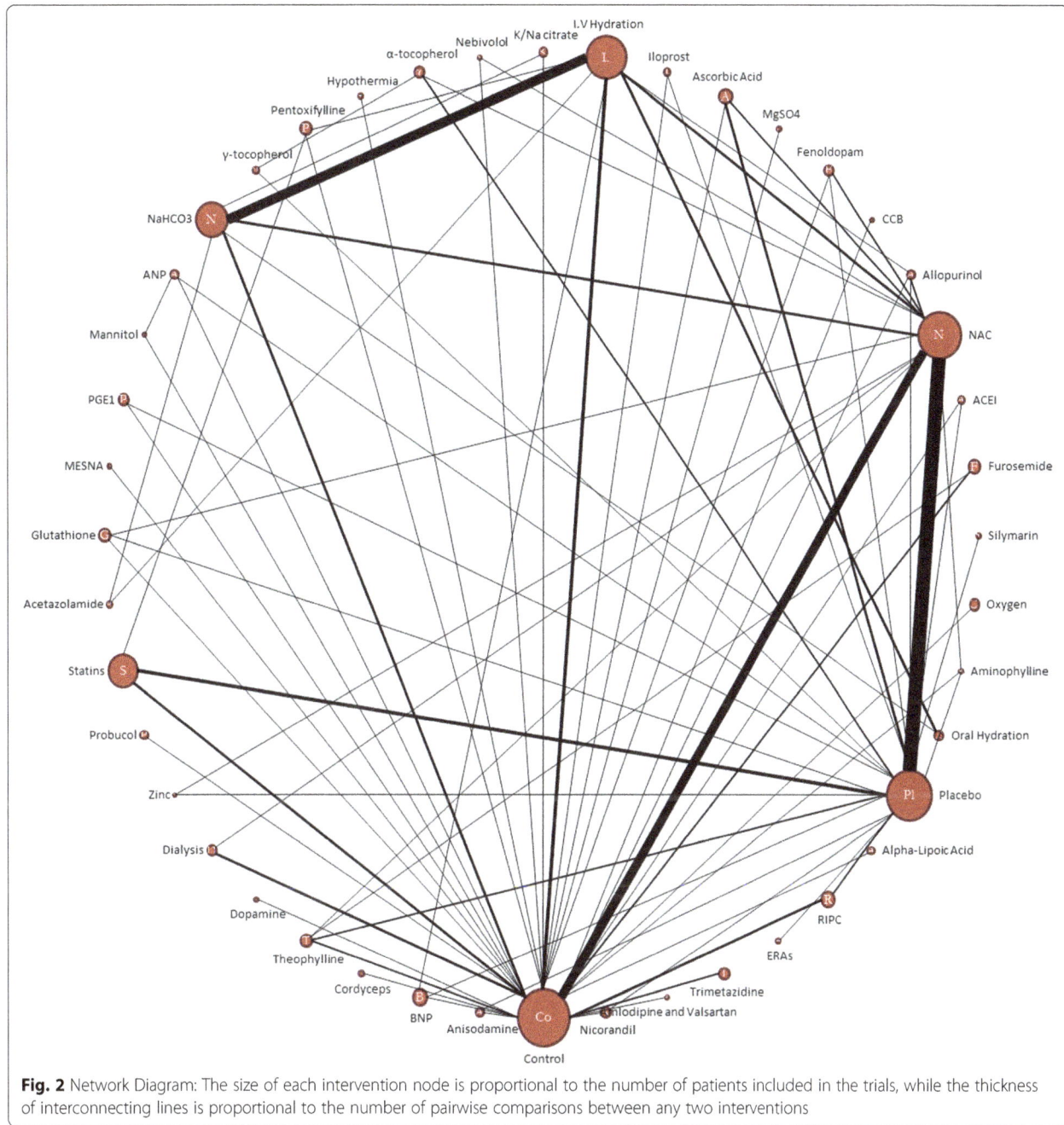

Fig. 2 Network Diagram: The size of each intervention node is proportional to the number of patients included in the trials, while the thickness of interconnecting lines is proportional to the number of pairwise comparisons between any two interventions

Sensitivity analysis

Flow chart for the main analyses and sub-analyses is included in Additional file 1. From the main analysis 200 RCTs we run sub-analysis that includes 184 RCTS in which we exclude all studies with zero values (*n* = 7). All figures and tables are included in Additional file 3.

The second analysis involved 173 RCTs after excluding studies reporting any use of hyperosmolar contrast media, the sub-analysis without zero values RCTs include 159 RCTS.

Trials with high baseline renal profile were in analysis 3 which includes 112 RCTs and sub-analysis for 105 RCTS. The 4th analysis includes 60 and 53 RCTs respectively. Analysis specifications, figures and tables provided in Additional file 5, Additional file 6 and Additional file 7.

When interpreting sub-analyses results in conventional direct pairwise comparisons the main effect results from the size of the excluded studies because there is no exclusion for interventions and they will always be present at both sides of the forest plot. This impact the overall diamond shape effect estimates size and confidence

Table 1 Interventions within Network Diagram

NO	Drug	Abbreviation	Patients
1	I.V Hydration	I.V	5136
2	Statins	Sta	3040
3	Furosemide	Fur	554
4	NAC	NAC	6095
5	Trimetazidine	Tri	352
6	NaHCO3	NaH	3393
7	PGE1	PGE	304
8	MgSO4	MgS	62
9	Pentoxifylline	Pen	438
10	Placebo	Pla	7044
11	Control	Con	9120
12	Allopurinol	All	204
13	BNP	BNP	744
14	Probucol	Pro	198
15	α-tocopherol	α-t	312
16	γ-tocopherol	γ-t	102
17	Oxygen	Oxy	346
18	Amlodipine and Valsartan	Aml	45
19	K/Na citrate	K/N	203
20	Nicorandil	Nic	291
21	Ascorbic Acid	Asc	552
22	Alpha-Lipoic Acid	Alp	139
23	Oral Hydration	Ora	254
24	Nebivolol	Neb	40
25	Anisodamine	Ani	192
26	RIPC	RIP	608
27	Theophylline	The	384
28	Hypothermia	Hyp	58
29	Glutathione	Glu	421
30	MESNA	MES	51
31	ACEI	AC	129
32	Aminophylline	Ami	45
33	Iloprost	Ilo	118
34	Acetazolamide	Ace	94
35	ANP	ANP	202
36	Zinc	Zin	18
37	Dialysis	Dia	293
38	Fenoldopam	Fe	333
39	ERAs	ER	77
40	CCB	CC	42
41	Dopamine	Do	48
42	Mannitol	Ma	35
43	Cordyceps	Co	88
44	Silymarin	Si	69

ACEI Angiotensin Converting-Enzyme Inhibitor, *ANP* Atrial Natriuretic Peptide, *BNP* B-Type Natriuretic Peptide, *CCB* Calcium Channels Blockers, *CI-AKI* Contrast Induced Acute Kidney Injury, *CIN* Contrast Induced Nephropathy, *ERAs* Endothelin Receptor Antagonism, *MESNA* 2-Mercaptoethane Sulfonate Sodium, *MgSo4* Magnesium Sulphate, *NAC* N-acetyl cysteine, *NaHco3* Sodium Bicarbonate, *PGE1* Prostaglandin E1, *RIPC* Remote Ischemic Preconditioning

Table 2 Network Characteristics

Characteristic	Number
Number of Interventions	44
Number of Studies	200
Total Number of Patients in Network	42,273
Total Number of Events in Network	4602
Total Possible Pairwise Comparisons	946
Total Number Pairwise Comparisons with Direct Data	81
Number of Two-arm Studies	179
Number of Multi-Arms Studies	21
Number of Studies with No Zero Events	184
Number of Studies With At Least One Zero Event	16
Number of Studies with All Zero Events	2

interval will either shift towards one treatment or touching the line of no effect indicating no superiority for any intervention. This is different in Network Meta-analysis in which we can see changes in connections dynamic (Network Diagram) and interventions numbers represented by node sizes and number of connections between them both can be affected or totally removed by the excluding studies. In the latter case the Network Diagram and characteristics of interventions and comparisons provide detailed visualization to help compare the main vs sub-analysis. In Additional file 3, Additional file 5, Additional file 6 and Additional file 7 we detailed all excluded studies, the affected interventions, Network Diagrams and the characteristics of the interventions and comparisons.

Assessment of consistency

An 'inconsistency plot' (Fig. 5) was generated to assess inconsistency. Inconsistency in network meta-analysis is similar to heterogeneity in conventional meta-analysis but consistency concerns the relation between the treatments whereas heterogeneity concerns the variation between trials within a pairwise comparison between two treatments. Inconsistency is caused by imbalances in the distribution of effect modifiers in the direct and indirect evidence. Effects modifiers in this large sample include but are not limited to patient factors, drug interactions, contrast media volume and type and renal function pre-intervention. Inevitably, some modifiers exist that cannot be completely eliminated in large multi-treatment network meta-analysis, leading to some inconsistency, indicating a need for careful interpretation of the results [301]. The consistency plot shows individual data points' posterior mean deviance contributions for the consistency model (horizontal axis) and the unrelated mean effects model (vertical axis) along with the line of equality. In our analysis, the main limitation is excel inability to handle a large amount of nodes. However, there should be a consideration

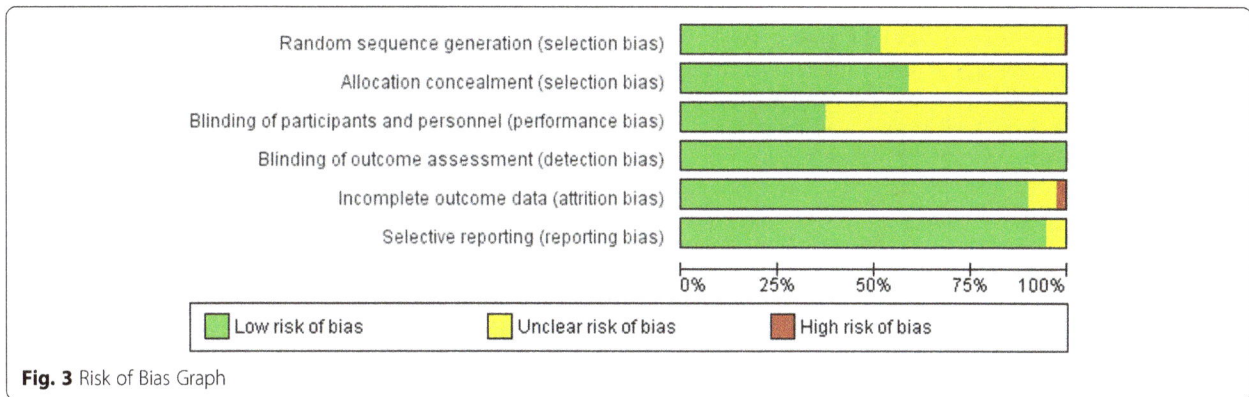

Fig. 3 Risk of Bias Graph

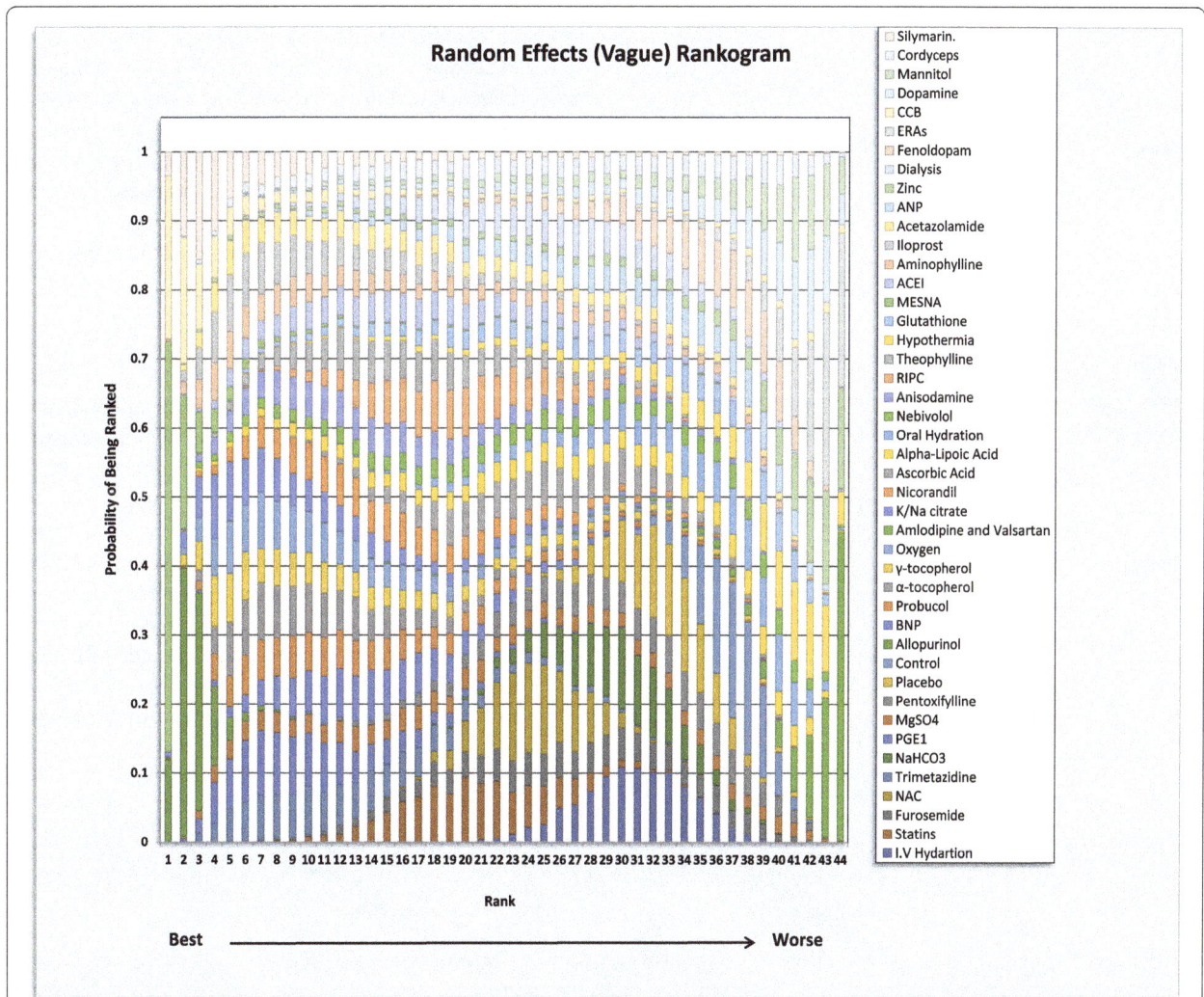

Fig. 4 Rankogram: ranking the interventions for the probability of being the best, the interventions are colour coded; the first column represents the chance of being first best and 2nd column is the chance of being 2nd best and so on. i.e. the first column represent the chance of being first best cmparing all interventions out of100% and the second represent the chance of being second best out of 100% up to last column in this case number 44 (nuber of interventions); the overall ranking for each treatment is the sum of scores through out the 44 compasrisons. The overall numerical value is presented in Table 3

Table 3 Interventions ranking the treatments names column follow the league table (which arranges the presentation of summary estimates by ranking the treatments in order of most pronounced impact on the outcome under consideration) the numerical values represents the cumulative results of the probability of being best in which the highest score is 1 or 100% (see Rankogram)

Treatment	SUCRA	Treatment	SUCRA
Allopurinol	0.9647	NaHCO3	0.3419
MESNA	0.9427	Pentoxifylline	0.3391
PGE1	0.7809	I.V Hydration	0.3124
α-tocopherol	0.7614	Placebo	0.2694
Oxygen	0.7527	Oral Hydration	0.2517
K/Na citrate	0.7469	Hypothermia	0.2021
Trimetazidine	0.7151	Control	0.1658
Probucol	0.7042	Amlodipine and Valsartan	0.05485
γ-tocopherol	0.689	ACEI	0.5783
BNP	0.6767	Aminophylline	0.6593
Anisodamine	0.6594	Iloprost	0.7481
Nicorandil	0.6442	Acetazolamide	0.6242
Theophylline	0.629	ANP	0.3291
RIPC	0.5692	Zinc	0.198
Statins	0.5497	Dialysis	0.4319
MgSO4	0.5177	Fenoldopam	0.2296
NAC	0.4592	ERAs	0.06734
Nebivolol	0.4543	CCB	0.7249
Ascorbic Acid	0.4433	Dopamine	0.1916
Alpha-Lipoic Acid	0.4322	Mannitol	0.1905
Furosemide	0.4027	Cordyceps	0.4459
Glutathione	0.3554	Silymarin	0.7934
Analysis	Random Effects (Vague)		

of individual pairwise comparisons effect estimates generated within the forest plot.

In GeMTC R analyses I^2 statistics and DIC was much smaller for Random effect indicating less heterogeneity compared with a fixed effect which is expected to provide the nature of the network. Detailed scores are presented in Additional file 1 while Gelman and Rubin's convergence diagnostics were added to corresponded analyses in Additional file 3, Additional file 5, Additional file 6 and Additional file 7.

In general, the main analysis reviled some interesting results with Allopurinol, Prostaglandin E1 (PGE1) & Oxygen were ranked high with good both statistical and clinical outcomes in relatively fewer number of studies comparing with other interventions studied in larger number of RCTs e.g. NAC, Statins, Hydration, NaHco3 and RIPC. The results were stable throughout different sub analysis considering the changes in network diagram being affected by excluded studies in all 7 networks. The model fitting and the consistency within the network was good considering the large size and it is understandable that it was better fitted in the 7 sub-groups analysis specially after excluding zero values studies. It is very important here to remember in network ranking is the probability of being the best within the interventions and we need to look at the forest plot for each comparison.

Discussion
Summary of evidence
This is a systematic review and network meta-analysis (multi-treatment comparison) of studies investigating methods for the prevention of contrast-induced nephropathy. We identified 200 eligible trials, of which 3 had 2 different arms and thus analysed separately. Data from a total of 42,273 patients undergoing 44 different interventions were included. Intravenous hydration (Nacl) was used as the reference treatment as there is a consensus supported by evidence accepting it as a method of prevention with no clear superiority for other I.V fluids [81]. in our network it was also included in many multiple arms

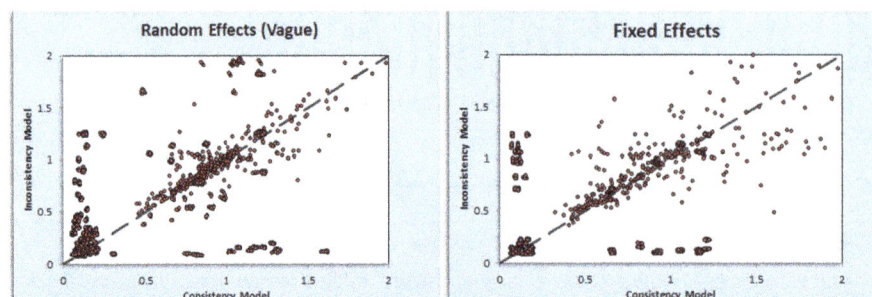

Fig. 5 Inconsistency Plot: Inconsistency is similar to heterogeneity in conventional meta-analysis, but consistency concerns the relation between the direct and indirect evidence. The consistency plot shows individual data points' posterior mean deviance contributions for the consistency model (horizontal axis) and the unrelated mean effects model (vertical axis) along with the line of equality

RCTs which make it statistically a very good comparator. While only randomized control trials were included, defining the outcome and inclusion criteria, help to minimize the number of effect modifiers at play in different studies, thus minimising inconsistency. However, the assumption of homogeneity should be accepted with caution in light of the large numbers of trials and patients included.

It is very important for readers more familiar with general probability measure in which the value one is assigned to the entire probability space to recognize that SUCRA use posterior probabilities for each treatment to be among the n - best options (cumulative probabilities) thus the sum add to > 1. The word best referred to the number of times that an intervention ranks first out of the total number of random samples [14] In Rankogram the first column represent the chance of being first best out of100% and the second represent the chance of being second best up to last column; the overall ranking for each treatment is the sum and that the reason each treatment probability is calculated out of 100%.

We can generally categorize the 44 ranked interventions in groups. The first group is high ranked interventions with relatively fewer number of studies and this group is mainly for further research consideration despite good design RCTs, good clinical outcomes, and our conscious effort to eliminate the effect of small node effect on the network and the fact we accommodate and accounted for the different in interventions size when calculating the probability but we cannot ignore that this may still play in favour of small studies and we think they deserve another look with larger well-designed trials, this group includes mainly Allopurinol, Prostaglandin E1 (PGE1) & Oxygen; Allopurinol a xanthine oxidase Inhibitor used for treatment of gout and management of hyperuricemia associated with chemotherapy and was assessed in 4 trials with 204 patients with recent published evidence suggesting some benefits [302] while PGE1 in 4 trails with total 304 patients. Interestingly Oxygen was highly ranked before and after exclusion of zero events studies and the total number of patients was 346 in 2 studies.

The scorned group is the middle group which included in decent number of studies and the interventions in this group with safe and or well tested profile can be used in patient care at the same time continuously evaluated and this group can include RIPC, Statins (which usually in use specially by cardiac and vascular patients), NAC, NaHco3, I.V hydration, Oral hydration and hypothermia. This group needed the physician to consult his local guidelines after evaluating each patient individually and some interventions like hypothermia is not applicable for all patients.

The sub-analyses in our network for was performed after excluding studies with zero events to eliminate favorable effect profile. It produced better statistical results and helped compare the results without the interventions involved in a small number of trials.

Research & Clinical impact

For health care providers, the results of this meta-analysis do not suggest changes to current clinical practice. The prevention methods assessed in large studies should be evaluated on a case-by-case basis, bearing in mind the comorbidities, clinical needs and prior risk factors of the individual patient with special consideration to national and local guidelines. Interventions with safe profile and supportive evidence from direct pair-wise meta-analysis can be considered as additional or second-line therapies for CA-AKI prevention. For clinical researchers, the highly-ranked treatments with relatively small number of trials merit further examonation in larger RCTs.

Limitations

One limitation of this meta-analysis is the exclusion of non-English language studies (n = 12). The inclusion of these studies may add to the supportive evidence for the use of some interventions, although the effect size of these trials is likely to be minimal in light of the sample sizes in question. Another limitation is the difference in contrast media used which may affect the outcomes; we excluded studies that used hyperosmolar contrast media to minimise this effect with some evidence suggesting similar CIN incidence for iso and low-osmolar CM in coronary angiography patients [303]. In large Network, another consideration is our inability to account for other possible effect modifiers, and our assumptions regarding homogeneity and similarity across a large number of studies thus it is important to look at each intervention ranking through the multiple analyses provided in the supplemnts.

While preparing this network meta-analysis a pairwise meta-analysis was published .comparing N-acetylcysteine, sodium bicarbonate, statins and ascorbic acid for CA-AKI reduction [304]. The data was obtained from controlled trials that used intravenous (IV) or intra-arterial contrast. The results of statins plus I.V saline vs I.V saline show clinically but not statistically significant difference. When comparing Sodium bicarbonate to I.V saline it was clinically better, but again the difference was not statistically significant. However Ascorbic acid was better both clinically and statistically vs I.V saline and show no such difference when compared with NAC. A similar result can be observed in our ranking table with 0.5497, 0.4433, 0.3419 and 0.3124 probability of being rank for statins, ascorbic acid, Sodium bicarbonate and I.V saline consequently. Although direct comparisons results were provided within forest plot in our network, we think the results from pair-wise reviews is important; the nature of conventional meta-analysis prevent utilization of multiple arms trials and creating indirect comparison but it can be used to look at sections of more comprehensive network-meta-analysis in addition to the fact that It is more flexible in terms of subgroup analysis and thus assessment of effects modifiers e.g. type of contrast media in this case.

Conclusion

This systematic review and network meta-analysis provide a comprehensive analysis of currently utilized CA-AKI prevention interventions. Results arising from this network identified some highly-ranked interventions throughout analyses and sub-analyses (e.g., Allopurinol, PGE1 & Oxygen) which were included in small number of trials and merit further examination on a larger scale in the context of a well-designed RCTs.

Additional files

Additional file 1: Analysis flow chart and statistical approach. (DOCX 125 kb)

Additional file 2: Studies characteristics. (DOCX 889 kb)

Additional file 3: Main Analysis 200–184 RCTs. (DOCX 46108 kb)

Additional file 4: Risk of Bias Table. (DOCX 1056 kb)

Additional file 5: Excluding hyperosmolar 173–159 RCTs. (DOCX 41962 kb)

Additional file 6: High Baseline Renal Profile 112–105 RCTs. (DOCX 32278 kb)

Additional file 7: Normal Baseline Renal Profile 60–53 RCTs. (DOCX 16081 kb)

Abbreviations

ACEI: Angiotensin Converting-Enzyme Inhibitor; ANP: Atrial Natriuretic Peptide; BNP: B-Type Natriuretic Peptide; CCB: Calcium Channels Blockers; CI-AKI: Contrast Induced Acute Kidney Injury; CIN: Contrast Induced Nephropathy; CM: Contrast Media; ERAs: Endothelin Receptor Antagonism; MESNA: 2-Mercaptoethane Sulfonate Sodium; MgSo4: Magnesium Sulphate; NAC: N-acetyl cysteine; NaHco3: Sodium Bicarbonate; PGE1: Prostaglandin E1; RCT: Randomise Control Trails; RIPC: Remote Ischemic Preconditioning

Acknowledgements

We acknowledge Ms. Geraldine Curtin and the staff in the James Hardiman library, NUI Galway, for their kind assistance in acquiring relevant papers and Information.

Funding

This research was funded by the National University of Ireland Galway.

Authors' contributions

KA: Study design, Literature search, figures, data collection, data Analysis, data interpretation and writing. TM: Critical appraisal, review and edit. RC Figures Editing: SM Figures Editing. MT Critical appraisal, review and edit. MK Methodology, statistical data analysis, data interpretation, review and edit. Professor SW: Methodology, literature search, data interpretation Critical appraisal, review, and edit. All authors read and approved the final manuscript.

Competing interests

The authors declare that they have no competing interests.

Author details

[1]Lambe Institute for Translational Research, Discipline of Surgery National University of Ireland, Galway, Republic of Ireland. [2]Department of Vascular surgery, Galway University Hospital, Galway, Republic of Ireland. [3]School of Population and Public Health, University of British Columbia, Scientist / Biostatistician, Centre for Health Evaluation and Outcome Sciences (CHEOS), St. Paul's Hospital, Vancouver, Canada. [4]HRB Clinical Research Facility Galway, Galway, Republic of Ireland.

References

1. Mohammed NM, Mahfouz A, Achkar K, Rafie IM, Hajar R. Contrast-induced nephropathy. Heart Views. 2013;14(3):106–16.
2. Goldfarb S, McCullough PA, McDermott J, Gay SB. Contrast-induced acute kidney injury: specialty-specific protocols for interventional radiology, diagnostic computed tomography radiology, and interventional cardiology. Mayo Clin Proc. 2009;84(2):170–9.
3. Goldenberg I, Matetzky S. Nephropathy induced by contrast media: pathogenesis, risk factors and preventive strategies. CMAJ. 2005;172(11):1461–71.
4. Castini D, Lucreziotti S, Bosotti L, Salerno Uriarte D, Sponzilli C, Verzoni A, et al. Prevention of contrast-induced nephropathy: a single center randomized study. Clin Cardiol. 2010;33(3):E63–8.
5. Maioli M, Toso A, Leoncini M, Gallopin M, Tedeschi D, Micheletti C, et al. Sodium bicarbonate versus saline for the prevention of contrast-induced nephropathy in patients with renal dysfunction undergoing coronary angiography or intervention. J Am Coll Cardiol. 2008;52(8):599–604.
6. Mehran R, Nikolsky E. Contrast-induced nephropathy: definition, epidemiology, and patients at risk. Kidney Int Suppl. 2006;100:S11–5.
7. Spargias K, Alexopoulos E, Kyrzopoulos S, Iokovis P, Greenwood DC, Manginas A, et al. Ascorbic acid prevents contrast-mediated nephropathy in patients with renal dysfunction undergoing coronary angiography or intervention. Circulation. 2004;110(18):2837–42.
8. Tumlin J, Stacul F, Adam A, Becker CR, Davidson C, Lameire N, et al. Pathophysiology of contrast-induced nephropathy. Am J Cardiol. 2006; 98(6A):14K–20K.
9. Wong PC, Li Z, Guo J, Zhang A. Pathophysiology of contrast-induced nephropathy. Int J Cardiol. 2012;158(2):186–92.
10. Ehrmann S, Aronson D, Hinson JS. Contrast-associated acute kidney injury is a myth: yes. Intensive Care Med. 2018;44(1):104–6.
11. Weisbord SD, du Cheryon D. Contrast-associated acute kidney injury is a myth: no. Intensive Care Med. 2018;44(1):107–9.
12. Thorlund K, Druyts E, Toor K, Jansen JP, Mills EJ. Incorporating alternative design clinical trials in network meta-analyses. Clin Epidemiol. 2015;7:29–35.
13. Salanti G, Higgins JP, Ades AE, Ioannidis JP. Evaluation of networks of randomized trials. Stat Methods Med Res. 2008;17(3):279–301.
14. Salanti G, Ades AE, Ioannidis JP. Graphical methods and numerical summaries for presenting results from multiple-treatment meta-analysis: an overview and tutorial. J Clin Epidemiol. 2011;64(2):163–71.
15. Hutton B, Salanti G, Caldwell DM, Chaimani A, Schmid CH, Cameron C, et al. The PRISMA extension statement for reporting of systematic reviews incorporating network meta-analyses of health care interventions: checklist and explanations. Ann Intern Med. 2015;162(11):777–84.
16. Brown S, Hutton B, Clifford T, Coyle D, Grima D, Wells G, et al. A Microsoft-excel-based tool for running and critically appraising network meta-analyses—an overview and application of NetMetaXL. Syst Rev. 2014;3:110.
17. Abaci O, Arat Ozkan A, Kocas C, Cetinkal G, Sukru Karaca O, Baydar O, et al. Impact of Rosuvastatin on contrast-induced acute kidney injury in patients at high risk for nephropathy undergoing elective angiography. Am J Cardiol. 2015;115(7):867–71.

18. Adolph E, Holdt-Lehmann B, Chatterjee T, Paschka S, Prott A, Schneider H, et al. Renal insufficiency following radiocontrast exposure trial (REINFORCE): a randomized comparison of sodium bicarbonate versus sodium chloride hydration for the prevention of contrast-induced nephropathy. Coron Artery Dis. 2008;19(6):413–9.

19. Akyuz S, Karaca M, Kemaloglu Oz T, Altay S, Gungor B, Yaylak B, et al. Efficacy of oral hydration in the prevention of contrast-induced acute kidney injury in patients undergoing coronary angiography or intervention. Nephron Clin Pract. 2014;128(1–2):95–100.

20. Albabtain MA, Almasood A, Alshurafah H, Alamri H, Tamim H. Efficacy of ascorbic acid, N-acetylcysteine, or combination of both on top of saline hydration versus saline hydration alone on prevention of contrast-induced nephropathy: a prospective randomized study. J Interv Cardiol. 2013;26(1):90–6.

21. Allaqaband S, Tumuluri R, Malik AM, Gupta A, Volkert P, Shalev Y, et al. Prospective randomized study of N-acetylcysteine, fenoldopam, and saline for prevention of radiocontrast-induced nephropathy. Catheter Cardiovasc Interv. 2002;57(3):279–83.

22. Amini M, Salarifar M, Amirbaigloo A, Masoudkabir F, Esfahani F. N-acetylcysteine does not prevent contrast-induced nephropathy after cardiac catheterization in patients with diabetes mellitus and chronic kidney disease: a randomized clinical trial. Trials. 2009;10:45.

23. Angoulvant D, Cucherat M, Rioufol G, Finet G, Beaune J, Revel D, et al. Preventing acute decrease in renal function induced by coronary angiography (PRECORD): a prospective randomized trial. Arch Cardiovasc Dis. 2009;102(11):761–7.

24. Aslanger E, Uslu B, Akdeniz C, Polat N, Cizgici Y, Oflaz H. Intrarenal application of N-acetylcysteine for the prevention of contrast medium-induced nephropathy in primary angioplasty. Coron Artery Dis. 2012;23(4):265–70.

25. Baker CS, Wragg A, Kumar S, De Palma R, Baker LR, Knight CJ. A rapid protocol for the prevention of contrast-induced renal dysfunction: the RAPPID study. J Am Coll Cardiol. 2003;41(12):2114–8.

26. Balderramo DC, Verdu MB, Ramacciotti CF, Cremona LS, Lemos PA, Orias M, et al. Renoprotective effect of high periprocedural doses of oral N-acetylcysteine in patients scheduled to undergo a same-day angiography. Rev Fac Cien Med Univ Nac Cordoba. 2004;61(2):13–9.

27. Baskurt M, Okcun B, Abaci O, Dogan GM, Kilickesmez K, Ozkan AA, et al. N-acetylcysteine versus N-acetylcysteine + theophylline for the prevention of contrast nephropathy. Eur J Clin Investig. 2009;39(9):793–9.

28. Berwanger O, Cavalcanti AB, Sousa AM, Buehler A, Castello-Junior HJ, Cantarelli MJ, et al. Acetylcysteine for the prevention of renal outcomes in patients with diabetes mellitus undergoing coronary and peripheral vascular angiography: a substudy of the acetylcysteine for contrast-induced nephropathy trial. Circ Cardiovasc Interv. 2013;6(2):139–45.

29. Bidram P, Roghani F, Sanei H, Hedayati Z, Golabchi A, Mousavi M, et al. Atorvastatin and prevention of contrast induced nephropathy following coronary angiography. J Res Med Sci. 2015;20(1):1–6.

30. Bilasy ME, Oraby MA, Ismail HM, Maklady FA. Effectiveness of theophylline in preventing contrast-induced nephropathy after coronary angiographic procedures. J Interv Cardiol. 2012;25(4):404–10.

31. Boscheri A, Weinbrenner C, Botzek B, Reynen K, Kuhlisch E, Strasser RH. Failure of ascorbic acid to prevent contrast-media induced nephropathy in patients with renal dysfunction. Clin Nephrol. 2007;68(5):279–86.

32. Boucek P, Havrdova T, Oliyarnyk O, Skibova J, Pecenkova V, Pucelikova T, et al. Prevention of contrast-induced nephropathy in diabetic patients with impaired renal function: a randomized, double blind trial of sodium bicarbonate versus sodium chloride-based hydration. Diabetes Res Clin Pract. 2013;101(3):303–8.

33. Brar SS, Shen AY, Jorgensen MB, Kotlewski A, Aharonian VJ, Desai N, et al. Sodium bicarbonate vs sodium chloride for the prevention of contrast medium-induced nephropathy in patients undergoing coronary angiography: a randomized trial. JAMA. 2008;300(9):1038–46.

34. Briguori C, Airoldi F, D'Andrea D, Bonizzoni E, Morici N, Focaccio A, et al. Renal insufficiency following contrast media administration trial (REMEDIAL): a randomized comparison of 3 preventive strategies. Circulation. 2007; 115(10):1211–7.

35. Briguori C, Colombo A, Airoldi F, Violante A, Castelli A, Balestrieri P, et al. N-acetylcysteine versus fenoldopam mesylate to prevent contrast agent-associated nephrotoxicity. J Am Coll Cardiol. 2004;44(4):762–5.

36. Briguori C, Manganelli F, Scarpato P, Elia PP, Golia B, Riviezzo G, et al. Acetylcysteine and contrast agent-associated nephrotoxicity. J Am Coll Cardiol. 2002;40(2):298–303.

37. Brueck M, Cengiz H, Hoeltgen R, Wieczorek M, Boedeker RH, Scheibelhut C, et al. Usefulness of N-acetylcysteine or ascorbic acid versus placebo to prevent contrast-induced acute kidney injury in patients undergoing elective cardiac catheterization: a single-center, prospective, randomized, double-blind, placebo-controlled trial. J Invasive Cardiol. 2013;25(6):276–83.

38. Burns KE, Priestap F, Martin C. N-acetylcysteine in critically ill patients undergoing contrast-enhanced computed tomography: a randomized trial. Clin Nephrol. 2010;74(4):323–6.

39. Carbonell N, Blasco M, Sanjuan R, Perez-Sancho E, Sanchis J, Insa L, et al. Intravenous N-acetylcysteine for preventing contrast-induced nephropathy: a randomised trial. Int J Cardiol. 2007;115(1):57–62.

40. Carbonell N, Sanjuan R, Blasco M, Jorda A, Miguel A. N-acetylcysteine: short-term clinical benefits after coronary angiography in high-risk renal patients. Rev Esp Cardiol. 2010;63(1):12–9.

41. Chen SL, Zhang J, Yei F, Zhu Z, Liu Z, Lin S, et al. Clinical outcomes of contrast-induced nephropathy in patients undergoing percutaneous coronary intervention: a prospective, multicenter, randomized study to analyze the effect of hydration and acetylcysteine. Int J Cardiol. 2008;126(3):407–13.

42. Cho R, Javed N, Traub D, Kodali S, Atem F, Srinivasan V. Oral hydration and alkalinization is noninferior to intravenous therapy for prevention of contrast-induced nephropathy in patients with chronic kidney disease. J Interv Cardiol. 2010;23(5):460–6.

43. Cicek M, Yildirir A, Okyay K, Yazici AC, Aydinalp A, Kanyilmaz S, et al. Use of alpha-lipoic acid in prevention of contrast-induced nephropathy in diabetic patients. Ren Fail. 2013;35(5):748–53.

44. Coyle LC, Rodriguez A, Jeschke RE, Simon-Lee A, Abbott KC, Taylor AJ. Acetylcysteine In Diabetes (AID): a randomized study of acetylcysteine for the prevention of contrast nephropathy in diabetics. Am Heart J. 2006; 151(5):1032 e9–12.

45. Durham JD, Caputo C, Dokko J, Zaharakis T, Pahlavan M, Keltz J, et al. A randomized controlled trial of N-acetylcysteine to prevent contrast nephropathy in cardiac angiography. Kidney Int. 2002;62(6):2202–7.

46. Dussol B, Morange S, Loundoun A, Auquier P, Berland Y. A randomized trial of saline hydration to prevent contrast nephropathy in chronic renal failure patients. Nephrol Dial Transplant. 2006;21(8):2120–6.

47. Dvorsak B, Kanic V, Ekart R, Bevc S, Hojs R. Ascorbic acid for the prevention of contrast-induced nephropathy after coronary angiography in patients with chronic renal impairment: a randomized controlled trial. Ther Apher Dial. 2013;17(4):384–90.

48. Efrati S, Dishy V, Averbukh M, Blatt A, Krakover R, Weisgarten J, et al. The effect of N-acetylcysteine on renal function, nitric oxide, and oxidative stress after angiography. Kidney Int. 2003;64(6):2182–7.

49. Er F, Nia AM, Dopp H, Hellmich M, Dahlem KM, Caglayan E, et al. Ischemic preconditioning for prevention of contrast medium-induced nephropathy: randomized pilot RenPro trial (renal protection trial). Circulation. 2012;126(3):296–303.

50. Erley CM, Duda SH, Rehfuss D, Scholtes B, Bock J, Muller C, et al. Prevention of radiocontrast-media-induced nephropathy in patients with pre-existing renal insufficiency by hydration in combination with the adenosine antagonist theophylline. Nephrol Dial Transplant. 1999;14(5):1146–9.

51. Erol T, Tekin A, Katircibasi MT, Sezgin N, Bilgi M, Tekin G, et al. Efficacy of allopurinol pretreatment for prevention of contrast-induced nephropathy: a randomized controlled trial. Int J Cardiol. 2013;167(4):1396–9.

52. Erturk M, Uslu N, Gorgulu S, Akbay E, Kurtulus G, Akturk IF, et al. Does intravenous or oral high-dose N-acetylcysteine in addition to saline prevent contrast-induced nephropathy assessed by cystatin C? Coron Artery Dis. 2014;25(2):111–7.

53. Ferrario F, Barone MT, Landoni G, Genderini A, Heidemperger M, Trezzi M, et al. Acetylcysteine and non-ionic isosmolar contrast-induced nephropathy—a randomized controlled study. Nephrol Dial Transplant. 2009;24(10):3103–7.

54. Firouzi A, Eshraghi A, Shakerian F, Sanati HR, Salehi N, Zahedmehr A, et al. Efficacy of pentoxifylline in prevention of contrast-induced nephropathy in angioplasty patients. Int Urol Nephrol. 2012;44(4):1145–9.

55. Firouzi A, Maadani M, Kiani R, Shakerian F, Sanati HR, Zahedmehr A, et al. Intravenous magnesium sulfate: new method in prevention of contrast-induced nephropathy in primary percutaneous coronary intervention. Int Urol Nephrol. 2015;47(3):521–5.

56. Fung JW, Szeto CC, Chan WW, Kum LC, Chan AK, Wong JT, et al. Effect of N-acetylcysteine for prevention of contrast nephropathy in patients with moderate to severe renal insufficiency: a randomized trial. Am J Kidney Dis. 2004;43(5):801–8.

57. Gare M, Haviv YS, Ben-Yehuda A, Rubinger D, Bdolah-Abram T, Fuchs S, et al. The renal effect of low-dose dopamine in high-risk patients undergoing coronary angiography. J Am Coll Cardiol. 1999;34(6):1682–8.

58. Geng W, Fu XH, Gu XS, Wang YB, Wang XC, Li W, et al. Preventive effects of anisodamine against contrast-induced nephropathy in type 2 diabetics with renal insufficiency undergoing coronary angiography or angioplasty. Chin Med J. 2012;125(19):3368–72.

59. Goldenberg I, Shechter M, Matetzky S, Jonas M, Adam M, Pres H, et al. Oral acetylcysteine as an adjunct to saline hydration for the prevention of contrast-induced nephropathy following coronary angiography. A randomized controlled trial and review of the current literature. Eur Heart J. 2004;25(3):212–8.

60. Gomes VO, Lasevitch R, Lima VC, Brito FS Jr, Perez-Alva JC, Moulin B, et al. Hydration with sodium bicarbonate does not prevent contrast nephropathy: a multicenter clinical trial. Arq Bras Cardiol. 2012;99(6):1129–34.

61. Gomes VO, Poli de Figueredo CE, Caramori P, Lasevitch R, Bodanese LC, Araujo A, et al. N-acetylcysteine does not prevent contrast induced nephropathy after cardiac catheterisation with an ionic low osmolality contrast medium: a multicentre clinical trial. Heart. 2005;91(6):774–8.

62. Gu GQ, Lu R, Cui W, Liu F, Zhang Y, Yang XH, et al. Low-dose furosemide administered with adequate hydration reduces contrast-induced nephropathy in patients undergoing coronary angiography. Cardiology. 2013;125(2):69–73.

63. Gulel O, Keles T, Eraslan H, Aydogdu S, Diker E, Ulusoy V. Prophylactic acetylcysteine usage for prevention of contrast nephropathy after coronary angiography. J Cardiovasc Pharmacol. 2005;46(4):464–7.

64. Gunebakmaz O, Kaya MG, Koc F, Akpek M, Kasapkara A, Inanc MT, et al. Does nebivolol prevent contrast-induced nephropathy in humans? Clin Cardiol. 2012;35(4):250–4.

65. Gupta RK, Kapoor A, Tewari S, Sinha N, Sharma RK. Captopril for prevention of contrast-induced nephropathy in diabetic patients: a randomised study. Indian Heart J. 1999;51(5):521–6.

66. Hafiz AM, Jan MF, Mori N, Shaikh F, Wallach J, Bajwa T, et al. Prevention of contrast-induced acute kidney injury in patients with stable chronic renal disease undergoing elective percutaneous coronary and peripheral interventions: randomized comparison of two preventive strategies. Catheter Cardiovasc Interv. 2012;79(6):929–37.

67. Han Y, Zhu G, Han L, Hou F, Huang W, Liu H, et al. Short-term rosuvastatin therapy for prevention of contrast-induced acute kidney injury in patients with diabetes and chronic kidney disease. J Am Coll Cardiol. 2014;63(1):62–70.

68. Hashemi M, Kharazi A, Shahidi S. Captopril for prevention of contrast induced nephropathy in patients undergoing coronary angiography: a double blind placebo controlled clinical trial. J Res Med Sci. 2005;10(5):305–8.

69. Heguilen RM, Liste AA, Payaslian M, Ortemberg MG, Albarracin LM, Bernasconi AR. N-acethyl-cysteine reduces the occurrence of contrast-induced acute kidney injury in patients with renal dysfunction: a single-center randomized controlled trial. Clin Exp Nephrol. 2013;17(3):396–404.

70. Heng AE, Cellarier E, Aublet-Cuvelier B, Decalf V, Motreff P, Marcaggi X, et al. Is treatment with N-acetylcysteine to prevent contrast-induced nephropathy when using bicarbonate hydration out of date? Clin Nephrol. 2008;70(6):475–84.

71. Hoole SP, Heck PM, Sharples L, Khan SN, Duehmke R, Densem CG, et al. Cardiac remote ischemic preconditioning in coronary stenting (CRISP stent) study: a prospective, randomized control trial. Circulation. 2009;119(6):820–7.

72. Hsu TF, Huang MK, Yu SH, Yen DH, Kao WF, Chen YC, et al. N-acetylcysteine for the prevention of contrast-induced nephropathy in the emergency department. Intern Med. 2012;51(19):2709–14.

73. Huber W, Schipek C, Ilgmann K, Page M, Hennig M, Wacker A, et al. Effectiveness of theophylline prophylaxis of renal impairment after coronary angiography in patients with chronic renal insufficiency. Am J Cardiol. 2003; 91(10):1157–62.

74. Inda-Filho AJ, Caixeta A, Manggini M, Schor N. Do intravenous N-acetylcysteine and sodium bicarbonate prevent high osmolal contrast-induced acute kidney injury? A randomized controlled trial. PLoS One. 2014; 9(9):e107602.

75. Investigators ACT. Acetylcysteine for prevention of renal outcomes in patients undergoing coronary and peripheral vascular angiography: main results from the randomized acetylcysteine for contrast-induced nephropathy trial (ACT). Circulation. 2011;124(11):1250–9.

76. Jaffery Z, Verma A, White CJ, Grant AG, Collins TJ, Grise MA, et al. A randomized trial of intravenous n-acetylcysteine to prevent contrast induced nephropathy in acute coronary syndromes. Catheter Cardiovasc Interv. 2012;79(6):921–6.

77. Jo SH, Kim SA, Kim HS, Han SJ, Park WJ, Choi YJ. Alpha-lipoic acid for the prevention of contrast-induced nephropathy in patients undergoing coronary angiography: the ALIVE study - a prospective randomized trial. Cardiology. 2013;126(3):159–66.

78. Jo SH, Koo BK, Park JS, Kang HJ, Cho YS, Kim YJ, et al. Prevention of radiocontrast medium-induced nephropathy using short-term high-dose simvastatin in patients with renal insufficiency undergoing coronary angiography (PROMISS) trial—a randomized controlled study. Am Heart J. 2008;155(3):499 e1–8.

79. Jo SH, Koo BK, Park JS, Kang HJ, Kim YJ, Kim HL, et al. N-acetylcysteine versus AScorbic acid for preventing contrast-induced nephropathy in patients with renal insufficiency undergoing coronary angiography NASPI study-a prospective randomized controlled trial. Am Heart J. 2009;157(3):576–83.

80. Jurado-Roman A, Hernandez-Hernandez F, Garcia-Tejada J, Granda-Nistal C, Molina J, Velazquez M, et al. Role of hydration in contrast-induced nephropathy in patients who underwent primary percutaneous coronary intervention. Am J Cardiol. 2015;115(9):1174–8.

81. Kama A, Yilmaz S, Yaka E, Dervisoglu E, Dogan NO, Erimsah E, et al. Comparison of short-term infusion regimens of N-acetylcysteine plus intravenous fluids, sodium bicarbonate plus intravenous fluids, and intravenous fluids alone for prevention of contrast-induced nephropathy in the emergency department. Acad Emerg Med. 2014;21(6):615–22.

82. Kay J, Chow WH, Chan TM, Lo SK, Kwok OH, Yip A, et al. Acetylcysteine for prevention of acute deterioration of renal function following elective coronary angiography and intervention: a randomized controlled trial. JAMA. 2003;289(5):553–8.

83. Kefer JM, Hanet CE, Boitte S, Wilmotte L, De Kock M. Acetylcysteine, coronary procedure and prevention of contrast-induced worsening of renal function: which benefit for which patient? Acta Cardiol. 2003;58(6):555–60.

84. Khoury Z, Schlicht JR, Como J, Karschner JK, Shapiro AP, Mook WJ, et al. The effect of prophylactic nifedipine on renal function in patients administered contrast media. Pharmacotherapy. 1995;15(1):59–65.

85. Kimmel M, Butscheid M, Brenner S, Kuhlmann U, Klotz U, Alscher DM. Improved estimation of glomerular filtration rate by serum cystatin C in preventing contrast induced nephropathy by N-acetylcysteine or zinc—preliminary results. Nephrol Dial Transplant. 2008;23(4):1241–5.

86. Kinbara T, Hayano T, Ohtani N, Furutani Y, Moritani K, Matsuzaki M. Efficacy of N-acetylcysteine and aminophylline in preventing contrast-induced nephropathy. J Cardiol. 2010;55(2):174–9.

87. Kitzler TM, Jaberi A, Sendlhofer G, Rehak P, Binder C, Petnehazy E, et al. Efficacy of vitamin E and N-acetylcysteine in the prevention of contrast induced kidney injury in patients with chronic kidney disease: a double blind, randomized controlled trial. Wien Klin Wochenschr. 2012;124(9–10):312–9.

88. Klima T, Christ A, Marana I, Kalbermatter S, Uthoff H, Burri E, et al. Sodium chloride vs. sodium bicarbonate for the prevention of contrast medium-induced nephropathy: a randomized controlled trial. Eur Heart J. 2012;33(16):2071–9.

89. Ko YG, Lee BK, Kang WC, Moon JY, Cho YH, Choi SH, et al. Preventive effect of pretreatment with intravenous nicorandil on contrast-induced nephropathy in patients with renal dysfunction undergoing coronary angiography (PRINCIPLE study). Yonsei Med J. 2013;54(4):957–64.

90. Koc F, Ozdemir K, Altunkas F, Celik A, Dogdu O, Karayakali M, et al. Sodium bicarbonate versus isotonic saline for the prevention of contrast-induced nephropathy in patients with diabetes mellitus undergoing coronary angiography and/or intervention: a multicenter prospective randomized study. J Investig Med. 2013;61(5):872–7.

91. Koc F, Ozdemir K, Kaya MG, Dogdu O, Vatankulu MA, Ayhan S, et al. Intravenous N-acetylcysteine plus high-dose hydration versus high-dose hydration and standard hydration for the prevention of contrast-induced nephropathy: CASIS—a multicenter prospective controlled trial. Int J Cardiol. 2012;155(3):418–23.

92. Koch JA, Plum J, Grabensee B, Modder U. Prostaglandin E1: a new agent for the prevention of renal dysfunction in high risk patients caused by radiocontrast media? PGE1 study group. Nephrol Dial Transplant. 2000;15(1):43–9.

93. Kong DG, Hou YF, Ma LL, Yao DK, Wang LX. Comparison of oral and intravenous hydration strategies for the prevention of contrast-induced nephropathy in patients undergoing coronary angiography or angioplasty: a randomized clinical trial. Acta Cardiol. 2012;67(5):565–9.

94. Kooiman J, Sijpkens YW, de Vries JP, Brulez HF, Hamming JF, van der Molen AJ, et al. A randomized comparison of 1-h sodium bicarbonate hydration versus standard peri-procedural saline hydration in patients with chronic kidney disease undergoing intravenous contrast-enhanced computerized tomography. Nephrol Dial Transplant. 2014;29(5):1029–36.

95. Kooiman J, Sijpkens YW, van Buren M, Groeneveld JH, Ramai SR, van der Molen AJ, et al. Randomised trial of no hydration vs. sodium bicarbonate hydration in patients with chronic kidney disease undergoing acute computed tomography-pulmonary angiography. J Thromb Haemost. 2014; 12(10):1658–66.

96. Kotlyar E, Keogh AM, Thavapalachandran S, Allada CS, Sharp J, Dias L, et al. Prehydration alone is sufficient to prevent contrast-induced nephropathy after day-only angiography procedures—a randomised controlled trial. Heart Lung Circ. 2005;14(4):245–51.

97. Kumar A, Bhawani G, Kumari N, Murthy KS, Lalwani V, Raju CN. Comparative study of renal protective effects of allopurinol and N-acetyl-cysteine on contrast induced nephropathy in patients undergoing cardiac catheterization. J Clin Diagn Res. 2014;8(12):HC03–7.

98. Kurnik BR, Allgren RL, Genter FC, Solomon RJ, Bates ER, Weisberg LS. Prospective study of atrial natriuretic peptide for the prevention of radiocontrast-induced nephropathy. Am J Kidney Dis. 1998;31(4):674–80.

99. Kurnik BR, Weisberg LS, Cuttler IM, Kurnik PB. Effects of atrial natriuretic peptide versus mannitol on renal blood flow during radiocontrast infusion in chronic renal failure. J Lab Clin Med. 1990;116(1):27–36.

100. Lavi S, D'Alfonso S, Diamantouros P, Camuglia A, Garg P, Teefy P, et al. Remote ischemic postconditioning during percutaneous coronary interventions: remote ischemic postconditioning-percutaneous coronary intervention randomized trial. Circ Cardiovasc Interv. 2014;7(2):225–32.

101. Lawlor DK, Moist L, DeRose G, Harris KA, Lovell MB, Kribs SW, et al. Prevention of contrast-induced nephropathy in vascular surgery patients. Ann Vasc Surg. 2007;21(5):593–7.

102. Lee SW, Kim WJ, Kim YH, Park SW, Park DW, Yun SC, et al. Preventive strategies of renal insufficiency in patients with diabetes undergoing intervention or arteriography (the PREVENT trial). Am J Cardiol. 2011;107(10):1447–52.

103. Lehnert T, Keller E, Gondolf K, Schaffner T, Pavenstadt H, Schollmeyer P. Effect of haemodialysis after contrast medium administration in patients with renal insufficiency. Nephrol Dial Transplant. 1998;13(2):358–62.

104. Leoncini M, Toso A, Maioli M, Tropeano F, Villani S, Bellandi F. Early high-dose rosuvastatin for contrast-induced nephropathy prevention in acute coronary syndrome: results from the PRATO-ACS study (protective effect of Rosuvastatin and antiplatelet therapy on contrast-induced acute kidney injury and myocardial damage in patients with acute coronary syndrome). J Am Coll Cardiol. 2014;63(1):71–9.

105. Li G, Yin L, Liu T, Zheng X, Xu G, Xu Y, et al. Role of probucol in preventing contrast-induced acute kidney injury after coronary interventional procedure. Am J Cardiol. 2009;103(4):512–4.

106. Li W, Fu X, Wang Y, Li X, Yang Z, Wang X, et al. Beneficial effects of high-dose atorvastatin pretreatment on renal function in patients with acute ST-segment elevation myocardial infarction undergoing emergency percutaneous coronary intervention. Cardiology. 2012;122(3):195–202.

107. Li WH, Li DY, Qian WH, Liu JL, Xu TD, Zhu H, et al. Prevention of contrast-induced nephropathy with prostaglandin E1 in high-risk patients undergoing percutaneous coronary intervention. Int Urol Nephrol. 2014;46(4):781–6.

108. Li XM, Cong HL, Li TT, He LJ, Zhou YJ. Impact of benazepril on contrast-induced acute kidney injury for patients with mild to moderate renal insufficiency undergoing percutaneous coronary intervention. Chin Med J. 2011;124(14):2101–6.

109. Ludwig U, Riedel MK, Backes M, Imhof A, Muche R, Keller F. MESNA (sodium 2-mercaptoethanesulfonate) for prevention of contrast medium-induced nephrotoxicity - controlled trial. Clin Nephrol. 2011;75(4):302–8.

110. Luo SJ, Zhou YJ, Shi DM, Ge HL, Wang JL, Liu RF. Remote ischemic preconditioning reduces myocardial injury in patients undergoing coronary stent implantation. Can J Cardiol. 2013;29(9):1084–9.

111. Luo Y, Wang X, Ye Z, Lai Y, Yao Y, Li J, et al. Remedial hydration reduces the incidence of contrast-induced nephropathy and short-term adverse events in patients with ST-segment elevation myocardial infarction: a single-center, randomized trial. Intern Med. 2014;53(20):2265–72.

112. MacNeill BD, Harding SA, Bazari H, Patton KK, Colon-Hernadez P, DeJoseph D, et al. Prophylaxis of contrast-induced nephropathy in patients undergoing coronary angiography. Catheter Cardiovasc Interv. 2003;60(4):458–61.

113. Maioli M, Toso A, Leoncini M, Micheletti C, Bellandi F. Effects of hydration in contrast-induced acute kidney injury after primary angioplasty: a randomized, controlled trial. Circ Cardiovasc Interv. 2011;4(5):456–62.

114. Malhis M, Al-Bitar S, Al-Deen ZK. The role of theophylline in prevention of radiocontrast media-induced nephropathy. Saudi J Kidney Dis Transpl. 2010;21(2):276–83.

115. Marenzi G, Assanelli E, Marana I, Lauri G, Campodonico J, Grazi M, et al. N-acetylcysteine and contrast-induced nephropathy in primary angioplasty. N Engl J Med. 2006;354(26):2773–82.

116. Marenzi G, Ferrari C, Marana I, Assanelli E, De Metrio M, Teruzzi G, et al. Prevention of contrast nephropathy by furosemide with matched hydration: the MYTHOS (induced diuresis with matched hydration compared to standard hydration for contrast induced nephropathy prevention) trial. JACC Cardiovasc Interv. 2012;5(1):90–7.

117. Marenzi G, Marana I, Lauri G, Assanelli E, Grazi M, Campodonico J, et al. The prevention of radiocontrast-agent-induced nephropathy by hemofiltration. N Engl J Med. 2003;349(14):1333–40.

118. Markota D, Markota I, Starcevic B, Tomic M, Prskalo Z, Brizic I. Prevention of contrast-induced nephropathy with Na/K citrate. Eur Heart J. 2013;34(30):2362–7.

119. Masuda M, Yamada T, Mine T, Morita T, Tamaki S, Tsukamoto Y, et al. Comparison of usefulness of sodium bicarbonate versus sodium chloride to prevent contrast-induced nephropathy in patients undergoing an emergent coronary procedure. Am J Cardiol. 2007;100(5):781–6.

120. Matejka J, Varvarovsky I, Vojtisek P, Herman A, Rozsival V, Borkova V, et al. Prevention of contrast-induced acute kidney injury by theophylline in elderly patients with chronic kidney disease. Heart Vessel. 2010;25(6):536–42.

121. Menting TP, Sterenborg TB, de Waal Y, Donders R, Wever KE, Lemson MS, et al. Remote ischemic preconditioning to reduce contrast-induced nephropathy: a randomized controlled trial. Eur J Vasc Endovasc Surg. 2015;50(4):527–32.

122. Merten GJ, Burgess WP, Gray LV, Holleman JH, Roush TS, Kowalchuk GJ, et al. Prevention of contrast-induced nephropathy with sodium bicarbonate: a randomized controlled trial. JAMA. 2004;291(19):2328–34.

123. Miao Y, Zhong Y, Yan H, Li W, Wang BY, Jin J. Alprostadil plays a protective role in contrast-induced nephropathy in the elderly. Int Urol Nephrol. 2013;45(4):1179–85.

124. Miner SE, Dzavik V, Nguyen-Ho P, Richardson R, Mitchell J, Atchison D, et al. N-acetylcysteine reduces contrast-associated nephropathy but not clinical events during long-term follow-up. Am Heart J. 2004;148(4):690–5.

125. Moore NN, Lapsley M, Norden AG, Firth JD, Gaunt ME, Varty K, et al. Does N-acetylcysteine prevent contrast-induced nephropathy during endovascular AAA repair? A randomized controlled pilot study. J Endovasc Ther. 2006;13(5):660–6.

126. Morikawa S, Sone T, Tsuboi H, Mukawa H, Morishima I, Uesugi M, et al. Renal protective effects and the prevention of contrast-induced nephropathy by atrial natriuretic peptide. J Am Coll Cardiol. 2009;53(12):1040–6.

127. Motohiro M, Kamihata H, Tsujimoto S, Seno T, Manabe K, Isono T, et al. A new protocol using sodium bicarbonate for the prevention of contrast-induced nephropathy in patients undergoing coronary angiography. Am J Cardiol. 2011;107(11):1604–8.

128. Ng TM, Shurmur SW, Silver M, Nissen LR, O'Leary EL, Rigmaiden RS, et al. Comparison of N-acetylcysteine and fenoldopam for preventing contrast-induced nephropathy (CAFCIN). Int J Cardiol. 2006;109(3):322–8.

129. Ochoa A, Pellizzon G, Addala S, Grines C, Isayenko Y, Boura J, et al. Abbreviated dosing of N-acetylcysteine prevents contrast-induced nephropathy after elective and urgent coronary angiography and intervention. J Interv Cardiol. 2004;17(3):159–65.

130. Oguzhan N, Cilan H, Sipahioglu M, Unal A, Kocyigit I, Kavuncuoglu F, et al. The lack of benefit of a combination of an angiotensin receptor blocker and calcium channel blocker on contrast-induced nephropathy in patients with chronic kidney disease. Ren Fail. 2013;35(4):434–9.

131. Oldemeyer JB, Biddle WP, Wurdeman RL, Mooss AN, Cichowski E, Hilleman DE. Acetylcysteine in the prevention of contrast-induced nephropathy after coronary angiography. Am Heart J. 2003;146(6):E23.

132. Onbasili AO, Yeniceriglu Y, Agaoglu P, Karul A, Tekten T, Akar H, et al. Trimetazidine in the prevention of contrast-induced nephropathy after coronary procedures. Heart. 2007;93(6):698–702.

133. Ozcan EE, Guneri S, Akdeniz B, Akyildiz IZ, Senaslan O, Baris N, et al. Sodium bicarbonate, N-acetylcysteine, and saline for prevention of radiocontrast-induced nephropathy. A comparison of 3 regimens for protecting contrast-induced nephropathy in patients undergoing coronary procedures. A single-center prospective controlled trial. Am Heart J. 2007;154(3):539–44.

134. Ozhan H, Erden I, Ordu S, Aydin M, Caglar O, Basar C, et al. Efficacy of short-term high-dose atorvastatin for prevention of contrast-induced nephropathy in patients undergoing coronary angiography. Angiology. 2010;61(7):711–4.

135. Pakfetrat M, Nikoo MH, Malekmakan L, Tabandeh M, Roozbeh J, Nasab MH, et al. A comparison of sodium bicarbonate infusion versus normal saline infusion and its combination with oral acetazolamide for prevention of contrast-induced nephropathy: a randomized, double-blind trial. Int Urol Nephrol. 2009;41(3):629–34.

136. Patti G, Ricottini E, Nusca A, Colonna G, Pasceri V, D'Ambrosio A, et al. Short-term, high-dose atorvastatin pretreatment to prevent contrast-induced nephropathy in patients with acute coronary syndromes undergoing percutaneous coronary intervention from the ARMYDA-CIN [atorvastatin for reduction of myocardial damage during angioplasty—contrast-induced nephropathy] trial. Am J Cardiol. 2011;108(1):1–7.

137. Poletti PA, Platon A, De Seigneux S, Dupuis-Lozeron E, Sarasin F, Becker CD, et al. N-acetylcysteine does not prevent contrast nephropathy in patients with renal impairment undergoing emergency CT: a randomized study. BMC Nephrol. 2013;14:119.

138. Qiao B, Deng J, Li Y, Wang X, Han Y. Rosuvastatin attenuated contrast-induced nephropathy in diabetes patients with renal dysfunction. Int J Clin Exp Med. 2015;8(2):2342–9.

139. Quintavalle C, Fiore D, De Micco F, Visconti G, Focaccio A, Golia B, et al. Impact of a high loading dose of atorvastatin on contrast-induced acute kidney injury. Circulation. 2012;126(25):3008–16.

140. Rahman MM, Haque SS, Rokeya B, Siddique MA, Banerjee SK, Ahsan SA, et al. Trimetazidine in the prevention of contrast induced nephropathy after coronary angiogram. Mymensingh Med J. 2012;21(2):292–9.

141. Rashid ST, Salman M, Myint F, Baker DM, Agarwal S, Sweny P, et al. Prevention of contrast-induced nephropathy in vascular patients undergoing angiography: a randomized controlled trial of intravenous N-acetylcysteine. J Vasc Surg. 2004;40(6):1136–41.

142. Reinecke H, Fobker M, Wellmann J, Becke B, Fleiter J, Heitmeyer C, et al. A randomized controlled trial comparing hydration therapy to additional hemodialysis or N-acetylcysteine for the prevention of contrast medium-induced nephropathy: the Dialysis-versus-diuresis (DVD) trial. Clin Res Cardiol. 2007;96(3):130–9.

143. Rohani A. Effectiveness of aminophylline prophylaxis of renal impairment after coronary angiography in patients with chronic renal insufficiency. Indian J Nephrol. 2010;20(2):80–3.

144. Sadat U, Walsh SR, Norden AG, Gillard JH, Boyle JR. Does oral N-acetylcysteine reduce contrast-induced renal injury in patients with peripheral arterial disease undergoing peripheral angiography? A randomized-controlled study. Angiology. 2011;62(3):225–30.

145. Saitoh T, Satoh H, Nobuhara M, Machii M, Tanaka T, Ohtani H, et al. Intravenous glutathione prevents renal oxidative stress after coronary angiography more effectively than oral N-acetylcysteine. Heart Vessel. 2011;26(5):465–72.

146. Sandhu C, Belli AM, Oliveira DB. The role of N-acetylcysteine in the prevention of contrast-induced nephrotoxicity. Cardiovasc Intervent Radiol. 2006;29(3):344–7.

147. Sanei H, Hajian-Nejad A, Sajjadieh-Kajouei A, Nazemzadeh N, Alizadeh N, Bidram P, et al. Short term high dose atorvastatin for the prevention of contrast-induced nephropathy in patients undergoing computed tomography angiography. ARYA Atheroscler. 2014;10(5):252–8.

148. Sar F, Saler T, Ecebay A, Saglam ZA, Ozturk S, Kazancioglu R. The efficacy of n-acetylcysteine in preventing contrast-induced nephropathy in type 2 diabetic patients without nephropathy. J Nephrol. 2010;23(4):478–82.

149. Savaj S, Savoj J, Jebraili I, Sezavar SH. Remote ischemic preconditioning for prevention of contrast-induced acute kidney injury in diabetic patients. Iran J Kidney Dis. 2014;8(6):457–60.

150. Sekiguchi H, Ajiro Y, Uchida Y, Ishida I, Otsuki H, Hattori H, et al. Oxygen pre-conditioning prevents contrast-induced nephropathy (OPtion CIN study). J Am Coll Cardiol. 2013;62(2):162–3.

151. Seyon RA, Jensen LA, Ferguson IA, Williams RG. Efficacy of N-acetylcysteine and hydration versus placebo and hydration in decreasing contrast-induced renal dysfunction in patients undergoing coronary angiography with or without concomitant percutaneous coronary intervention. Heart Lung. 2007;36(3):195–204.

152. Shehata M. Impact of trimetazidine on incidence of myocardial injury and contrast-induced nephropathy in diabetic patients with renal dysfunction undergoing elective percutaneous coronary intervention. Am J Cardiol. 2014;114(3):389–94.

153. Shehata M, Hamza M. Impact of high loading dose of atorvastatin in diabetic patients with renal dysfunction undergoing elective percutaneous coronary intervention: a randomized controlled trial. Cardiovasc Ther. 2015;33(2):35–41.

154. Shyu KG, Cheng JJ, Kuan P. Acetylcysteine protects against acute renal damage in patients with abnormal renal function undergoing a coronary procedure. J Am Coll Cardiol. 2002;40(8):1383–8.

155. Solomon R, Werner C, Mann D, D'Elia J, Silva P. Effects of saline, mannitol, and furosemide to prevent acute decreases in renal function induced by radiocontrast agents. N Engl J Med. 1994;331(21):1416–20.

156. Spargias K, Adreanides E, Demerouti E, Gkouziouta A, Manginas A, Pavlides G, et al. Iloprost prevents contrast-induced nephropathy in patients with renal dysfunction undergoing coronary angiography or intervention. Circulation. 2009;120(18):1793–9.

157. Spargias K, Adreanides E, Giamouzis G, Karagiannis S, Gouziouta A, Manginas A, et al. Iloprost for prevention of contrast-mediated nephropathy in high-risk patients undergoing a coronary procedure. Results of a randomized pilot study. Eur J Clin Pharmacol. 2006;62(8):589–95.

158. Stone GW, McCullough PA, Tumlin JA, Lepor NE, Madyoon H, Murray P, et al. Fenoldopam mesylate for the prevention of contrast-induced nephropathy: a randomized controlled trial. JAMA. 2003;290(17):2284–91.

159. Stone GW, Vora K, Schindler J, Diaz C, Mann T, Dangas G, et al. Systemic hypothermia to prevent radiocontrast nephropathy (from the COOL-RCN randomized trial). Am J Cardiol. 2011;108(5):741–6.

160. Tamura A, Goto Y, Miyamoto K, Naono S, Kawano Y, Kotoku M, et al. Efficacy of single-bolus administration of sodium bicarbonate to prevent contrast-induced nephropathy in patients with mild renal insufficiency undergoing an elective coronary procedure. Am J Cardiol. 2009;104(7):921–5.

161. Tanaka A, Suzuki Y, Suzuki N, Hirai T, Yasuda N, Miki K, et al. Does N-acetylcysteine reduce the incidence of contrast-induced nephropathy and clinical events in patients undergoing primary angioplasty for acute myocardial infarction? Intern Med. 2011;50(7):673–7.

162. Tasanarong A, Piyayotai D, Thitiarchakul S. Protection of radiocontrast induced nephropathy by vitamin E (alpha tocopherol): a randomized controlled pilot study. J Med Assoc Thail. 2009;92(10):1273–81.

163. Tasanarong A, Vohakiat A, Hutayanon P, Piyayotai D. New strategy of alpha- and gamma-tocopherol to prevent contrast-induced acute kidney injury in chronic kidney disease patients undergoing elective coronary procedures. Nephrol Dial Transplant. 2013;28(2):337–44.

164. Tepel M, van der Giet M, Schwarzfeld C, Laufer U, Liermann D, Zidek W. Prevention of radiographic-contrast-agent-induced reductions in renal function by acetylcysteine. N Engl J Med. 2000;343(3):180–4.

165. Thiele H, Hildebrand L, Schirdewahn C, Eitel I, Adams V, Fuernau G, et al. Impact of high-dose N-acetylcysteine versus placebo on contrast-induced nephropathy and myocardial reperfusion injury in unselected patients with ST-segment elevation myocardial infarction undergoing primary percutaneous coronary intervention. The LIPSIA-N-ACC (Prospective, Single-Blind, Placebo-Controlled, Randomized Leipzig Immediate PercutaneouS Coronary Intervention Acute Myocardial Infarction N-ACC) Trial. J Am Coll Cardiol. 2010;55(20):2201–9.

166. Toso A, Maioli M, Leoncini M, Gallopin M, Tedeschi D, Micheletti C, et al. Usefulness of atorvastatin (80 mg) in prevention of contrast-induced nephropathy in patients with chronic renal disease. Am J Cardiol. 2010;105(3):288–92.

167. Traub SJ, Mitchell AM, Jones AE, Tang A, O'Connor J, Nelson T, et al. N-acetylcysteine plus intravenous fluids versus intravenous fluids alone to prevent contrast-induced nephropathy in emergency computed tomography. Ann Emerg Med. 2013;62(5):511–20 e25.

168. Trivedi HS, Moore H, Nasr S, Aggarwal K, Agrawal A, Goel P, et al. A randomized prospective trial to assess the role of saline hydration on the development of contrast nephropathy. Nephron Clin Pract. 2003;93(1):C29–34.

169. Tumlin JA, Wang A, Murray PT, Mathur VS. Fenoldopam mesylate blocks reductions in renal plasma flow after radiocontrast dye infusion: a pilot trial in the prevention of contrast nephropathy. Am Heart J. 2002;143(5):894–903.

170. Vasheghani-Farahani A, Sadigh G, Kassaian SE, Khatami SM, Fotouhi A, Razavi SA, et al. Sodium bicarbonate in preventing contrast nephropathy in patients at risk for volume overload: a randomized controlled trial. J Nephrol. 2010;23(2):216–23.

171. Vasheghani-Farahani A, Sadigh G, Kassaian SE, Khatami SM, Fotouhi A, Razavi SA, et al. Sodium bicarbonate plus isotonic saline versus saline for prevention of contrast-induced nephropathy in patients undergoing coronary angiography: a randomized controlled trial. Am J Kidney Dis. 2009;54(4):610–8.

172. Vogt B, Ferrari P, Schonholzer C, Marti HP, Mohaupt M, Wiederkehr M, et al. Prophylactic hemodialysis after radiocontrast media in patients with renal insufficiency is potentially harmful. Am J Med. 2001;111(9):692–8.

173. Wang A, Holcslaw T, Bashore TM, Freed MI, Miller D, Rudnick MR, et al. Exacerbation of radiocontrast nephrotoxicity by endothelin receptor antagonism. Kidney Int. 2000;57(4):1675–80.

174. Wang Y, Fu X, Wang X, Jia X, Gu X, Zhang J, et al. Protective effects of anisodamine on renal function in patients with ST-segment elevation myocardial infarction undergoing primary percutaneous coronary intervention. Tohoku J Exp Med. 2011;224(2):91–7.

175. Webb JG, Pate GE, Humphries KH, Buller CE, Shalansky S, Al Shamari A, et al. A randomized controlled trial of intravenous N-acetylcysteine for the prevention of contrast-induced nephropathy after cardiac catheterization: lack of effect. Am Heart J. 2004;148(3):422–9.

176. Weisberg LS, Kurnik PB, Kurnik BR. Dopamine and renal blood flow in radiocontrast-induced nephropathy in humans. Ren Fail. 1993;15(1):61–8.

177. Wrobel W, Sinkiewicz W, Gordon M, Wozniak-Wisniewska A. Oral versus intravenous hydration and renal function in diabetic patients undergoing percutaneous coronary interventions. Kardiol Pol. 2010;68(9):1015–20.

178. Xu X, Zhou Y, Luo S, Zhang W, Zhao Y, Yu M, et al. Effect of remote ischemic preconditioning in the elderly patients with coronary artery disease with diabetes mellitus undergoing elective drug-eluting stent implantation. Angiology. 2014;65(8):660–6.

179. Yamanaka T, Kawai Y, Miyoshi T, Mima T, Takagaki K, Tsukuda S, et al. Remote ischemic preconditioning reduces contrast-induced acute kidney injury in patients with ST-elevation myocardial infarction: a randomized controlled trial. Int J Cardiol. 2015;178:136–41.

180. Yang K, Liu W, Ren W, Lv S. Different interventions in preventing contrast-induced nephropathy after percutaneous coronary intervention. Int Urol Nephrol. 2014;46(9):1801–7.

181. Yavari V, Ostovan MA, Kojuri J, Afshariani R, Hamidian Jahromi A, Roozbeh J, et al. The preventive effect of pentoxifylline on contrast-induced nephropathy: a randomized clinical trial. Int Urol Nephrol. 2014;46(1):41–6.

182. Yeganehkhah MR, Iranirad L, Dorri F, Pazoki S, Akbari H, Miryounesi M, et al. Comparison between three supportive treatments for prevention of contrast-induced nephropathy in high-risk patients undergoing coronary angiography. Saudi J Kidney Dis Transpl. 2014;25(6):1217–23.

183. Yin L, Li G, Liu T, Yuan R, Zheng X, Xu G, et al. Probucol for the prevention of cystatin C-based contrast-induced acute kidney injury following primary or urgent angioplasty: a randomized, controlled trial. Int J Cardiol. 2013; 167(2):426–9.

184. Zhang J, Fu X, Jia X, Fan X, Gu X, Li S, et al. B-type natriuretic peptide for prevention of contrast-induced nephropathy in patients with heart failure undergoing primary percutaneous coronary intervention. Acta Radiol. 2010;51(6):641–8.

185. Zhao K, Lin Y, Li YJ, Gao S. Efficacy of short-term cordyceps sinensis for prevention of contrast-induced nephropathy in patients with acute coronary syndrome undergoing elective percutaneous coronary intervention. Int J Clin Exp Med. 2014;7(12):5758–64.

186. Zhou L, Chen H. Prevention of contrast-induced nephropathy with ascorbic acid. Intern Med. 2012;51(6):531–5.

187. Abouzeid SM, ElHossary HE. Na/K citrate versus sodium bicarbonate in prevention of contrast-induced nephropathy. Saudi J Kidney Dis Transpl. 2016;27(3):519–25.

188. Arabmomeni M, Najafian J, Abdar Esfahani M, Samadi M, Mirbagher L. Comparison between theophylline, N-acetylcysteine, and theophylline plus N-acetylcysteine for the prevention of contrast-induced nephropathy. ARYA Atheroscler. 2015;11(1):43–9.

189. Balbir Singh G, Ann SH, Park J, Chung HC, Lee JS, Kim ES, et al. Remote ischemic preconditioning for the prevention of contrast-induced acute kidney injury in diabetics receiving elective percutaneous coronary intervention. PLoS One. 2016;11(10):e0164256.

190. Chong E, Poh KK, Lu Q, Zhang JJ, Tan N, Hou XM, et al. Comparison of combination therapy of high-dose oral N-acetylcysteine and intravenous sodium bicarbonate hydration with individual therapies in the reduction of contrast-induced nephropathy during cardiac catheterisation and percutaneous coronary intervention (CONTRAST): a multi-Centre, randomised, controlled trial. Int J Cardiol. 2015;201:237–42.

191. Eshraghi A, Naranji-Sani R, Pourzand H, Vojdanparast M, Morovatfar N, Ramezani J, et al. Pentoxifylline and prevention of contrast-induced nephropathy: is it efficient in patients with myocardial infarction undergoing coronary angioplasty? ARYA atheroscler[Internet]. 2017;12(5):1–5 Available from: http://onlinelibrary.wiley.com/o/cochrane/clcentral/articles/737/CN-01298737/frame.html.

192. Fan Y, Wei Q, Cai J, Shi Y, Zhang Y, Yao L, et al. Preventive effect of oral nicorandil on contrast-induced nephropathy in patients with renal insufficiency undergoing elective cardiac catheterization. Heart Vessel. 2016; 31(11):1776–82.

193. Healy DA, Feeley I, Keogh CJ, Scanlon TG, Hodnett PA, Stack AG, et al. Remote ischemic conditioning and renal function after contrast-enhanced CT scan: a randomized trial. Clin Invest Med. 2015;38(3):E110–8.

194. Izani WMW, Darus Z, Yusof Z. Oral N-acetylcysteine in prevention of contrast induced nephropathy following coronary angiogram. Int Med J [Internet]. 2008;15(5):353–61 Available from: http://onlinelibrary.wiley.com/o/cochrane/clcentral/articles/905/CN-00754905/frame.html.

195. Kai Z, Yongjian L, Sheng G, Yu L. Effect of Dongchongxiacao (Cordyceps) therapy on contrast-induced nephropathy in patients with type 2 diabetes and renal insufficiency undergoing coronary angiography. J Tradit Chin Med. 2015;35(4):422–7.

196. Khosravi A, Dolatkhah M, Hashemi HS, Rostami Z. Preventive effect of atorvastatin (80 mg) on contrast-induced nephropathy after angiography in high-risk patients: double-blind randomized clinical trial. Nephrourol Mon. 2016;8(3):e29574.

197. Liu J, Xie Y, He F, Gao Z, Hao Y, Zu X, et al. Recombinant brain natriuretic peptide for the prevention of contrast-induced nephropathy in patients with chronic kidney disease undergoing nonemergent percutaneous coronary intervention or coronary angiography: a randomized controlled trial. Biomed Res Int. 2016;2016:5985327.

198. Liu W, Ming Q, Shen J, Wei Y, Li W, Chen W, et al. Trimetazidine prevention of contrast-induced nephropathy in coronary angiography. Am J Med Sci. 2015;350(5):398–402.

199. Minoo F, Lessan-Pezeshki M, Firouzi A, Nikfarjam S, Gatmiri SM, Ramezanzade E. Prevention of contrast-induced nephropathy with oxygen supplementation: a randomized controlled trial. Iran J Kidney Dis. 2016;10(5):291–8.

200. Nawa T, Nishigaki K, Kinomura Y, Tanaka T, Yamada Y, Kawasaki M, et al. Continuous intravenous infusion of nicorandil for 4 hours before and 24 hours after percutaneous coronary intervention protects against contrast-induced nephropathy in patients with poor renal function. Int J Cardiol. 2015;195:228–34.

201. Nijssen EC, Rennenberg RJ, Nelemans PJ, Essers BA, Janssen MM, Vermeeren MA, et al. Prophylactic hydration to protect renal function from intravascular iodinated contrast material in patients at high risk of contrast-induced nephropathy (AMACING): a prospective, randomised, phase 3, controlled, open-label, non-inferiority trial. Lancet. 2017;389(10076):1312–22.

202. Rezaei Y, Khademvatani K, Rahimi B, Khoshfetrat M, Arjmand N, Seyyed-Mohammadzad MH. Short-term high-dose vitamin E to prevent contrast medium-induced acute kidney injury in patients with chronic kidney disease undergoing elective coronary angiography: a randomized placebo-controlled trial. J Am Heart Assoc. 2016;5(3):e002919.

203. Sadineni R, Karthik KR, Swarnalatha G, Das U, Taduri G. N-acetyl cysteine versus allopurinol in the prevention of contrast nephropathy in patients with chronic kidney disease: a randomized controlled trial. Indian J Nephrol. 2017;27(2):93–8.

204. Sedighifard Z, Roghani F, Bidram P, Harandi SA, Molavi S. Silymarin for the prevention of contrast-induced nephropathy: a placebo-controlled clinical trial. Int J Prev Med. 2016;7:23.

205. Solomon R, Gordon P, Manoukian SV, Abbott JD, Kereiakes DJ, Jeremias A, et al. Randomized trial of bicarbonate or saline study for the prevention of contrast-induced nephropathy in patients with CKD. Clin J Am Soc Nephrol. 2015;10(9):1519–24.

206. Sun C, Zhi J, Bai X, Li X, Xia H. Comparison of the efficacy of recombinant human brain natriuretic peptide with saline hydration in preventing contrast-induced nephropathy in patients undergoing coronary angiography with or without concomitant percutaneous coronary intervention. Int J Clin Exp Med. 2015;8(8):14166–72.

207. Wang C, Wang W, Ma S, Lu J, Shi H, Ding F. Reduced glutathione for prevention of renal outcomes in patients undergoing selective coronary angiography or intervention. J Interv Cardiol. 2015;28(3):249–56.

208. Xu RH, Ma GZ, Cai ZX, Chen P, Zhu ZD, Wang WL. Combined use of hydration and alprostadil for preventing contrast-induced nephropathy following percutaneous coronary intervention in elderly patients. Exp Ther Med. 2013;6(4):863–7.

209. Zagidullin NS, Dunayeva AR, Plechev VV, Gilmanov AZ, Zagidullin SZ, Er F, et al. Nephroprotective effects of remote ischemic preconditioning in coronary angiography. Clin Hemorheol Microcirc. 2017;65(3):299–307.

210. Droppa M, Desch S, Blase P, Eitel I, Fuernau G, Schuler G, et al. Impact of N-acetylcysteine on contrast-induced nephropathy defined by cystatin C in

patients with ST-elevation myocardial infarction undergoing primary angioplasty. Clin Res Cardiol. 2011;100(11):1037–43.

211. Huber W, Ilgmann K, Page M, Hennig M, Schweigart U, Jeschke B, et al. Effect of theophylline on contrast material-nephropathy in patients with chronic renal insufficiency: controlled, randomized, double-blinded study. Radiology. 2002;223(3):772–9.

212. Marenzi G, Bartorelli AL. Hemofiltration in the prevention of radiocontrast agent induced nephropathy. Minerva Anestesiol. 2004;70(4):189–91.

213. Masuda M, Yamada T, Okuyama Y, Morita T, Sanada S, Furukawa Y, et al. Sodium bicarbonate improves long-term clinical outcomes compared with sodium chloride in patients with chronic kidney disease undergoing an emergent coronary procedure. Circ J. 2008;72(10):1610–4.

214. Zhang J, Li Y, Tao GZ, Chen YD, Hu TH, Cao XB, et al. Short-term rosuvastatin treatment for the prevention of contrast-induced acute kidney injury in patients receiving moderate or high volumes of contrast media: a sub-analysis of the TRACK-D study. Chin Med J. 2015;128(6):784–9.

215. Sketch MH Jr, Whelton A, Schollmayer E, Koch JA, Bernink PJ, Woltering F, et al. Prevention of contrast media-induced renal dysfunction with prostaglandin E1: a randomized, double-blind, placebo-controlled study. Am J Ther. 2001;8(3):155–62.

216. Acikel S, Muderrisoglu H, Yildirir A, Aydinalp A, Sade E, Bayraktar N, et al. Prevention of contrast-induced impairment of renal function by short-term or long-term statin therapy in patients undergoing elective coronary angiography. Blood Coagul Fibrinolysis. 2010;21(8):750–7.

217. Allie DE, Lirtzman MD, Wyatt CH, Keller VA, Mitran EV, Hebert CJ, et al. Targeted renal therapy and contrast-induced nephropathy during endovascular abdominal aortic aneurysm repair: results of a feasibility pilot trial. J Endovasc Ther. 2007;14(4):520–7.

218. Assadi F. Acetazolamide for prevention of contrast-induced nephropathy: a new use for an old drug. Pediatr Cardiol. 2006;27(2):238–42.

219. Avci E, Yesil M, Bayata S, Postaci N, Arikan E, Cirit M. The role of nebivolol in the prevention of contrast-induced nephropathy in patients with renal dysfunction. Anadolu Kardiyol Derg. 2011;11(7):613–7.

220. Awal A, Ahsan SA, Siddique MA, Banerjee S, Hasan MI, Zaman SM, et al. Effect of hydration with or without n-acetylcysteine on contrast induced nephropathy in patients undergoing coronary angiography and percutaneous coronary intervention. Mymensingh Med J. 2011; 20(2):264–9.

221. Azmus AD, Gottschall C, Manica A, Manica J, Duro K, Frey M, et al. Effectiveness of acetylcysteine in prevention of contrast nephropathy. J Invasive Cardiol. 2005;17(2):80–4.

222. Bader BD, Berger ED, Heede MB, Silberbaur I, Duda S, Risler T, et al. What is the best hydration regimen to prevent contrast media-induced nephrotoxicity? Clin Nephrol. 2004;62(1):1–7.

223. Barrett BJ, Parfrey PS, Vavasour HM, McDonald J, Kent G, Hefferton D, et al. Contrast nephropathy in patients with impaired renal function: high versus low osmolar media. Kidney Int. 1992;41(5):1274–9.

224. Boccalandro F, Amhad M, Smalling RW, Sdringola S. Oral acetylcysteine does not protect renal function from moderate to high doses of intravenous radiographic contrast. Catheter Cardiovasc Interv. 2003;58(3):336–41.

225. Brar SS, Aharonian V, Mansukhani P, Moore N, Shen AY, Jorgensen M, et al. Haemodynamic-guided fluid administration for the prevention of contrast-induced acute kidney injury: the POSEIDON randomised controlled trial. Lancet. 2014;383(9931):1814–23.

226. Briguori C. Renalguard system in high-risk patients for contrast-induced acute kidney injury. Minerva Cardioangiol. 2012;60(3):291–7.

227. Briguori C, Colombo A, Violante A, Balestrieri P, Manganelli F, Paolo Elia P, et al. Standard vs double dose of N-acetylcysteine to prevent contrast agent associated nephrotoxicity. Eur Heart J. 2004;25(3):206–11.

228. Briguori C, Visconti G, Focaccio A, Airoldi F, Valgimigli M, Sangiorgi GM, et al. Renal insufficiency after contrast media administration trial II (REMEDIAL II): RenalGuard system in high-risk patients for contrast-induced acute kidney injury. Circulation. 2011;124(11):1260–9.

229. Buyukhatipoglu H, Sezen Y, Yildiz A, Bas M, Kirhan I, Ulas T, et al. N-acetylcysteine fails to prevent renal dysfunction and oxidative stress after noniodine contrast media administration during percutaneous coronary interventions. Pol Arch Med Wewn. 2010;120(10):383–9.

230. Clavijo LC, Pinto TL, Kuchulakanti PK, Torguson R, Chu WW, Satler LF, et al. Effect of a rapid intra-arterial infusion of dextrose 5% prior to coronary angiography on frequency of contrast-induced nephropathy in high-risk patients. Am J Cardiol. 2006;97(7):981–3.

231. Deray G, Bellin MF, Boulechfar H, Baumelou B, Koskas F, Baumelou A, et al. Nephrotoxicity of contrast media in high-risk patients with renal insufficiency: comparison of low- and high-osmolar contrast agents. Am J Nephrol. 1991;11(4):309–12.

232. Dorval JF, Dixon SR, Zelman RB, Davidson CJ, Rudko R, Resnic FS. Feasibility study of the RenalGuard balanced hydration system: a novel strategy for the prevention of contrast-induced nephropathy in high risk patients. Int J Cardiol. 2013;166(2):482–6.

233. Drager LF, Andrade L, Barros de Toledo JF, Laurindo FR, Machado Cesar LA, Seguro AC. Renal effects of N-acetylcysteine in patients at risk for contrast nephropathy: decrease in oxidant stress-mediated renal tubular injury. Nephrol Dial Transplant. 2004;19(7):1803–7.

234. Erley CM, Duda SH, Schlepckow S, Koehler J, Huppert PE, Strohmaier WL, et al. Adenosine antagonist theophylline prevents the reduction of glomerular filtration rate after contrast media application. Kidney Int. 1994;45(5):1425–31.

235. Frank H, Werner D, Lorusso V, Klinghammer L, Daniel WG, Kunzendorf U, et al. Simultaneous hemodialysis during coronary angiography fails to prevent radiocontrast-induced nephropathy in chronic renal failure. Clin Nephrol. 2003;60(3):176–82.

236. Gandhi MR, Brown P, Romanowski CA, Morcos SK, Campbell S, el Nahas AM, et al. The use of theophylline, an adenosine antagonist in the prevention of contrast media induced nephrotoxicity. Br J Radiol. 1992;65(777):838.

237. Goo JJ, Kim JJ, Kang JH, Kim KN, Byun KS, Kim MK, et al. Effect of renin-angiotensin-system blockers on contrast-medium-induced acute kidney injury after coronary angiography. Korean J Intern Med. 2014;29(2):203–9.

238. Han S, Li XM, Mohammed Ali LA, Fu NK, Jin DX, Cong HL. Effect of short-term different statins loading dose on renal function and CI-AKI incidence in patients undergoing invasive coronary procedures. Int J Cardiol. 2013; 168(5):5101–3.

239. Harris KG, Smith TP, Cragg AH, Lemke JH. Nephrotoxicity from contrast material in renal insufficiency: ionic versus nonionic agents. Radiology. 1991; 179(3):849–52.

240. Hoffmann U, Fischereder M, Kruger B, Drobnik W, Kramer BK. The value of N-acetylcysteine in the prevention of radiocontrast agent-induced nephropathy seems questionable. J Am Soc Nephrol. 2004;15(2):407–10.

241. Hoshi T, Sato A, Kakefuda Y, Harunari T, Watabe H, Ojima E, et al. Preventive effect of statin pretreatment on contrast-induced acute kidney injury in patients undergoing coronary angioplasty: propensity score analysis from a multicenter registry. Int J Cardiol. 2014;171(2):243–9.

242. Huber W, Eckel F, Hennig M, Rosenbrock H, Wacker A, Saur D, et al. Prophylaxis of contrast material-induced nephropathy in patients in intensive care: acetylcysteine, theophylline, or both? A randomized study. Radiology. 2006;239(3):793–804.

243. Huber W, Jeschke B, Page M, Weiss W, Salmhofer H, Schweigart U, et al. Reduced incidence of radiocontrast-induced nephropathy in ICU patients under theophylline prophylaxis: a prospective comparison to series of patients at similar risk. Intensive Care Med. 2001;27(7):1200–9.

244. Igarashi G, Iino K, Watanabe H, Ito H. Remote ischemic pre-conditioning alleviates contrast-induced acute kidney injury in patients with moderate chronic kidney disease. Circ J. 2013;77(12):3037–44.

245. Katholi RE, Taylor GJ, McCann WP, Woods WT Jr, Womack KA, McCoy CD, et al. Nephrotoxicity from contrast media: attenuation with theophylline. Radiology. 1995;195(1):17–22.

246. Kaya A, Kurt M, Tanboga IH, Isik T, Ekinci M, Aksakal E, et al. Rosuvastatin versus atorvastatin to prevent contrast induced nephropathy in patients undergoing primary percutaneous coronary intervention (ROSA-cIN trial). Acta Cardiol. 2013;68(5):489–94.

247. Khanal S, Attallah N, Smith DE, Kline-Rogers E, Share D, O'Donnell MJ, et al. Statin therapy reduces contrast-induced nephropathy: an analysis of contemporary percutaneous interventions. Am J Med. 2005;118(8):843–9.

248. Kini AA, Sharma SK. Managing the high-risk patient: experience with fenoldopam, a selective dopamine receptor agonist, in prevention of radiocontrast nephropathy during percutaneous coronary intervention. Rev Cardiovasc Med. 2001;2(Suppl 1):S19–25.

249. Kolonko A, Wiecek A, Kokot F. The nonselective adenosine antagonist theophylline does prevent renal dysfunction induced by radiographic contrast agents. J Nephrol. 1998;11(3):151–6.

250. Kramer BK, Preuner J, Ebenburger A, Kaiser M, Bergner U, Eilles C, et al. Lack of renoprotective effect of theophylline during aortocoronary bypass surgery. Nephrol Dial Transplant. 2002;17(5):910–5.

251. Krasuski RA, Beard BM, Geoghagan JD, Thompson CM, Guidera SA. Optimal timing of hydration to erase contrast-associated nephropathy: the OTHER CAN study. J Invasive Cardiol. 2003;15(12):699–702.

252. Kristeller JL, Zavorsky GS, Prior JE, Keating DA, Brady MA, Romaldini TA, et al. Lack of effectiveness of sodium bicarbonate in preventing kidney injury in patients undergoing cardiac surgery: a randomized controlled trial. Pharmacotherapy. 2013;33(7):710–7.

253. Lassnigg A, Donner E, Grubhofer G, Presterl E, Druml W, Hiesmayr M. Lack of renoprotective effects of dopamine and furosemide during cardiac surgery. J Am Soc Nephrol. 2000;11(1):97–104.

254. Lee PT, Chou KJ, Liu CP, Mar GY, Chen CL, Hsu CY, et al. Renal protection for coronary angiography in advanced renal failure patients by prophylactic hemodialysis. A randomized controlled trial. J Am Coll Cardiol. 2007;50(11):1015–20.

255. Majumdar SR, Kjellstrand CM, Tymchak WJ, Hervas-Malo M, Taylor DA, Teo KK. Forced euvolemic diuresis with mannitol and furosemide for prevention of contrast-induced nephropathy in patients with CKD undergoing coronary angiography: a randomized controlled trial. Am J Kidney Dis. 2009;54(4):602–9.

256. Marenzi G, Bartorelli AL, Lauri G, Assanelli E, Grazi M, Campodonico J, et al. Continuous veno-venous hemofiltration for the treatment of contrast-induced acute renal failure after percutaneous coronary interventions. Catheter Cardiovasc Interv. 2003;58(1):59–64.

257. Miller HI, Dascalu A, Rassin TA, Wollman Y, Chernichowsky T, Iaina A. Effects of an acute dose of L-arginine during coronary angiography in patients with chronic renal failure: a randomized, parallel, double-blind clinical trial. Am J Nephrol. 2003;23(2):91–5.

258. Mueller C, Buerkle G, Buettner HJ, Petersen J, Perruchoud AP, Eriksson U, et al. Prevention of contrast media-associated nephropathy: randomized comparison of 2 hydration regimens in 1620 patients undergoing coronary angioplasty. Arch Intern Med. 2002;162(3):329–36.

259. Neumayer HH, Junge W, Kufner A, Wenning A. Prevention of radiocontrast-media-induced nephrotoxicity by the calcium channel blocker nitrendipine: a prospective randomised clinical trial. Nephrol Dial Transplant. 1989;4(12):1030–6.

260. Recio-Mayoral A, Chaparro M, Prado B, Cozar R, Mendez I, Banerjee D, et al. The Reno-protective effect of hydration with sodium bicarbonate plus N-acetylcysteine in patients undergoing emergency percutaneous coronary intervention: the RENO Study. J Am Coll Cardiol. 2007;49(12):1283–8.

261. Rosenstock JL, Bruno R, Kim JK, Lubarsky L, Schaller R, Panagopoulos G, et al. The effect of withdrawal of ACE inhibitors or angiotensin receptor blockers prior to coronary angiography on the incidence of contrast-induced nephropathy. Int Urol Nephrol. 2008;40(3):749–55.

262. Schwab SJ, Hlatky MA, Pieper KS, Davidson CJ, Morris KG, Skelton TN, et al. Contrast nephrotoxicity: a randomized controlled trial of a nonionic and an ionic radiographic contrast agent. N Engl J Med. 1989;320(3):149–53.

263. Shavit L, Korenfeld R, Lifschitz M, Butnaru A, Slotki I. Sodium bicarbonate versus sodium chloride and oral N-acetylcysteine for the prevention of contrast-induced nephropathy in advanced chronic kidney disease. J Interv Cardiol. 2009;22(6):556–63.

264. Shemirani H. Pourrmoghaddass M. a randomized trial of saline hydration to prevent contrast-induced nephropathy in patients on regular captopril or furosemide therapy undergoing percutaneous coronary intervention. Saudi J Kidney Dis Transpl. 2012;23(2):280–5.

265. Shin DH, Choi DJ, Youn TJ, Yoon CH, Suh JW, Kim KI, et al. Comparison of contrast-induced nephrotoxicity of iodixanol and iopromide in patients with renal insufficiency undergoing coronary angiography. Am J Cardiol. 2011;108(2):189–94.

266. Sochman J, Krizova B. Prevention of contrast agent-induced renal impairment in patients with chronic renal insufficiency and heart disease by high-dose intravenous N-acetylcysteine: a pilot-ministudy. Kardiol Pol. 2006;64(6):559–64 discussion 65-6.

267. Spangberg-Viklund B, Berglund J, Nikonoff T, Nyberg P, Skau T, Larsson R. Does prophylactic treatment with felodipine, a calcium antagonist, prevent low-osmolar contrast-induced renal dysfunction in hydrated diabetic and nondiabetic patients with normal or moderately reduced renal function? Scand J Urol Nephrol. 1996;30(1):63–8.

268. Staniloae CS, Doucet S, Sharma SK, Katholi RE, Mody KR, Coppola JT, et al. N-acetylcysteine added to volume expansion with sodium bicarbonate does not further prevent contrast-induced nephropathy: results from the cardiac angiography in renally impaired patients study. J Interv Cardiol. 2009;22(3):261–5.

269. Stegmayr BG, Brannstrom M, Bucht S, Crougneau V, Dimeny E, Ekspong A, et al. Low-dose atorvastatin in severe chronic kidney disease patients: a randomized, controlled endpoint study. Scand J Urol Nephrol. 2005;39(6):489–97.

270. Sterner G, Frennby B, Kurkus J, Nyman U. Does post-angiographic hemodialysis reduce the risk of contrast-medium nephropathy? Scand J Urol Nephrol. 2000;34(5):323–6.

271. Stevens MA, McCullough PA, Tobin KJ, Speck JP, Westveer DC, Guido-Allen DA, et al. A prospective randomized trial of prevention measures in patients at high risk for contrast nephropathy: results of the PRINCE Study Prevention of Radiocontrast Induced Nephropathy Clinical Evaluation. J Am Coll Cardiol. 1999;33(2):403–11.

272. Tamai N, Ito S, Nakasuka K, Morimoto K, Miyata K, Inomata M, et al. Sodium bicarbonate for the prevention of contrast-induced nephropathy: the efficacy of high concentration solution. J Invasive Cardiol. 2012;24(9):439–42.

273. Taylor AJ, Hotchkiss D, Morse RW, McCabe JPREPARED. Preparation for angiography in renal dysfunction: a randomized trial of inpatient vs outpatient hydration protocols for cardiac catheterization in mild-to-moderate renal dysfunction. Chest. 1998;114(6):1570–4.

274. Torigoe K, Tamura A, Watanabe T, Kadota J. 20-hour preprocedural hydration is not superior to 5-hour preprocedural hydration in the prevention of contrast-induced increases in serum creatinine and cystatin C. Int J Cardiol. 2013;167(5):2200–3.

275. Ueda H, Yamada T, Masuda M, Okuyama Y, Morita T, Furukawa Y, et al. Prevention of contrast-induced nephropathy by bolus injection of sodium bicarbonate in patients with chronic kidney disease undergoing emergent coronary procedures. Am J Cardiol. 2011;107(8):1163–7.

276. Weinstein JM, Heyman S, Brezis M. Potential deleterious effect of furosemide in radiocontrast nephropathy. Nephron. 1992;62(4):413–5.

277. Xinwei J, Xianghua F, Jing Z, Xinshun G, Ling X, Weize F, et al. Comparison of usefulness of simvastatin 20 mg versus 80 mg in preventing contrast-induced nephropathy in patients with acute coronary syndrome undergoing percutaneous coronary intervention. Am J Cardiol. 2009;104(4):519–24.

278. Carraro M, Stacul F, Collari P, Toson D, Zucconi F, Torre R, et al. Contrast media nephrotoxicity: urinary protein and enzyme pattern in patients with or without saline infusion during digital subtracting angiography. Contrib Nephrol. 1993;101:251–4.

279. Shakeryan F, Sanati H, Fathi H, Firouzi A, Zahedmehr A, Valizadeh G, et al. Evaluation of combination therapy with vitamin C and pentoxifylline on preventing kidney failure secondary to intravenous contrast material in coronary angioplasty. Iranian Heart J. 2013:17–21.

280. Berger ED, Bader BD, Bosker J, Risler T, Erley CM. Contrast media-induced kidney failure cannot be prevented by hemodialysis. Dtsch Med Wochenschr. 2001;126(7):162–6.

281. Koch JA, Sketch M, Brinker J, Bernink PJ. Prostaglandin E1 for prevention of contrast medium-induced kidney dysfunction. Rofo. 1999;170(6):557–63.

282. Cao S, Wang P, Cui K, Zhang L, Hou Y. Atorvastatin prevents contrast agent-induced renal injury in patients undergoing coronary angiography by inhibiting oxidative stress. Nan Fang Yi Ke Da Xue Xue Bao. 2012;32(11):1600–2.

283. Chen GL, Su JZ. Atorvastatin attenuated contrast induced renal function damage. Zhonghua Xin Xue Guan Bing Za Zhi. 2009;37(5):389–93.

284. Hui H, Li K, Li Z, Wang J, Gao M, Han X. Protective effect of amlodipine against contrast agent-induced renal injury in elderly patients with coronary heart disease. Nan Fang Yi Ke Da Xue Xue Bao. 2012;32(11):1580–3.

285. Wang ZL, Liu M, Zhang YQ. The prevention of denhong injection on contrast-induced renal impairment after percutaneous coronary intervention. Zhongguo Zhong Xi Yi Jie He Za Zhi. 2011;31(12):1611–4.

286. Yin L, Li GP, Liu T, Liu HM, Chen X, He M, et al. Role of probucol in preventing contrast induced acute kidney injury after coronary interventional procedure: a randomized trial. Zhonghua Xin Xue Guan Bing Za Zhi. 2009;37(5):385–8.

287. Zhou X, Jin YZ, Wang Q, Min R, Zhang XY. Efficacy of high dose atorvastatin on preventing contrast induced nephropathy in patients underwent coronary angiography. Zhonghua Xin Xue Guan Bing Za Zhi. 2009;37(5):394–6.

288. Diez T, Bagilet D, Ramos M, Jolly H, Diab M, Marcucci R, et al. Evaluation of two methods to avoid the nephropathy associated with radiologic contrast. Medicina (B Aires). 1999;59(1):55–8.

289. El Mahmoud R, Le Feuvre C, Le Quan Sang KH, Helft G, Beygui F, Batisse JP, et al. Absence of nephro-protective effect of acetylcysteine in patients with chronic renal failure investigated by coronary angiography. Arch Mal Coeur Vaiss. 2003;96(12):1157–61.

290. Toprak O, Cirit M, Bayata S, Yesil M, Aslan SL. The effect of pre-procedural captopril on contrast-induced nephropathy in patients who underwent coronary angiography. Anadolu Kardiyol Derg. 2003;3(2):98–103.

291. Vallero A, Cesano G, Pozzato M, Garbo R, Minelli M, Quarello F, et al. Contrast nephropathy in cardiac procedures: no advantages with prophylactic use of N-acetylcysteine (NAC). G Ital Nefrol. 2002;19(5):529–33.

292. Chen H, Wu H, He Q, Chen H, Mao Y. Comparison of sodium bicarbonate and sodium chloride as strategies for preventing contrast nephropathy [abstract no: SU-PO1046]. J Am Soc Nephrol : JASN. 2007:817A–8A.

293. Grygier M, Janus M, Araszkiewicz A, Kowal J, Mularek-Kubzdela T, Olasinska-Wisniewska A, et al. Combined treatment with ascorbic acid and N-acetylcysteine prevents contrast-induced nephropathy in high-risk patients with acute myocardial infarction undergoing percutaneous coronary intervention. Eur heart J. 2011:954–5.

294. Habib M, Hillis A, Hamad A. Low dose of N-acetylcysteine plus ascorbic acid versus hydration with (saline 0.9%) for prevention of contrast-induced nephropathy in patients undergoing coronary angiography. Int J Cardiol. 2013:S81–S.

295. Lin M, Sabeti M, Iskandar E, Malhotra N, Pham PT, Pham PC. Prevention of contrast nephropathy with sodium bicarbonate [abstract no: PUB591]. J Am Soc Nephrol : JASN. 2007:959a–60a.

296. Lukas R, Eren A, Keller F, Jehle P. Prevention of contrast nephropathy (cnp) with hydratation and furosemide (fs) [abstract]. Nephrol Dial Transplant. 1999:A73–A.

297. Moreyra A, Natarajan MK, Doucet S, Sharma SK, Staniloae CS, Katholi RE. Contrast nephropathy in patients with chronic kidney disease undergoing either diagnostic or interventional procedures [abstract no:TCT-313]. Am J Cardiol. 2007:124L–L.

298. Ray DS, Srinivas V. Role of n-acetyl cysteine in prevention of contrast nephropathy in patients of diabetic renal failure: a prospective study [abstract]. Nephrol Dial Transplant. 2003:664.

299. Saidin R, Zainudin S, Kong NCT, Maskon O, Saaidin NF, Shah SA. Intravenous sodium bicarbonate versus normal saline infusion as prophylaxis against contrast nephropathy in patients with chronic kidney disease undergoing coronary angiography or angioplasty [abstract no: F-SA-DS911]. Journal of the American Society of Nephrology : JASN. 2006:766A–A.

300. Andrew Lewington RM, Hoefield R, Sutton A, Smith D, Downes M. Prevention of Contrast Induced Acute Kidney Injury (CI-AKI). In: Adult. Patients. The Renal Association, British Cardiovascular Intervention Society and The Royal College of Radiologists; 2013.

301. Dias S, Welton NJ, Sutton AJ, Caldwell DM, Lu G, Ades AE. Evidence synthesis for decision making 4: inconsistency in networks of evidence based on randomized controlled trials. Med Decis Mak. 2013;33(5):641–56.

302. Zhang JZ, Kang XJ, Gao Y, Zheng YY, Wu TT, Li L, et al. Efficacy of alprostadil for preventing of contrast-induced nephropathy: a meta-analysis. Sci Rep. 2017;7(1):1045.

303. Feldkamp T, Baumgart D, Elsner M, Herget-Rosenthal S, Pietruck F, Erbel R, et al. Nephrotoxicity of iso-osmolar versus low-osmolar contrast media is equal in low risk patients. Clin Nephrol. 2006;66(5):322–30.

304. Subramaniam RM, Suarez-Cuervo C, Wilson RF, Turban S, Zhang A, Sherrod C, et al. Effectiveness of prevention strategies for contrast-induced nephropathy: a systematic review and meta-analysis. Ann Intern Med. 2016;164(6):406–16.

22

Study protocol: mycophenolate mofetil as maintenance therapy after rituximab treatment for childhood-onset, complicated, frequently-relapsing nephrotic syndrome or steroid-dependent nephrotic syndrome: a multicenter double-blind, randomized, placebo-controlled trial (JSKDC07)

Tomoko Horinouchi[1], Mayumi Sako[2], Koichi Nakanishi[3], Kenji Ishikura[4], Shuichi Ito[5], Hidefumi Nakamura[6], Mari Saito Oba[7], Kandai Nozu[1] and Kazumoto Iijima[1]* (iD)

Abstract

Background: Idiopathic nephrotic syndrome (INS) is the most common chronic glomerular disease in children. Approximately 80–90% of patients with childhood INS have steroid-sensitive nephrotic syndrome (SSNS), and can obtain remission with steroid therapy, while the remainder have steroid-resistant nephrotic syndrome (SRNS). Furthermore, approximately 50% of children with SSNS develop frequently-relapsing nephrotic syndrome (FRNS) or steroid-dependent nephrotic syndrome (SDNS). Children with FRNS/SDNS are usually treated with immunosuppressive agents such as cyclosporine, cyclophosphamide, or mizoribine in Japan. However, 10–20% of children receiving immunosuppressive agents still show frequent relapse and/or steroid dependence during or after treatment, which is defined as complicated FRNS/SDNS. Furthermore, 30% of SRNS patients who obtain remission after additional treatments such as cyclosporine also turn out to be complicated FRNS/SDNS. For such complicated FRNS/SDNS patients, rituximab (RTX) is currently used; however, recurrence after RTX treatment also remains an open issue. Because long-term use of existing immunosuppressive drugs has limitations, development of a novel treatment for maintenance therapy after RTX is desirable. Mycophenolate mofetil (MMF) is an immunosuppressive drug with fewer side effects than cyclosporine or cyclophosphamide. Importantly, recent studies have reported the efficacy of MMF in children with nephrotic syndrome.

(Continued on next page)

* Correspondence: iijima@med.kobe-u.ac.jp
[1]Department of Pediatrics, Kobe University Graduate School of Medicine, 5-1 Kusunoki-cho 7 chome, Chuo-ku, Kobe 650-0017, Japan
Full list of author information is available at the end of the article

(Continued from previous page)

Methods: We conduct a multicenter, double-blind, randomized, placebo-controlled trial to evaluate the efficacy and safety of MMF after RTX therapy in children with complicated FRNS/SDNS. Patients are allocated to either RTX plus MMF treatment group, or RTX plus placebo treatment group. For the former group, MMF is administered at a dose of 1000–1200 mg/m²/day (maximum 2 g/day) twice daily for 17 months after RTX treatment. The primary endpoint is time-to-treatment failure (development of frequent relapses, steroid dependence or steroid resistance).

Discussion: The results will provide important data on the use of MMF as maintenance therapy after RTX to prevent complicated FRNS/SDNS patients from declining into treatment failure. In future, MMF in conjunction with RTX treatment may permit increased duration of remission in 'complicated' FRNS/SDNS cases.

Keywords: Mycophenolate mofetil, rituximab., frequently-relapsing nephrotic syndrome., steroid-dependent nephrotic syndrome., steroid-sensitive nephrotic syndrome., multicenter, double-blind, randomized, placebo-controlled trial.

Background

Childhood-onset idiopathic nephrotic syndrome (INS) is the most common glomerular disease which occurs in more than 2 cases/100,000 children [1]. Notably, in Japan, the estimated incidence of INS is 6.49 cases/100,000 children annually [2]. Minimal change nephrotic syndrome is the most common form of the disorder, for which steroid therapy is effective for most patients [3]. Eighty to 90 % of patients achieve remission with the administration of steroids (steroid-sensitive nephrotic syndrome; SSNS) while 10–20% of patients suffer from steroid-resistant nephrotic syndrome (SRNS) which does not achieve remission with the administration of steroids [4].

Those who respond well rarely progress to end stage renal disease, but up to 50% of SSNS cases develop frequently-relapsing nephrotic syndrome (FRNS) [5]. FRNS is defined as at least four relapses per year or at least two within 6 months of the initial presentation (Table 2) [6]. A total of 50–60% of children with FRNS develop two consecutive relapses during tapering or within 14 days of stopping steroid therapy, this is termed steroid-dependent nephrotic syndrome (SDNS) (Table 2) [3, 6]. Treatment with immunosuppressive drugs is carried out to avoid the steroid-specific adverse event because each relapse requires a large dose of steroids. The Kidney Disease: Improving Global Outcomes Clinical Practice Guideline for Glomerulonephritis recommends alkylating agents, such as cyclophosphamide or chlorambucil, levamisole, calcineurin inhibitors, including cyclosporine or tacrolimus, and mycophenolate mofetil (MMF) as corticosteroid-sparing agents for children with FRNS/SDNS [7]. The clinical practice guidelines for pediatric idiopathic nephrotic syndrome (2013) recommend cyclosporine, cyclophosphamide, and mizoribine as immunosuppressive drugs for FRNS/SDNS [6]. Most children with FRNS/SDNS are effectively treated with

these recommended immunosuppressant drugs; however, at least 10–20% of children receiving immunosuppressive agents still show frequent relapses or steroid dependence after treatment (complicated FRNS/SDNS). Additionally, some patients with SRNS develop steroid-sensitive frequent relapses or steroid dependence after achievement of complete remission by immunosuppressive therapies including calcineurin inhibitors (complicated FRNS/SDNS). A 5-year follow-up study of cyclosporine treatment in children with SRNS showed that 7 of 31 (23%) patients developed frequent relapses under immunosuppressive therapy after achievement of complete remission [8]. Meanwhile, the total dosage of cyclophosphamide is restricted due to gonadal toxicity and late-onset carcinogenicity, and we cannot use cyclosporine exclusively because cyclosporine can cause chronic nephrotoxicity as a side effect. However, discontinuation of cyclosporine often results in frequent relapses again [9, 10].

In that context, there have been many reports that rituximab (RTX), a monoclonal antibody directed against the CD20 differentiation antigen expressed on the surface of B cells, is effective and safe in children with complicated FRNS/SDNS [11–13]. Recently, RTX has been used for complicated FRNS/SDNS, although some cases tend to relapse after the recovery of B cell counts [14–16]. In addition, the safety of long-term B cell suppression caused by repeated administration of RTX in children whose immune system is developing is unknown. Therefore, a new maintenance therapy to prevent the relapse after RTX treatment is urgently needed.

Mycophenolate mofetil (MMF) is an immunosuppressant which selectively blocks de novo purine synthesis, a pathway crucial for both B and T lymphocytes, and has been used for various autoimmune diseases and as immunosuppressive therapy after organ transplantation [17–20]. In addition, it is reported that MMF is effective in childhood-onset nephrotic syndrome [21–30]. Our group has conducted a pilot study and reported that maintenance therapy with MMF after a single dose of RTX in complicated SDNS significantly prolonged the relapse-free period compared with RTX monotherapy [31]. Thus, MMF is a promising drug for maintenance therapy after RTX, however a prospective randomized clinical trial is still needed. [32] Therefore, we conduct a multicenter, double-blind, randomized, placebo-controlled trial to evaluate the efficacy and safety of MMF after RTX therapy in children with complicated FRNS/SDNS.

Methods/design

A flow chart of the study design is shown in Fig. 1.

Aim

The aim of this trial is to investigate whether RTX plus MMF combination therapy is superior to RTX alone for the maintenance of remission after RTX treatment in children with complicated FRNS/SDNS.

Study design and patients

We conduct a multicenter, double-blind, randomized, placebo-controlled trial to assess the efficacy and safety of MMF after RTX therapy in children with complicated FRNS/SDNS (Fig. 1, Table 2 [6]). In total, 80 patients from 27 institutions in Japan will be enrolled in this study. We will diagnose NS and remission and relapse according to the International Study of Kidney Disease in Children (ISKDC) [6, 33]. Patients who are aged between 1 and 18 years old at the time of onset of idiopathic nephrotic syndrome and are aged 2 years or above at the time of registration are eligible if they fall into the complicated FRNS/SDNS category.

Inclusion and exclusion criteria are as follows:
Inclusion criteria:

1. Diagnosed as INS according to the ISKDC criteria.
2. The initial onset of INS is at between 1 and 18 years of age, and the patient is 2 years of age or older at assignment.
3. Patients meeting one of the following criteria:
   1) Diagnosed with frequent relapse or steroid dependence and once again diagnosed with frequent relapse or steroid dependence after completion of immunosuppressive drug therapy (cyclosporine, cyclophosphamide, or mizoribine, etc.).

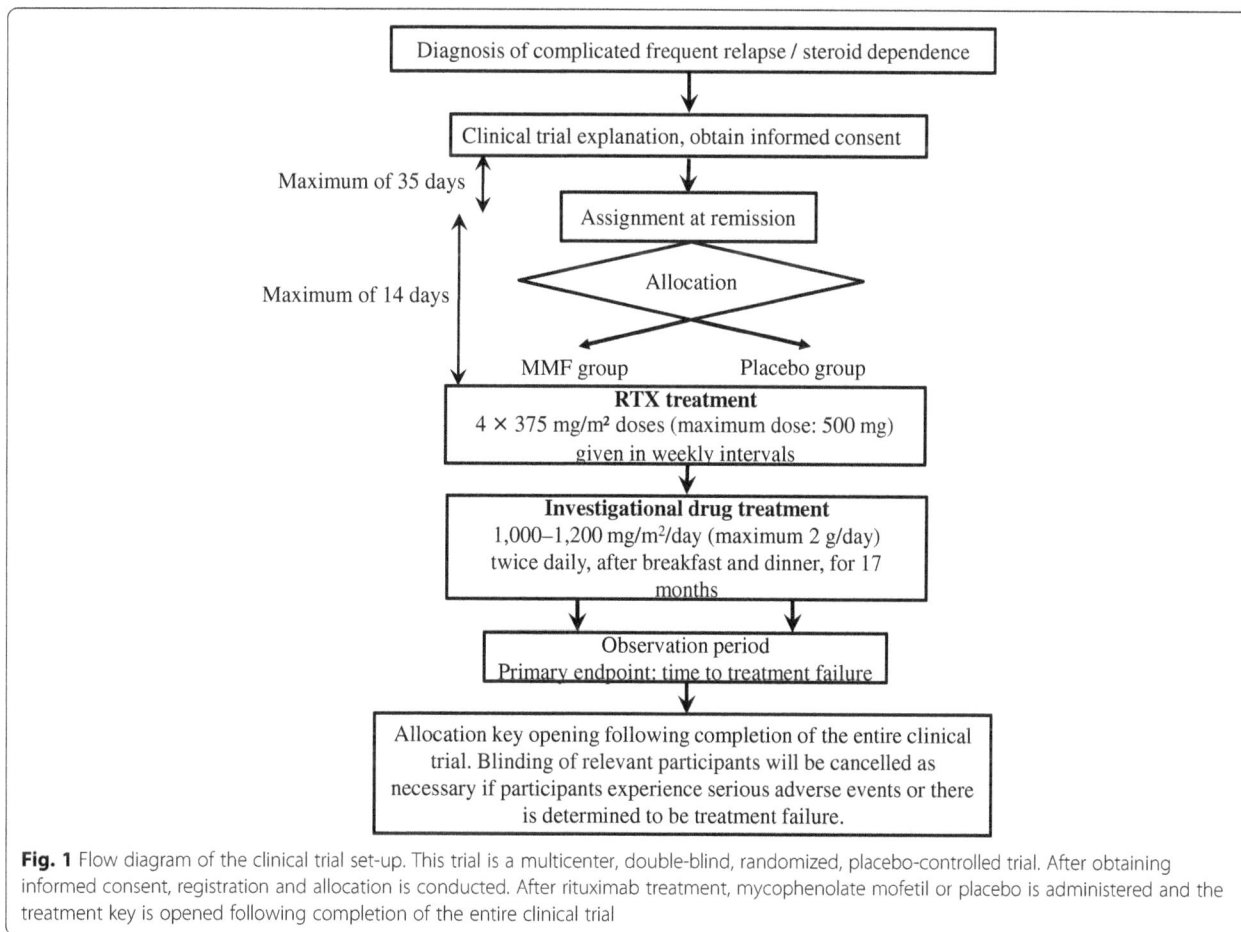

Fig. 1 Flow diagram of the clinical trial set-up. This trial is a multicenter, double-blind, randomized, placebo-controlled trial. After obtaining informed consent, registration and allocation is conducted. After rituximab treatment, mycophenolate mofetil or placebo is administered and the treatment key is opened following completion of the entire clinical trial

2) Diagnosed with frequent relapse or steroid dependence and once again diagnosed with frequent relapse or steroid dependence during immunosuppressive drug therapy (cyclosporine, cyclophosphamide, or mizoribine, etc.).

3) Diagnosed with steroid resistance following the onset of INS and diagnosed with frequent relapse or steroid dependence during or after the completion of immunosuppressive drug therapy (cyclosporine alone or combination of cyclosporine and methylprednisolone, etc.).

4. Patients with records of the nearest preceding 3 relapses.

5. Patients in whom steroid sensitivity is observed during treatment of relapse immediately prior to assignment.

6. Patients in whom ≥5 CD20-positive cells/μL are observed in the peripheral blood.

7. Patients who can be hospitalized overnight on the first day of rituximab administration.

8. Written informed consent.

Exclusion criteria:

1. Patients who have been diagnosed with nephritic-NS, such as IgA nephropathy, prior to assignment or in whom secondary NS is suspected.

2. Patients who have used a monoclonal antibody other than rituximab.

3. Patients meeting one of the following infection criteria:
   1) Presence or history of severe infections within 6 months prior to assignment.
   2) Presence or history of opportunistic infections within 6 months prior to assignment.
   3) Presence of active tuberculosis.
   4) Patients with a history of tuberculosis or in whom tuberculosis is suspected.
   5) Presence or history of active hepatitis B or hepatitis C or hepatitis B virus carrier.
   6) Presence of human immunodeficiency virus (HIV) infection.

4. Presence or history of angina pectoris, cardiac failure, myocardial infarction, or serious arrhythmia (findings observed under Grade 4 of the Common Terminology Criteria for Adverse Events (CTCAE)).

5. Presence or history of autoimmune diseases or vascular purpura.

6. Presence or history of malignant tumor.

7. History of organ transplantation.

8. History of drug allergies to methylprednisolone, acetaminophen, or d-chlorpheniramine maleate.

9. Uncontrollable hypertension.

10. Deteriorated kidney function, e.g. estimated glomerular filtration rate (GFR) < 60 mL/min/1.73 m^2.

11. Having received a live vaccine within 4 weeks prior to enrollment.

12. Patients showing one of the following abnormal clinical laboratory values:
    1) Leukocytes < 3000/μL.
    2) Neutrophils < 1500/μL.
    3) Platelets < 50,000/μL.
    4) Alanine aminotransferase (ALT) > 2.5× upper limit of normal value.
    5) Aspartate aminotransferase (AST) > 2.5× upper limit of normal value.
    6) Positive for hepatitis B surface (HBs) antigen, HBs antibody, hepatitis B core (HBc) antibody, or HCV antibody.
    7) Positive for HIV antibody.

13. Patients who do not agree with contraception during the study period.

14. Women during pregnancy or breast-feeding.

15. Judged inappropriate for this study by the treating or study physicians.

Randomization

Patients are randomly assigned to either RTX plus MMF, or RTX plus placebo group at an approximate ratio of 1:1 using the following allocation adjustment factors; medical institution, age, treatment history (presence or absence of immunosuppressive drug administration at the relapse immediately prior to enrollment, presence or absence of steroid administration at the relapse immediately prior to enrollment), interval between the last 3 relapses, presence or absence of history of SRNS.

Patients, their guardians, treating physicians, and individuals assessing outcomes and analyzing data are blinded to the patients' assigned treatment. Apart from the data-monitoring committee, all treating physicians and other investigators remain blinded to the trial results until follow-ups are completed.

Procedures
Observation period
The observation period is from the date the first dose of RTX is administered (day 1) to the date MMF administration is finished (day 505).

Dosage regimen
RTX and the investigational drug (MMF or placebo) are administered in this trial. The dosage regimen is shown in Fig. 2. For the RTX plus MMF combination group, RTX is administered as 4 × 375 mg/m^2 doses (maximum dose: 500 mg) given at weekly intervals and MMF is additionally administered at a dose of 1000–1200 mg/m^2/day (maximum 2 g/day) twice daily after breakfast

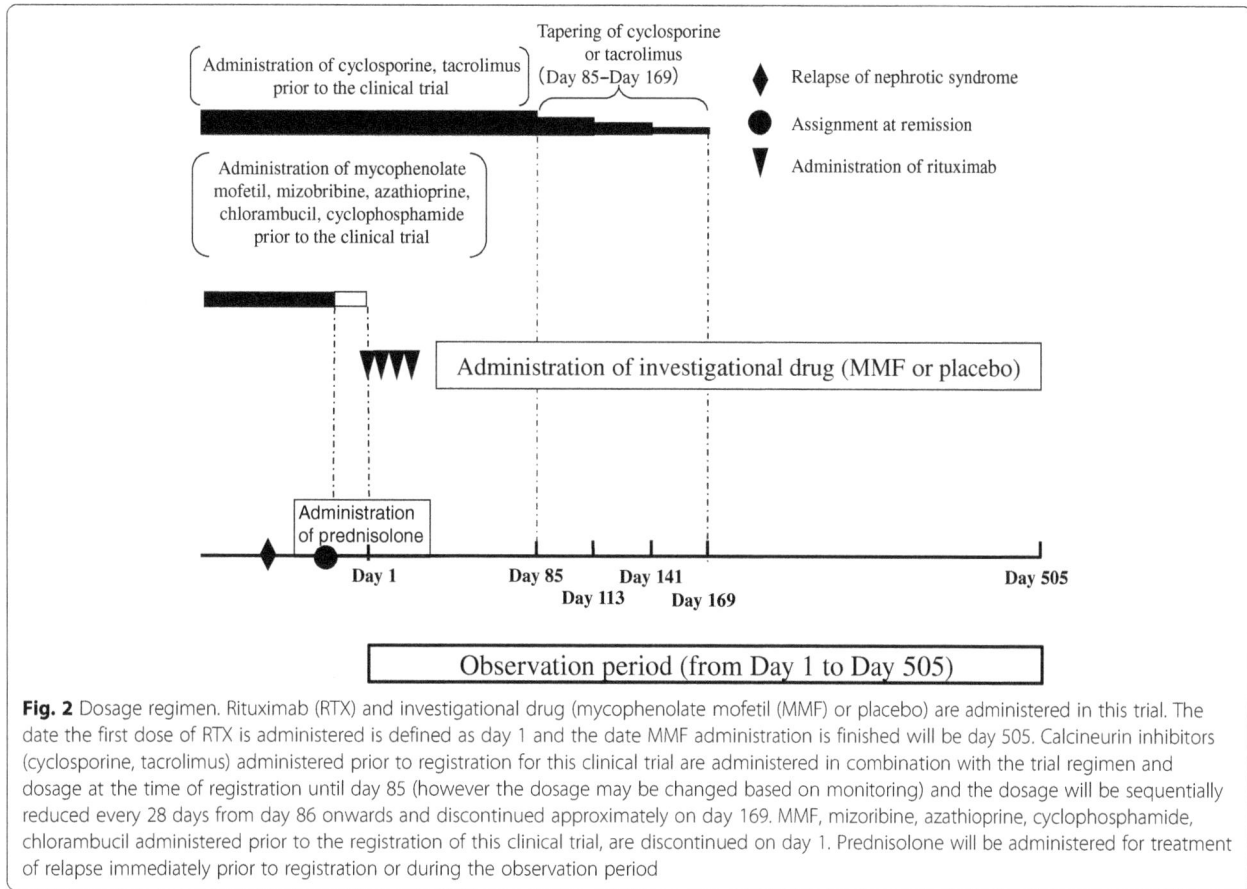

Fig. 2 Dosage regimen. Rituximab (RTX) and investigational drug (mycophenolate mofetil (MMF) or placebo) are administered in this trial. The date the first dose of RTX is administered is defined as day 1 and the date MMF administration is finished will be day 505. Calcineurin inhibitors (cyclosporine, tacrolimus) administered prior to registration for this clinical trial are administered in combination with the trial regimen and dosage at the time of registration until day 85 (however the dosage may be changed based on monitoring) and the dosage will be sequentially reduced every 28 days from day 86 onwards and discontinued approximately on day 169. MMF, mizoribine, azathioprine, cyclophosphamide, chlorambucil administered prior to the registration of this clinical trial, are discontinued on day 1. Prednisolone will be administered for treatment of relapse immediately prior to registration or during the observation period

and dinner, continued for 17 months after RTX treatment. For the RTX plus placebo group, RTX is administered as 4× 375 mg/m^2 doses (maximum dose: 500 mg) given at weekly intervals and the placebo is administered in place of MMF.

The investigational drug can be begun at half the dose and increased to the defined dose in the absence of adverse reactions within 3 months. If patients cannot accept the full dose due to of adverse events, the doctors in attendance can decide the dose reduction. To prevent infusion reactions, patients receive a premedication with methylprednisolone, oral acetaminophen, oral d-chlorpheniramine maleate approximately 30 min prior to the administration of each dose of RTX [11].

Prednisolone treatment for relapse at screening and during the study period

Participants receiving prednisolone for relapse at screening continue receiving the drug, taking 60 mg/m^2 orally three times a day (maximum of 80 mg per day or 60 mg per day, depending on the institution policy) for 4 weeks. Participants with relapse not receiving prednisolone at screening receive the same dose until 3 days after complete remission is achieved. After 4 weeks (in

patients who received prednisolone at screening) or from 3 days after complete remission (in patients who did not receive prednisolone at screening), patients take 60 mg/m^2 prednisolone in the morning on alternate days (maximum 80 mg per day or 60 mg per day) for 2 weeks, then 30 mg/m^2 on alternate days (maximum 40 mg per day or 30 mg per day) for 2 weeks, and then 15 mg/m^2 on alternate days (maximum 20 mg per day or 15 mg per day) for 2 weeks. When patients have relapses during the study period, they receive 60 mg/m^2 oral prednisolone three times a day (maximum 60 mg per day) until 3 days after complete remission is obtained, then take 60 mg/m^2 prednisolone in the morning on alternate days (maximum 60 mg per day) for 2 weeks, then 30 mg/m^2 on alternate days (maximum 30 mg per day) for 2 weeks, and then 15 mg/m^2 on alternate days (maximum 15 mg per day) for 2 weeks.

Concomitant dugs and combination therapy

In the event patients are receiving a calcineurin inhibitor (cyclosporine or tacrolimus) at screening, tapering of the drug begins at day 86, with discontinuation by day 169; the dosage will be sequentially reduced every 28 days from day 86 onwards and discontinued on approximately day 169 (Fig. 2). If patients were taking any other immunosuppressive agents (MMF, mizoribine, azathioprine, cyclophosphamide or chlorambucil), these drugs are discontinued by the beginning of RTX administration (day 1) (Fig. 2).

Trimethoprim-sulfamethoxazole is administered from the beginning of RTX treatment (day 1) until the date on which peripheral blood B cell recovery (≥ 5 cells/µL) is confirmed for the prevention of *Pneumocystis jirovecii* infection.

Combination therapy with the following drugs and treatment are prohibited during the clinical trial period.

1. Commercially available rituximab.
2. Immunosuppressive drugs or alkylating agents with an immunosuppressive effect except in the following cases.
    1) In the case "cyclosporine, tacrolimus, cyclophosphamide, mizoribine, MMF or chlorambucil" continues to be used from prior to the start of the clinical trial.
    2) In the case treatment failure is determined.

Live vaccines
The discontinuation of investigational drug administration

Investigators are to discontinue the administration of investigational drugs to participants to whom any of the following circumstances apply:

(1) If treatment failure (FRNS, SDNS, or SRNS) is observed during the observation period.
(2) If prohibited drug 1.2. (see above) is used as a treatment for nephrotic syndrome.
(3) If the participant or legal representative requests discontinuation of the administration of the investigational drug.
(4) If the investigators determine the continuation of investigational drug administration to be difficult for any other reason such as the occurrence of adverse events.
(5) If the participant becomes pregnant.

Visit schedule

During the clinical trial period, investigators carry out observations, examinations, and surveys in accordance with the prescribed schedule. The visit schedule is shown in Table 1. Study visits occur every week during the RTX administration period, every 1 month during the first 6 month of the investigational drug administration period, and every 2 month, thereafter. Urine samples and blood samples are taken every visit.

Allocation key opening

To maintain blinding, the "allocation codes" will be disclosed after the entire clinical trial is completed and all data and determination secured. However, if any of the following circumstances apply, the allocation code of the patient will be urgently disclosed.

(1) The participant experiences a serious adverse event that leads to death or is life-threatening.
(2) The participant experiences another serious adverse event and it is determined the information is essential in considering the relevant patient's treatment.
(3) There is determined to be treatment failure (FRNS, SDNS or SRNS).
(4) The participant becomes pregnant and discontinues the administration of investigational drug.

Outcomes

The primary endpoint is defined as the time-to-treatment failure (development of frequent relapses, steroid dependence or steroid resistance). Diagnosis of FRNS, SDNS, and SRNS is based on relapse dates according to the ISKDC (Table 2). The secondary end points are time to relapse, relapse rate, time to FRNS, time to SDNS, time to SRNS, total steroid dose, peripheral blood B cell depletion period and adverse events. Adverse events are recorded throughout the trial period and assessed using CTCAE.

Statistical analyses

The primary aim of this study is to examine the superiority of RTX plus MMF combination therapy compared with RTX monotherapy in extending the duration to treatment failure. Based on a previous study, we hypothesize a 1-year event rate of 40% in the RTX treatment group and expect the RTX plus MMF treatment to decrease that to 20%. The planned sample size is 80 patients: 37 patients in each group will be needed to have 80% power for a log-rank test with a 5% significance level, under an assumption of proportional hazard rates, 3 years accrual, and one-and-a-half years follow-up. To allow for withdrawal of consent after participation in the study or loss to follow-up, we set the study size to 80 participants in total. The power calculation was performed using SAS version 9.3 (SAS Institute Inc., Cary, NC, USA). As a primary analysis, time-to-treatment failure is summarized using the Kaplan-Meier method and results compared using the log-rank test. The hazard ratios with 95% confidence intervals are estimated using Cox proportional hazard model. Secondary endpoints including time to relapse, time to FRNS, time to SDNS, time to SRNS, and B cell depletion period will be analyzed in the same manner as the primary endpoint. Model based analysis will be

Table 1 Clinical trial schedule

	Screening period	Observation period (Rituximab administration period)				Observation period (Investigational drug administration period)												Relapse	Investigation drug discontinuation	Follow-up period
Day	Within 35 days	1	8	15	22	29	57	85	113	141	169	225	281	337	393	449	505			36/48 month Clinical trial discontinuation
Visit		1	2	3	4	5	6	7	8	9	10	11	12	13	14	15	16			
Obtaining informed consent	○																			
Medical examination	○	○	○	○	○	○	○	○	○	○	○	○	○	○	○	○	○	○	○	
Investigation drug administration		○	○	○	○	○	○	○	○	○	○	○	○	○	○	○	○	○	○	
Background survey	○																			
Concomitant drug survey	○	○	○	○	○	○	○	○	○	○	○	○	○	○	○	○	○	○	○	
Height/weight	○	○	○	○	○	○	○	○	○	○	○	○	○	○	○	○	○	○	△	○
Blood pressure	○	○	○	○	○	○	○	○	○	○	○	○	○	○	○	○	○	○	△	○
Pulse, body temperature	○	○	○	○	○	○					○			○					△	
Pregnancy test	○																			
HIV, HCV, HBV[a]	○																			
Electrocardiogram	○															○		△	△	
Chest X-ray	○																○	△	△	
Relapse evaluation		○	○	○	○	○	○	○	○	○	○	○	○	○	○	○	○	○	○	○
Adverse event evaluation		○	○	○	○	○	○	○	○	○	○	○	○	○	○	○	○	○	○	○
After treatment																			○	○
Hematological examination	○	○	○	○	○	○	○	○	○	○	○	○	○	○	○	○	○	○	△	
Immunoglobulin examination		○					○		○		○		○	○		○	○	○	△	
Estimated glomerular filtration rate	○	○			○	○			○		○		○	○		○	○	○	○	
Urinalysis	○	○	○	○	○	○	○	○	○	○	○	○	○	○	○	○	○	○	○	○
Peripheral blood B cell count	○	○	○	○	○	○	○	○	○	○	○	○	○	○	○	○	○	○	○	□

△: Conduct if possible
□: Conduct until the peripheral blood B cell recovery (≥ 5/μL) is confirmed
[a] *HIV* human immunodeficiency virus, *HCV* hepatitis C virus, *HBV* hepatitis B virus

Table 2 Definitions [6]

A. *Nephrotic syndrome*	The presence of a urine protein-to-creatinine ratio of 1.8 or above and serum albumin of 2.5 g/dL or below.
B. *Complicated nephrotic syndrome*	A patient that fulfills any of the following criteria is deemed to suffer from complicated nephrotic syndrome: (1) Diagnosed with frequent relapse or steroid dependence and once again diagnosed with frequent relapse or steroid dependence after completion of immunosuppressive drug therapy (cyclosporine, cyclophosphamide, mizoribine, etc.) (2) Diagnosed with frequent relapse or steroid dependence and once again diagnosed with frequent relapse or steroid dependence during immunosuppressive drug therapy (cyclosporine, cyclophosphamide, mizoribine, etc.) (3) Diagnosed with steroid resistance and diagnosed with frequent relapse or steroid dependence during or after the completion of immunosuppressive drug therapy (cyclosporine or combination of cyclosporine and methylprednisolone, etc.)
C. *Remission*	Negative protein on urine dipstick in the first morning urine for 3 consecutive days.
D. *Steroid sensitivity*	When the daily administration of prednisolone at 60 mg/m^2/day leads to remission within 4 weeks.
E. *Relapse*	Protein 2+ or above detected by urine dipstick in the first morning urine for 3 consecutive days and prednisolone treatment is required.
F. *Frequent relapse*	Two or more relapses within 6 months after initial remission or 4 or more relapses within any 12-month period.
G. *Steroid dependence*	Two consecutive relapses during the reduction of steroid therapy or within 2 weeks of discontinuation of steroid therapy.
H. *Steroid resistance*	When the daily administration of prednisolone at 60 mg/m^2/day does not lead to remission within 4 weeks.

performed as needed. Relapse rate will be compared by permutation testing. Total steroid dose will be compared with the Wilcoxon test.

Discussion

The purpose of this trial is to examine its safety and assess whether RTX plus MMF combination therapy is superior to RTX plus placebo for the maintenance of remission after RTX treatment in children with complicated FRNS/SDNS. Recently, RTX dramatically altered the treatment of complicated FRNS/SDNS [34]. Some patients can attain a 'steroid-free period' and/or 'cyclosporine-free period', while some cases tend to relapse after the recovery of B cell counts [14–16]. However, MMF has recently been focused on as a new treatment for childhood-onset nephrotic syndrome [21–30]. MMF is an immunosuppressive agent whose mechanism is similar to mizoribine in its inhibitory effect on the de novo pathway of nucleic acid synthesis [35]. In addition, we previously found that SDNS patients who do not relapse after RTX treatment were taking MMF [14]. Therefore, upon receiving the results of a pilot study, [31] we initiated a multicenter, double-blind, randomized, placebo-controlled trial to assess the efficacy and safety of MMF after RTX therapy in children with complicated FRNS/SDNS.

At present, there is a consensus that after RTX treatment, we do not use immunosuppressants until patients lapse into FRNS/SDNS again. Although the efficacy of MMF was shown in the pilot study, MMF is not an established treatment for maintenance therapy after RTX. Thus, it is reasonable to set the control group as immunosuppressant free. Simultaneously, we must pay

careful attention so as not to restrict the chance for appropriate treatment in participants. To rescue the patients who fall into treatment failure, we are setting an urgent key open system. If a patient falls into FRNS, SDNS, or SRNS, the allocation code will be opened immediately and treatment conducted using immunosuppressants as soon as possible.

For complicated FRNS/SDNS patients, long-term treatment and multiple side effects are major issues. Current immunosuppressants such as calcineurin inhibitors, cyclophosphamide, mizoribine, and RTX have certainly helped patients, but existing treatments are not optimal. If we can demonstrate that MMF is safe and able to attain the long remission used for maintenance therapy after RTX, we will reduce the total dose of steroids, calcineurin inhibitors, and improve the quality of life in patients with complicated FRNS/SDNS. However, a limitation is that we cannot know the long-term prognosis of patients just by this trial, of which the observational period is just 18 months. In addition, MMF may not be curative like other existing treatments. Therefore, we must investigate the long-term prognosis of MMF in conjunction with RTX treatment while the discovery of treatments with a curative mechanism is also anticipated.

In conclusion, we conduct a multicenter, double-blind, randomized, placebo-controlled trial to evaluate the efficacy and safety of MMF after RTX therapy in children with complicated FRNS/SDNS. Results from this study may impact the management of pediatric complicated FRNS/SDNS patients. Improvement in quality of life will be accomplished by long-term remission, which should be of great benefit to both children with complicated FRNS/SDNS and their families.

Abbreviations
CTCAE: Common Terminology Criteria for Adverse Events.; FRNS: Frequently-relapsing nephrotic syndrome; INS: Idiopathic nephrotic syndrome; ISKDC: International Study of Kidney Disease in Children; MMF: Mycophenolate mofetil; RTX: Rituximab; SDNS: Steroid-dependent nephrotic syndrome; SRNS: Steroid-resistant nephrotic syndrome

Acknowledgements
The authors are grateful to all the members of Japanese Study Group for Kidney Disease in Children for their help. We thank Simon Teteris, PhD, from the Edanz Group (https://www.edanzediting.com), for editing the English text of a draft of this manuscript.

Funding
The trial is supported by a grant from the Ministry of Health, Labor and Welfare, Japan (H25-iryogijutsu-ippan-008), and by the Japan Agency for Medical Research and Development (AMED) under grant number 151k0201021h0003 and 18lk0201082h0001. This study protocol has undergone peer-review by the funding bodies.

Authors' contributions
Kli, KaN, and MS are responsible for the study concept and management of the study. MS, KoN, Kls, SI, and HN contributed to study design. MSO is responsible for statistical analysis. TH and Kli wrote the first draft of this manuscript; all co-authors critically reviewed and revised the initial draft and approved the final version of the manuscript.

Competing interests
Mayumi Sako has received a consulting fee from Zenyaku Kogyo Co. Ltd. Koichi Nakanishi has received lecture fees from Novartis Pharma K.K. Kenji Ishikura has received a grant from Chugai Pharmaceutical Co., Ltd. and Pfizer Japan Inc. and a lecture fee from Zenyaku Kogyo Co. Ltd. Kandai Nozu has received lecture fees from Chugai Pharmaceutical Co., Ltd. Kazumoto Iijima has received lecture fees and/or consulting fees from Chugai Pharmaceutical Co., Ltd., Zenyaku Kogyo Co. Ltd., Takeda Pharmaceutical Co., Ltd., Novartis Pharma K.K., Kyowa Hakko Kirin Co. Ltd.
MMF is provided by Chugai Pharmaceutical Co., Ltd. The sponsor approved the study protocol, but had no role in data collection, data analysis and drafting or approving the present manuscript.

Author details
[1]Department of Pediatrics, Kobe University Graduate School of Medicine, 5-1 Kusunoki-cho 7 chome, Chuo-ku, Kobe 650-0017, Japan. [2]Division for Clinical Trials, Department of Clinical Research Promotion, Clinical Research Center, National Center for Child Health and Development, Tokyo, Japan. [3]Department of Child Health and Welfare (Pediatrics), Graduate School of Medicine, University of the Ryukyus, Okinawa, Japan. [4]Division of Nephrology and Rheumatology, National Center for Child Health and Development, Tokyo, Japan. [5]Department of Pediatrics, Graduate School of Medicine, Yokohama City University, Yokohama, Japan. [6]Clinical Research Center, National Center for Child Health and Development, Tokyo, Japan. [7]Department of Medical Statistics, Toho University, Tokyo, Japan.

References
1. Eddy AA, Symons JM. Nephrotic syndrome in childhood. Lancet. 2003; 362(9384):629–39.
2. Kikunaga K, Ishikura K, Terano C, Sato M, Komaki F, Hamasaki Y, Sasaki S, Iijima K, Yoshikawa N, Nakanishi K, et al. High incidence of idiopathic nephrotic syndrome in East Asian children: a nationwide survey in Japan (JP-SHINE study). Clin Exp Nephrol. 2017;21(4):651–7.
3. Schulman SL, Kaiser BA, Polinsky MS, Srinivasan R, Baluarte HJ. Predicting the response to cytotoxic therapy for childhood nephrotic syndrome: superiority of response to corticosteroid therapy over histopathologic patterns. J Pediatr. 1988;113(6):996–1001.
4. Koskimies O, Vilska J, Rapola J, Hallman N. Long-term outcome of primary nephrotic syndrome. Arch Dis Child. 1982;57(7):544–8.
5. Tarshish P, Tobin JN, Bernstein J, Edelmann CM Jr. Prognostic significance of the early course of minimal change nephrotic syndrome: report of the international study of kidney disease in children. J Am Soc Nephrol. 1997; 8(5):769–76.
6. Ishikura K, Matsumoto S, Sako M, Tsuruga K, Nakanishi K, Kamei K, Saito H, Fujinaga S, Hamasaki Y, Chikamoto H, et al. Clinical practice guideline for pediatric idiopathic nephrotic syndrome 2013: medical therapy. Clin Exp Nephrol. 2015;19(1):6–33.
7. Kidney Disease: Improving Global Outcomes (KDIGO) Glomerulonephritis Work Group. Chapter 3: steroid-sensitive nephrotic syndrome in children. Kidney Int Suppl. 2012;2(2):163–71.
8. Hamasaki Y, Yoshikawa N, Nakazato H, Sasaki S, Iijima K, Nakanishi K, Matsuyama T, Ishikura K, Ito S, Kaneko T, et al. Prospective 5-year follow-up of cyclosporine treatment in children with steroid-resistant nephrosis. Pediatr Nephrol (Berlin, Germany). 2013;28(5):765–71.
9. Inoue Y, Iijima K, Nakamura H, Yoshikawa N. Two-year cyclosporin treatment in children with steroid-dependent nephrotic syndrome. Pediatr Nephrol (Berlin, Germany). 1999;13(1):33–8.
10. Iijima K, Hamahira K, Tanaka R, Kobayashi A, Nozu K, Nakamura H, Yoshikawa N. Risk factors for cyclosporine-induced tubulointerstitial lesions in children with minimal change nephrotic syndrome. Kidney Int. 2002;61(5):1801–5.
11. Iijima K, Sako M, Nozu K, Mori R, Tuchida N, Kamei K, Miura K, Aya K, Nakanishi K, Ohtomo Y, et al. Rituximab for childhood-onset, complicated, frequently relapsing nephrotic syndrome or steroid-dependent nephrotic syndrome: a multicentre, double-blind, randomised, placebo-controlled trial. Lancet. 2014;384(9950):1273–81.
12. Benz K, Dotsch J, Rascher W, Stachel D. Change of the course of steroid-dependent nephrotic syndrome after rituximab therapy. Pediatr Nephrol (Berlin, Germany). 2004;19(7):794–7.
13. Ravani P, Magnasco A, Edefonti A, Murer L, Rossi R, Ghio L, Benetti E, Scozzola F, Pasini A, Dallera N, et al. Short-term effects of rituximab in children with steroid- and calcineurin-dependent nephrotic syndrome: a randomized controlled trial. Clin J Am Soc Nephrol. 2011;6(6):1308–15.
14. Kamei K, Ito S, Nozu K, Fujinaga S, Nakayama M, Sako M, Saito M, Yoneko M, Iijima K. Single dose of rituximab for refractory steroid-dependent nephrotic syndrome in children. Pediatr Nephrol (Berlin, Germany). 2009;24(7):1321–8.
15. Fujinaga S, Hirano D, Nishizaki N, Kamei K, Ito S, Ohtomo Y, Shimizu T, Kaneko K. Single infusion of rituximab for persistent steroid-dependent minimal-change nephrotic syndrome after long-term cyclosporine. Pediatr Nephrol (Berlin, Germany). 2010;25(3):539–44.
16. Guigonis V, Dallocchio A, Baudouin V, Dehennault M, Hachon-Le Camus C, Afanetti M, Groothoff J, Llanas B, Niaudet P, Nivet H, et al. Rituximab treatment for severe steroid- or cyclosporine-dependent nephrotic syndrome: a multicentric series of 22 cases. Pediatr Nephrol (Berlin, Germany). 2008;23(8):1269–79.
17. The Tricontinental Mycophenolate Mofetil Renal Transplantation Study Group. A blinded, randomized clinical trial of mycophenolate mofetil for the prevention of acute rejection in cadaveric renal transplantation. Transplantation. 1996;61(7):1029–37.
18. Vanrenterghem Y. The use of mycophenolate mofetil (Cellcept) in renal transplantation. Contrib Nephrol. 1998;124:64–9 discussion 69-75.
19. Chan TM, Li FK, Tang CS, Wong RW, Fang GX, Ji YL, Lau CS, Wong AK, Tong MK, Chan KW, et al. Efficacy of mycophenolate mofetil in patients with diffuse proliferative lupus nephritis. Hong Kong-Guangzhou nephrology study group. N Engl J Med. 2000;343(16):1156–62.

20. Lau KK, Jones DP, Hastings MC, Gaber LW, Ault BH. Short-term outcomes of severe lupus nephritis in a cohort of predominantly African-American children. Pediatr Nephrol (Berlin, Germany). 2006;21(5):655–62.

21. Afzal K, Bagga A, Menon S, Hari P, Jordan SC. Treatment with mycophenolate mofetil and prednisolone for steroid-dependent nephrotic syndrome. Pediatr Nephrol (Berlin, Germany). 2007;22(12):2059–65.

22. Bagga A, Hari P, Moudgil A, Jordan SC. Mycophenolate mofetil and prednisolone therapy in children with steroid-dependent nephrotic syndrome. Am J Kidney Dis. 2003;42(6):1114–20.

23. Barletta GM, Smoyer WE, Bunchman TE, Flynn JT, Kershaw DB. Use of mycophenolate mofetil in steroid-dependent and -resistant nephrotic syndrome. Pediatr Nephrol (Berlin, Germany). 2003;18(8):833–7.

24. Fujinaga S, Ohtomo Y, Hirano D, Nishizaki N, Someya T, Ohtsuka Y, Kaneko K, Shimizu T. Mycophenolate mofetil therapy for childhood-onset steroid dependent nephrotic syndrome after long-term cyclosporine: extended experience in a single center. Clin Nephrol. 2009;72(4):268–73.

25. Fujinaga S, Ohtomo Y, Umino D, Takemoto M, Shimizu T, Yamashiro Y, Kaneko K. A prospective study on the use of mycophenolate mofetil in children with cyclosporine-dependent nephrotic syndrome. Pediatr Nephrol (Berlin, Germany). 2007;22(1):71–6.

26. Gellermann J, Querfeld U. Frequently relapsing nephrotic syndrome: treatment with mycophenolate mofetil. Pediatr Nephrol (Berlin, Germany). 2004;19(1):101–4.

27. Hogg RJ, Fitzgibbons L, Bruick J, Bunke M, Ault B, Baqi N, Trachtman H, Swinford R. Mycophenolate mofetil in children with frequently relapsing nephrotic syndrome: a report from the southwest pediatric nephrology study group. Clin J Am Soc Nephrol. 2006;1(6):1173–8.

28. Mendizabal S, Zamora I, Berbel O, Sanahuja MJ, Fuentes J, Simon J. Mycophenolate mofetil in steroid/cyclosporine-dependent/resistant nephrotic syndrome. Pediatr Nephrol (Berlin, Germany). 2005;20(7):914–9.

29. Okada M, Sugimoto K, Yagi K, Yanagida H, Tabata N, Takemura T. Mycophenolate mofetil therapy for children with intractable nephrotic syndrome. Pediatr Int. 2007;49(6):933–7.

30. Ulinski T, Dubourg L, Said MH, Parchoux B, Ranchin B, Cochat P. Switch from cyclosporine a to mycophenolate mofetil in nephrotic children. Pediatr Nephrol (Berlin, Germany). 2005;20(4):482–5.

31. Ito S, Kamei K, Ogura M, Sato M, Fujimaru T, Ishikawa T, Udagawa T, Iijima K. Maintenance therapy with mycophenolate mofetil after rituximab in pediatric patients with steroid-dependent nephrotic syndrome. Pediatr Nephrol (Berlin, Germany). 2011;26(10):1823–8.

32. Filler G, Huang SH, Sharma AP. Should we consider MMF therapy after rituximab for nephrotic syndrome? Pediatr Nephrol (Berlin, Germany). 2011; 26(10):1759–62.

33. Abramowicz M, Barnett HL, Edelmann CM Jr, Greifer I, Kobayashi O, Arneil GC, Barron BA, Gordillo PG, Hallman N, Tiddens HA. Controlled trial of azathioprine in children with nephrotic syndrome. A report for the international study of kidney disease in children. Lancet. 1970;1(7654):959–61.

34. Iijima K, Sako M, Nozu K. Rituximab for nephrotic syndrome in children. Clin Exp Nephrol. 2017;21(2):193–202.

35. Allison AC, Eugui EM. Immunosuppressive and other effects of mycophenolic acid and an ester prodrug, mycophenolate mofetil. Immunol Rev. 1993;136:5–28.

23

Renal outcomes of STOP-IgAN trial patients in relation to baseline histology (MEST-C scores)

Judith Isabel Schimpf[1†], Till Klein[1,2†], Christina Fitzner[3], Frank Eitner[4], Stefan Porubsky[5,6], Ralf-Dieter Hilgers[3], Jürgen Floege[1], Hermann-Josef Groene[5] and Thomas Rauen[1]*

Abstract

Background: The Oxford classification of IgA nephropathy (IgAN) defines histologic criteria (MEST-C) that provide prognostic information based on the kidney biopsy. There are few data on the predictive impact of this classification in randomized clinical trial settings.

Methods: We performed an exploratory analysis of MEST-C scores in 70 available renal biopsies from 162 randomized STOP-IgAN trial participants and correlated the results with clinical outcomes. Analyses were performed by researchers blinded to the clinical outcome of the patients. Biopsies had been obtained 6.5 to 95 (median 9.4) months prior to randomization.

Results: Mesangial hypercellularity (M1) associated with higher annual eGFR-loss during the 3-year trial (M1: -5.06 ± 5.17 ml/min/1.73 m^2, M0: -0.79 ± 4.50 ml/min/1.73 m^2, $p = 0.002$). An M0-score additionally showed a weak association with full clinical remission, whereas the percentage of patients losing ≥ 15 ml/min/1.73 m^2 over the 3-year trial phase was higher among those scored as M1. Among patients with additional immunosuppression, ESRD occurred more frequently in patients when tubulointerstitial fibrosis (T1/2) was present (T1/2 = 33%, T0 = 0%, $p = 0.008$). In patients receiving supportive care only, ESRD frequencies were similar (T1/2 = 18%, T0 = 7%, $p = 0.603$). At randomization, eGFR was significantly lower when tubulointerstitial fibrosis was present (T1/2: 45.2 ± 15.7 ml/min/1.73 m^2, T0: 74.6 ± 28.2 ml/min/1.73 m^2, $p < 0.0001$). Endocapillary hypercellularity (E), and glomerular segmental sclerosis (S) were not associated with any clinical outcome parameter. In the analyzed cohort, patients with glomerular crescents (C1/2 scores) in their biopsies were more likely to develop ESRD during the 3-year trial phase, but this trend was only significant in patients under supportive care.

Conclusions: This secondary analysis of STOP-IgAN biopsies indicates that M1, T1/2 and C1/2 scores associate with worse renal outcomes.

Keywords: IgA nephropathy, IgAN, MEST-C, Oxford classification, STOP-IgAN

Background

IgA nephropathy (IgAN) is the most common form of primary glomerulonephritis, presenting with a wide range of clinical features, pathological findings and variable progression of disease [1, 2]. In 2009, the Oxford classification, based on pathological characteristics in IgAN renal biopsies, was introduced to improve individual risk prediction for disease progression. Mesangial hypercellularity (M), endocapillary proliferation (E), segmental glomerulosclerosis or adhesions (S), tubular atrophy and interstitial fibrosis (T) were identified as significant variables predicting renal outcome independent of clinical features [3, 4]. Numerous retrospective analyses aimed to validate these parameters and assessed their predictivity [5–13]. However, these studies did not provide concordant results. Whereas the T-score is consistently accepted as a parameter with high prognostic

---

* Correspondence: trauen@ukaachen.de
†Judith Isabel Schimpf and Till Klein contributed equally to this work.
[1]Division of Nephrology and Clinical Immunology, RWTH Aachen University, Pauwelsstr. 30, 52074 Aachen, Germany
Full list of author information is available at the end of the article

relevance, the predictive value of M, E and S lesions remains controversial, which might be largely due to differences in patient selection criteria, treatment and outcome measures as well as inter-investigator variability in biopsy assessment [14]. Nonetheless, combination of MEST scores with clinical data at the time of biopsy, i.e. renal function, the degree of proteinuria and arterial hypertension, provided a comparable predictive power as monitoring clinical data over a 2-year period [15]. In 2017, the presence of glomerular crescents (C) was added as a fifth parameter to the revised Oxford classification [16], mainly based on a multicentric analysis of more than 3000 IgAN patients [17].

Despite the continuous improvement in histological characterization and tools to predict disease progression in IgAN patients, optimal therapeutic management on IgAN remains a matter of ongoing debate. There is widely accepted consensus on the essential role of blood pressure and proteinuria control using renin-angiotensin system (RAS) blocking agents. A number of recent randomized clinical trials investigated whether systemic or local immunosuppression on top of comprehensive supportive measures, particularly in patients at risk for a progressive disease course, provides further renal benefits [18–20]. Of note, none of these studies used histologic criteria for trial eligibility and/or patient stratification. Among these trials, STOP-IgAN was the first to evaluate the value of additional systemic immunosuppression in IgAN patients with optimized supportive care. The trial was initiated in 2006, when the Oxford classification was not yet published, and applied a novel, two-phase study design in which 379 patients with biopsy-proven IgAN were enrolled into a 6 months run-in phase of optimizing supportive care measures in accordance with the current KDIGO guidelines [21]. Subsequently, a homogenous high-risk group of 162 patients with persistent proteinuria above 0.75 g/day despite optimized supportive care was randomized to either continue on supportive care (SUP arm) or to receive additional immunosuppression (IMM arm) during a 3-year study phase. Additional immunosuppression induced more full clinical remissions, defined as preserved renal function and proteinuria below 0.2 g/g creatinine at the end of the study phase. However, the overall course of renal function and end-stage renal disease (ESRD) rates were not significantly different between the two arms [20].

Since the Oxford classification of IgAN was introduced in 2009, when our trial had already been initiated, we aimed to collect and re-analyze renal biopsies from randomized STOP-IgAN trial participants using the MEST-C score and to align these criteria with renal outcome data, in particular the two primary end points of the trial, i.e. (1) full remission defined as urinary protein-creatinine ratio < 0.2 g/g and an eGFR-decrease less than 5 ml/min/1.73m^2 and (2) an eGFR-loss ≥15 ml/min/1.73m^2 during the trial phase.

Methods

Study design

The study protocol and results of STOP-IgAN have been published previously [20, 22]. Briefly, all eligible patients with biopsy-proven IgAN ($n = 337$) entered a 6-months run-in phase with comprehensive optimization of supportive treatment measures. One-hundred-sixty-two patients at high risk for disease progression (i.e. those with a persistent proteinuria > 0.75 g/d, but less than 3.5 g/d, despite optimized supportive care) were then randomized into the following 3-year trial phase and were assigned to either continue on supportive therapy alone or to receive additional immunosuppression.

The Oxford classification of IgAN was introduced in 2009, when the STOP-IgAN trial had already been initiated. Thus, the original trial protocol was amended in 2009 and allowed to retrieve all available original renal biopsies from randomized trial participants. Written informed consent for re-assessment of available kidney biopsies was obtained from all patients included in this secondary substudy.

Study population

This secondary analysis reports data from 87 of the original 162 randomized trial patients. Seventeen biopsies showed less than 8 glomeruli and thus could not be assessed based on the MEST-C criteria. Thirty-two of the remaining 70 patients received supportive care (SUP arm) and 38 patients received immunosuppression in addition to supportive care (IMM arm) during the 3-year study phase (Fig. 1).

Microscopic analyses

Before enrollment into the STOP-IgAN trial, all patients underwent renal biopsy that was analyzed by a nephropathologist (H.J.G. or one of the pathologists listed in the Acknowledgements). Because of the heterogeneity of the pathology criteria and the high inter-individual examiner bias described in the original publication of the Oxford MEST classification [4], for the present secondary analysis pathology scoring was performed by only one examiner (T.K.), who had been trained and who was subsequently supervised through random control of achieved results obtained from 20 biopsies (i.e. 29% of all biopsies) by two experienced nephropathologists (H.J.G. and S.P.). Concordance rate between MEST-C scoring through T.K. and the one obtained by H.J.G. and S.P. was > 90%. T.K. was blinded to clinical data and previous nephropathologists' reports. Available renal biopsies were retrieved and analyzed in 2011

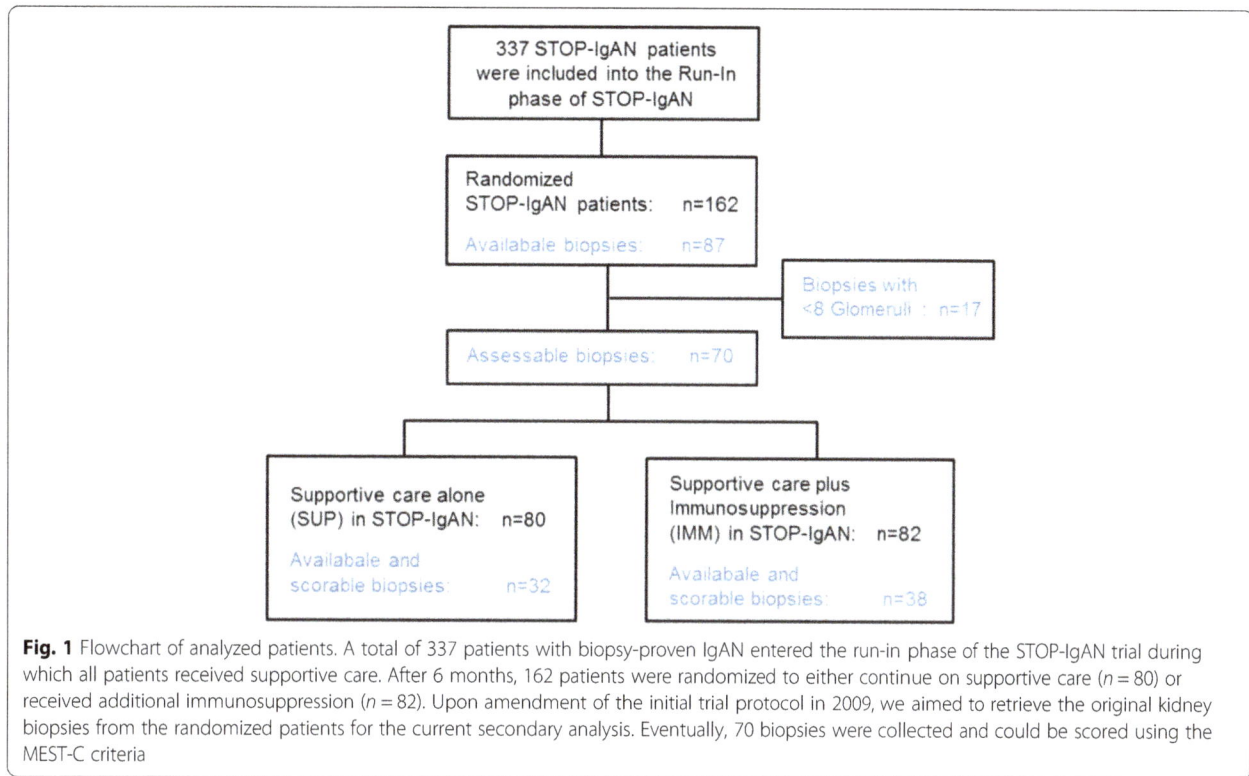

Fig. 1 Flowchart of analyzed patients. A total of 337 patients with biopsy-proven IgAN entered the run-in phase of the STOP-IgAN trial during which all patients received supportive care. After 6 months, 162 patients were randomized to either continue on supportive care ($n = 80$) or received additional immunosuppression ($n = 82$). Upon amendment of the initial trial protocol in 2009, we aimed to retrieve the original kidney biopsies from the randomized patients for the current secondary analysis. Eventually, 70 biopsies were collected and could be scored using the MEST-C criteria

according to the current Oxford classification of IgAN using the MEST-C criteria [16]. MEST-C criteria consisted of mesangial hypercellularity (M0: < 50% of glomeruli showing hypercellularity; M1: > 50% of glomeruli showing hypercellularity), endocapillary hypercellularity (E0: absent; E1: present when 3 capillary tubes in two glomeruli showed endocapillary hypercellularity), segmental glomerulosclerosis (S0: absent; S1: present) and tubular atrophy, interstitial fibrosis or interstitial inflammation (T0:< 25%; T1: 25–50%; T2:> 50% of cortical area involved).

The original Oxford classification study as well as the previous validation studies assessed the T-score by visual estimation of the percentage of cortical area involved. Based on these investigations, the T-score is consistently accepted as a histological lesion referring to high prognostic significance [10]. In this study, we used a virtual microscope tool (MIRAX Viewer) to encircle the pathologic lesions in the cortical area and then putting it in relation to the entire cortical area. Thus, we intended to improve the validity of the T-score and to reduce the inter-individual and intra-individual examiner variation to a minimum (Fig. 2).

Crescents were not yet part of the original Oxford classification in 2009 since their prognostic relevance was uncertain at that time, however it was already suggested to also add this information to the biopsy reports. Crescents were then officially introduced in the latest

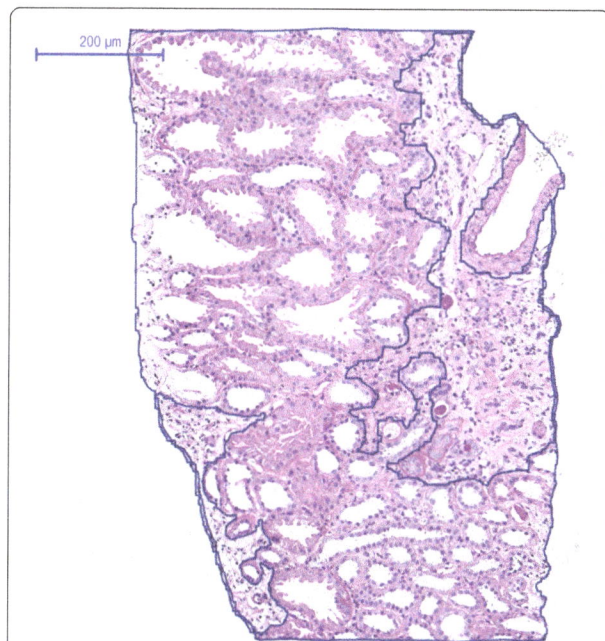

Fig. 2 Quantitative morphometry of the T-score in kidney biopsies. In contrast to semiquantitative analyses of tubular atrophy and interstitial fibrosis (T-score) in previous validation studies of the Oxford MEST-C classification, we assessed the T-score of by quantitative morphometry of the tubulointerstitial area using a virtual microscope tool (MIRAX Viewer). The pathologic lesions in the cortical area were encircled and then put in relation to the entire cortical area

update of the IgA Nephropathy Classification Working Group [16]. In a prescient fashion, the presence of cellular and fibrocellular crescents was also noted and evaluated in our analyses (C0: no crescents, C1: crescents in < 25% of glomeruli, C2: crescents in > 25% of glomeruli).

Statistical analysis

Data are presented as means ± standard deviations for continuous variables and as counts percentages. Association between MEST-C scores and continuous parameters are analyzed by Satterthwaite t-test. MEST-C scores and binary parameters are analyzed by *Fisher's exact* tests. The statistical test results are reported by *p*-values. Because of the small sample size, we conducted an explorative statistical analysis only. Consequently, the term "significance" was not used in the statistical confirmatory meaning (by comparison with a significance level). Furthermore, association of selected exploratory variables to renal outcome was evaluated by bivariate analyses (t-test and *Fisher's exact* test) assuming no confounding factors. Occurrence of the two primary STOP-IgAN endpoints (i.e. achievement of full clinical remission and eGFR-loss ≥15 ml/min/1.73 m^2) and ESRD was analyzed and visualized by Kaplan-Meier curves using the time of randomization as the starting point. Survival analyses

using uni- and multivariate Cox regression (adjusting for GFR and proteinuria at baseline and the treatment arm) were performed as sensitivity analyses to assess the interrelationship between individual MEST scores and these endpoints. For the C-score, Cox regression was not justified since the proportional hazards assumption was not met here. Statistical analyses were performed with SAS (Version 9.4, SAS Institute Inc., Cary, NC, USA).

Results

Baseline characteristics of biopsied patients

Among the 162 randomized patients entering the 3-year trial phase, we obtained 87 biopsies. Seventeen biopsies contained fewer than 8 glomeruli and therefore could not be analyzed. Seventy biopsies (43%) fulfilled the required quality criteria proposed for performing the Oxford MEST-C scoring. Of these, 32 were from patients randomized to the SUP arm and 38 to the IMM arm (Fig. 1). Demographic and clinical characteristics of this sub-cohort at the time of enrollment (i.e. at the beginning of the 6-month Run-In phase) are outlined in Table 1 and were similar to the entire study cohort [20]. Time between initial biopsies and trial enrollment ranged between from 6.5 to 95 months (median

Table 1 Patient characteristics at the start of the run-in phase and patients with primary endpoints at the end of the 3-year trial phase

	All (SUP + IMM)	Supportive Care (SUP)	Supportive Care plus Immunosuppression (IMM)
	(N = 70)	(N = 32)	(N = 38)
Patient characteristics:			
Female sex -%	17	13	21
Smoker -%	19	19	18
Age –yr	43.4 ± 13.6	48.2 ± 10.8	39.3 ± 14.5
Body-mass index	28.0 ± 5.0	29.0 ± 4.8	27.3 ± 5.1
Blood pressure- mmHg			
Systolic	131 ± 14	135 ± 16	127 ± 12
Diastolic	82 ± 11	86 ± 11	79 ± 10
Serum creatinine -mg/dl	1.4 ± 0,5	1.5 ± 0.5	1.3 ± 0.5
eGFR-ml/min/1.73m^2	67 ± 28	61 ± 25	73 ± 30
Creatinine clearance - ml/min	82 ± 34 (N = 60)	80 ± 30 (N = 28)	84 ± 37 (N = 32)
Daily urinary protein excretion - g/day	2.3 ± 1.3	2.4 ± 1.3	2.2 ± 1.3
Urinary protein-creatinine ratio - g/g	1.4 ± 0.8 (N = 60)	1.4 ± 0.8 (N = 28)	1.4 ± 0.8 (N = 32)
Cholesterol - mg/dl	210 ± 44 (N = 67)	208 ± 37 (N = 29)	211 ± 48 (N = 38)
Primary endpoints:			
Full clinical remission[a]	8	2	6
eGFR-loss ≥15 ml/min	23	11	12
ESRD[b]	8	4	4

[a]urinary protein-creatinine ratio < 0.2 g/g and an eGFR decrease of < 5 ml/min/1.73m^2
[b]end-stage renal disease

9.4 months), however only 6% of patients were biopsied more than 3 years before trial enrollment.

Pathology score distribution

Among the randomized patients followed through the 3-year trial phase, 26% had diffuse mesangial hypercellularity (M1), 17% endocapillary hypercellularity (E1), 91% segmental glomerulosclerosis (S1) and 41% tubular atrophy and interstitial fibrosis (T1/T2). Consistent with the VALIGA cohort [6] T2 lesions were rare (only in 4% of analyzed patients), therefore T1 and T2 lesions were combined to facilitate subsequent statistical analyses. The same procedure was applied to the glomerular crescent scores C1 and C2 (only 7% had a C2-score), resulting in 31% of biopsies showing crescents (C1/C2) (Table 2).

Within the analyzed sub-cohort baseline eGFR was significantly lower in patients with T1/T2 scores as compared to those with a T0-score (T1/2: 45 ± 16 ml/min/1.73 m^2 vs. T0: 75 ± 28 ml/min/1.73 m^2, $p < 0.0001$; Table 3). Mean baseline proteinuria levels did not differ between the T0 and the T1/2 group. Moreover, no obvious differences in eGFR, occurence of microhematuria and proteinuria were observed in the M, S, E and C categories.

Association between MEST-C scores and clinical outcome data

Patients with an M1-score had fewer full clinical remissions (M1: 0%vs. M0: 17%, $p = 0.099$; Table 4) and a

Table 3 Association between MEST-C score and baseline eGFR in STOP-IgAN patients

	Mean eGFR[a,b]	p-value
Mesangial hypercellularity		0.674
M0	62 ± 26	
M1	65 ± 34	
Endocapillary hypercellularity		0.308
E0	64 ± 27	
E1	53 ± 34	
Segmental glomerulosclerosis		0.422
S0	74 ± 34	
S1	61 ± 27	
Tubular atrophy/Interstitial fibrosis		< 0.0001
T0	75 ± 28	
T1/2	45 ± 16	
Crescents		0.815
C0	62 ± 29	
C1/2	64 ± 25	

[a] end of the 6-month run-in phase
[b] ml/min/1.73m^2

higher incidence of eGFR-loss ≥15 ml/min/1.73m^2 during the trial phase (M1: 50%vs. M0: 27%, $p = 0.092$), yet these trends did not reach the level of statistical significance. There were no differences in remission rates between individuals in the different study arms, neither in patients under supportive care (M1: 0%, M0: 9%, $p = 1.0$,

Table 2 MEST-C score distribution in STOP-IgAN patients

	All (SUP + IMM)	Supportive Care (SUP)	Supportive Care plus Immunosuppression (IMM)
	(N = 70)	(N = 32)	(N = 38)
Mesangial hypercellularity			
M0	52 (74%)	24 (75%)	28 (74%)
M1	18 (26%)	8 (25%)	10 (26%)
Endocapillary hypercellularity			
E0	58 (83%)	27 (84%)	31 (82%)
E1	12 (17%)	5 (16%)	7 (18%)
Segmental glomeruloscerlosis			
S0	6 (9%)	3 (9%)	3 (8%)
S1	64 (91%)	29 (91%)	35 (92%)
Tubular atrophy/Interstitial fibrosis			
T0	41 (59%)	15 (47%)	26 (68%)
T1	26 (37%)	17 (53%)	9 (24%)
T2	3 (4%)	0 (0%)	3 (8%)
Crescents			
C0	48 (69%)	24 (75%)	24 (63%)
C1	17 (24%)	7 (22%)	10 (26%)
C2	5 (7%)	1 (3%)	4 (11%)

Table 4 Association between M-, T- and C- scores and clinical outcome in STOP-IgAN patients (available cases analysis)

	M0 events/ total	M1 events/ total	p-value	T0 events/ total	T1/2 events/ total	p-value	C0 events/ total	C1/2 events/ total	p-value
Full clinical remission[a]	8/48 (17%)	0/17 (0%)	0.099	6/39 (15%)	2/26 (8%)	0.460	4/45 (9%)	4/20 (20%)	0.238
GFR-loss ≥15 ml/min	14/51 (27%)	9/18 (50%)	0.092	11/40 (28%)	12/29 (41%)	0.302	16/47 (34%)	7/22 (32%)	1.000
ESRD[b]	7/51 (14%)	1/18 (6%)	0.671	1/40 (3%)	7/29 (24%)	0.008	4/47 (9%)	4/22 (18%)	0.255
Disappearance of microhematuria	11/34 (32%)	3/15 (20%)	n.d.[c]	10/29 (35%)	4/20 (20%)	n.d.[c]	10/34 (29%)	4/15 (27%)	1.000
Absolute annual GFR change (ml/min/1.73m^2)	-0.79 ± 4.50	-5.06 ± 5.17	0.002	-2.05 ± 5.40	-2.01 ± 4.54	0.362	-2.66 ± 5.02	-0.82 ± 5.02	0.131

[a]urinary protein-creatinine ratio < 0.2 g/g and an eGFR decrease of < 5 ml/min/1.73m^2
[b]end-stage renal disease
[c]not determined (due to the low total numbers of available data points in this category, $n = 49$)

Table 5), nor in patients under additional immunosuppression (M1: 0%, M0: 23%, $p = 0.304$, Table 5). Mean annual GFR loss was significantly higher for patients in the M1 group than for those in the M0 group (M0: -0.79 ± 4.50 ml/min/1.73 m^2 vs. M1-5.06 ± 5.17 ml/min/1.73 m^2, $p = 0.002$).

In our cohort, T1/2-scores did not correlate with full clinical remission or eGFR-loss rates during the trial phase, however, T1/2 was significantly associated with ESRD development (T1/2: 24% vs. T0: 3%, $p = 0.008$). This association was exclusively observed in patients under additional immunosuppression (T1/2: 44% vs. T0: 0%, p = 0.008), but not among those under supportive treatment (T1/2: 18% vs. T0: 7%, $p = 0.603$). Mean baseline eGFR in the four patients under additional immunosuppression with an T1/2 score who developed ESRD was 47 ± 15 ml/min/1.73 m^2 and among the three patients with an T1/2 in the supportive care group 51 ± 8 ml/min/1.73 m^2. Urinary protein-creatinine ratios did not differ between these subcohorts ($1,7 \pm 0,8$ g/g for both).

ESRD occurred more frequently in patients with glomerular crescents (C1/C2) than in patients with a C0-score (C1/2: 18% vs. C0: 9%, $p = 0.255$), whereas this trend was only significant in patients receiving supportive therapy (C1/2: 38% vs. C0: 4%, $p = 0.039$, Table 5). Accordingly, eGFR-loss rates of at least 15 ml/min/1.73m^2 did not correlate with crescents in patients

receiving supportive therapy (C1/2: 63% vs. C0: 25%, $p = 0.088$) nor in those receiving additional immunosuppression (C1/2: 15% vs. C0: 43%, $p = 0.084$, Table 5). Occurrence of primary trial endpoints (full clinical remission and eGFR-loss ≥15 ml/min/1.73m^2) and ESRD over the 3-year trial phase in the individual MEST-C subgroups was also visualized in Kaplan-Meier curves (Figs. 3, 4 and 5). Sensitivity analyses including uni- and multivariate Cox regression analyses entirely confirmed the previous trends for the MEST criteria as the only significant association in our cohort was observed for the T-score and ESRD development ($p = 0.02$ in the univariate Cox regression model; $p = 0.01$ in the multivariate Cox regression adjusting for GFR and proteinuria at baseline and the treatment arm).

Endocapillary hypercellularity (E) and segmental glomerular sclerosis (S) did not correlate with any of the other analyzed clinical outcome parameters. Disappearance of microhematuria did not correlate with any of the MEST-C criteria.

In our cohort, thrombotic microangiopathy (TMA) lesions were screened in randomly selected biopsies and were observed in only 2–4% of biopsies at maximum.

Discussion

All randomized clinical trials (RCTs) that evaluated therapeutic strategies in IgAN patients, of course

Table 5 Association between M-, T- and C- scores and clinical outcome in the two treatment arms of the STOP-IgAN trial (available cases analysis)

		M0 events/ total	M1 events/ total	T0 events/ total	T1/2 events/ total	C0 events/ total	C1/2 events/ total
Full clinical remission[a]	SUP[c]	2/22 (9%)	0/8 (0%)	2/15 (13%)	0/15 (0%)	1/23 (4%)	1/7 (14%)
	IMM[d]	6/26 (23%)	0/9 (0%)	4/24 (17%)	2/11 (18%)	3/22 (14%)	3/13 (23%)
GFR-loss ≥15 ml/min	SUP	7/24 (29%)	4/8 (50%)	4/15 (27%)	7/17 (41%)	6/24 (25%)	5/8 (63%)
	IMM	7/27 (26%)	5/10 (50%)	7/25 (28%)	5/12 (42%)	10/23 (43%)	2/14 (15%)
ESRD[b]	SUP	3/24 (13%)	1/8 (13%)	1/15 (7%)	3/17 (18%)	1/24 (4%)	3/8 (38%)
	IMM	4/27 (15%)	0/10 (0%)	0/25 (0%)	4/12 (33%)	3/23 (13%)	1/14 (7%)

[a]urinary protein-creatinine ratio < 0.2 g/g and an eGFR decrease of < 5 ml/min/1.73m^2
[b]end-stage renal disease
[c]patients under supportive treatment during the 3-year trial phase
[d]patients under additional immunosuppression during the 3-year trial phase

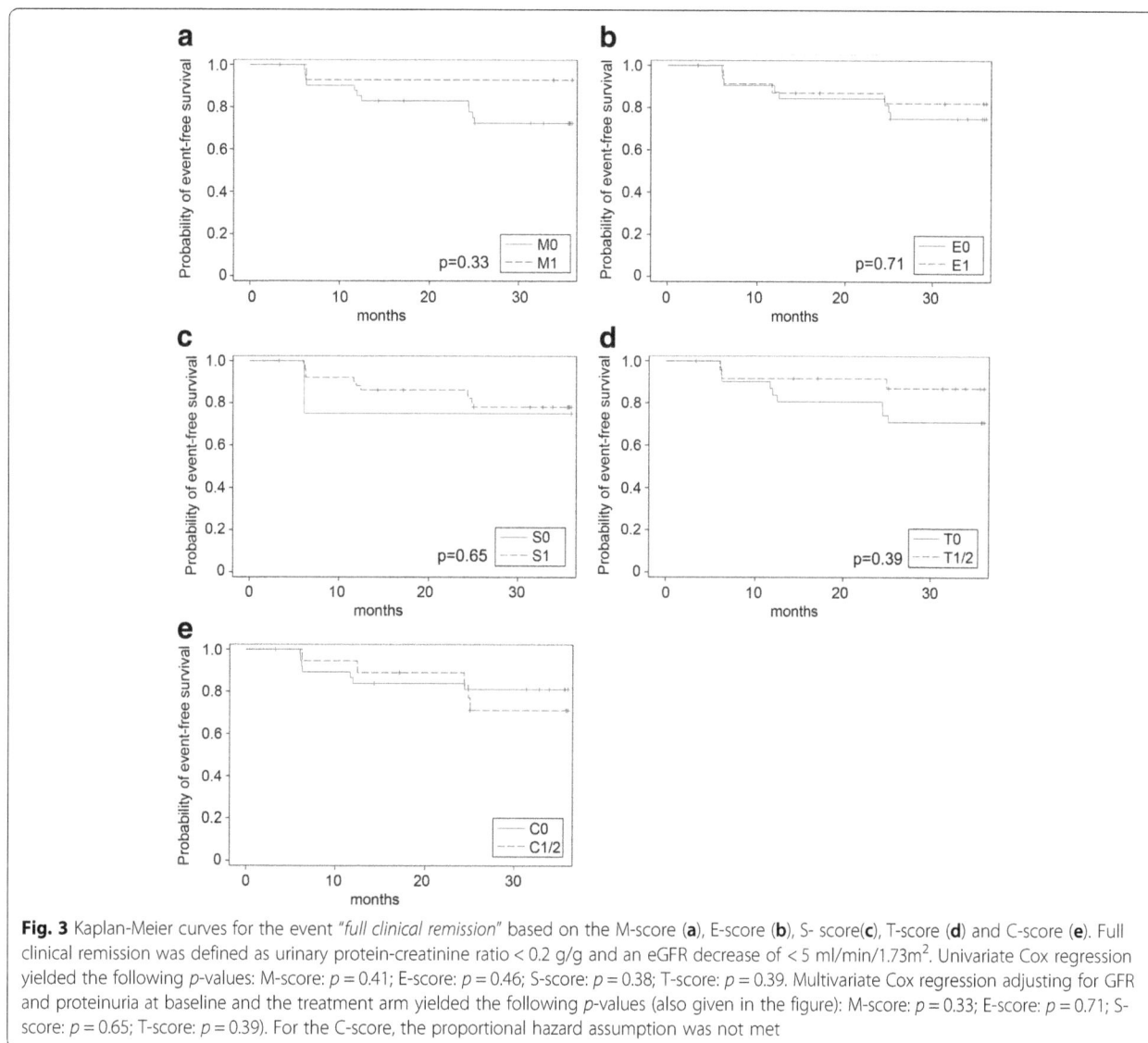

Fig. 3 Kaplan-Meier curves for the event *"full clinical remission"* based on the M-score (**a**), E-score (**b**), S- score(**c**), T-score (**d**) and C-score (**e**). Full clinical remission was defined as urinary protein-creatinine ratio < 0.2 g/g and an eGFR decrease of < 5 ml/min/1.73m^2. Univariate Cox regression yielded the following *p*-values: M-score: $p = 0.41$; E-score: $p = 0.46$; S-score: $p = 0.38$; T-score: $p = 0.39$. Multivariate Cox regression adjusting for GFR and proteinuria at baseline and the treatment arm yielded the following *p*-values (also given in the figure): M-score: $p = 0.33$; E-score: $p = 0.71$; S-score: $p = 0.65$; T-score: $p = 0.39$. For the C-score, the proportional hazard assumption was not met

required a renal biopsy as an eligibility criterion to confirm the diagnosis of IgAN. However, none of these trials, including the most recent ones [18–20], applied pre-defined histological features such as the MEST-C parameters for patient selection or stratification nor did these trials prospectively analyze renal outcomes in individual histological subgroups. In this regard, STOP-IgAN is no exception which is not surprising since the first version of the Oxford classification was published when STOP-IgAN was already recruiting patients [3, 4].

Here, we present an exploratory analysis from a representative STOP-IgAN subcohort [20] that includes 43% of randomized patients with available and sufficient biopsies that were scored based on the current MEST-C classification.

Baseline eGFR was significantly lower in patients with T1/2 scores as compared to those with T0. This is not

surprising since tubular atrophy and interstitial fibrosis are hallmark features of irreversible kidney damage and markers of advanced stages of renal disease regardless of the underlying pathology. Our data confirm older studies that tubulointerstitial damage in IgAN exhibits a very close association with renal function [23]. Retrospective data from the European VALIGA cohort that included more than 1100 IgAN patients suggested that the T-score was consistently predictive for poor renal outcomes, also in patients with a baseline GFR below 30 ml/min/1.73m^2 [6]. Notably, patients with such low renal function at enrollment had been excluded in STOP-IgAN and other randomized controlled trials. A large cohort of Korean IgAN patients also exhibited a significant correlation between T-scores and eGFR at the time of the biopsy [8]. In line with this, STOP-IgAN patients with biopsies showing T1/2 scores had a lower

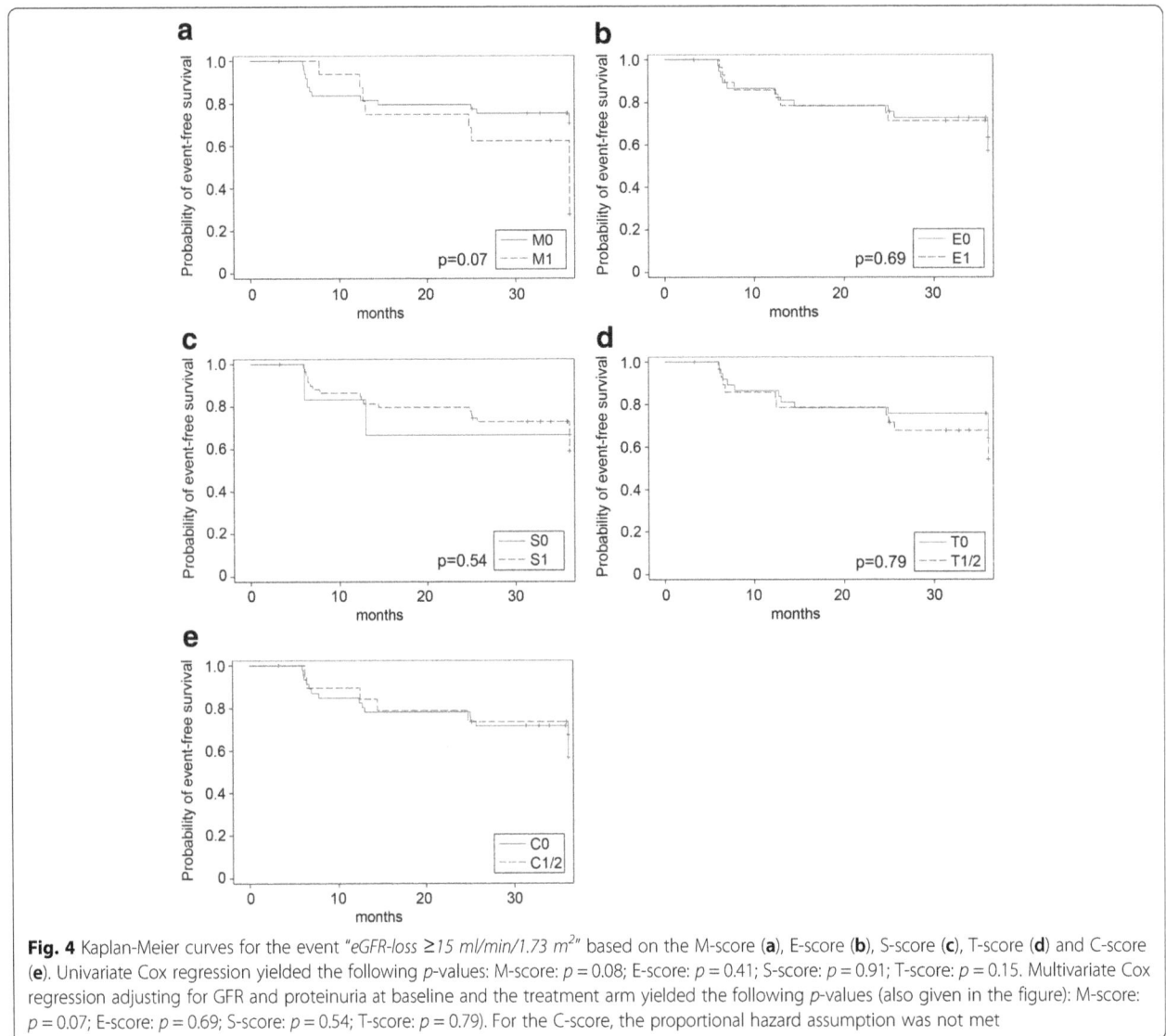

Fig. 4 Kaplan-Meier curves for the event "*eGFR-loss* ≥*15 ml/min/1.73 m²*" based on the M-score (**a**), E-score (**b**), S-score (**c**), T-score (**d**) and C-score (**e**). Univariate Cox regression yielded the following p-values: M-score: $p = 0.08$; E-score: $p = 0.41$; S-score: $p = 0.91$; T-score: $p = 0.15$. Multivariate Cox regression adjusting for GFR and proteinuria at baseline and the treatment arm yielded the following p-values (also given in the figure): M-score: $p = 0.07$; E-score: $p = 0.69$; S-score: $p = 0.54$; T-score: $p = 0.79$. For the C-score, the proportional hazard assumption was not met

mean baseline eGFR as compared to the the whole study cohort and were more likely to progress to end-stage renal disease (ESRD). Subgroup-analyses showed that T1/2-scores were only predictive for ESRD among patients who received additional immunosuppression and not in those under supportive care albeit only eight patients in the present subcohort (11%) developed ESRD (four patients in each treatment arm). Although the present secondary analysis only included 70 IgAN patients, it is worth noting that unlike many preceding clinical trials, all STOP-IgAN patients received RAS-blocking agents in a standardized fashion [20], i.e. dose titration based on proteinuria and blood pressure levels. To our knowledge, the current analysis from the STOP-IgAN cohort is the first one suggesting a potential interaction between tubular atrophy/interstitial fibrosis and immunosuppression. Lv et al. had pooled renal outcome data from 16 retrospective cohort studies comprising more than 3800 IgAN patients and found that the presence of a T1/2 score heralded an increased risk for ESRD development (HR 3.2; 95%-CI 1.8–5.6; $p < 0.001$) [10]. In general, T-scoring has proven to be a valuable predictor in nearly all validation studies [14].

In contrast, the predictive impact of endocapillary hypercellularity (E-score) is a matter of ongoing debate. In the above cited VALIGA cohort, the E-score was not predictive in the entire population or various subgroups [6]. Similar results were reported in the meta-analysis of Lv et al. [10]. However, other studies suggested that endocapillary lesions might respond to immunosuppressive therapy: a subgroup analysis from the original Oxford classification study revealed that the annual GFR-loss was significantly higher in patients scored as E1 as compared to those with E0, however only in patients without immunosuppression and not among those receiving immunosuppression [3]. Along these lines, a

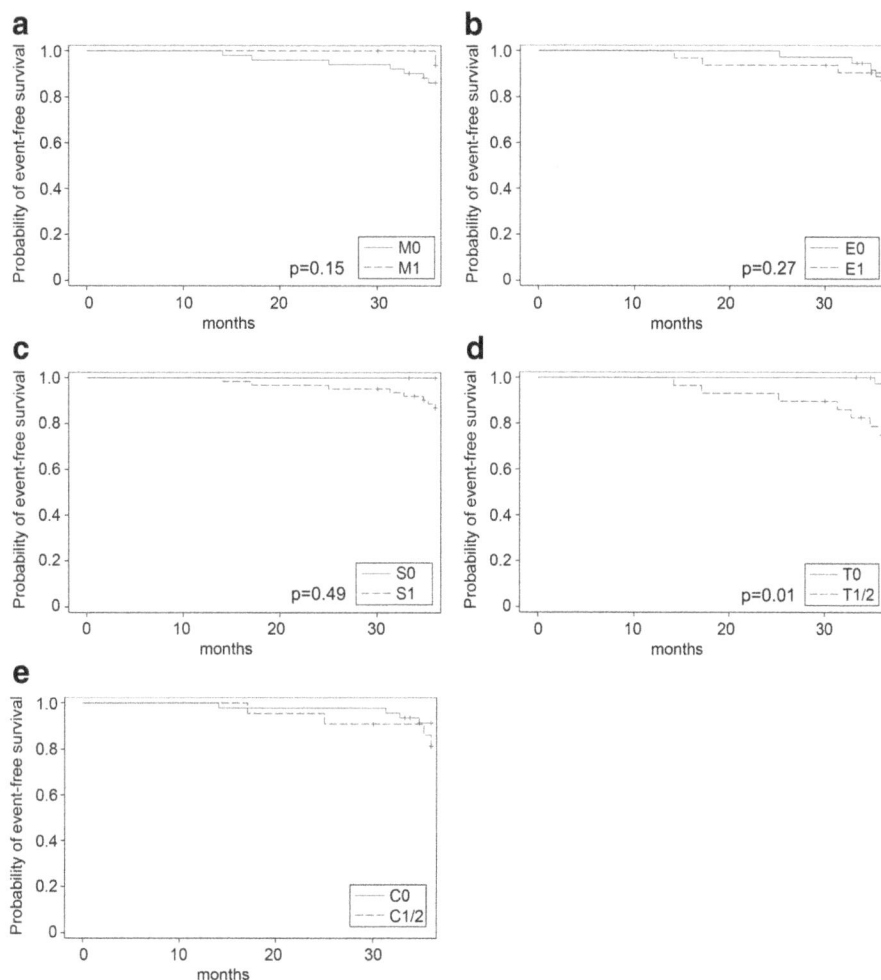

Fig. 5 Kaplan-Meier curves for the event "ESRD development" based on the M-score (**a**), E-score (**b**), S-Sscore (**c**), T-score (**d**) and C-score (**e**). Univariate Cox regression yielded the following p-values: M-score: $p = 0.32$; E-score: $p = 0.96$; S-score: $p = 0.90$; T-score: $p = 0.02$. Multivariate Cox regression adjusting for GFR and proteinuria at baseline and the treatment arm yielded the following p-values (also given in the figure): M-score: $p = 0.15$; E-score: $p = 0.27$; S-score: $p = 0.49$; T-score: $p = 0.01$. For the C-score, the proportional hazard assumption was not met

recently published, single-center study confirmed an E1-score as an independent predictor for ESRD in patients who did not receive immunosuppression [24]. In contrast to these studies, in STOP IgAN patients E-scoring did not predict any measured outcome.

Mesangial hypercellularity (M-score) is considered a very sensitive pathology marker in predicting disease progression [6, 25]. In accordance with the VALIGA cohort [6], STOP-IgAN patients with an M1-score had a significantly higher annual loss of renal function than patients scored as M0. However, M-scoring did not show a significant association with the percentage of patients losing > 15 ml/min/1.73 m^2 of GFR and ESRD occurrence. The reason for this might relate to the limited observation time of 3 years only and the overall low number of ESRD events in the analyzed subcohort. Furthermore, the predictive value of M-scoring might be abandoned if patients receive immunosuppressive

therapy [6] and indeed in our subgroup of immunosuppressed STOP-IgAN patients (IMM arm), the M-score was not validated as an independent risk factor. Previous cohort analyses suggest that in IgAN patients at more advanced disease stages M-scoring is no longer predictive [5, 7]. Further studies are needed to evaluate the relationship between supportive and/or immunosuppressive therapy and mesangial hypercellularity as a disease predictor.

Crescents have been introduced as the C-score only very recently in the revised Oxford classification [16]. This was based on several observations from smaller studies and a large IgAN cohort pooled from four previous analyses [17]. The latter found that patients with glomeruli containing crescents had a worse renal outcome than those without crescents. In the STOP-IgAN subcohort, analyzed patients displaying glomerular crescents in their biopsies were more likely to lose at least

15 ml/min/1.73m^2 of GFR or to develop ESRD during the 3-year trial phase. This trend was only significant among patients under supportive care and not in those under additional immunosuppression. This might indicate that the cellular proliferative component in the extracapillary space is responsive to immunosuppressive therapy [17, 26]. Whether in fact immunosuppression has beneficial effects on active crescentic lesions and results in subsequent GFR improvement is an intriguing hypothesis that needs to be evaluated in future studies.

We did not find evidence for frequent thrombotic microangiopathy (TMA) lesions in the biopsies from our STOP-IgAN subcohort. At maximum, we observed 2–4% TMA lesions in our patients contrasting data from a French single-center study reporting > 50% of such lesions [27], however our findings are consistent with data from other cohorts [28].

Compared to numerous preceding studies that aimed to validate the original Oxford classification, our study has several strengths. First, we applied a novel morphometric tool to more reliably quantify the degree of tubulointerstitial damage. The original Oxford Classification study as well as the subsequent validation studies only assessed the T-score by rough visual estimation of the involved cortical area [3, 4, 16]. Given its high prognostic significance on renal outcome, our approach might help to improve the validity of the T-score and minimize the inter- and intra-individual examiner variation. Furthermore, to our knowledge, this is the first validation study assessing all five parameters of the updated Oxford classification of IgAN including the presence of crescents in a prospective clinical trial.

Limitations of this secondary analysis include its *post-hoc* character and the variable intervals between time point of kidney biopsy and study enrollment (between 6.5 and 95 months), however only 6% of the biopsies were performed more than 3 years before trial enrollment. It might well be that with progressing disease course between kidney biopsy and trial enrollment, active renal lesions such as E- or C-lesions might transform into more chronic pathological manifestations. Thus, our study bares a certain "observational gap" between the actual biopsy and the time of trial inclusion. However, given the overall very slow annual decline of renal function, even in IgAN patients under supportive therapy only (approx. −1,5 ml/min/1.73m^2 per year), we consider this relatively short median time span of 9.4 months not relevant with respect to the chosen renal outcome parameters. Since the original Oxford classification was published in 2009, when STOP-IgAN was already recruiting patients, these histopathological characteristics were not "state of the art" at the time of enrollment and had to be obtained *ex post*. However, the histological analyses described here were performed blindly with regard to clinical trial data. Nowadays, IgAN kidney biopsies are reported based on the updated Oxford criteria in a standardized fashion [16]. The number of kidney biopsies to which the current MEST-C criteria were applicable was limited to 43% of randomized STOP-IgAN patients. Unfortunately, it was not feasible to obtain biopsies from all randomized patients, in part, because in the STOP-IgAN trial protocol, original biopsies were not requested to be delivered to the central trial coordinator. However, with regard to baseline renal function, proteinuria and other major patient characteristics the analyzed subcohort was representative for the entire STOP-IgAN population [20]. Nevertheless, given this sample size our *post-hoc* analysis was not sufficiently powered to determine interrelationships between histopathological scores and treatment effects. Moreover, because of the small sample size, we conducted an explorative statistical analysis only.

Conclusions

We applied the current Oxford classification to 70 randomized STOP-IgAN patients, either receiving immunosuppressive or supportive therapy only. Mesangial hypercellularity associated with a more rapid annual decline of eGFR, whereas the degree of tubular atrophy and interstitial fibrosis was predictive for ESRD, particularly in patients under immunosuppressive therapy. Since approximately one third of IgAN patients progresses to ESRD over 20–40 years [29], it is of outmost importance to identify patients early who are at risk for a progressive disease course. M1- as well as T1/2 and C1/C2 scores in the kidney biopsy might serve as valuable parameters to identify such high-risk candidates.

Abbreviations
eGFR: Estimated glomerular filtration rate; ESRD: End-stage renal disease; IgAN: Immunoglobulin A nephropathy; IMM arm: Patients under additional immunosuppression on top of optimized supportive care in the STOP-IgAN trial; KDIGO: Kidney Disease Improving Global Outcomes; MEST-C: (M)esangial hypercellularity, (E)ndocapillary hypercellularity, (S)egmental glomerulosclerosis, (T)ubular atrophy and interstitial fibrosis, (C)rescents; RAS: Renin-angiotensin system; SUP arm: Patients under optimized supportive care in the STOP-IgAN trial; TMA: Thrombotic microangiopathy; VALIGA study: European VALidation Study of the Oxford Classification of IGA Nephropathy

Acknowledgements
We are grateful to all study participants and trials centers for their contribution to this work. We are grateful to K. Amann (Erlangen, Germany), U. Helmchen (Hamburg, Germany), R. Waldherr (Heidelberg, Germany), H. Lobeck (Potsdam, Germany) to provide the original kidney biopsies for the present re-evaluation following the updated Oxford MEST-C classification.

Funding
The STOP-IgAN trial was funded through the German Federal Ministry of Education and Research (GFVT01044604). There was no third-party funding for the current secondary subanalysis.

Authors' contributions

The study was designed by JF, FE, RDH and TR All biopsies were analyzed by TK who was intensively trained and supervised by HJG and SP Statistical analyses were performed by JS, CF and RDH. TK wrote the entire manuscript. JS, JF and TR edited the manuscript text. The final manuscript version was approved by all listed authors.

Competing interests

J. Floege has received consultant honoraria from Omeros, USA and Pharmalink, Sweden, and investigator fees from Anthera Pharmaceuticals Inc., USA. The other authors declare no competing financial interests.

Author details

[1]Division of Nephrology and Clinical Immunology, RWTH Aachen University, Pauwelsstr. 30, 52074 Aachen, Germany. [2]Department of Intensive Care, RWTH Aachen University, Aachen, Germany. [3]Department of Medical Statistics, RWTH Aachen University, Aachen, Germany. [4]Bayer AG, Wuppertal, Germany. [5]Cellular and Molecular Pathology, German Cancer Research Center, Heidelberg, Germany. [6]Institute of Pathology, University Medical Centre Mannheim, Mannheim, Germany.

References

1. Barratt J, Feehally J. IgA nephropathy. J Am Soc Nephrol. 2005;16:2088–97.
2. Wyatt RJ, Julian BA. IgA nephropathy. N Engl J Med. 2013;368:2402–14.
3. Cattran DC, Coppo R, Cook HT, Feehally J, Roberts IS, Troyanov S, et al. The Oxford classification of IgA nephropathy: rationale, clinicopathological correlations, and classification. Kidney Int. 2009;76:534–45.
4. Roberts IS, Cook HT, Troyanov S, Alpers CE, Amore A, Barratt J, et al. The Oxford classification of IgA nephropathy: pathology definitions, correlations, and reproducibility. Kidney Int. 2009;76:546–56.
5. Alamartine E, Sauron C, Laurent B, Sury A, Seffert A, Mariat C. The use of the Oxford classification of IgA nephropathy to predict renal survival. Clin J Am Soc Nephrol. 2011;6:2384–8.
6. Coppo R, Troyanov S, Bellur S, Cattran D, Cook HT, Feehally J, et al. Validation of the Oxford classification of IgA nephropathy in cohorts with different presentations and treatments. Kidney Int. 2014;86:828–36.
7. Herzenberg AM, Fogo AB, Reich HN, Troyanov S, Bavbek N, Massat AE, et al. Validation of the Oxford classification of IgA nephropathy. Kidney Int. 2011; 80:310–7.
8. Kang SH, Choi SR, Park HS, Lee JY, Sun IO, Hwang HS, et al. The Oxford classification as a predictor of prognosis in patients with IgA nephropathy. Nephrol Dial Transplant. 2012;27:252–8.
9. Lee H, Yi SH, Seo MS, Hyun JN, Jeon JS, Noh H, et al. Validation of the Oxford classification of IgA nephropathy: a single-center study in Korean adults. Korean J Intern Med. 2012;27:293–300.
10. Lv J, Shi S, Xu D, Zhang H, Troyanov S, Cattran DC, et al. Evaluation of the Oxford classification of IgA nephropathy: a systematic review and meta-analysis. Am J Kidney Dis. 2013;62:891–9.
11. Moriyama T, Nakayama K, Iwasaki C, Ochi A, Tsuruta Y, Itabashi M, et al. Severity of nephrotic IgA nephropathy according to the Oxford classification. Int Urol Nephrol. 2012;44:1177–84.
12. Shi SF, Wang SX, Jiang L, Lv JC, Liu LJ, Chen YQ, et al. Pathologic predictors of renal outcome and therapeutic efficacy in IgA nephropathy: validation of the oxford classification. Clin J Am Soc Nephrol. 2011;6:2175–84.
13. Yau T, Korbet SM, Schwartz MM, Cimbaluk DJ. The Oxford classification of IgA nephropathy: a retrospective analysis. Am J Nephrol. 2011;34:435–44.
14. Roberts IS. Oxford classification of immunoglobulin a nephropathy: an update. Curr Opin Nephrol Hypertens. 2013;22:281–6.
15. Barbour SJ, Espino-Hernandez G, Reich HN, Coppo R, Roberts IS, Feehally J, et al. The MEST score provides earlier risk prediction in IgA nephropathy. Kidney Int. 2016;89(1):167–75.
16. Trimarchi H, Barratt J, Cattran DC, Cook HT, Coppo R, Haas M, et al. Oxford classification of IgA nephropathy 2016: an update from the IgA nephropathy classification working group. Kidney Int. 2017;91:1014–21.
17. Haas M, Verhave JC, Liu ZH, Alpers CE, Barratt J, Becker JU, et al. A multicenter study of the predictive value of crescents in IgA nephropathy. J Am Soc Nephrol. 2017;28:691–701.
18. Fellstrom BC, Barratt J, Cook H, Coppo R, Feehally J, de Fijter JW, et al. Targeted-release budesonide versus placebo in patients with IgA nephropathy (NEFIGAN): a double-blind, randomised, placebo-controlled phase 2b trial. Lancet. 2017;389:2117–27.
19. Lv J, Zhang H, Wong MG, Jardine MJ, Hladunewich M, Jha V, et al. Effect of Oral methylprednisolone on clinical outcomes in patients with IgA nephropathy: the TESTING randomized clinical trial. JAMA. 2017;318:432–42.
20. Rauen T, Eitner F, Fitzner C, Sommerer C, Zeier M, Otte B, et al. Intensive supportive care plus immunosuppression in IgA nephropathy. N Engl J Med. 2015;373:2225–36.
21. KDIGO Clinical Practice Guideline for Glomerulonephritis. Kidney Int. 2012; 2(Suppl 2):209–10.
22. Eitner F, Ackermann D, Hilgers RD, Floege J. Supportive versus immunosuppressive therapy of progressive IgA nephropathy (STOP) IgAN trial: rationale and study protocol. J Nephrol. 2008;21:284–9.
23. Vleming LJ, de Fijter JW, Westendorp RG, Daha MR, Bruijn JA, van Es LA. Histomorphometric correlates of renal failure in IgA nephropathy. Clin Nephrol. 1998;49:337–44.
24. Chakera A, MacEwen C, Bellur SS, Chompuk LO, Lunn D, Roberts ISD. Prognostic value of endocapillary hypercellularity in IgA nephropathy patients with no immunosuppression. J Nephrol. 2016;29:367–75.
25. Reich HN, Troyanov S, Scholey JW, Cattran DC. Remission of proteinuria improves prognosis in IgA nephropathy. J Am Soc Nephrol. 2007;18: 3177–83.
26. Kuppe C, van RC, Leuchtle K, Kabgani N, Vogt M, Van ZM, et al. Investigations of glucocorticoid action in GN. J Am Soc Nephrol. 2017;28: 1408–20.
27. El KK, Hill GS, Karras A, Jacquot C, Moulonguet L, Kourilsky O, et al. A clinicopathologic study of thrombotic microangiopathy in IgA nephropathy. J Am Soc Nephrol. 2012;23:137–48.
28. Chang A, Kowalewska J, Smith KD, Nicosia RF, Alpers CE. A cliniopathologic study of thrombotic microangiopathy in the setting of IgA nephropathy. Clin Nephrol. 2006;66:397–404.
29. Lai KN, Tang SC, Schena FP, Novak J, Tomino Y, Fogo AB, et al. IgA nephropathy. Nat Rev Dis Primers. 2016;2:16001.

Permissions

The contributors of this book come from diverse backgrounds, making this book a truly international effort. This book will bring forth new frontiers with its revolutionizing research information and detailed analysis of the nascent developments around the world.

We would like to thank all the contributing authors for lending their expertise to make the book truly unique. They have played a crucial role in the development of this book. Without their invaluable contributions this book wouldn't have been possible. They have made vital efforts to compile up to date information on the varied aspects of this subject to make this book a valuable addition to the collection of many professionals and students.

This book was conceptualized with the vision of imparting up-to-date information and advanced data in this field. To ensure the same, a matchless editorial board was set up. Every individual on the board went through rigorous rounds of assessment to prove their worth. After which they invested a large part of their time researching and compiling the most relevant data for our readers.

The editorial board has been involved in producing this book since its inception. They have spent rigorous hours researching and exploring the diverse topics which have resulted in the successful publishing of this book. They have passed on their knowledge of decades through this book. To expedite this challenging task, the publisher supported the team at every step. A small team of assistant editors was also appointed to further simplify the editing procedure and attain best results for the readers.

Apart from the editorial board, the designing team has also invested a significant amount of their time in understanding the subject and creating the most relevant covers. They scrutinized every image to scout for the most suitable representation of the subject and create an appropriate cover for the book.

The publishing team has been an ardent support to the editorial, designing and production team. Their endless efforts to recruit the best for this project, has resulted in the accomplishment of this book. They are a veteran in the field of academics and their pool of knowledge is as vast as their experience in printing. Their expertise and guidance has proved useful at every step. Their uncompromising quality standards have made this book an exceptional effort. Their encouragement from time to time has been an inspiration for everyone.

The publisher and the editorial board hope that this book will prove to be a valuable piece of knowledge for researchers, students, practitioners and scholars across the globe.

List of Contributors

J. Schikowski, M. Ladrière, M. Kessler and L. Frimat
Service de Néphrologie et Transplantation rénale, CHRU Nancy Brabois, Vandoeuvre-les-, Nancy, France

S. Girerd
Service de Néphrologie et Transplantation rénale, CHRU Nancy Brabois, Vandoeuvre-les-, Nancy, France INSERM, Centre d'Investigations Cliniques Plurithématique 1433, Université de Lorraine, CHRU de Nancy and F-CRIN INI-CRCT, Nancy, France

N. Girerd and K. Duarte
INSERM, Centre d'Investigations Cliniques Plurithématique 1433, Université de Lorraine, CHRU de Nancy and F-CRIN INI-CRCT, Nancy, France

H. Busby
Service d'Anatomie pathologique, CHRU Nancy Brabois, Vandoeuvre-lès-Nancy, France

N. Gambier
Service de Pharmacologie-Toxicologie, CHRU Nancy Brabois, Vandoeuvre-lès-Nancy, France

A. Aarnink
5Laboratoire d'Histocompatibilité, CHRU Nancy Brabois, Vandoeuvre-lès-Nancy, France

Xi Tang, Xinrui Li and Ping Fu
Kidney Research Laboratory, Division of Nephrology, National Clinical Research Center for Geriatrics, West China Hospital, Sichuan University, No. 37, Guoxue Alley, Chengdu, Sichuan, People's Republic of China610041

Yan Yang
Kidney Research Laboratory, Division of Nephrology, National Clinical Research Center for Geriatrics, West China Hospital, Sichuan University, No. 37, Guoxue Alley, Chengdu, Sichuan, People's Republic of China610041
Department of Nephrology, The First People's Hospital of Changzhou, The Third Affiliated Hospital of Soochow University, Changzhou, Jiangsu, People's Republic of China213000

Qiang Wei and Shi Qiu
Department of Urology, Institute of Urology, West China Hospital, Sichuan University, Chengdu, Sichuan, People's Republic of China

Linghui Deng
Stroke Clinical Research Unit, Department of Neurology, West China Hospital, Sichuan University, Chengdu, Sichuan, People's Republic of China

Michele F. Eisenga, Adry Diepenbroek, Stephan J. L. Bakker and Casper F. M. Franssen
Department of Nephrology, University Medical Center Groningen, University of Groningen, Hanzeplein 1, Groningen 9713GZ, The Netherlands

Jesse M. G. Hofman
Department of Nephrology, University Medical Center Groningen, University of Groningen, Hanzeplein 1, Groningen 9713GZ, The Netherlands
Department of Internal Medicine, Division of Nephrology, University Medical Center Groningen, Hanzeplein 1, 9713GZ Groningen, The Netherlands

Ilja M. Nolte
Department of Epidemiology, University Medical Center Groningen, University of Groningen, Hanzeplein 1, Groningen 9713GZ, The Netherlands

Bastiaan van Dam
Department of Internal Medicine, Medical Center Alkmaar, Wilhelminalaan 12, 1815JD Alkmaar, The Netherlands

Ralf Westerhuis
Dialysis Center Groningen, Hanzeplein 1, Groningen 9713GZ, The Netherlands

Carlo A. J. M. Gaillard
Department of Internal Medicine and Dermatology, University Medical Center Utrecht, University of Utrecht, Heidelberglaan 100, 3584CX Utrecht, The Netherlands

Shashidhar Cherukuri
Royal Wolverhampton Hospital, Renal Services, Wolverhampton, England

Maria Bajo
Hospital Universitario La Paz, Servicio de Nefrologia, Madrid, Spain

Giacomo Colussi
Niguarda Hospital, Nefrologia – Centro Trapianti Rene, Milan, Italy

Roberto Corciulo
Policlinic University, Azienda Ospedaliero-Universitaria Consorziale Policlinico, Bari, Italy

Hafedh Fessi
Hôpital Tenon, Service de Néphrologie et Dialyses, Paris, France

Maxence Ficheux
CHR Clémenceau, Service Néphrologie-Hémodialyse-Transplantation, Caen, France

Maria Slon
Hospital de Navarra, Servicio de Nefrologia, Pamplona, Spain

Eric Weinhandl
NxStage Medical, Inc., 350 Merrimack Street, Lawrence, MA 01843, USA
Department of Pharmaceutical Care and Health Systems, University of Minnesota, Minneapolis, MN, USA

Natalie Borman
Queen Alexandra Hospital, Wessex Kidney Centre, Portsmouth, England

Mehedi Hasan, Ipsita Sutradhar and Rajat Das Gupta
Centre for Non-Communicable Diseases and Nutrition, BRAC James P Grant School of Public Health, BRAC University, 5th Floor (Level-6), icddrb Building, 68 Shahid Tajuddin Ahmed Sarani, Mohakhali, Dhaka 1212, Bangladesh

Malabika Sarker
Centre for Science of Implementation and Scale-Up, Centre for Non-Communicable Diseases and Nutrition, BRAC James P Grant School of Public Health, BRAC University, Dhaka, Bangladesh
Adjunct Research Faculty, Institute of Public Health, Heidelberg University, Heidelberg, Germany

Jeppe B. Rosenbaek, Erling B. Pedersen and Jesper N. Bech
University Clinic in Nephrology and Hypertension, Regional Hospital West Jutland and Aarhus University, Laegaardvej 12J, DK-7500 Holstebro, Denmark

Julia Arnold, Khai Ping Ng, Paul Cockwell and Charles Ferro
Department of Nephrology, University Hospitals Birmingham, Birmingham B15 2WB, UK

Don Sims
Department of Stroke, University Hospitals Birmingham, Birmingham, UK

Paramjit Gill
Institute of Applied Health Research, College of Medical and Dental Sciences, University of Birmingham, Birmingham, UK
Warwick Medical School, University of Warwick, Coventry, UK

Guanhong Li, Yubing Wen, Xuemei Li and Ruitong Gao
Division of Nephrology, Department of Internal Medicine, Peking Union Medical College Hospital, Chinese Academy of Medical Sciences and Peking Union Medical College, NO.1, Shuaifuyuan, Dongcheng District, Beijing 100730, China.

Wei Wu, Xinyao Zhang and Yuan Huang
Department of Clinical Laboratory, Peking Union Medical College Hospital, Chinese Academy of Medical Sciences and Peking Union Medical College, Beijing, China

Jarcy Zee, Junhui Zhao, Lalita Subramanian, Bruce M. Robinson and Ronald L. Pisoni
Arbor Research Collaborative for Health, 340 E. Huron Street Suite 300, Ann Arbor, MI 48104, USA

Francesca Tentori
Arbor Research Collaborative for Health, 340 E. Huron Street Suite 300, Ann Arbor, MI 48104, USA
Vanderbilt University Medical Center, Nashville, TN, USA

Erica Perry
University of Michigan Health System, Ann Arbor, MI, USA

Nicole Bryant, Margie McCall, Yanko Restovic and Delma Torres
Advisory panel, Ann Arbor, MI, USA
Vanderbilt University Medical Center, Nashville, TN, USA

Arushi Kansal
Department of Nephrology, Monash Health, Clayton, Victoria 3168, Australia

Andy K.H. Lim and John Kanellis
Department of Nephrology, Monash Health, Clayton, Victoria 3168, Australia
Department of Medicine, Monash University, Clayton, Victoria 3168, Australia

Sang Soo Kim, Hye Won Lee, Eun Soon Jung, Min Young Lee, Miyeun Han, Harin Rhee, Eun Young Seong and Sang Heon Song
Biomedical Research Institute and Department of Internal Medicine, Pusan National University Hospital, Gudeok-ro 179 Seo-gu, Busan 49241, Republic of Korea

Il Young Kim, Dong Won Lee and Soo Bong Lee
Research Institute for Convergence of Biomedical Science and Technology and Department of Internal Medicine, Pusan National Universityv Yangsan Hospital, Yangsan, Gyeongsangnamdo, Republic of Korea

Sun Sik Bae
MRC for Ischemic Tissue Regeneration, Medical Research Institute, and Department of Pharmacology, Pusan National University School of Medicine, Yangsan, Republic of Korea

Hong Koo Ha
Biomedical Research Institute and Department of Urology, Pusan National University Hospital, Busan, Republic of Korea

David H. Lovett
The Department of Medicine, San Francisco Department of Veterans Affairs Medical Center, University of California San Francisco, California, USA

Yuuta Hara, Kosuke Sonoda, Koji Hashimoto, Kazuaki Fuji, Yosuke Yamada and Yuji Kamijo
Department of Nephrology, Shinshu University School of Medicine, 3-1-1 Asahi, Matsumoto, Nagano 390-8621, Japan

Jutta Dierkes, Helene Dahl, Natasha Lervaag Welland and Kristina Sandnes
Department of Clinical Medicine, Center for Nutrition, University of Bergen, Jonas Lies vei 68, 5021 Bergen, Norway

Hans-Peter Marti
Department of Clinical Medicine, Center for Nutrition, University of Bergen, Jonas Lies vei 68, 5021 Bergen, Norway
Department of Nephrology, Haukeland University Hospital, Jonas Lies vei 65, 5021 Bergen, Norway

Kristin Sæle and Ingegjerd Sekse
Department of Nephrology, Haukeland University Hospital, Jonas Lies vei 65, 5021 Bergen, Norway

Alain Michel
CHU Pontchaillou, Service de néphrologie, 2 rue H Le Guilloux, 35033 Rennes cedex, France

Cécile Vigneau
CHU Pontchaillou, Service de néphrologie, 2 rue H Le Guilloux, 35033 Rennes cedex, France
Université de Rennes 1, 2 av prof L Bernard, 35000 Rennes, France

Inserm (Institut national de la santé et de la recherche médicale), IRSET, U1085, SFR Biosit, 9 Avenue du Professeur Léon Bernard, 35000 Rennes, France

Adelaide Pladys
EHESP, Département d'Epidémiologie et de Bio-statistiques, Rennes, France
Université Rennes 1, UMR CNRS 6290, Rennes, France

Sahar Bayat
EHESP, Département d'Epidémiologie et de Bio-statistiques, Rennes, France
EA MOS EHESP, Rennes, France

Cécile Couchoud
Registre REIN, Agence de la biomédecine, La Plaine Saint Denis, France

Thierry Hannedouche
Faculté de médecine de Strasbourg, Hôpitaux universitaires de Strasbourg, 1 place de l'Hôpital, 67091 Strasbourg cedex, France

Clint Douglas
School of Nursing, Queensland University of Technology, Victoria Park Rd, Kelvin Grove, Brisbane, QLD 4059, Australia

Kathryn Havas
School of Nursing, Queensland University of Technology, Victoria Park Rd, Kelvin Grove, Brisbane, QLD 4059, Australia
NHMRC Chronic Kidney Disease Centre for Research Excellence, University of Queensland, St Lucia, Australia

Ann Bonner
School of Nursing, Queensland University of Technology, Victoria Park Rd, Kelvin Grove, Brisbane, QLD 4059, Australia
NHMRC Chronic Kidney Disease Centre for Research Excellence, University of Queensland, St Lucia, Australia
Visiting Research Fellow, Kidney Health Service, Metro North Hospital and Health Service, Brisbane, Australia

A. D. Fialla and O. B. Schaffalitzky de Muckadell
Department of Gastroenterology and Hepatology, Odense University Hospital, Sdr Boulevard, 5000 Odense C 29 Odense, Denmark

H. C. Thiesson
Department of Nephrology, Odense University Hospital, Odense, Denmark

P. Bie
Cardiovascular and Renal Research, University of Southern Denmark, Odense, Denmark

Hao-Yu Wang, Wen-Rui Shi and Ying-Xian Sun
Department of Cardiology, The First Hospital of China Medical University, 155 Nanjing North Street, Heping District, Shenyang 110001, China

Xin Yi
2Department of Cardiovascular Medicine, Beijing Moslem Hospital, Beijing 100054, China

Shu-Ze Wang
Department of Computational Medicine and Bioinformatics, University of Michigan, 100 Washtenaw Avenue, Ann Arbor, MI 48109, USA

Si-Yuan Luan
West China School of Medicine, Sichuan University, #37 Guoxue Alley, Chengdu 610041, China

Aaltje Y. Adema, Camiel L. M. de Roij van Zuijdewijn and Piet M. Ter Wee
Department of Nephrology, VU University Medical Center, De Boelelaan 1117, 1081, HV, Amsterdam, The Netherlands

Marc G. Vervloet
Department of Nephrology, VU University Medical Center, De Boelelaan 1117, 1081, HV, Amsterdam, The Netherlands
Amsterdam Cardiovascular Sciences (ACS), Amsterdam, The Netherlands

Joost G. Hoenderop
2Department of Physiology, Radboud University Medical Center Nijmegen, Nijmegen, The Netherlands

Martin H. de Borst
Department of Internal Medicine, Division of Nephrology, University Medical Center Groningen, Groningen, The Netherlands.

Annemieke C. Heijboer
Department of Clinical Chemistry, VU University Medical Center, Amsterdam, The Netherlands.

Anneleen Pletinck, Wim Van Biesen, Clement Dequidt and Sunny Eloot
Nephrology Division, Ghent University Hospital, C. Heymanslaan 10, 9000 Ghent, Belgium

Sara Campbell and G. Venkat-Raman
Wessex Kidney Centre, Queen Alexandra Hospital, Portsmouth Hospitals NHS Trust, Southwick Hill Road, Cosham, Portsmouth PO6 3LY, UK

Christine Gast
Wessex Kidney Centre, Queen Alexandra Hospital, Portsmouth Hospitals NHS Trust, Southwick Hill Road, Cosham, Portsmouth PO6 3LY, UK
Human Genetics and Genomic Medicine, Faculty of Medicine, University of Southampton, Southampton, UK

Eleanor G. Seaby, Sarah Ennis and Reuben J. Pengelly
Human Genetics and Genomic Medicine, Faculty of Medicine, University of Southampton, Southampton, UK

Anthony Marinaki and Monica Arenas-Hernandez
Purine Research Laboratory, Guys and St Thomas' NHS Foundation Trust, London, UK

Daniel P. Gale
UCL Centre for Nephrology, Royal Free Hospital, London, UK

Thomas M. Connor
Oxford Kidney Unit, Churchill Hospital, Oxford, UK

David J. Bunyan
Wessex Regional Genetics Laboratory, Salisbury NHS Foundation Trust, Salisbury, UK

Kateřina Hodaňová, Martina Živná and Stanislav Kmoch
Research Unit for Rare Diseases, Department of Pediatrics and Adolescent Medicine, First Faculty of Medicine, Charles University Prague, Prague, Czech Republic

Terri McVeigh, Raminta Cerneviciute and Sara Mohamed
Lambe Institute for Translational Research, Discipline of Surgery National University of Ireland, Galway, Republic of Ireland

Khalid Ahmed
Lambe Institute for Translational Research, Discipline of Surgery National University of Ireland, Galway, Republic of Ireland
Department of Vascular surgery, Galway University Hospital, Galway, Republic of Ireland

Stewart Walsh
Lambe Institute for Translational Research, Discipline of Surgery National University of Ireland, Galway, Republic of Ireland
Department of Vascular surgery, Galway University Hospital, Galway, Republic of Ireland
HRB Clinical Research Facility Galway, Galway, Republic of Ireland

Mohammad Tubassam
Department of Vascular surgery, Galway University Hospital, Galway, Republic of Ireland

Mohammad Karim
School of Population and Public Health, University of British Columbia, Scientist / Biostatistician, Centre for Health Evaluation and Outcome Sciences (CHEOS), St. Paul's Hospital, Vancouver, Canada

Tomoko Horinouchi, Kandai Nozu and Kazumoto Iijima
Department of Pediatrics, Kobe University Graduate School of Medicine, 5-1 Kusunoki-cho 7 chome, Chuo-ku, Kobe 650-0017, Japan

Mayumi Sako
Division for Clinical Trials, Department of Clinical Research Promotion, Clinical Research Center, National Center for Child Health and Development, Tokyo, Japan

Koichi Nakanishi
Department of Child Health and Welfare (Pediatrics), Graduate School of Medicine, University of the Ryukyus, Okinawa, Japan

Kenji Ishikura
Division of Nephrology and Rheumatology, National Center for Child Health and Development, Tokyo, Japan

Shuichi Ito
Department of Pediatrics, Graduate School of Medicine, Yokohama City University, Yokohama, Japan

Hidefumi Nakamura
Clinical Research Center, National Center for Child Health and Development, Tokyo, Japan

Mari Saito Oba
Department of Medical Statistics, Toho University, Tokyo, Japan

Judith Isabel Schimpf, Jürgen Floege and Thomas Rauen
Division of Nephrology and Clinical Immunology, RWTH Aachen University, Pauwelsstr. 30, 52074 Aachen, Germany

Till Klein
Division of Nephrology and Clinical Immunology, RWTH Aachen University, Pauwelsstr. 30, 52074 Aachen, Germany
Department of Intensive Care, RWTH Aachen University, Aachen, Germany

Christina Fitznera and Ralf-Dieter Hilgers
Department of Medical Statistics, RWTH Aachen University, Aachen, Germany

Frank Eitner
Bayer AG, Wuppertal, Germany

Hermann-Josef Groene
Cellular and Molecular Pathology, German Cancer Research Center, Heidelberg, Germany

Stefan Porubsky
Cellular and Molecular Pathology, German Cancer Research Center, Heidelberg, Germany
Institute of Pathology, University Medical Centre Mannheim, Mannheim, Germany

Index

www.ingramcontent.com/pod-product-compliance
Lightning Source LLC
Chambersburg PA
CBHW080506200326
41458CB00012B/4102